CLINICAL HANDBOOK
FOR THE
DIAGNOSIS AND
TREATMENT
OF
PEDIATRIC
MOOD DISORDERS

CLINICAL HANDBOOK
FOR THE
DIAGNOSIS AND
TREATMENT
OF
PEDIATRIC
MOOD DISORDERS

EDITED BY

Manpreet Kaur Singh, M.D., M.S.

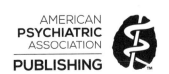

AMERICAN
PSYCHIATRIC
ASSOCIATION
PUBLISHING™

If you wish to buy 50 or more copies of the same title, please go to www.appi.org/specialdiscounts for more information.

Copyright © 2019 American Psychiatric Association Publishing

ALL RIGHTS RESERVED

First Edition
Manufactured in the United States of America on acid-free paper
23   22   21   20   19   5   4   3   2   1

American Psychiatric Association Publishing
800 Maine Avenue SW
Suite 900
Washington, DC 20024-2812
www.appi.org

Library of Congress Cataloging-in-Publication Data
Names: Singh, Manpreet Kaur, editor.
Title: Clinical handbook for the diagnosis and treatment of pediatric mood disorders
   / edited by Manpreet Kaur Singh.
Description: First edition. | Washington, D.C. : American Psychiatric Association
   Publishing, [2019] | Includes bibliographical references and index.
Identifiers: LCCN 2019011531 (print) | LCCN 2019012801 (ebook) |
   ISBN 9781615372553 (ebook) | ISBN 9781615371747 (pbk. : alk. paper)
Subjects: | MESH: Mood Disorders—diagnosis | Mood Disorders—therapy |
   Child Behavior Disorders—diagnosis | Child Behavior Disorders—therapy |
   Child | Adolescent
Classification: LCC RJ506.D4 (ebook) | LCC RJ506.D4 (print) | NLM WM 171
   | DDC 618.92/8527—dc23
LC record available at https://lccn.loc.gov/2019011531

British Library Cataloguing in Publication Data
A CIP record is available from the British Library.

Contents

Part 1
Diagnosis

Part 2

Treatment

Part 3
Appendixes:
Resources and Readings and
Quick Reference Facts

Contributors

Daniel Azzopardi-Larios, M.D.
Volunteer Program Coordinator, Kings County Hospital Center, Brooklyn, New York

Michele Berk, Ph.D.
Assistant Professor, Department of Child and Adolescent Psychiatry, Stanford University, Stanford, California

Boris Birmaher, M.D.
Endowed Chair in Early Onset Bipolar Disorder; Director, Child and Adolescent Bipolar Spectrum Services (CABS); Professor of Psychiatry, Western Psychiatric Institute and Clinic, Pittsburgh, Pennsylvania

Julie Carbray, Ph.D.
Clinical Professor of Psychiatry and Nursing, Institute for Juvenile Research, Department of Psychiatry, University of Illinois at Chicago, Chicago, Illinois

Gabrielle A. Carlson, M.D.
Professor of Psychiatry and Pediatrics, Stony Brook University School of Medicine, Putnam Hall-South Campus, Stony Brook, New York

Stephanie Clarke, Ph.D.
Clinical Instructor, Department of Child and Adolescent Psychiatry, Stanford University School of Medicine, Stanford, California

Paul E. Croarkin, D.O., M.S.
Associate Professor of Psychiatry; Division Chair, Child and Adolescent Psychiatry; Director, Mayo Clinic Depression Center, Mayo Clinic College of Medicine and Science, Rochester, Minnesota

Kathryn R. Cullen, M.D.
Associate Professor and Child and Adolescent Psychiatry Division Head, Department of Psychiatry and Behavioral Sciences, University of Minnesota Medical School, Minneapolis, Minnesota

Melissa P. DelBello, M.D., M.S.
Professor of Psychiatry and Pediatrics and Dr. Stanley and Mickey Kaplan Professor and Chair, Department of Psychiatry and Behavioral Neuroscience, University of Cincinnati College of Medicine, Cincinnati, Ohio

Daniel P. Dickstein, M.D.
Director, PediMIND Program, Bradley Hospital; Associate Professor, Brown University Departments of Psychiatry and of Human Behavior and Pediatrics, East Providence, Rhode Island

Rasim Somer Diler, M.D.
Director, Inpatient Child and Adolescent Bipolar Spectrum Services (In-CABS); Co-Director, Child and Adolescent Bipolar Spectrum Services (CABS); Associate Professor of Psychiatry, Western Psychiatric Institute and Clinic, Pittsburgh, Pennsylvania

Cathryn A. Galanter, M.D.
Visiting Associate Professor, State University of New York Downstate, Brooklyn, New York

Raghu Gandhi, M.D.
Child and Adolescent Psychiatry Fellow, Department of Psychiatry and Behavioral Sciences, University of Minnesota Medical School, Minneapolis, Minnesota

Danella Hafeman, M.D., Ph.D.
Assistant Professor, Department of Psychiatry, University of Pittsburgh, Pittsburgh, Pennsylvania

Nadia Jassim, M.F.A.
School Mental Health Team, Division of Child and Adolescent Psychiatry, Lucile Packard Children's Hospital at Stanford, Stanford University School of Medicine, Stanford, California

Shashank V. Joshi, M.D.
Associate Professor and Director, School Mental Health Team, Division of Child and Adolescent Psychiatry, Lucile Packard Children's Hospital at Stanford, Stanford University School of Medicine, Stanford, California

Gyung-Mee Kim, M.D., Ph.D.
Associate Professor, Department of Psychiatry, College of Medicine, Inje University Haeundae Paik Hospital, Busan, Republic of Korea

Tiffany Lei, B.S.
Medical Student, School of Medicine, University of California, Irvine, California

Amber C. May, M.D.
Chief Fellow, Division of Child and Adolescent Psychiatry, Institute for Juvenile Research, Department of Psychiatry, University of Illinois at Chicago, Chicago, Illinois

David J. Miklowitz, Ph.D.
Professor and Director of Child and Adolescent Mood Disorder Program, Department of Psychiatry, Semel Institute, UCLA School of Medicine, Los Angeles, California

M. Melissa Packer, M.A.
Lab Manager, Stanford Pediatric Emotion and Resilience Lab, Department of Psychiatry and Behavioral Sciences, Stanford University, Stanford, California

Luis R. Patino, M.D., M.Sc.
Assistant Professor of Clinical Medicine, Department of Psychiatry and Behavioral Neuroscience, University of Cincinnati College of Medicine, Cincinnati, Ohio

Mani N. Pavuluri, M.D., Ph.D.
Director, Brain and Wellness Institute, Adult, Adolescent and Child Psychiatry, Chicago, Illinois

Erica Ragan, Ph.D.
Clinical Assistant Professor, Department of Child and Adolescent Psychiatry, Stanford University School of Medicine, Stanford, California

Uma Rao, M.D.
Professor of Psychiatry and Human Behavior, and Pediatrics; Vice Chair for Child and Adolescent Psychiatry; Fellow, Center for the Neurobiology of Learning and Memory, University of California, Irvine, California; Director of Education and Research in Psychiatry, Children's Hospital of Orange County, Irvine, California

Pilar Santamarina, Ph.D.
Clinical Psychologist, Department of Child and Adolescent Psychiatry and Psychology, Institut Clinic of Neurociències, Hospital Clínic, Barcelona, Spain

Manpreet Kaur Singh, M.D., M.S.
Associate Professor and Director of the Pediatric Mood Disorders Program, Department of Psychiatry and Behavioral Sciences, Stanford University School of Medicine, Stanford, California

Meredith Spada, M.D.
Child and Adolescent Psychiatry Fellow, University of Pittsburgh Medical Center, Western Psychiatric Hospital, Pittsburgh, Pennsylvania

Anna Van Meter, Ph.D.
Assistant Professor, The Feinstein Institute for Medical Research, Manhasset, New York; The Zucker Hillside Hospital, Department of Psychiatry Research, Glen Oaks, New York; Hofstra Northwell School of Medicine, Department of Psychiatry and Molecular Medicine, Hempstead, New York

Sally M. Weinstein, Ph.D.
Assistant Professor of Clinical Psychology, Institute for Juvenile Research, Department of Psychiatry, University of Illinois at Chicago

Isheeta Zalpuri, M.D.
Clinical Assistant Professor, Department of Psychiatry and Behavioral Sciences, Stanford University School of Medicine, Stanford, California

Disclosures of Competing Interests

The following contributors to this book have indicated a financial interest in or other affiliation with a commercial supporter, a manufacturer of a commercial product, a provider of a commercial service, a nongovernmental organization, and/or a government agency, as listed below:

Boris Birmaher, M.D.—*Research support:* National Institute of Mental Health; *Royalties:* American Psychiatric Association, Random House, UpToDate

Gabrielle A. Carlson, M.D.—*Research support:* Patient-Centered Outcomes Research Institute, National Institute of Mental Health; the author's spouse is on Data Safety Monitoring Board for Lundbeck and Pfizer

Paul E. Croarkin, D.O., M.S.—*Research support/funding:* Mayo Clinic Foundation, National Institutes of Health (grant R01 MH113700), Pfizer; *Equipment support:* Neuronetics; *Supplies and genotyping services:* Assurex (for investigator-initiated studies); *Paid consultant:* Procter & Gamble; *Other:* Primary investigator for a multicenter study funded by Neuronetics; site primary investigator for a study funded by NeoSync

Melissa P. DelBello, M.D., M.S.—*Research support:* Assurex, Johnson & Johnson, Lundbeck, National Institute of Mental Health, Patient-Centered Outcomes Research Institute (PCORI), Pfizer, Sunovion; *Consultant/Advisory board/Honoraria/Speaker's bureau:* Allergan, Assurex CMEology, Johnson & Johnson, Lundbeck, Neuronetics, Pfizer, Sunovion, Supernus.

Cathryn A. Galanter, M.D.—*Research subcontract:* Patient-Centered Outcomes Research Institute (PCORI); *Book royalties:* American Psychiatric Association Publishing; *Other:* The Resource for Advancing Children's Health (REACH) Institute, Mini-Fellowship in Primary Pediatric Psychopharmacology (PPP), Steering Committee and Faculty

Shashank V. Joshi, M.D.—*Advisory board:* National Center for School Mental Health

David J. Miklowitz, Ph.D.—*Research support: Research funding:* AIM for Mental Health, Attias Foundation, Danny Alberts Foundation, Deutsch Foundation, Kayne Foundation, Max Gray Foundation, National Institute of Mental Health; *Book royalties:* Guilford Press, John Wiley & Sons

Manpreet Kaur Singh, M.D., M.S.—*Research support:* Allergan, Brain and Behavior Research Foundation, Johnson & Johnson, National Institutes of Health, Neuronetics, Stanford Maternal Child Health Research Institute; *Consultant/Advisory board:* Google X, Limbix, Sunovion

Anna Van Meter, Ph.D.—*Research support:* American Psychological Foundation

Sally M. Weinstein, Ph.D.—*Research support:* National Heart, Lung, and Blood Institute (grant 1R01HL123797; PI: Molly Martin); work was also supported by the Young Investigator Award YIG-1-140-11 from the American Foundation for Suicide Prevention (PI: Weinstein) and the National Institutes of Mental Health (NIMH; K23 grant MH079935; PI: West); *Book royalties:* American Psychiatric Association Publishing

Isheeta Zalpuri, M.D.—*Research support:* Johnson & Johnson; National Institute of Mental Health

The following contributors to this book have indicated no competing interests to disclose:

Daniel Azzopardi-Larios, M.D.
Michele Berk, Ph.D.
Stephanie Clarke, Ph.D.
Kathryn R. Cullen, M.D.
Raghu Gandhi, M.D.
Gyung-Mee Kim, M.D., Ph.D.

Tiffany Lei, B.S.
M. Melissa Packer, M.A.
Mani N. Pavuluri, M.D., Ph.D.
Uma Rao, M.D.
Pilar Santamarina, Ph.D.

Foreword

Depression is the number one public health morbidity problem in the world. Although we know a great deal about depression, most clinicians may not realize that mood disorders commonly begin in childhood or adolescence. Despite the importance of early recognition, until now there has been no available definitive reference for the diagnosis and treatment of mood disorders in youth. In the past two decades alone, we have made significant gains in our understanding of mood disorders in youth and their underlying etiologies. With advancements in technology and novel tools in neuroscience, we now understand how the brain develops and are forming an understanding of how psychopathology impacts normal brain development. *Clinical Handbook for the Diagnosis and Treatment of Pediatric Mood Disorders* is an essential resource, synthesizing the available body of evidence now established in this field. Using a developmental neuroscience perspective, this book provides a foundation from which novel methods of studying the characteristics and impact of mood disorders across the life span can emerge.

Youth with mood disorders experience a number of challenges that can delay their ability to receive appropriate diagnosis and treatment. With increased recognition that mood disorders occur and are common in youth today, any such delays can have rippling consequences that may affect transitions into adulthood or last a lifetime. Dr. Singh assembled a team of leading experts in pediatric mood disorders with the charge to provide the most contemporary approaches to diagnosing and treating youth with mood disorders. The book takes a head-on approach to the challenges experienced by youth today, providing practical and evidence-based solutions to problems such as varying presentations of mood symptoms across development, co-occurring conditions, polypharmacy, and the complex course and outcome frequently observed when mood disorders start in childhood. The text consists of 16 chapters spanning basic and clinical neuroscience, preventive strategies, and current and emerging somatic and psychosocial treatments for patients. It leverages empirical knowledge to allow clear delineation, definition, and treatment of mood symptoms in ever more effective ways, providing exceptional teaching on complex topics.

The book balances a synthesis of evidence-based knowledge with case-based examples and historical perspectives to engage readers about the clinical relevance of the concepts covered. The teaching is comprehensive yet usable, with knowledge drawn from multiple disciplines but presented in an understandable format. It encourages using a collaborative team-based approach to address the complexities associated with pediatric-onset mood disorders. The book will appeal to learners along a wide continuum, from the novice seeking a jump start in working with youth populations to the experienced clinician interested in brushing up on the most state-of-the-art evidence.

This handbook is a readable, timely guide to the clinical assessment and management of the mood disorders, addressing the increasing demand for clinicians to provide evidence-based care and helping to translate the rapid advances in neuroscience into real-world clinical practice. It is a must for anyone interested in pediatric mood disorders.

Alan F. Schatzberg, M.D.
Kenneth T. Norris Jr. Professor of Psychiatry and Behavioral Sciences
Director, Stanford Mood Disorders Center
Department of Psychiatry and Behavioral Sciences
Stanford University School of Medicine
Stanford, California

Preface

Mood disorders are increasingly being diagnosed and treated in youth with improved awareness that these disorders commonly have their onset in childhood and adolescence. We have learned much about mood disorders from the experience of adults with these disorders, around two-thirds of whom report symptom onset in childhood or adolescence and, on average, suffer a decade or more with symptoms before receiving an accurate diagnosis or adequate treatment. This lag in identification and treatment has resulted in progression of the severity of mood disorders, often making it even more challenging to treat these conditions. Contextualizing the early roots of mood disorders is imperative not just for clinicians working with children and adolescents but also for clinicians providing treatment for adults. Emerging evidence also suggests that in youth offspring of parents with mood disorders, there is an increased risk of developing mood and other psychiatric conditions compared with the general population, and that there may be a differential response to psychotropic medications (toward increased side effects) based on this family risk. Moreover, clinicians and trainees frequently have questions about how to investigate common risk factors for developing lifelong mood problems. Inspired by these questions, we assembled a team of experts in child psychiatry to write a handbook for a wide readership of trainees and professionals interested in understanding pediatric-onset mood disorders.

The first of its kind, this handbook strives to deliver a readable contemporary guide to the assessment and management of childhood-onset mood disorders. Despite the increasing prevalence of mood disorders in youth, there are no available clinical handbooks for mental health professionals and trainees to use as a reference in this field. This book is intended to fill this critical gap, with expert reviews provided by clinicians and researchers who are proven leaders in this field. Our goal in writing it was to provide both an up-to-date resource that captures the rapid and dramatic advances in the field and an evidence-based framework that permits easy integration into practice.

The handbook includes controlled treatment trials and U.S. Food and Drug Administration–approved interventions for pediatric mood disorders, taking into account more than a decade of clinical research and clinical treatment experience by clinicians practicing in North America and abroad. The format, approach, and style balance evidence-based practice with a breadth of clinical experience to provide the most up-to-date ways of understanding and treating mood disorders with onset in childhood. Because of rapid advancements in the field and in our understanding of brain development, we used a developmental framework whenever possible. This book has three major scientific, clinical, and teaching objectives:

- **The scientific mission.** The mechanisms underlying risk for developing a lifelong mood disorder or how a child responds to treatment for a mood disorder are largely unknown. However, since the development and application of novel scientific tools to better understand brain function and behavior, the field has seen dramatic and accelerated advances in recent years. A number of researchers are now conducting and reporting on prospective longitudinal observations of youth with mood disorders or at risk for such disorders through the course of their neurodevelopment and as they transition into adulthood. These longitudinal studies are pivotal and will increase the field's capacity to predict which youth are most liable to suffer from lifelong mood disorders and which youth are most likely to respond to treatment. These scientific advancements pose a challenge for clinicians to remain abreast of the latest research, to integrate it into their practice, and to educate patients about the relative impact and relevance of the research on their health and well-being. With a strong movement in medicine toward evidence-based practices, clinicians and patients alike are seeking guidance from contemporary observational and intervention studies to guide clinical best practices and to usher in the development of novel treatments that will outperform the current standard of care and lead to optimal long-term outcomes.
- **The clinical mission.** More than 300 million individuals worldwide live with depression, representing an increase of more than 18% from 2005 to 2015 (World Health Organization 2017). Depression has now become the leading cause of ill health and disability worldwide. Although there are known effective treatments, fewer than half of individuals affected receive such treatments, frequently because of lack of support for people with mental disorders and a fear of stigma. This handbook

will provide tangible solutions to real-world clinical challenges in being able to engage pediatric patients and families in safe and effective treatments for mood disorders. It will also provide stepwise and developmentally informed strategies and timelines for starting, maintaining, and discontinuing treatments in youth experiencing mood disorders.

- **The teaching mission.** This handbook addresses the critical unmet educational need of a definitive clinical handbook in the diagnosis and management of pediatric-onset mood disorders. The handbook offers "one-stop shopping" for anyone interested in bridging the latest evidence base with personal clinical experiences to guide the diagnosis and treatment of a spectrum of mood disorders in youth. We aspire to reach a broad audience of learners by providing authoritative and accessible information that is relevant and applicable to real-world clinical practice. This book is intended for mental and primary care health professionals and trainees from diverse clinical training backgrounds, providing evidence-based guidelines that can easily be translated into real-world clinical practice. We hope this book will be a useful compendium to clinicians in training, serving as a resource for expert consultation or to augment their learning in their clinical and academic settings. It will also provide professionals with the practical information needed to balance benefits, risks, and alternatives to state-of-the-art treatment approaches. To optimize learning, the authors have made liberal use of case examples and graphical formats to illustrate, explain, and summarize chapter content, and the text is supplemented by an appendix of resources for those interested in expanding their knowledge and quick reference facts for treating pediatric mood disorders.

Finally, given what is known and what remains to be learned in this field, we provide the best practical wisdom available with humility that our knowledge and practice are continually evolving.

Manpreet Kaur Singh, M.D., M.S.

Reference

World Health Organization: Depression and Other Common Mental Disorders: Global Health Estimates. Geneva, World Health Organization, 2017

Acknowledgments

There are many people to thank along the journey to develop this handbook. The chapter authors and coauthors deserve special appreciation for their expertise, exceptional teaching, and service to the field. Without this village of talented clinician-scholars, this handbook would not have been possible. The editorial staff at American Psychiatric Association (APA) Publishing—and, in particular, John McDuffie—have my appreciation for their careful reading, technical skill, and support. Dr. Laura Roberts deserves special mention for her encouragement and confidence in the project, as a leader both at APA Publishing and in our Department of Psychiatry and Behavioral Sciences at Stanford. We also appreciate the insights and feedback provided by our colleagues and trainees at Stanford and from around the world. Their feedback helps us see our blind spots and makes us better educators. Marianne Thompson, a kindred childhood friend and accomplished artist, provided the cover art. A special thanks to my parents, Baljeet and Pashaura, for walking the walk, and to my husband, Mandeep, my mother-in-law, Jagdish, and our three children, Kirpa, Himmet, and Ganeev, for their unwavering support on the home front to ensure that this handbook received the time and care needed to make it as good as it could be.

Last, but certainly not least, this project was inspired by the youth and families we evaluate and treat every day, who challenge us to ask the following fundamental questions that, in turn, drive our efforts: What will generations to come say about us? Did we seize the possibilities of our time? Did we answer why sustained sadness is experienced in childhood and continues into adulthood for some but not others? Did we drive science forward as far as it could go to benefit the many and not just the few? We hope this handbook inspires you to be curious about youth who present with mood symptoms and to consider how your efforts today might create hope for youth tomorrow.

Manpreet Kaur Singh, M.D., M.S.

Part 1
DIAGNOSIS

1

Principles of Assessment of Mood Disorders in Childhood

Manpreet Kaur Singh, M.D., M.S.

It has been 4 months since Blue broke up with his girlfriend. They dated until his fifteenth birthday, when Blue discovered that she was flirting with another guy in his class on social media. Blue was heartbroken when they ended their steady relationship, crying every day and having trouble sleeping. After a couple of weeks, he felt better, convincing himself that he was better off without her and could now spend more time focusing on his schoolwork. A month later, Blue started to feel down again, initially for a few days at a time, and then eventually more frequently, to the point at which he would snap at his friends and family nearly every day. Much like his mom, he viewed the glass as half empty, and he spent most of nearly every day in a low mood. It would take him 2–3 hours to fall asleep most nights, and several times a week he found himself awoken from sleep by a nightmare or needing to use the bathroom. He would feel tired the next day from fitful sleep and would drag himself out of bed, frequently missing his first period in school. Blue spent most of the time watching videos on the

Internet or listening to heavy metal music in his room. He no longer enjoyed wrestling, playing the saxophone, or hanging out with his friends over the weekend. Instead, he would sneak junk food into his room, and sometimes he would get high with edible marijuana brownies to escape from his troubles. Candy would lift him out of a low mood for just enough time for him to start his homework, but then he would get distracted, look at himself in the mirror, feel guilty for overeating, and fall back into a slump. Consequently, his grades started to fall, and his teachers expressed concern. After several weeks, Blue started to feel hopeless that he wouldn't be able to catch up in school and wondered whether he would be better off dead. This thought scared him, so he asked his mom to take him to his pediatrician.

What principles apply for the initial assessment of Blue? In the pediatrician's busy practice, what questions can be asked and what assessments can be conducted to determine whether Blue's condition can be managed in a primary care setting? How would the pediatrician know when to refer Blue to more specialized care? How does she determine whether Blue has depression or another psychiatric disorder, or is adjusting to his breakup from his girlfriend? How does she determine whether his mood symptoms are secondary to an underlying medical condition or due to recreational drug use? This chapter will aim to provide introductory answers to these questions, which will be elaborated on in specialized ways throughout this handbook.

Even with the burgeoning field of neuroscience and multiple valid screening and assessment tools, the gold-standard approach to the diagnosis of mood disorders in youth is still the clinical interview, ideally one involving multiple informants. Clinicians in a variety of settings can ask simple but key questions to assess for mood symptoms in youth and to determine severity, as well as how these symptoms relate to a child's day-to-day functioning. Once a core low or elevated mood symptom is endorsed, its persistence, associated factors, and functional impact can help a clinician efficiently decide whether it falls within the scope of his or her practice. Underlying neurophysiological contributors such as anemia, altered thyroid function, and vitamin D and lead levels can all be assessed with a single blood draw while referrals for more in-depth evaluations are being considered. Furthermore, asking youth about recreational drug use individually and directly is generally preferred over urine toxicology screening in an outpatient setting. This underscores the point that because no validated diagnostic biomarkers or confirmatory tests for mood disorders yet exist, healthcare providers must rely on clinical criteria and diagnostic acumen to diagnose these conditions early and accurately.

Because symptoms of mood disorders may resemble and co-occur with other conditions or psychiatric problems, a comprehensive assessment of endorsed symptoms as well as pertinent positive and negative symptoms will likely yield the most accurate primary and secondary diagnoses, which may merit a more in-depth interview or referral to a mental health professional. Indeed, life problems such as a relationship breakup, academic stress, or bullying can trigger and perpetuate mood symptoms. One goal of a careful diagnostic assessment is to help a patient cultivate insight about what factors contribute to triggering, perpetuating, or alleviating mood symptoms. Helping the patient describe symptoms in his or her own words supports this goal and establishes an early alliance between the patient and clinician for the purpose of understanding mood symptoms and their impact and for collaboratively monitoring these symptoms as they evolve with treatment.

Children and adolescents may experience a spectrum of mood symptoms, which in early stages of development may be ill-defined diagnostically and may change over time. For example, the most common first episode in bipolar disorder is a depressive episode that, when treated with an antidepressant, may trigger mania or mania-like symptoms. To ensure that the full spectrum of mood disorders is considered at any and all clinical evaluations of a child presenting with mood symptoms, all index mood symptoms, including sad mood, anhedonia, and irritability for major depressive disorder (MDD) and explosive irritability and euphoria for bipolar disorder, should be considered and explored. Index mood symptoms are solicited in the patient's own words first, followed by secondary or "Criterion B" symptoms of depression and mania as defined in DSM-5 (American Psychiatric Association 2013).

In MDD, S-I-G-E-C-A-P-S remains a popular mnemonic, where *S* generally stands for sleep abnormalities (insomnia or hypersomnia; initial/middle/terminal), *I* for diminished interest or pleasure in the things youth normally find to be fun, *G* for guilt or self-blame, *E* for low energy, *C* for concentration difficulties or poor decision making, *A* for appetite changes (increases or decreases with corresponding weight changes), *P* for psychomotor agitation or retardation, and *S* for suicidal ideation or related behavior. A major depressive episode requires at least 2 weeks of an index depressed mood and four additional Criterion B symptoms. In bipolar disorder, index euphoria on a daily basis for over 50% of the day for at least a week is accompanied by at least three additional symptoms (four if the index mood is explosive irritability) and is captured in the mnemonic D-I-G-F-A-S-T, where *D* stands for distractibility or motor hyperactivity, *I* for increased goal-directed activity, *G* for grandiosity, *F* for flight of ideas and racing thoughts, *A* for accelerated speech, *S* for decreased *need* for sleep, and *T* for "trouble," or engagement with impulsive risk-taking or hypersexual behaviors that have the potential for dangerous consequences for the patient or others. In youth, general examples of high-risk behaviors include staying out all night, spending a lot of money, and taking trips unexpectedly. Adolescents might report that during a manic episode, they got involved in relationships quickly, had a lot of one-night stands, or drove recklessly. Preadolescents might also report that they jumped from elevated places, went on long trips without planning or supervision, played serious pranks in school, or engaged in inappropriate sexual behavior during mania. These symptoms manifest differently depending on age and should therefore be contextualized developmentally.

Establishing the timeline of onset and offset of mood symptoms early in the interview allows a clinician to quickly and easily rule in or rule out a major mood disorder such as bipolar I disorder or MDD. The clinician can then proceed systematically down a list of potential diagnoses of exclusion and co-occurring conditions. Unfortunately, clinicians in naturalistic and often busy clinical settings tend to underuse DSM, frequently not collecting sufficient information to establish a correct diagnosis for most psychiatric disorders (Nakash et al. 2015). Moreover, research diagnostic assessments and clinical evaluations have only low to moderate agreement (Rettew et al. 2009). Missing diagnostic information may result in poor reliability and clinical decision making (Jensen-Doss et al. 2014), delaying effective treatment or resulting in the implementation of inappropriate, costly, or potentially harmful treatments. Thus, accurate and effective diagnostic skills can prevent adverse clinical and financial outcomes at multiple levels.

Indeed, efforts to systematically evaluate clinicians' assessment processes in naturalistic settings may help to identify the best diagnostic probes to use in clinical practice to improve diagnostic accuracy and efficiency. For the busy clinician, access to a toolkit of feasible assessments that are integrated into practice and supported by billing structures may facilitate use of more systematic approaches to making a diagnosis. Several measurement-based care solutions are being developed by for-profit and not-for-profit organizations to try to improve real-time clinical decision making, enhance reimbursement, and optimize resource utilization in behavioral health. Because measurement-based care is still emerging, data to demonstrate its efficacy in improving diagnostic accuracy and treatment outcomes are still pending. What follows is a brief summary of some well-validated structured clinical interviews and clinical and self-report rating scales we have used frequently in research and in clinical practice. Validity measurements for these assessments are widely available, but there is no substitute for personal experience for becoming proficient at conducting these assessments and determining their utility in measuring symptom severity or treatment response or predicting long-term outcome.

Structured and Semi-structured Clinical Interviews

The gold-standard method for evaluating for a pediatric mood disorder is to use structured or semi-structured clinical interviews. Researchers and clinicians use this method for its systematic approach to ruling in and ruling out a psychiatric diagnosis, and such assessments serve as benchmarks for comparisons with other methods of deriving a psychiatric diagnosis, including self-, parent-, or teacher-administered instruments or observations. Although the specificity of a mood disorder diagnosis remains high between a structured clinical interview and a self-administered instrument, the sensitivity decreases, so the most reliable method of identifying cases of MDD remains the structured clinical interview (Martin et al. 2017). Importantly, a family history of depression increases the chances of a more reliable diagnosis from a structured interview than from a self-administered rating, suggesting some advantage of having a family member with depression to improve reliable reporting of depressive symptoms (Verweij et al. 2011). On the other hand, sometimes parents affected by mood disorder symptoms experience an attribution bias, projecting symptoms onto their children or other family members. When there is a misattribution, this can cause undue stress in a family and consequent overdiagnosis and treatment seeking in youth who are otherwise well adapted. A systematic assessment of mood and other psychopathology in parents can provide important context for how symptoms are reported in a child. Thus, for all youth presenting with mood symptoms, a family history of mood and other psychiatric disorders not only informs risk and prognostic factors but also contextualizes the potential for informant bias.

There are two main disadvantages of using a structured clinical interview: 1) the time that it takes to train on and conduct these interviews, and 2) the cost associated with having an expert rater conduct these interviews. In contrast, studies have shown that patients have a high acceptance of and satisfaction with structured interviews even when their clinicians estimate that patients' acceptance would be lower than it actually is (Bruchmüller et al. 2011). Anecdotal feedback frequently given by patients who receive both a clinical psychiatric interview and a research-based structured diagnostic interview suggests that the latter makes them feel heard and increases their confidence that an accurate diagnosis is being made. Structured interviews abidingly attempt to comprehensively capture all symptoms experienced, with follow-up clarifying questions posed to determine levels of associated impairment. Such interviews can increase the number of diagnoses ascribed to a patient but reduce the number of non-specific (e.g., "unspecified"; formerly "not otherwise specified") diagnoses given (Matuschek et al. 2016).

Several structured clinical interviews have been validated for youth with mood disorders across the age spectrum (Table 1–1). The relative strengths and limitations of the most commonly used interview instruments have been reviewed by Leffler et al. (2015), who suggest that in order to choose the most appropriate instrument for diagnostic decision making and treatment planning, the clinician begin the interview with a bio-psycho-socio-cultural history, to increase the success and reliability of the diagnostic interview. In the young child, the Preschool Age Psychiatric Assessment (PAPA) has been validated for administration to parents of youth between 2 and 7 years of age (Egger et al. 2006). This parent interview has proven useful both to characterize symptom manifestations of mood disorders in very young children (Luby and Belden 2008) and to predict future patterns of psychopathology in school-age children (Dougherty et al. 2015; Kertz et al. 2017) and adolescents (Finsaas et al. 2018; Luby et al. 2014). As demonstrated by systematic prospective follow-up using age-appropriate structured clinical interviews, preschool-onset depression is no longer considered a developmentally transient syndrome; rather, it is thought to be a chronic and recurrent syndrome that may evolve and warrant observation over time.

In school-age children 6 years and older, trained interviewers assess for the presence or absence of a psychiatric disorder by semi-structured diagnostic interviews administered separately to youth and their parents (about the youth). Interviews from which to choose include the Kiddie Schedule for Affective Disorders and Schizophrenia (for School-Age Children)—Present and Lifetime Version (K-SADS-PL; Kaufman et al. 1997); the mood sections of the Washington University (St. Louis) Kiddie Schedule for Affective Disorders and Schizophrenia (WASH-U K-SADS; Geller et al. 2001), for more detailed questions about the nature and course of childhood-onset mood disorders; and the Mini International Neuropsychiatric Interview for Children and Adolescents (MINI-KID; Sheehan et al. 2010). The latest version of the K-SADS-PL combines dimensional and categorical assessment approaches to diagnose current and past episodes of psychopathology in children and adolescents according to DSM-5 criteria. Probes included in the interview illustrate ways to elicit information but are not intended to be recited verbatim; thus, the interview is considered semi-structured. Rather, the interviewer is encouraged to adjust the probes to the developmental level of the child, and to use language provided by the parent and child when asking about specific symptoms. Parent and child ratings may be optimally obtained separately, and summary ratings are achieved by including all sources of information (i.e., parent, child, school, chart, or other). The order of administration may vary case by case, but in general, it is recommended that the interviewer conduct the parent interview first for preadolescents and the child interview first for adolescents. When discrepancies between sources of information arise, the rater uses clinical judgment to determine the final summary score, and possibly probes the informants further about discrepant information.

Mood disorders frequently run in families. Although systematic and quantitative data on familial aggregation of mood disorders are still emerging (Fears et al. 2014), it is well recognized that offspring of parents who are both affected by mood disorders are far more likely to have a mood disorder compared with families in which only one parent is affected (Goodwin and Jamison 1990). The Structured Clinical Interview for DSM-5 (SCID-5; First et al. 2016) and a family history interview such as the Family Interview for Genetic Studies (FIGS; Maxwell 1982) or the Family History—Research Diagnostic Criteria (FH-RDC; Andreasen et al. 1977) may be administered in order to assess parental and other family history of mood and other psychiatric disorders. Both the FIGS and the FH-RDC start with a pedigree drawing, which can be a great way to organize and stratify family history loading based on first-, second-, and other degree-relative psychiatric family histories. Any clinical encounter of a youth with mood symptoms should assess for mood symptoms and disorders (specifically bipolar and depressive disorders), suicide completions, sudden death, substance use, and schizophrenia in family members. This information can then be used both diagnostically and for treatment planning.

To track psychiatric symptoms in youth over time, the Longitudinal Interval Follow-up Evaluation (LIFE; Keller et al. 1987) provides a weekly prospective assessment of mood, psychotic, and other psychiatric symptoms tracked on a week-by-week basis using this instrument's Psychiatric Status Rating (PSR) scales. The PSR scales assign numeric values that can be operationally linked to DSM criteria, with assessment made in the interview and then translated into ratings for each week of the follow-up period. The ratings reflect symptom severity and impairment during an episode and capture periods of recurrence or recovery. For mood disorders,

TABLE 1–1. Structured and semi-structured clinical interviews for pediatric mood disorders

Clinical interview	Age validated for use	Description
Preschool Age Psychiatric Assessment (PAPA; Egger et al. 2006)	2–7 years	Structured assessment used to interview parents about preschool-age youth down to age 2 for DSM-related mood and other psychiatric symptoms and disorders
Kiddie Schedule for Affective Disorders and Schizophrenia—Present and Lifetime Version (K-SADS-PL; Kaufman et al. 1997)	6–17 years	Semi-structured interview that combines dimensional and categorical assessment approaches to diagnose current and past episodes of psychopathology in children and adolescents using DSM criteria
Washington University (St. Louis) Kiddie Schedule for Affective Disorders and Schizophrenia (WASH-U K-SADS; Geller et al. 2001)	6–17 years	Specialized and expanded semi-structured interview for the diagnosis of mood disorders; sometimes combined with the K-SADS-PL to provide a complete assessment of all current and past psychopathologies
Mini International Neuropsychiatric Interview for Children and Adolescents (MINI-KID; Sheehan et al. 2010)	6–17 years	A short, structured diagnostic interview for DSM and ICD-10 psychiatric disorders in children and adolescents; standard version assesses the 30 most common and clinically relevant disorders or disorder subtypes in pediatric mental health; tracking yields a quantitative score that can be used to monitor treatment response over time

TABLE 1–1. Structured and semi-structured clinical interviews for pediatric mood disorders *(continued)*

Clinical interview	Age validated for use	Description
Structured Clinical Interview for DSM-5 (SCID-5; First et al. 2016)	18 years and over	A semi-structured interview guide to making the major DSM-5 diagnoses in adults; it is administered by a clinician or trained mental health professional who is familiar with the DSM-5 classification and diagnostic criteria; the interview subjects may be either psychiatric or general medical patients—or individuals who do not identify themselves as patients, such as participants in a community survey of mental illness or family members of psychiatric patients
Family Interview for Genetic Studies (FIGS; Maxwell 1982)	All ages	Interview used to assess psychopathology in all first- and second-degree relatives
Family History—Research Diagnostic Criteria (FH-RDC; Andreasen et al. 1977)	All ages	Interview used to assess psychopathology in all first- and second-degree relatives
Longitudinal Interval Follow-up Evaluation (LIFE; Keller et al. 1987)	All ages	Interview used to longitudinally track mood and other psychiatric symptoms; the LIFE interview provides a weekly longitudinal assessment of mood and psychotic symptoms and suicidal ideation

scores on the PSR scales may range from 1 for no symptoms to 2–4 for varying levels of subthreshold symptoms and impairment to 5–6 for presentations that meet full criteria with high levels of symptom severity and functional impairment. A consensus score between parents and children is established after each of them is interviewed individually.

The LIFE and other commonly used structured and semi-structured interviews are summarized in Table 1–1.

Clinician-Administered Instruments

Clinician-administered rating scales can provide objective assessments of time-varying and dimensionally scaled mood symptoms and their response to treatment. Clinical rating scales are available for depression; mania; suicide; co-occurring conditions such as anxiety and attention deficit/hyperactivity disorder (ADHD); and global functioning. Scales commonly used for the assessment of pediatric depression and mania are summarized below (see Table 1–2 for brief descriptions of these assessments and other assessments used in clinical practice.)

The Children's Depression Rating Scale—Revised (CDRS-R; Poznanski et al. 1984) is a clinician-administered interview conducted with parents and children separately to capture depression symptom severity and its impact on multiple areas of functioning. The CDRS-R has several advantages over self-report measures of depression: 1) it provides the presence or resolution of a comprehensive list of depressive symptoms that may have meaningful associations with neurobiological function (e.g., brain imaging measures), 2) it contextualizes depressive symptoms in terms of levels of severity and impact on daily function, 3) it only takes 10–15 minutes to complete, 4) it is empirically derived and validated and has been used widely as a primary outcome measure for clinical trials in youth with mood disorders (Mayes et al. 2010) and has been found to be preferable to adult depression rating scales (Jain et al. 2007), 5) it is administered to both parent and child and allows for clinician observation of symptoms to provide multi-informant data, and 6) it generates a raw score and a scaled T score normed for a population of youth with accompanying interpretation about the likelihood of a depressive disorder or the need for diagnostic confirmation. These features provide some advantages that are appealing for implementation into clinical practice once adapted.

Symptoms of hypomania and mania are commonly assessed by using the clinician-rated Young Mania Rating Scale (YMRS; Young et al. 1978). The YMRS has 11 items, with total scores ranging from 0 (no manic symptoms) to 60 (severely manic). Manic symptoms are rated on a scale of

0 to 4, with some item scores doubled to weight their clinical importance or low base rate (i.e., irritability, speech, thought content, and disruptive/aggressive behavior). The YMRS and other pediatric mania severity scales (e.g., Child Mania Rating Scale; C-MRS) have demonstrated good reliability and discriminant validity to distinguish bipolar spectrum disorders from unipolar depression (Yee et al. 2006) and commonly co-occurring conditions such as ADHD (Pavuluri et al. 2006). Moreover, the YMRS has been used as the primary mania severity outcome measure in clinical trials evaluating the efficacy of pharmacological interventions for mood stabilization.

The YMRS and CDRS-R provide dimensionally useful summary scores for mania and depression severity that can be tracked over time. The summary scores, although informative clinically, may represent a combination of heterogeneous clinical constructs (Isa et al. 2014) that may or may not map onto single or specific biological targets. Neuroscience tools such as multimodal magnetic resonance imaging (MRI) have emerged in the last 20 years that hold increasing promise for advancing mechanistic understanding of how aberrant structure and function in brain regions contribute to the onset, persistence, and recurrence of mood symptoms and episodes from childhood, adolescence, and in transition to adulthood. Taken together, these studies have consistently shown that altered interactions between prefrontal and subcortical brain regions are central to mood disorders, resulting in dysfunctional regulation or imbalance of emotion and cognitive processes. However, there is still much to be learned about these processes over the course of development, and MRI is still a research rather than a diagnostic or clinical tool. Indeed, more work is needed to translate the clinically meaningful experience and observation of depression and mania into measurable biological units. Nevertheless, clinician-based assessments have demonstrated utility in research and clinical practice.

Self-Administered Instruments

Self-administered instruments may be more time- and cost-efficient compared with clinically administered interviews and rating scales and, when completed in earnest by youth, can give patients the opportunity to share their experience with mood symptoms without confrontation. This may be particularly useful for patients with impairments in social functioning due to mood disorders (e.g., anxious depression), or in a busy clinical practice when time for clinical assessments is limited. For example, many primary care offices use the Patient Health Questionnaire–9 (PHQ-9), which scores each of the nine DSM criteria for depression as 0 ("not at all") to

TABLE 1–2. Clinician-administered mood symptom severity assessments

Clinical assessment	Age validated for use	Description
Children's Depression Rating Scale—Revised (CDRS-R; Poznanski et al. 1984)	6–17 years	A scale used to evaluate depressive symptoms based on DSM criteria; core symptoms of depression are rated according to CDRS-R criteria and anchors; in research, these questions are administered by trained raters separately to youth and children
Young Mania Rating Scale (YMRS; Young et al. 1978)	4–17 years	A scale used to dimensionally assess mania severity; symptoms of hypomania and mania are assessed using the clinician-rated YMRS; the YMRS has 11 items, with total scores ranging from 0 (no manic symptoms) to 60 (severely manic); manic symptoms are rated on a 0–4 scale, with some item scores doubled to weigh for their clinical importance and low base rate; the YMRS has been used as a clinician-rated instrument in juvenile bipolar disorder and has demonstrated good reliability and good ability to discriminate bipolar spectrum disorders from attention-deficit/hyperactivity disorder; study clinicians will assess symptoms using this scale at every visit and will enter scores on the case report form
Columbia–Suicide Severity Rating Scale (C-SSRS; Posner et al. 2011)	5–17 years	Clinician-rated measure used to assess lifetime suicide severity symptoms; C-SSRS has 18 items with yes/no responses and quantified number and lethality of attempts

TABLE 1–2.   Clinician-administered mood symptom severity assessments (*continued*)

Clinical assessment	Age validated for use	Description
Clinical Global Impression—Severity (CGI-S) and —Improvement (CGI-I; Busner and Targum 2007)	All ages	Readily understood, practical measurement tool that can easily be administered by a clinician in a busy clinical practice setting; functions as a stand-alone assessment of the clinician's view of the patient's global functioning prior to and after initiation of a study medication; provides an overall clinician-determined summary measure that takes into account knowledge of the patient's history, psychosocial circumstances, symptoms, behavior, and impact of the symptoms on the patient's ability to function
Children's Global Assessment Scale (CGAS; Shaffer et al. 1983)	6–17 years	A rating of functioning in which a child is given a single score between 1 and 100, based on a clinician's assessment of a range of aspects related to the child's psychological and social functioning; the score puts the youth in one of 10 categories that range from "extremely impaired" (1–10) to "doing very well" (91–100)

3 ("nearly every day") and has been validated for use in pediatric primary care (Allgaier et al. 2012). Similarly, efforts to screen for pediatric-onset mania have been described that involve administering parents a 10-item version of the General Behavioral Inventory (GBI) in an outpatient setting (Youngstrom et al. 2008). However, when measured against gold-standard clinical interviews, self-administered instruments either underestimate or overestimate the probability of a psychiatric diagnosis. For example, children who score at or near the clinical thresholds at which sensitivity and specificity are optimized are unlikely to meet criteria for psychopathology on gold-standard interviews (Sheldrick et al. 2015). Thus, self-administered scales and other instruments used to screen for depression should be interpreted probabilistically, with consideration of where an individual may fall along a continuum of positive scores, rather than used to categorically assign a diagnosis. Thus, because of varying degrees of accuracy and reliability, youth who screen positive for depression should be followed up with a comprehensive clinical evaluation whenever possible. Some commonly used self-report instruments for pediatric mood disorders are summarized in Table 1–3.

Early and accurate detection and treatment of pediatric-onset mood disorders may reduce the severity, chronicity, and treatment-resistant characteristics commonly observed in these disorders in adulthood (Chang et al. 2006). Differential diagnosis of mood disorders in children and adolescents, however, is especially challenging. First, there is a significant overlap in mood symptoms and other psychiatric disorders, notably ADHD and anxiety disorders. Second, mood symptoms in youth are often overlooked unless they cause clear functional impairment. Third, in certain stages of development, parents tend to be more reliable reporters of mood symptoms than are children, yet some clinicians rely exclusively on child report. Finally, a "backlash" against the possible overdiagnosis of certain mood disorders in youth (e.g., bipolar disorder) may cause some clinicians to err on the side of using "unspecified" diagnoses, or they may have doubts about the significance of the mood symptoms (Safer et al. 2015). These issues may adversely affect the reliability of diagnosis of mood disorders in routine clinical practice.

Mood disorders are increasing in prevalence in youth and are treatable. Effective management of mood symptoms begins with a careful multi-informant assessment that is bio-psycho-social-culturally informed and continually updated as a child grows. With early detection and timely intervention, perhaps children experiencing mood disorders early in life can grow to never experience a serious mood episode as adults.

TABLE 1–3. Self-administered mood assessments

Self- or parent-rated assessment	Age validated for use	Description
Patient Health Questionnaire–9 (PHQ-9; Kroenke et al. 2001)	11–17 years	A self-administered diagnostic instrument for depression that scores each of the nine DSM criteria as 0 ("not at all") to 3 ("nearly every day")
10-item mania assessment from the Parent General Behavior Inventory (P-GBI; Youngstrom et al. 2008)	5–17 years	A brief (10-item) instrument used to assess for parent-reported mania in outpatients presenting with a variety of different DSM diagnoses, including frequent comorbid conditions; parents most notice elated mood, high energy, irritability, and rapid changes in mood and energy as the prominent features of juvenile bipolar disorder
Child Behavior Checklist (CBCL) (Achenbach and Rescorla 2001) (includes Youth Self-Report [YSR])	6–18 years	A 113-item parent report of a child's behavior containing eight subscales: aggressive behavior, anxious/depressed, attention problems, rule-breaking behavior, somatic complaints, social problems, thought problems, and withdrawn/depressed; the Youth Self-Report is the corresponding behavior checklist completed by youth down to age 6
How I Feel (HIF; Walden et al. 2003)	8–12 years	A 30-item child self-report measure of emotion and arousal assessing the frequency and intensity of positive and negative emotion, and positive and negative emotion control; children are asked to rate how true each item is for him or her using a 5-point Likert scale (1= "not at all true of me" to 5= "very true of me")

TABLE 1–3.   Self-administered mood assessments *(continued)*

Self- or parent-rated assessment	Age validated for use	Description
Snaith-Hamilton Pleasure Scale (SHAPS; Snaith et al. 1995)	Down to age 14 years (Leventhal et al. 2015)	A 14-item self-rated scale of hedonic function; items on the SHAPS may be scored from 1 to 4 (1 = "strongly disagree" to 4 = "strongly agree")
Behavioral Inhibition–Behavioral Activation Scale (BIS-BAS; De Decker et al. 2017)	5–17 years	A 40-item checklist assessing behavioral inhibition and activation in youth; children are asked to rate how true each item is for them on a 4-point Likert scale (1 = "very true for me" to 4 = "very false for me")

References

Achenbach TM, Rescorla LA: Manual for the ASEBA School-Age Forms and Profiles: An Integrated System of Multi-informant Assessment. Burlington, VT, University of Vermont, Research Center for Children, Youth, and Families, 2001

Allgaier A-K, Pietsch K, Frühe B, et al: Screening for depression in adolescents: validity of the Patient Health Questionnaire in pediatric care. Depress Anxiety 29(10):906–913, 2012 22753313

American Psychiatric Association: Diagnostic and Statistical Manual of Mental Disorders, 5th Edition. Arlington, VA, American Psychiatric Association, 2013

Andreasen NC, Endicott J, Spitzer RL, et al: The family history method using diagnostic criteria: reliability and validity. Arch Gen Psychiatry 34(10):1229–1235, 1977 911222

Bruchmüller K, Margraf J, Suppiger A, et al: Popular or unpopular? Therapists' use of structured interviews and their estimation of patient acceptance. Behav Ther 42(4):634–643, 2011 22035992

Busner J, Targum SD: The clinical global impressions scale: applying a research tool in clinical practice. Psychiatry (Edgmont) 4(7):28–37, 2007 20526405

Chang K, Howe M, Gallelli K, et al: Prevention of pediatric bipolar disorder: integration of neurobiological and psychosocial processes. Ann N Y Acad Sci 1094:235–247, 2006 17347355

De Decker A, Verbeken S, Sioen I, et al: BIS/BAS scale in primary school children: parent-child agreement and longitudinal stability. Behav Change 34(2):98–116, 2017

Dougherty LR, Smith VC, Bufferd SJ, et al: Preschool irritability predicts child psychopathology, functional impairment, and service use at age nine. J Child Psychol Psychiatry 56(9):999–1007, 2015 26259142

Egger HL, Erkanli A, Keeler G, et al: Test-retest reliability of the Preschool Age Psychiatric Assessment (PAPA). J Am Acad Child Adolesc Psychiatry 45(5):538–549, 2006 16601400

Fears SC, Service SK, Kremeyer B, et al: Multisystem component phenotypes of bipolar disorder for genetic investigations of extended pedigrees. JAMA Psychiatry 71(4):375–387, 2014 24522887

Finsaas MC, Bufferd SJ, Dougherty LR, et al: Preschool psychiatric disorders: homotypic and heterotypic continuity through middle childhood and early adolescence. Psychol Med Jan 16, 2018 [Epub ahead of print] 29335030

First MB, Williams J, Karg R, et al: Structured Clinical Interview for DSM-5—Clinician Version (SCID-5-CV). Arlington, VA, American Psychiatric Association, 2016

Geller B, Zimerman B, Williams M, et al: Reliability of the Washington University in St. Louis Kiddie Schedule for Affective Disorders and Schizophrenia (WASH-U-KSADS) mania and rapid cycling sections. J Am Acad Child Adolesc Psychiatry 40(4):450–455, 2001 11314571

Goodwin FK, Jamison K: Manic-Depressive Illness. New York, Oxford University Press, 1990

Isa A, Bernstein I, Trivedi M, et al: Childhood depression subscales using repeated sessions on Children's Depression Rating Scale—Revised (CDRS-R) scores. J Child Adolesc Psychopharmacol 24(6):318–324, 2014 25137188

Jain S, Carmody TJ, Trivedi MH, et al: A psychometric evaluation of the CDRS and MADRS in assessing depressive symptoms in children. J Am Acad Child Adolesc Psychiatry 46(9):1204–1212, 2007 17712244

Jensen-Doss A, Youngstrom EA, Youngstrom JK, et al: Predictors and moderators of agreement between clinical and research diagnoses for children and adolescents. J Consult Clin Psychol 82(6):1151–1162, 2014 24773574

Kaufman J, Birmaher B, Brent D, et al: Schedule for Affective Disorders and Schizophrenia for School-Age Children—Present and Lifetime version (K-SADS-PL): initial reliability and validity data. J Am Acad Child Adolesc Psychiatry 36(7):980–988, 1997 9204677

Keller MB, Lavori PW, Friedman B, et al: The Longitudinal Interval Follow-up Evaluation: a comprehensive method for assessing outcome in prospective longitudinal studies. Arch Gen Psychiatry 44(6):540–548, 1987 3579500

Kertz SJ, Sylvester C, Tillman R, et al: Latent class profiles of anxiety symptom trajectories from preschool through school age. J Clin Child Adolesc Psychol Mar 20, 2017 [Epub ahead of print] 28318338

Kroenke K, Spitzer RL, Williams JB: The PHQ-9: validity of a brief depression severity measure. J Gen Intern Med 16(9):606–613, 2001 11556941

Leffler JM, Riebel J, Hughes HM: A review of child and adolescent diagnostic interviews for clinical practitioners. Assessment 22(6):690–703, 2015 25520212

Leventhal AM, Unger JB, Audrain-McGovern J, et al: Measuring anhedonia in adolescents: a psychometric analysis. J Pers Assess 97(5):506–514, 2015 25893676

Luby JL, Belden AC: Clinical characteristics of bipolar vs. unipolar depression in preschool children: an empirical investigation. J Clin Psychiatry 69(12):1960–1969, 2008 19192470

Luby JL, Gaffrey MS, Tillman R, et al: Trajectories of preschool disorders to full DSM depression at school age and early adolescence: continuity of preschool depression. Am J Psychiatry 171(7):768–776, 2014 24700355

Martin J, Streit F, Treutlein J, et al: Expert and self-assessment of lifetime symptoms and diagnosis of major depressive disorder in large-scale genetic studies in the general population: comparison of a clinical interview and a self-administered checklist. Psychiatr Genet 27(5):187–196, 2017 28731911

Matuschek T, Jaeger S, Stadelmann S, et al: Implementing the K-SADS-PL as a standard diagnostic tool: effects on clinical diagnoses. Psychiatry Res 236:119–124, 2016 26724908

Maxwell E: Manual for the FIGS. Rockville, MD, Clinical Neurogenetics Branch, Intramural Research Program, National Institute of Mental Health, 1982

Mayes TL, Bernstein IH, Haley CL, et al: Psychometric properties of the Children's Depression Rating Scale—Revised in adolescents. J Child Adolesc Psychopharmacol 20(6):513–516, 2010 21186970

Nakash O, Nagar M, Kanat-Maymon Y: Clinical use of the DSM categorical diagnostic system during the mental health intake session. J Clin Psychiatry 76(7):e862–e869, 2015 26231013

Pavuluri MN, Henry DB, Devineni B, et al: Child Mania Rating Scale: development, reliability, and validity. J Am Acad Child Adolesc Psychiatry 45(5):550–560, 2006 16601399

Posner K, Brown GK, Stanley B, et al: The Columbia–Suicide Severity Rating Scale: initial validity and internal consistency findings from three multisite studies with adolescents and adults. Am J Psychiatry 168(12):1266–1277, 2011 22193671

Poznanski EO, Grossman JA, Buchsbaum Y, et al: Preliminary studies of the reliability and validity of the Children's Depression Rating Scale. J Am Acad Child Psychiatry 23(2):191–197, 1984 6715741

Rettew DC, Lynch AD, Achenbach TM, et al: Meta-analyses of agreement between diagnoses made from clinical evaluations and standardized diagnostic interviews. Int J Methods Psychiatr Res 18(3):169–184, 2009 19701924

Safer DJ, Rajakannan T, Burcu M, et al: Trends in subthreshold psychiatric diagnoses for youth in community treatment. JAMA Psychiatry 72(1):75–83, 2015 25426673

Shaffer D, Gould MS, Brasic J, et al: A children's global assessment scale (CGAS). Arch Gen Psychiatry 40(11):1228–1231, 1983 6639293

Sheehan DV, Sheehan KH, Shytle RD, et al: Reliability and validity of the Mini International Neuropsychiatric Interview for Children and Adolescents (MINI-KID). J Clin Psychiatry 71(3):313–326, 2010 20331933

Sheldrick RC, Benneyan JC, Kiss IG, et al: Thresholds and accuracy in screening tools for early detection of psychopathology. J Child Psychol Psychiatry 56(9):936–948, 2015 26096036

Snaith RP, Hamilton M, Morley S, et al: A scale for the assessment of hedonic tone: the Snaith-Hamilton Pleasure Scale. Br J Psychiatry 167(1):99–103, 1995 7551619

Verweij KHW, Derks EM, Hendriks EJE, et al: The influence of informant characteristics on the reliability of family history interviews. Twin Res Hum Genet 14(3):217–220, 2011 21623650

Walden TA, Harris VS, Catron TF: How I Feel: a self-report measure of emotional arousal and regulation for children. Psychol Assess 15(3):399–412, 2003 14593841

Yee AM, Algorta GP, Youngstrom EA, et al: Unfiltered administration of the YMRS and CDRS-R in a clinical sample of children. J Am Acad Child Adolesc Psychiatry 44(6):992–1007, 2006 24885078

Young RC, Biggs JT, Ziegler VE, et al: A rating scale for mania: reliability, validity and sensitivity. Br J Psychiatry 133:429–435, 1978 728692

Youngstrom EA, Frazier TW, Demeter C, et al: Developing a 10-item mania scale from the Parent General Behavior Inventory for children and adolescents. J Clin Psychiatry 69(5):831–839, 2008 18452343

2

DSM-5 Diagnosis of Mood Disorders in Children and Adolescents

Anna Van Meter, Ph.D.

Sasha is in fifth grade. Her parents report that she has been struggling psychologically for the past 18 months. In third grade, she exhibited significant anxiety; she did not want to be separated from her mother, she worried excessively about what her peers thought of her, and she was convinced she would fail out of school. She started seeing a psychiatrist, who prescribed fluoxetine to treat her anxiety. Her symptoms of anxiety improved; however, about 6 months later, she started struggling socially, and both she and her parents say that her mood has been "depressed" since then. Her parents report that Sasha is often withdrawn and prefers to be alone in her room. They say that she is irritable, snapping at other people, and frequently becomes "enraged" when things don't go her way. For example, when her mother told Sasha she had to wear a coat over her Halloween costume because of cold temperatures, Sasha cut the arm off her coat with a pair of scissors and refused to go trick-or-treating. Sasha's irritability has also contributed to her social problems; her teacher reported that

Sasha screamed at a classmate who wouldn't make room for her at the lunch table and pushed his lunch tray to the floor. Other children were upset by her actions and avoid her now. At home, Sasha argues frequently with her brother and parents but spends the majority of her time alone in her room. Her parents report that she has "completely taken over the family" and that everyone "walks on eggshells to avoid setting her off."

Sasha acknowledges that she gets mad easily, but she also says that she feels "sad" a lot of the time. She says that the past year has been "horrible" and reports feeling as though "everyone's against" her. She reports that it is difficult for her to fall asleep, often taking an hour or more, during which time she feels like "all the bad stuff from the day comes rushing back." Sasha says that on the mornings after she can't fall asleep, she feels very tired and argues with her mother about getting up for school. Sasha also reports that she thinks about death frequently and wonders "what happens after we die," but denies any thoughts about wanting to be dead herself.

Sasha cannot recall a time when she felt much better than usual or experienced elated mood out of proportion to the situation. Similarly, her parents report that she occasionally gets happy and excited when working on an art project, but that her elevated moods never seem concerning or too intense. Additionally, when these happy moods occur, they tend to be relatively brief, lasting only an hour or two over the course of the day. She is never "up" or happy for an entire day. Neither Sasha nor her parents report periods of increased energy or agitation, either. However, Sasha's parents report that she can be "pretty grandiose" and often talks about how life will be when she is a "famous artist." Sasha also has a strong interest in sex; her mother reports that she asks "tons of questions" and that she occasionally acts in provocative ways—for example, demanding that her brother's friend teach her how to French-kiss. On a mania rating scale, Sasha's mother rates her as a 9, out of a possible 30, putting her in the mild-to-neutral risk category.

Sasha's diagnostic picture is complicated; she is impaired by multiple symptoms, including depressed mood, anxiety, and poor social functioning. And she is significantly impacting her family with her frequent temper outbursts. She endorses depressed mood, irritability, insomnia, and morbid ideation, but this falls short of the five symptoms necessary for a diagnosis of major depression. Additionally, her mood brightens considerably on occasion, and she has some other mild symptoms of hypomania. However, given her age, it is not entirely clear whether her grandiosity and interest in sex are outside the bounds of a typically developing preadolescent. Her temper outbursts seem like they could be indicative of oppositional defiant disorder (ODD), but rather than being defiant and breaking rules, Sasha is described by her parents as "ultrasensitive," with her outbursts mostly triggered by some sense of injustice or perceived slight.

Although an argument could be made for comorbid persistent depressive disorder and ODD, a more parsimonious diagnosis is disruptive mood dysregulation disorder (DMDD). Her mood is dysphoric and irritable most of the day, nearly every day, and according to both Sasha and her parents, it has been that way for about a year. She is also experiencing temper outbursts in multiple settings, multiple times a week, that are unusual for her age and out of proportion to the situation at hand. Although hypomania is an exclusionary criterion for DMDD, her symptoms are very brief and intermittent and are not adequate to justify a bipolar spectrum diagnosis. Because bipolar disorder often begins with a depressive episode, these symptoms should be monitored closely, and if they become more severe or last longer, the diagnosis should be revisited.

As we can see with Sasha, the diagnosis of mood disorders in youth can be challenging; complicating factors include developmental considerations and the line between normal and abnormal moods in youth; the need to establish episodicity; and symptom overlap with other childhood disorders. Discrepancies in youth and caregiver reports can also lead to ambiguity when the clinician is working to establish whether diagnostic criteria have been met. Although these factors can add "noise" to the diagnostic process, focusing on DSM criteria and using tools that facilitate this approach (as described in Chapter 1, "Principles of Assessment of Mood Disorders in Childhood") can provide structure and improve diagnostic reliability and validity.

The majority of research on which DSM-5 (American Psychiatric Association 2013) is based was conducted with adults, and as such, the criteria do not always reflect the particular challenges of working with youth. However, subsequent research has shown that the DSM criteria for depression and bipolar disorder, when applied in youth populations, lead to valid and reliable diagnoses (Yorbik et al. 2004; Youngstrom et al. 2008). And although DSM criteria are imperfect, they provide consistency, which facilitates appropriate treatment and prognostication. In this chapter, we outline the DSM criteria for each mood disorder, highlighting developmental considerations and details important to differential diagnosis.

Major Depressive Disorder

Major depressive disorder (MDD) is an episodic illness; the onset of symptoms must coincide with a change in functioning, and an adequate number of symptoms must be present concurrently to constitute an episode. The episode, during which the youth must have depressed/low or irritable mood plus at least four additional symptoms, must last at least 2 weeks to meet criteria for MDD. There is some evidence that in children, depressive episodes may be shorter, on average, than in adults, and recommendations have been made for reducing the duration criterion for very young children (Luby et al. 2009b). However, other research suggests that, on average, depressive episodes in youth do meet the DSM duration criteria (Birmaher et al. 2004), and given the option of an other specified depressive disorder diagnosis, there is no strong rationale for giving an MDD diagnosis if the duration criterion has not been met.

Establishing episodicity for a diagnosis of MDD can be difficult. Particularly in young children, caregivers may have the sense that the child has "always" been depressed or had low mood. Asking about how the child was doing at memorable events (e.g., holidays, school starting) can help to establish the onset/offset of mood episodes. Understanding the episodicity can be particularly important when one is trying to distinguish between a diagnosis of depression and another, more chronic presentation such as anxiety, attention-deficit/hyperactivity disorder (ADHD), or persistent depressive disorder.

The inclusion of irritable mood as an A criterion is specific to youth; because young people may not have the vocabulary or emotional awareness to articulate sadness, depressed mood is often expressed with anger/irritability. Depressed youth can be very sensitive, and families may describe going to great effort to avoid provoking an irritable outburst. Because irritability can significantly impact people around the youth, other signs of depression may go unnoticed. This can negatively impact the diagnostic process; if the presenting complaint is irritability, a diagnosis of ODD or another problem behavior–based diagnosis may be made incorrectly if other depressive symptoms are not fully assessed and ruled out.

The other primary symptoms of MDD include diminished interest in activities or an inability to enjoy things, excessive appetite/weight gain or decreased appetite/weight loss (which in children can also manifest as failure to grow as expected), sleep disturbance (hypersomnia or insomnia), psychomotor agitation or retardation, feelings of worthlessness or guilt, difficulty concentrating or indecisiveness, and recurrent morbid thoughts about death or suicide (Table 2–1). Many youth with MDD may also have somatic complaints such as headache or stomachache or exhibit very low energy, though these do not constitute specific criteria. A common presentation of MDD in youth is lethargy coupled with lack of interest in activities that the child normally would enjoy or low engagement and withdrawal from pleasurable events. Children may be disinterested in their peers or family activities and show little enthusiasm. In some children with depression, anxiety may also play a role; rumination is common and can impact sleep, contributing to insomnia. Youth may also experience hypersomnia and feel tired despite getting adequate sleep at night; youth with hypersomnia may be difficult to wake in the morning and may fall asleep in class or at other inopportune times.

Youth with depression can be inclined to blame themselves for negative things that occur, such as an argument between parents. There can also be a tendency to hold oneself to unrealistic standards and to be very self-critical when these standards are not met—for example, expecting perfect grades and becoming despondent when perfection is not achieved. Unfortunately, the poor concentration associated with depression can make it more difficult for youth to meet their obligations, whether these entail completing homework assignments or doing chores as instructed. This creates more opportunities for criticism, which can further exacerbate depressed mood.

In some cases, youth with depression may express thoughts related to death or suicide, suggesting that they wish they had never been born or expressing that their family would be better off if they were dead. Although suicide is not prevalent in children or adolescents, it is one of the most common causes of death among youth, and recent data suggest that rates are increasing among school-age girls (Centers for Disease Control and Prevention 2015). Any expression related to suicide should be taken seriously and comprehensively assessed—repeatedly, if necessary—to rule out imminent risk.

Depression can occur in very young children (Luby et al. 2009a) but becomes more common as youth age. Individuals whose depression has an early onset, prior to puberty, may be more likely to have a severe course of illness, with frequent recurrences and fewer days well. Depression in postpubertal youth is twice as common in females compared with males, likely because of a greater accumulation of risk factors in females, including societal expectations, life stressors, and coping style (Nolen-Hoeksema and Girgus 1994; Salk et al. 2016, 2017). Although the criteria used to diagnose depression are the same in adults and children (with the exception of irritable mood counting toward the diagnosis only in children), there can be some differences in symptoms. For example, children with depression are more likely than adolescents or adults to report somatic complaints and are less likely to experience hopelessness and dysphoria (Avenevoli et al. 2008). In contrast, adolescents are more likely than children to experience suicidal ideation or to attempt suicide, to experience hypersomnia, and to have weight loss (Yorbik et al. 2004).

There is evidence to suggest that in the United States, ethnic minority youth are at higher risk for depression than their white peers (Anderson and Mayes 2010). However, inconsistencies in the prevalence rates reported across studies and methodological issues (e.g., relying on self-reported symp-

TABLE 2–1. DSM-5 criteria for a major depressive episode

Criterion	Details	Special considerations
A. Two-week period that represents a change from previous functioning during which youth experiences depressed or irritable mood or loss of interest or pleasure. *Plus* five (or more) additional symptoms (see "Details") that are present most of the day, nearly every day, during the same 2-week period.	Depressed or irritable mood (as reported by the youth or observed by others)	Irritability can often be misattributed to externalizing disorders. When irritable mood is prominent, depression should be considered.
	Decreased interest or enjoyment in all, or almost all, activities	Youths' interests can shift frequently, so it may be that an activity that was formerly enjoyable no longer is. However, if most things fail to engage the youth's interest (including peers), the extent of the decreased interest is clinically significant.
	Significant, unintentional weight loss or weight gain or failure to meet expected weight gains with growth	Weight changes can be related to somatic symptoms that youth often have when depressed; frequent complaints of stomachaches or headaches may also be indicative of depressed mood.

TABLE 2–1. DSM-5 criteria for a major depressive episode *(continued)*

Criterion	Details	Special considerations
A. Two-week period that represents a change from previous functioning during which youth experiences depressed or irritable mood or loss of interest or pleasure. *Plus* five (or more) additional symptoms (see "Details") that are present most of the day, nearly every day, during the same 2-week period. *(continued)*	Insomnia or hypersomnia	Many youth resist going to bed, but insomnia is only considered when the youth is in bed and wants to fall asleep but cannot. This should be distinguished from decreased need for sleep, which is when the youth cannot fall asleep but has good energy the next day despite a short sleep. Additionally, many youth—especially teenagers—are tired during the day. Being tired after not getting enough sleep the night before must be distinguished from hypersomnia, which is when the youth feels very tired, and even dozes off during the day, despite sleeping 8 or more hours at night.
	Psychomotor agitation or retardation as observed by others	Restlessness and agitation should be a change—if a youth is chronically fidgety and restless, this might be more consistent with ADHD.
	Fatigue or loss of energy	The feelings of low energy/being tired must be inconsistent with the amount of sleep and exercise the youth is getting.

TABLE 2–1.   DSM-5 criteria for a major depressive episode (*continued*)

Criterion	Details	Special considerations
A. Two-week period that represents a change from previous functioning during which youth experiences depressed or irritable mood or loss of interest or pleasure. *Plus* five (or more) additional symptoms (see "Details") that are present most of the day, nearly every day, during the same 2-week period. (*continued*)	Feelings of worthlessness or excessive or inappropriate guilt	Youth with depression may hold themselves to high, even unrealistic, standards that they inevitably fail to meet. This can lead to feelings of worthlessness. Even if the perceived "failure" is in a specific domain (e.g., athletics, academics), youth may generalize this to all aspects of their lives. Youth may also take responsibility for things that are far outside their control and feel guilty when others struggle.
	Diminished ability to think or concentrate, or indecisiveness	Poor concentration or indecisiveness must be distinguished from characteristics of ADHD or anxiety, which would have a more chronic presentation.
	Recurrent thoughts of death (not just fear of dying), recurrent suicidal ideation with or without a plan, or a suicide attempt or a specific plan for dying by suicide	Youth may not express a desire to hurt themselves (even if they are having suicidal thoughts) but may instead talk about wishing they had never been born or say that their families would be better off without them. Carefully assessing for suicidal thoughts is important in youth who have mood disturbance.

TABLE 2–1.　DSM-5 criteria for a major depressive episode *(continued)*

Criterion	Details	Special considerations
B. The symptoms cause clinically significant distress or impairment in functioning.		Some people are able to function adequately while depressed but will experience a significant decline in quality of life. Youth who are depressed may still perform well in school, but it is important to pay attention to how their engagement may have changed in other aspects of their lives.
C. The episode is not attributable to the physiological effects of a substance or another medical condition.		Youth may be more hesitant than adults to disclose the use of substances, and caregivers may be unaware of substance use. In cases in which there is a very dramatic, sudden change, it is worth testing for substances that could be implicated in the presenting symptoms.

Note.　ADHD=attention-deficit/hyperactivity disorder.

Source.　Adapted from American Psychiatric Association: *Diagnostic and Statistical Manual of Mental Disorders,* 5th Edition. Arlington, VA, American Psychiatric Association. Copyright 2013, American Psychiatric Association. Used with permission.

toms, not controlling for socioeconomic status) make it difficult to draw con-clusions from these findings. Relatedly, there is inconsistent evidence that ethnic minority youth may be more likely to express depressed mood through oppositional or somatic symptoms (Stewart et al. 2012). Despite these in-consistencies, it is helpful to keep in mind that ethnic minority youth may be more likely to have significant risk factors for depression (e.g., poverty, trau-matic events) and that ethnic minority families may be less likely to seek men-tal health services. Consequently, ethnic minority youth with depression may be more likely to present at primary care or school; screening for depression in these settings can help identify youth who would not otherwise get help.

When caregivers do bring their children for treatment, it is usually re-lated to externalizing rather than internalizing symptoms, which means that many youth with depression are not diagnosed or treated. Youth with depression, particularly those who do not have irritable mood, may come across as withdrawn but otherwise not "problematic," in terms of behavior. Youth with irritable mood may come to the clinic but are often misdiag-nosed with an externalizing disorder, as described earlier. If the youth has a comorbid disorder, as close to half of depressed youth do (Ford et al. 2003; Rohde et al. 1991), the likelihood of a missed depression diagnosis is even higher. ADHD and anxiety are particularly common among youth with depression and may exacerbate depressed mood by interfering with a youth's cognitive and behavioral functioning. This highlights the impor-tance of conducting a comprehensive clinical interview and following up with appropriate assessment tools to ensure that depression is not missed.

The course of MDD can vary widely, but the majority of both children and adolescents who have an episode of depression will recover. Of those who recover, about 40% will experience a new episode of depression (Birmaher et al. 2004). Once depression has recurred, another depressive episode becomes increasingly likely. Unlike some childhood disorders, de-pression is generally homotypic, meaning that if a child has depression, she or he is more likely to have depression as an adult (relative to another disorder), although the specific symptoms may shift over time (Carballo et al. 2011; Ormel et al. 2015; Shankman et al. 2009).

Persistent Depressive Disorder

Persistent depressive disorder (PDD) is a new diagnosis in DSM-5, one that consolidates the prior DSM-IV diagnoses of dysthymic disorder and chronic major depression into a single diagnosis. For criteria for PDD to be met, youth must experience depressed or irritable mood, plus two or more additional symptoms, for at least a year. During the symptomatic year, the youth cannot have been symptom-free for more than 2 months. Youth with symptoms that meet criteria for an episode of major depression that lasts for a year (or longer) would be given a diagnosis of PDD with major depressive episode(s). Although for youth with relatively mild symptoms, this change in the diagnostic criteria is unlikely to affect treatment, for those who have chronic major depression, the change could minimize the extent of their impairment.

In addition to depressed or irritable mood, the other symptoms of PDD include appetite changes (increased/decreased), sleep disturbance (insomnia or hypersomnia), low energy or fatigue, poor self-esteem, poor concentration or difficulty making decisions, and feelings of hopelessness. Although there is overlap between PDD symptoms and the symptoms of MDD, there are also some important differences; poor self-esteem and feelings of hopelessness are only criteria for PDD, whereas anhedonia, physical agitation or retardation, feelings of worthlessness or guilt, and thoughts of death are specific to MDD. Because of these differences, it is possible that a youth would have depressed mood and two additional symptoms of MDD (but not of PDD) for a year. This would result in a diagnosis of other specified depressive disorder. The diagnoses of PDD and MDD are not mutually exclusive. If a youth has a year during which she or he has symptoms that meet criteria for PDD and later has a major depressive episode, the youth would carry both diagnoses—this is sometimes referred to as "double depression."

The onset of PDD can be more insidious than would be typical of MDD, so although a change in functioning must be associated with the onset of symptoms to meet diagnostic criteria, it can be more difficult to establish the onset of the episode than it might be with MDD. Additionally, because of the chronic nature of PDD, youth and their caregivers may express that they have "always" been depressed, or caregivers may attribute the low mood to temperament rather than to a mental illness that can be treated. Failure to identify PDD can also be related to comorbid disorders that may obscure diagnosis; the majority of youth with PDD also have anxiety and/or externalizing disorders (Masi et al. 2001). Accurate diagnosis of PDD is important because youth who have PDD are at increased risk for developing an episode of major depression, and research suggests that treating the PDD can help to prevent the more severe symptoms associated with MDD (Kovacs et al. 1994; Shankman et al. 2009).

Adjustment Disorder With Depressed Mood

If depressed mood begins within 3 months following a stressor—for example, parents' divorce, school change, or move—and causes impairment and/or distress that is out of proportion to the situation, a diagnosis of adjustment disorder with depressed mood would be appropriate. In these cases, the markers of depressed mood may include sadness and feelings of hopelessness. When the stressor or its consequences resolve, the depressed mood is expected to lift within 6 months. However, in some situations, the adjustment disorder may become persistent if the stressor is not resolved (e.g., ongoing abuse, long-term absence of a parent because of military deployment). If a child's symptoms are severe enough to warrant a diagnosis of MDD, this diagnosis should be made, rather than adjustment disorder, even if a specific stressor precipitated the symptoms. Similarly, it should be noted that although the symptoms of grief typically differ from depression in some ways (e.g., grief is associated with more mood reactivity and less self-criticism), and previous versions of DSM have excluded cases of bereavement from the diagnosis of MDD, a change was made in DSM-5, which states that "the presence of a major depressive episode in addition to the normal response to a significant loss should also be carefully considered" (American Psychiatric Association 2013, p. 161).

Other Specified/Unspecified Depressive Disorder

The other specified/unspecified categories are used when a child experiences impairment due to depressed mood and associated symptoms but does not have symptoms that meet criteria for another depressive disorder. For example, if an individual experienced depressed mood, insomnia, lack of interest, psychomotor agitation, and suicidal ideation for 10 days, this would fall short of the duration criterion for an episode of major depression and, consequently, she would be diagnosed with other specified depressive disorder. Or, as described above, in some cases, an individual may have symptoms of depression lasting over a year, but not two symptoms that are specific to PDD; in this case the individual would also receive an "other specified" diagnosis. The central distinguishing characteristic between *unspecified* and *other specified* is whether the clinician indicates why the criteria for another depressive disorder were not met (e.g., unspecified is too few symptoms to constitute an episode of MDD). It is important for the clinician to assess for symptoms consistent with MDD and PDD (and other depressive disorders outside the scope of this chapter, including premenstrual dysphoric disorder and substance-induced depressive disorder) before considering this diagnostic classification. For a quick guide on differentiating between mood disorder types, see Table 2–2.

Disruptive Mood Dysregulation Disorder

Disruptive mood dysregulation disorder is a new diagnosis to DSM-5, based on past research on severe mood dysregulation and temper dysregulation with dysphoria. DMDD is classified as a depressive disorder, but its presentation is primarily irritable. DMDD was introduced in DSM-5 as a diagnostic "home" for youth with extreme irritability and tantrums, who—some worried—were at risk of being misdiagnosed with bipolar disorder (Fristad et al. 2016; Margulies et al. 2012). The criteria for DMDD include persistent angry or irritable mood for at least a year (with no more than 3 months during that year symptom-free) and frequent (three or more times per week), severe temper tantrums that are developmentally inappropriate and out of proportion to the situation and that occur across multiple settings.

Research suggests that in as many as 90% of youth with symptoms that meet criteria for DMDD, the symptoms could also meet criteria for ODD (Copeland et al. 2013; Mayes et al. 2016); however, a youth cannot be diagnosed with both. The main differentiating factor between the two disorders is chronic angry/irritable mood, which would indicate a diagnosis of DMDD rather than ODD. Bipolar spectrum disorders are also mutually exclusive with DMDD—if the child has had four or more symptoms of mania lasting a full day at any time, a diagnosis of DMDD cannot be made. When DMDD is compared with other specified bipolar disorder, the presence of manic symptoms and a family history of bipolar disorder are the primary distinctions between the two groups (Fristad et al. 2016). A choice must also be made between DMDD and intermittent explosive disorder; although the tantrum behavior might be similar in the two disorders, the mood between tantrums does not have to be irritable for a diagnosis of intermittent explosive disorder, and the duration criterion for intermittent explosive disorder is only 3 months.

Results from the first studies designed to evaluate DMDD specifically are now being published; there is substantial debate about the validity of

TABLE 2–2. Quick guide to differentiating between childhood mood disorders

	Episode of depression; ≥2 weeks	Depressive symptoms, no episode	Episode of mania; ≥7 days or hospitalized	Episode of hypomania; 4 days, no impairment	Manic symptoms, no episode	Extreme irritability	Chronic presentation
Major depressive disorder	●	O	■	■	■	O	O
Persistent depressive disorder	O	●	■	■	■	O	●
DMDD	O	O	■	■	O	●	●
Adjustment disorder w/ depressed mood	O	In response to a stressor	O	O	O	O	O
Other specified depressive disorder	O	●	■	■	■	O	O
Bipolar I disorder	O	O	●	O	O	O	O
Bipolar II disorder	●	O	■	●	O	O	O
Cyclothymic disorder	■	●	■	■	●	O	●
Other specified bipolar disorder	■	O	■	O	●	O	O

Note. ●=inclusion; ■=exclusion; O =could be present; does not affect diagnosis (manic symptoms lasting more than a day would exclude DMDD). DMDD= disruptive mood dysregulation disorder.

this diagnosis (Is it stable over time? Does it identify a unique group of youth? Does it inform treatment?), and this work should help to clarify the clinical role DMDD will play moving forward.

Bipolar I Disorder

Bipolar I disorder is characterized by one or more episodes of mania. For criteria for a manic episode to be met, a youth or adolescent must experience elevated, expansive, or irritable mood most of the day, nearly every day, for at least a week. During this time, the individual must also have abnormally and persistently increased activity or energy, plus at least three additional manic symptoms (described below), unless the predominant mood state is irritable, in which case, four additional symptoms are necessary. The duration criterion of 1 week may be disregarded if the symptoms are severe enough to warrant hospitalization; in these cases, treatment may prevent the symptoms from persisting a week despite clear evidence that the individual was manic. Relatedly, if there are psychotic symptoms in conjunction with other manic symptoms, the episode would be defined as mania.

Other symptoms of mania include grandiosity or excessive self-esteem, decreased need for sleep, pressured speech or increased talkativeness, flight of ideas or a sense that one's thoughts are racing out of control, distractibility, increased goal-directed activity or physical agitation (restlessness activity absent a goal), and involvement in activities that are likely to result in negative consequences (Table 2–3). In order for these symptoms to be applied toward a diagnosis of mania, onset of the symptoms must represent a clear change in functioning and the symptoms must co-occur. For example, if a youth had elated mood for several days that abated and later developed grandiosity for a brief period of time, these symptoms would not constitute an episode because they did not occur at the same time. Relatedly, if a youth had long been distractible and restless and later developed elated mood and grandiosity, only the symptoms of elated mood and grandiosity would be applied toward a bipolar diagnosis because the distractibility and restlessness are chronic and do not represent a change in functioning. Instead, these symptoms might indicate a comorbid condition.

A life chart can help the clinician determine episodicity. For example, the Longitudinal Interval Follow-up Evaluation (LIFE; Keller et al. 1987) assesses multiple symptom domains on a week-by-week basis, which can be very helpful for understanding whether symptoms tend to begin and end at the same time. It can also be helpful to choose a memorable event (e.g., a birthday, start of school, a vacation) and ask what, if any, symptoms

TABLE 2–3.   DSM-5 criteria for a manic or hypomanic episode

Criterion	Details	Special considerations
A. A period of abnormally and persistently elevated, expansive, or irritable mood *and* abnormally and persistently increased activity or energy, lasting at least 1 week and present most of the day, nearly every day (or any duration if hospitalization is necessary).		In hypomania, the duration criterion is only 4 days.
B. During the period of mood disturbance and increased energy or activity, three (or more) additional symptoms (four if the mood is only irritable; see right) are present to a significant degree and represent a noticeable change from usual behavior.	Inflated self-esteem or grandiosity	Must be considered in the developmental context; youth often have unrealistic ambitions; to meet criteria there must be a distinct change.
	Decreased need for sleep (e.g., feels rested after only 3 hours of sleep)	Important to differentiate from not wanting to sleep or insomnia; in [hypo]mania the youth will be fully awake/energetic after an objectively brief sleep.
	More talkative than usual or pressure to keep talking	Many youth speak rapidly, especially when excited; note whether this is a change and whether it persists across situations.
	Flight of ideas or subjective experience that thoughts are racing	It may be difficult to follow the youth in conversation due to excessive, unusual tangents. The youth may complain of having too much going on in his or her head.
	Distractibility	It is important to establish a change; many youth are distractible, and distractibility can also be associated with attention-deficit/hyperactivity disorder or depression.

TABLE 2–3.   DSM-5 criteria for a manic or hypomanic episode (*continued*)

Criterion	Details	Special considerations
B. During the period of mood disturbance and increased energy or activity, three (or more) additional symptoms (four if the mood is only irritable; see right) are present to a significant degree and represent a noticeable change from usual behavior. (*continued*)	Increase in goal-directed activity (either socially, at work or school, or sexually) or psychomotor agitation	Youth may take on new interests to an almost obsessional degree or express great interest in many new things, jumping from one project to another. Agitation can include pacing, squirming around, and so forth. This must be a change from the individual's usual degree of psychomotor activity.
	Excessive involvement in activities that have a high potential for painful consequences	Youth often do things that show poor judgment; to qualify as a symptom, this behavior should show a new degree of impulsivity or clear disregard for rules, values, or personal safety.
C. The mood disturbance is sufficiently severe to cause marked impairment in social functioning or to necessitate hospitalization to prevent harm to self or others, or there are psychotic features.		This criterion applies *only* to mania; hypomania is not associated with marked impairment. If there is a need for hospitalization or there are psychotic features, the correct diagnosis is mania.
D. The episode is not attributable to the physiological effects of a substance or another medical condition.		Youth may be more hesitant than adults to disclose the use of substances, and caregivers may be unaware of substance use. In cases in which there is a very dramatic, sudden change, it is worth testing for substances that could be implicated in the presenting symptoms.

Source.   Adapted from American Psychiatric Association: *Diagnostic and Statistical Manual of Mental Disorders*, 5th Edition. Arlington, VA, American Psychiatric Association. Copyright 2013, American Psychiatric Association. Used with permission.

the youth was experiencing at that time. This event, and the symptoms present at that time, are marked on a paper. This is the beginning of the life chart; moving forward in time, the clinician then inquires about other events and whether symptoms had their onset or remitted at that point, and marks these in a sequential way on the paper. This approach helps families remember key details about the child's symptoms and functioning over time, and the life chart can be helpful to refer back to as the youth progresses in treatment.

There has been debate about the diagnosis of mania in youth; this debate has focused on the following points: 1) whether irritable mood is adequate, or whether, because of the prevalence of irritability in youth, elated mood should be required; 2) whether distinct episodes are necessary, and if they are, whether the 7-day criterion should be required; 3) whether to count nonspecific symptoms, such as distractibility, toward diagnoses of both mania and a comorbid condition; 4) whether mania is qualitatively different in youth than in adults; and 5) how to handle discrepant symptom reports from youth and caregiver. Although the phenomenology of mania in youth can be different from what might be more typical in adults, research has shown consistently that reliable, valid diagnoses can be made using DSM criteria without modification (Youngstrom 2009; Youngstrom et al. 2008). Additionally, taking a hierarchical approach to diagnosis (counting each symptom toward only one diagnosis) is less likely to result in unnecessary diagnoses and associated treatments (Youngstrom et al. 2003).

The requirement of persistently increased activity or energy as an A criterion for mania is new to DSM-5 and has raised some questions because similar language (increase in goal-directed activity—either socially, at work or school, or sexually—or psychomotor agitation) is used to describe additional B symptom criteria. Although it is not clear from DSM, experts in the field seem to agree that a single symptom or change in functioning should only be counted once. However, because there are different ways that an individual could exhibit increased energy, goal-directed activity, or psychomotor agitation, this set of symptoms could be counted toward both the A and B criteria if there are two distinct symptoms (e.g., increased goal-directed activity *and* psychomotor agitation).

As with depression, because mania is episodic, it is important to establish that the symptoms begin at the same time. In youth, it can be difficult to distinguish some symptoms of mania from symptoms of other childhood disorders (e.g., ODD, ADHD) and from normal childhood behaviors. For example, in an adult, a proclamation by a patient that he is sure to be elected president in the next election would be evidence of grandiosity, but in a child, this type of goal is encouraged. Consequently, it is especially important to determine whether the symptom represents a change in functioning. Relatedly, assessing the intensity of the symptom can be helpful in distinguishing typical from concerning behavior; taking an interest in learning a foreign language is not unusual, but staying up all night to practice speaking the language and to plan a trip to its country of origin is not. The quality of a symptom might also be somewhat different across different disorders; many youth with ADHD have trouble settling down and initiating sleep at night; however, if they stay up late, they are typically difficult to rouse in the morning. In contrast, a child with decreased need for sleep will go to bed very late and wake up at an early hour, full of energy, despite only having slept a few hours.

Establishing episodes can also help with differential diagnosis. For example, distractibility is a criterion both for mania and for ADHD. However, ADHD is a chronic childhood disorder, and distractibility is expected to persist across settings and over the course of months or years without intervention. In contrast, the distractibility that is present in mania will come and go in conjunction with other symptoms. This distinction can be murky when bipolar disorder and ADHD are comorbid, as is commonly seen (Singh et al. 2006).

Many, but not all, youth who experience mania will also have one or more episodes of depression. The criteria to diagnose bipolar depression are the same as the criteria used to diagnose unipolar depression. There are some symptoms that may be more representative of bipolar depression than of unipolar depression (these are described below in the section on bipolar II disorder). In most cases, an episode of depression will predate the first episode of mania (see, e.g., Zeschel et al. 2013). Consequently, when the clinician is assessing a youth for depression, it is good practice to inquire about symptoms of mania and about family history of bipolar disorder, because the presence of either of these would indicate that a future episode of hypomania or mania is more likely and could influence treatment decisions (Axelson et al. 2015).

In the course of bipolar I disorder, some youth may experience what was referred to as a "mixed episode" in DSM-IV-TR (American Psychiatric Association 2000) and is now denoted with the "mixed features" specifier. A mixed features specifier is assigned when an individual has symptoms that simultaneously meet criteria for both mania and major depression. During these episodes, the individual is likely to be extremely agitated, with dysphoric mood and hopelessness, coupled with high energy. Judgment may be particularly impaired, as the person is likely to be ruminative and distracted and, in many cases, sleep deprived. Suicide risk is especially high when mood is mixed, as the youth may have suicidal thoughts precipitated by his or her depressed mood, and the energy to act on those thoughts (Birmaher et al. 2009; Goldstein et al. 2005).

Bipolar II Disorder

Youth with symptoms that meet criteria for bipolar II disorder must have one or more episodes of major depression, along with one or more episodes of hypomania. Hypomania is the diagnosis for manic symptoms that fail to meet either the duration or severity criterion for mania—the same number of symptoms (three if mood is elated; four if mood is irritable) is required. The duration criteria for hypomania is 4 consecutive days, but this has been described as arbitrary, and some suggest that a 2-day requirement would better capture this presentation (Akiskal et al. 2000). However, for criteria for bipolar II disorder to be met, hypomanic symptoms must represent a change in functioning that is observable by others, a hypomanic episode will not necessarily be impairing, and, in some cases, the individual may feel more productive, energetic, or creative during this time. Because people often feel better than usual while hypomanic—and consequently do not seek treatment—these episodes can go undetected, resulting in misdiagnosis if the individual later presents with an episode of depression. As mentioned earlier, when a youth has depressed mood, it is prudent to inquire about times in the past when he or she may have had more energy, been more excitable, or been otherwise different from his or her usual self. If the manic symptoms last more than 4 days, require hospitalization, or include psychosis, a diagnosis of bipolar I disorder is appropriate. Additionally, if criteria for mania have *ever* been met, a diagnosis of bipolar I disorder remains, even if future episodes are hypomanic in nature. It is not uncommon, after a period of episodes of depression and hypomania, for a youth to experience an episode of mania. In this case, the diagnosis would be updated to bipolar I disorder (Birmaher et al. 2009). Sometimes, a youth will have one or more episodes of depression and manic symptoms that do not meet criteria for a hypomanic or manic episode. If the manic symptoms cause a change in functioning, this presentation (depression with manic symptoms) would be consistent with a diagnosis of other specified bipolar disorder (see below).

An episode of bipolar depression may be indistinguishable from an episode of unipolar depression, and the diagnostic criteria are the same. However, bipolar depression is more often associated with "atypical" symptoms than is unipolar depression (Bowden 2001; Van Meter et al. 2013a). These include increased appetite and weight gain, hypersomnia, a feeling of heaviness in one's limbs, and mood reactivity, which is when an individual's mood will brighten temporarily in response to positive events. Another atypical feature is rejection sensitivity, in which the individual has a long-standing pattern of fear about interpersonal abandonment, which causes impairment in social relationships (Diler et al. 2017).

Depressive episodes tend to be more common and last longer (by definition) than hypomanic episodes. Depressive episodes also tend to be associated with more distress and impairment (Van Meter et al. 2013a); this is likely due, at least in part, to the fact that bipolar depression tends to respond less well (relative to both unipolar depression and mania) to pharmacological intervention (McClellan et al. 2007).

Suicide is a serious risk among all subtypes of bipolar disorder, and assessing for suicidal thoughts should be done regularly. Because of its predominantly depressed presentation, bipolar II disorder might be more strongly associated with suicide risk than the other subtypes. More than 50% of youth with bipolar disorder report suicidal ideation, and nearly a quarter will attempt. The combination of depressed mood and [hypo]manic energy can be particularly dangerous. Evidence suggests that periods during which an individual is switching between mood polarities are the times at which suicide risk is highest (Hauser et al. 2013).

Cyclothymic Disorder

Cyclothymic disorder is a chronic presentation of both depressive and manic symptoms. Youth with symptoms that meet criteria for cyclothymic disorder must be symptomatic for at least a year, during which time they must not have been symptom-free for more than 2 months. The symptoms of depression must be impairing but fall short of ever meeting criteria for an episode of major depression. Similarly, the manic symptoms must be noticeable and represent a change in functioning but cannot ever meet the criteria for an episode of mania or hypomania. Youth with cyclothymic disorder are characterized by significant irritable mood and struggle interpersonally; because their symptoms are chronic, they may be less able to initiate and maintain friendships than youth with disorders on the bipolar spectrum who experience periods of wellness (Van Meter et al. 2016).

It is not uncommon for mood symptoms in youth to fluctuate significantly, lasting only a day or two, but recurring frequently, or lasting just a few hours, but across many days in a row. Determining whether these symptoms meet criteria for an episode—and a diagnosis of bipolar I or II disorder—is one of the main challenges associated with diagnosing pediatric bipolar spectrum disorders. Cyclothymic disorder is very rarely diagnosed, in part because it is difficult to ascertain whether symptoms have been present for a year (and sometimes they may not have been present for a year yet) and to establish that an episode of hypomania or depression has not occurred. More than with other bipolar subtypes, it may be necessary to follow a case for some time before making a definitive cyclothymic disorder diagnosis. There is some evidence that this diagnosis may have a different course than other specified bipolar disorder (described below), so, although it may require a more detail-oriented assessment, focused on determining both the long-term presence of symptoms and the absence of severe episodes (life charting can be very helpful with this), there may be prognostic implications. Specifically, there are preliminary data suggesting that youth with cyclothymic disorder may be less likely than youth with other specified bipolar disorder to develop a manic or depressive episode over time (Van Meter et al. 2017). However, this does not mean that these youth are less impaired; in fact, the more chronic nature of their symptoms can be just as impairing as the shorter duration and greater severity of symptoms seen in the other bipolar sub-types. Youth with cyclothymic disorder are also very likely to have significant comorbidity and may respond less well to treatment than youth with bipolar I disorder, in particular (Van Meter et al. 2013b).

Other Specified/Unspecified Bipolar and Related Disorder

Some youth experience impairing symptoms of mania that do not meet the criteria for any other subtype of bipolar disorder. In these situations, it is appropriate to make a diagnosis of other specified or unspecified bipolar disorder. For example, in some cases, youth will have bursts of manic symptoms that last only a day or two, or that happen several days in a row, but only for an hour or two and never to the extent that hospitalization is necessary. Other presentations that would warrant this diagnosis include those in which there are only two or three symptoms of mania that co-occur, rather than the minimum of four symptoms (including elevated mood) required by DSM-5. Someone who experiences repeated episodes of hypomania but does not have an episode of depression would also receive this diagnosis, although this is not often seen clinically.

In many research studies (e.g., Birmaher et al. 2009; Findling et al. 2013), the threshold for an other specified diagnosis has been operationalized as requiring either a sufficient number of symptoms of inadequate duration or too few symptoms that do last the requisite 4 or 7 days. Although it is not necessary to follow these operationalized criteria in a clinical setting, there is a risk of overdiagnosis when the clinician relies on the other specified criteria; because many of the symptoms of mania (e.g., distractibility, increased energy, irritability) are common to other childhood disorders, if close attention is not paid to episodicity (Do the symptoms begin and end around the same time?) and change in functioning, a bipolar diagnosis could be given inappropriately. There are also numerous occurrences of two diagnoses being given (e.g., ADHD and other specified bipolar disorder) when one would be more appropriate, often because of symptoms being double counted. If a child presents with extremely irritable mood, rule breaking and defiance toward her parents, multiple tantrums per week, plus rapid speech, distractibility, and excessive energy, a clinician could justify diagnoses of ODD (loses temper, is in angry mood, argues with adults, defies rules), other specified bipolar disorder (irritable mood, rapid speech, distractibility, high energy), and even ADHD (distractible, energetic, irritable). It is possible for a youth to have multiple comorbidities, but before adding an additional diagnosis, it is prudent to determine whether one diagnosis could suffice. Did these symptoms occur all at once? If not, have the required symptoms for a diagnosis of ODD been present for at least 6 months? If so, are there enough additional symptoms that started together to constitute an episode of hypomania? If it is determined that the tantrums, irritable mood, and rule breaking are due to ODD, and the distractibility, rapid speech, and high energy are due to bipolar disorder, is there any evidence that an additional diagnosis of ADHD makes sense? Were these symptoms present at an early age in a chronic, milder form? It may be that three diagnoses best describe the youth's presentation and will inform the best treatment approach, but in many cases a "less is more" approach will adequately capture the presentation and inform treatment without unnecessarily burdening the child and family. Diagnoses can always be added as the child is followed and a better understanding of his or her symptoms is gained. However, once a diagnosis is given, it typically sticks.

Clinical Pearls

- If the presenting problem includes mood disturbance, assess for lifetime history of both depression and mania.

- Pay attention to episodes! Many symptoms of mood disorders overlap with symptoms of other childhood disorders; figuring out when specific symptoms started is key to making a differential diagnosis and establishing the episodicity of mood disorders. Using a life chart can be very helpful for this.

- Look for a change in functioning. People's moods shift naturally, and many symptoms of depression and mania exist on a continuum with typical mood states. Learning about the child's history and whether a mood or behavior is unusual for him or her is essential to accurately diagnosing these heterogeneous disorders.

- Approach diagnosis in a hierarchical way. If you have determined that there is an episodic presentation and change in functioning, consider whether a mood disorder diagnosis can account for most or all of the youth's symptoms. If there are remaining symptoms that are chronic in nature or are not consistent with a mood disorder diagnosis, evaluate whether a comorbid diagnosis is necessary. If symptoms are not episodic, consider non–mood disorder diagnoses first.

References

Akiskal HS, Bourgeois ML, Angst J, et al: Re-evaluating the prevalence of and diagnostic composition within the broad clinical spectrum of bipolar disorders. J Affect Disord 59 (suppl 1):S5–S30, 2000 11121824

American Psychiatric Association: Diagnostic and Statistical Manual of Mental Disorders, 4th Edition, Text Revision. Washington, DC, American Psychiatric Association, 2000

American Psychiatric Association: Diagnostic and Statistical Manual of Mental Disorders, 5th Edition. Arlington, VA, American Psychiatric Association, 2013

Anderson ER, Mayes LC: Race/ethnicity and internalizing disorders in youth: a review. Clin Psychol Rev 30(3):338–348, 2010 20071063

Avenevoli S, Knight E, Kessler RC, et al: Epidemiology of depression in children and adolescents, in Handbook of Depression in Children and Adolescents. Edited by Abela JRZ, Hankin BL. New York, Guilford, 2008, pp 6–32

Axelson D, Goldstein B, Goldstein T, et al: Diagnostic precursors to bipolar disorder in offspring of parents with bipolar disorder: a longitudinal study. Am J Psychiatry 172(7):638–646, 2015 25734353

Birmaher B, Williamson DE, Dahl RE, et al: Clinical presentation and course of depression in youth: does onset in childhood differ from onset in adolescence? J Am Acad Child Adolesc Psychiatry 43(1):63–70, 2004 14691361

Birmaher B, Axelson D, Goldstein B, et al: Four-year longitudinal course of children and adolescents with bipolar spectrum disorders: the Course and Outcome of Bipolar Youth (COBY) study. Am J Psychiatry 166(7):795–804, 2009 19448190

Bowden CL: Strategies to reduce misdiagnosis of bipolar depression. Psychiatr Serv 52(1):51–55, 2001 11141528

Carballo JJ, Muñoz-Lorenzo L, Blasco-Fontecilla H, et al: Continuity of depressive disorders from childhood and adolescence to adulthood: a naturalistic study in community mental health centers. Prim Care Companion CNS Disord 13(5):PCC.11m01150, 2011 22295270

Centers for Disease Control and Prevention: Youth Suicide. Injury Prevention and Control: Division of Violence Prevention, 2015

Copeland WE, Angold A, Costello EJ, et al: Prevalence, comorbidity, and correlates of DSM-5 proposed disruptive mood dysregulation disorder. Am J Psychiatry 170(2):173–179, 2013 23377638

Diler RS, Goldstein TR, Hafeman D, et al: Distinguishing bipolar depression from unipolar depression in youth: preliminary findings. J Child Adolesc Psychopharmacol 27(4):310–319, 2017 28398819

Findling RL, Jo B, Frazier TW, et al: The 24-month course of manic symptoms in children. Bipolar Disord 15(6):669–679, 2013 23799945

Ford T, Goodman R, Meltzer H: The British Child and Adolescent Mental Health Survey 1999: the prevalence of DSM-IV disorders. J Am Acad Child Adolesc Psychiatry 42(10):1203–1211, 2003 14560170

Fristad MA, Wolfson H, Algorta GP, et al; LAMS Group: Disruptive mood dysregulation disorder and bipolar disorder not otherwise specified: fraternal or identical twins? J Child Adolesc Psychopharmacol 26(2):138–146, 2016 26859630

Goldstein TR, Birmaher B, Axelson D, et al: History of suicide attempts in pediatric bipolar disorder: factors associated with increased risk. Bipolar Disord 7(6):525–535, 2005 16403178

Hauser M, Galling B, Correll CU: Suicidal ideation and suicide attempts in children and adolescents with bipolar disorder: a systematic review of prevalence and incidence rates, correlates, and targeted interventions. Bipolar Disord 15(5):507–523, 2013 23829436

Keller MB, Lavori PW, Friedman B, et al: The Longitudinal Interval Follow-up Evaluation: a comprehensive method for assessing outcome in prospective longitudinal studies. Arch Gen Psychiatry 44(6):540–548, 1987 3579500

Kovacs M, Akiskal HS, Gatsonis C, et al: Childhood-onset dysthymic disorder: clinical features and prospective naturalistic outcome. Arch Gen Psychiatry 51(5):365–374, 1994 8179460

Luby JL, Belden AC, Pautsch J, et al: The clinical significance of preschool depression: impairment in functioning and clinical markers of the disorder. J Affect Disord 112(1–3):111–119, 2009a 18486234

Luby JL, Si X, Belden AC, et al: Preschool depression: homotypic continuity and course over 24 months. Arch Gen Psychiatry 66(8):897–905, 2009b 19652129

Margulies DM, Weintraub S, Basile J, et al: Will disruptive mood dysregulation disorder reduce false diagnosis of bipolar disorder in children? Bipolar Disord 14(5):488–496, 2012 22713098

Masi G, Favilla L, Mucci M, et al: Depressive symptoms in children and adolescents with dysthymic disorder. Psychopathology 34(1):29–35, 2001 11150928

Mayes SD, Waxmonsky JD, Calhoun SL, et al: Disruptive Mood dysregulation disorder symptoms and association with oppositional defiant and other disorders in a general population child sample. J Child Adolesc Psychopharmacol 26(2):101–106, 2016 26745442

McClellan J, Kowatch R, Findling RL; Work Group on Quality Issues: Practice parameter for the assessment and treatment of children and adolescents with bipolar disorder. J Am Acad Child Adolesc Psychiatry 46(1):107–125, 2007 17195735

Nolen-Hoeksema S, Girgus JS: The emergence of gender differences in depression during adolescence. Psychol Bull 115(3):424–443, 1994 8016286

Ormel J, Raven D, van Oort F, et al: Mental health in Dutch adolescents: a TRAILS report on prevalence, severity, age of onset, continuity and co-morbidity of DSM disorders. Psychol Med 45(2):345–360, 2015 25066533

Rohde P, Lewinsohn PM, Seeley JR: Comorbidity of unipolar depression, II: comorbidity with other mental disorders in adolescents and adults. J Abnorm Psychol 100(2):214–222, 1991 2040773

Salk RH, Petersen JL, Abramson LY, et al: The contemporary face of gender differences and similarities in depression throughout adolescence: development and chronicity. J Affect Disord 205:28–35, 2016 27391269

Salk RH, Hyde JS, Abramson LY: Gender differences in depression in representative national samples: meta-analyses of diagnoses and symptoms. Psychol Bull 143(8):783–822, 2017 28447828

Shankman S, Lewinsohn P, Klein D, et al: Subthreshold conditions as precursors for full syndrome disorders: a 15-year longitudinal study of multiple diagnostic classes. J Child Psychol Psychiatry 50(12):1485–1494, 2009 19573034

Singh MK, DelBello MP, Kowatch RA, et al: Co-occurrence of bipolar and attention-deficit hyperactivity disorders in children. Bipolar Disord 8(6):710–720, 2006 17156157

Stewart SM, Simmons A, Habibpour E: Treatment of culturally diverse children and adolescents with depression. J Child Adolesc Psychopharmacol 22(1):72–79, 2012 22251021

Van Meter AR, Henry DB, West AE: What goes up must come down: the burden of bipolar depression in youth. J Affect Disord 150(3):1048–1054, 2013a 23768529

Van Meter A, Youngstrom E, Demeter C, et al: Examining the validity of cyclothymic disorder in a youth sample: replication and extension. J Abnorm Child Psychol 41(3):367–378, 2013b 22968491

Van Meter A, Youngstrom E, Freeman A, et al: Impact of irritability and impulsive aggressive behavior on impairment and social functioning in youth with cyclothymic disorder. J Child Adolesc Psychopharmacol 26(1):26–37, 2016 26835744

Van Meter AR, Youngstrom EA, Birmaher B, et al: Longitudinal course and characteristics of cyclothymic disorder in youth. J Affect Disord 215:314–322, 2017 28365522

Yorbik O, Birmaher B, Axelson D, et al: Clinical characteristics of depressive symptoms in children and adolescents with major depressive disorder. J Clin Psychiatry 65(12):1654–1659, quiz 1760–1761, 2004 15641870

Youngstrom E: Definitional issues in bipolar disorder across the life cycle. Clinical Psychological Science and Practice 16(2):140–160, 2009

Youngstrom EA, Findling RL, Calabrese JR: Who are the comorbid adolescents? Agreement between psychiatric diagnosis, youth, parent, and teacher report. J Abnorm Child Psychol 31(3):231–245, 2003 12774858

Youngstrom EA, Birmaher B, Findling RL: Pediatric bipolar disorder: validity, phenomenology, and recommendations for diagnosis. Bipolar Disord 10 (1 Pt 2):194–214, 2008 18199237

Zeschel E, Correll CU, Haussleiter IS, et al: The bipolar disorder prodrome revisited: is there a symptomatic pattern? J Affect Disord 151(2):551–560, 2013 23932736

3

Addressing Clinical Diagnostic Challenges in Pediatric Mood Disorders

HISTORICAL, CONCEPTUAL, AND PRACTICAL CONSIDERATIONS

Gabrielle A. Carlson, M.D.

Historical Considerations

Depression

Most central to diagnostic challenges in recognizing mood disorders has been that our understanding of mood disorders varies between clinicians and researchers. Research efforts have tried to identify the essence of depression, and in that pursuit, various categorical classifications have been developed in an attempt to produce homogeneous groups with reliable diagnoses. A review of the history of the attempts to classify depression is instructive. Volumes have been written about whether depression is a binary or a unitary phenomenon. Kraepelin (1913) was the first to propose what was taken to be a unitary concept and offered that melancholia (severe and usually recurrent depression) and circular psychoses be subsumed under one category, namely manic-depressive psychosis. He was most concerned with separating manic depression from dementia praecox. It was Leonhard, many years later (1957), who examined recurrent, severe depressions and recognized that some of the depressions were punctuated by manic episodes and that those suffering from depression had family members who were similarly afflicted. That conclusion gave rise to the "bipolar" disorder versus nonbipolar depression (i.e., those without manic episodes) classification that we currently employ. Thus, much has been written about distinguishing the depression of bipolar disorder from the depression of nonbipolar disorder, without conclusive results (Cardoso de Almeida and Phillips 2013).

Those who contend depression has two subtypes distinguish melancholia (autonomous, severe, endogenous, and sometimes psychotic depression) from nonmelancholic or reactive depressions (Taylor and Fink 2008). They can literally quote the Bible! Mark Altschule, in 1967, cited a passage from St. Paul's Second Letter to the Corinthians, chapter 7, verse 10: "For godly sorrow worketh repentance to salvation not to be repented of, but the sorrow [i.e., sadness or depression] of the world worketh death." This was interpreted by medieval theologians as meaning there were two kinds of depression, the one "from God" and the other "of the world," and provided a provenance for the "endogenous or melancholic/reactive," or "psychotic/neurotic," distinctions.

Endogenous/melancholic depressions are characterized by affect disproportionate to stressors, unremitting apprehension and morbid statements, blunted emotional responses, nonreactive mood, and pervasive anhedonia despite improved circumstances. Such depressions have psychomotor disturbance such as slowed thought, movement, and speech or spontaneous agitation, including stereotypic movements, cognitive impairment, and vegetative dysfunction. If psychosis is present, nihilistic convictions of hopelessness, guilt, sin, and ruin prevail (Parker et al. 2010). There are often cortisol abnormalities associated with endogenous depressions, as demonstrated by abnormal dexamethasone suppression test (DST) results (Fink and Taylor 2007). Individuals with nonmelancholic depressions are younger, are less severely ill, have anxiety comorbidities, and have reactive moods. Nonendogenous depressions are felt to be psychological or characterological and much more heterogeneous. There are convincing data that electroconvulsive therapy and tricyclic antidepressants treat melancholic depression more effectively than selective serotonin reuptake inhibitors and are less effective in treating nonmelancholic depression, giving that form of depression specificity. However, electroconvulsive therapy is not applicable to most people with depression (Fink and Taylor 2007).

DSM-III (American Psychiatric Association 1980) rejected the binary view of depression, as did subsequent editions. The reasoning is beyond the scope of this review. However, it is this author's opinion that the committee gave up trying to decide about types of depression, developed diagnostic criteria, and announced that if the criteria are met, the disorder is present. Kendler (2016) has made the point that there were many symptoms left out of the criteria and that restricting the symptoms would thwart future efforts to study phenomenology because the information collected on psychopathology was limited. That is especially true for children and teens, whose descriptors were never part of the thinking about mood disorders. The other point was that the criteria themselves became the disorder and may have changed the configuration of clinical depression. The question, then, is whether children have the kinds of depressions adults have (e.g., melancholia) and whether the mood issues germane to children are captured in the criteria (Whalen et al. 2017).

A review of the history of "childhood depression" is germane to the discussion above. In an important paper in 1966, Dr. Herbert Rie summarized the state of childhood depression by stating the following: "A survey of the literature yields two indisputable facts. First, childhood depression and disorders which represent it or emulate it are rarely discussed." He then listed all of the important texts and journals that omitted the term "depression" when discussing children. Two divergent conclusions emerge: One is that depression cannot exist on theoretical grounds of inadequate ego development (and thus that it is an intrinsic developmental impossibility), and the other is that depressive symptoms differ from those in adulthood. In fact, he said there are an "unbelievable variety of symptoms which have been identified as pathognomonic of childhood depression" and are called "depressive equivalents."

Rie goes on to say: "In the apparent absence of a consistent definition of childhood depression, manifestations of adult clinical depression are reexamined in order to clarify what the presumed disorder is not." He then quotes a 1959 paper by an adult psychiatrist, Heinz Lehmann, on adult depression:

> The characteristic symptoms [of depression or melancholia] are: a sad, despairing mood; decrease of mental productivity and reduction of drive; retardation or agitation in the field of expressive motor responses. These

might be called the primary symptoms of depression....The group of secondary symptoms comprises: feelings of hopelessness; hypochondriacal preoccupations; feelings of depersonalization; obsessive-compulsive behavior; ideas of self-accusation and self-depreciation; nihilistic delusions; paranoid delusions; hallucinations; suicidal ruminations and tendencies.... Sometimes, however, the patient's appearance is deceiving and our diagnosis then depends entirely on the evaluation of a single symptom, which is possibly the most essential of all, namely the patient's verbal description of his mood or feelings. (Lehmann 1959, quoted in Rie 1966, pp. 655–656)

Rie (1966) then concludes:

[I]n view of the child's relatively greater difficulty in maintaining independently a consistent self-representation and his often rather inadequate ability in representing his internal states verbally, this latter observation may have implications for differential diagnosis in childhood.

What this paper suggests is that the absence of childhood depression in the literature of the early to mid–twentieth century was due not to blindness to the fact that children (and it is unclear if this includes adolescents) become unhappy or even depressed, but rather to the fact that they do not have "melancholia" with all of the attendant psychoanalytic theories that explained the occurrence of melancholia in adults. Those theories emphasized that some intrinsic deficit in the person rather than something extrinsic in the environment caused melancholia to occur. When children did get depressed, the depressive psychopathology was likely overshadowed by other things called "depressive equivalents," or what we call comorbidities. In those cases, Rie was hard-pressed to know how the authors writing about such equivalents could conclude the child was depressed. Suffice it to say, the field was in a stalemate.

The real impetus to identify depression in children emerged with the recognition that antidepressants (tricyclic antidepressants and monoamine oxidase inhibitors) helped adults with depression, and thus it was hoped that they would be similarly helpful in children. Frommer (1967) in England, for instance, reported a crossover trial of phenelzine and phenobarbitone in children ages 9–15 years with either phobic or depressive symptoms. Phenelzine was more effective than the comparator, phenobarbitone. Her description of the children in the group with mood disorders was that "they were weepy, irritable, had temper outbursts, and some displayed seriously antisocial behavior. A few complained of actually being depressed, and one boy made suicidal threats. More came from emotionally deprived homes or had been upset by death or loss in other ways of both parents" (p. 730). In other words, her subjects did not look melancholic, they had multiple comorbidities and "depressive equivalents," and most came from stressful life circumstances.

Although there was interest initially in identifying children with true, adult-type endogenous/melancholic/sometimes psychotic depression, attempts to do so revealed low rates. Following on adult studies, there were efforts to validate childhood depression with the DST given that the hypothalamic-pituitary-adrenal axis is known to become increasingly dysregulated from child to adult manifestations of depression. However, dexamethasone nonsuppression in children and adolescents could not even distinguish subjects with major depressive disorder (MDD) from those without the disorder with a useful positive predictive value (Casat and Powell 1988; Casat et al. 1989). Although Rush et al. (1996) felt that the DST's sensitivity of 46.2% and specificity of 89.9% differentiating endogenous from nonendogenous major depressive episodes in adults was robust, there appeared to be little universal support for maintaining a specific melancholic/endogenous depression. DSM's continued "atheoretical" position has been the result.

Predictors of depression in children, beginning with preschool-age children, include stress/conflict, parenting practices, and neglect (Whalen et al. 2017). In that regard, childhood depression is "reactive" rather than "endogenous." However, recognition that extrinsic factors are important to depression in children goes back to Robert Burton in his 1621 book, *The Anatomy of Melancholy*. Burton stated:

> A principal cause, bad parents, step-mothers, Tutors, Masters, Teachers, too rigorous and too severe, or too remiss or indulgent on the other side, are often fountains and furthers of this disease. Parents and such as have the tuition and oversight of children, offend many times in that they are too stern, always threatening, chiding, brawling, whipping, or striking; by meanes of which their poore children are so disheartened and cowed that they never after have any courage, or a merry houre in their lives, or take pleasure in any thing. (Burton 1621/2000)

One conclusion that we can draw, then, is not that children cannot manifest psychological distress in distressing circumstances, but that the distress they manifest is not really melancholic depression as it was understood for many years. What has changed is that much of what we call depression in children and adults is this response to distress. That does not make this depression invalid or insignificant. Studies of disease burden reflect this kind of depression. However, the broadening of what is included in depression may explain why treatments that were once said to have been effective are now not much better than placebo. The diagnostic challenge has been trying to figure out how to capture the essence of melancholic/endogenous/psychotic depression.

Bipolar Disorder

The history of our understanding of bipolar disorder evolved from recognizing the relation between what we call depression and what we call mania (e.g., Falret's *folie circulaire* in 1894). This was followed by Kraepelin's separating schizophrenia from manic-depressive "insanity." Recognition of manic depression as distinct from other forms of depression—that is, the potential importance of polarity rather than recurrence—was addressed by German, Swiss, and Scandinavian psychiatrists in the 1950s and 1960s (see Carlson and Glovinsky 2009 for review). Dunner et al. (1976) recommended distinguishing patients with recurrent depression and hypomania from those with mania, thus beginning the concept of the bipolar spectrum. Finally, the World Health Organization's U.S./U.K. study of manic depression and schizophrenia highlighted the importance of both a systematic approach to diagnosis and some level of agreement as to what the symptoms and behaviors of the disorders should be (Gurland et al. 1970). As noted earlier, the subsequent emergence of DSM-III opened the Pandora's box of multiple comorbidities as well as established diagnoses based on symptoms rather than longitudinal course.

Reports of children (adolescents, actually) with the same conditions usually followed each major conceptual shift, although it was clear that these cases were very rare. For instance, there is a nice description of a 13-year-old in 1898 that highlights manic-depressive cyclicity (Carlson and Glovinsky 2009):

> He was a dull child, and had been so often punished at school, on account of his slow progress, that he became deeply melancholy and tried to kill himself. The melancholy alternated with mania, in which he whistled and sang day and night, tore his clothes, and was filthy in his habits. (p. 259)

After Kraepelin's 1920 publication, there were reports of adolescents with recurrent depressive episodes and some reports of those with mania, but again, they were rare. There was an attempt in the mid-1950s to broaden the concept of manic depression, which was ended by a literature search that found very few cases of classic manic depression before age 12. After DSM-III, the issue of affective storms and distinguishing mania from attention-deficit/hyperactivity disorder (ADHD) began in earnest, culminating in the description of a unique form of prepubertal bipolar disorder characterized by severe, explosive outbursts, which had otherwise lost its diagnostic home when DSM-III eliminated emotion dysregulation from its definition (Carlson and Glovinsky 2009; Carlson and Klein 2014). In 2000, the National Institute of Mental Health had a Bipolar Roundtable (National Institute of Mental Health 2001), after which the concept of different bipolar "phenotypes" was born. One of those, severe mood dysregulation, provided an alternative set of criteria for chronically irritable and explosive children to be studied along with children with more classic bipolar disorder (Leibenluft et al. 2003). Although this approach has not solved the problem of whether there is a unique form of bipolar disorder in general or specifically in younger children, it has provided a way to examine the issue further.

Diagnostic issues for bipolar disorder continue to include distinguishing 1) pathological mood fluctuations from normal (or at least developmental) mood lability, 2) highs and lows (which represent a change in behavior) from a baseline state in which mood fluctuations are part of the person's personality, 3) symptoms of mania from other developmental conditions in which irritability or silly moods occur (e.g., ADHD), 4) severe, frantic manic agitation from catastrophic anxiety or severe agitated depression, and 5) severe psychosis related to mania from that related to schizophrenia. Finally, when manic depression/bipolar disorder was defined, there was no developmental information available to modify (or not) the criteria. Thus, the question of how symptoms and behaviors felt to be basic to the definition of mania or depression apply to children of different ages remains unanswered.

Criteria for mania remained largely unchanged between 1980 and the publication of DSM-5. A number of refinements took place with the 2013 iteration, most of which eliminated the ambiguities that led to the bipolar controversy in youth. Thus, episodes are more clearly defined. Symptoms must occur most of the day, every day. Symptoms overlapping with comorbid conditions must intensify so that the episode of mania represents a clearly different change from the person's premorbid self. Dr. Leibenluft's proposal to distinguish episodic from chronic irritability by calling the latter "severe mood dysregulation" (Leibenluft et al. 2003) became the template for the condition now called "disruptive mood dysregulation disorder" (DMDD). The decision was made intentionally to prevent children with severe temper outbursts from being automatically diagnosed with bipolar disorder. Although the intent was noble, it is not entirely clear which children the condition identifies or whether it will be successful in "saving" children from a false diagnosis of bipolar disorder (Margulies et al. 2012).

DMDD is defined by chronic irritability, punctuated by outbursts that are out of proportion to the trigger that started them. The irritability, which persists between outbursts, and outbursts themselves must occur in multiple settings (to eliminate the possibility that they are a localized problem), have lasted at least a year, and not be better explained by another mood disorder (which is better understood and treated). DMDD is not diagnosed before age 6 or after age 18, and onset should be before age 10. If the child has both oppositional defiant disorder and DMDD, the latter diagnosis takes precedence.

One of the biggest problems with the diagnosis is that irritability has two components that are confounded in the diagnosis. One aspect is how the person feels (grouchy, angry, sad, easily annoyed, loses temper); the other component is what the person does when angry, which can be verbal and/or physical aggression. Severity of the former is stated in terms of frequency; the latter should be characterized in terms of level of aggression (Carlson and Klein 2018).

Measurement Issues

Measurement issues emerge from the question of what makes up a mood disorder. As we know, diagnosis has been particularly challenging because we do not have a way to validate the information we obtain. We need to obtain information from multiple sources, some of whom are more verbal or better informed than others. We also need to know what besides the mood disorder should be measured (i.e., what other developmental or behavioral issues are occurring). We address these issues in several ways: drawing on clinical experience with the conditions we diagnose and treat; obtaining information in a standardized way by asking comprehensive questions to multiple sources; obtaining rating scales that provide scores that have been studied in large populations and thus have norms; and doing other tests where they exist to provide additional information (e.g., cognitive, language, learning disabilities testing; appropriate blood chemistries).

With respect to mood disorders, there are also diagnostic challenges, because, like most conditions, these disorders exist as continuums or dimensions, representing a range of symptoms from negligible to severe. The dimensional approach to symptomatology, which has always been acknowledged in children, has also been adopted in DSM-5. One explanation given for rejecting the binary view of depression was that melancholia was felt by many to be a difference in the degree of depression, not the kind of depression.

For mood disorders, among the best-studied dimensional "diagnosis" is the Child Behavior Checklist (CBCL) "bipolar"/"dysregulation" phenotype, which was initially described by Biederman and colleagues (see, e.g., Biederman et al. 1995). These authors first claimed that the delinquency, aggressive behavior, somatic complaints, anxiety, and thought problems with T scores over 70 predicted children with mania. After several meta-analyses, the profile was refined to elevations in anxiety/depression, attention, and aggression (Faraone et al. 2005). This profile has been studied extensively and appears to have genetic, longitudinal, and clinical utility (Althoff et al. 2012). In terms of clinical utility (the subject of this chapter), for instance, we reported on two samples of 6-year-olds who appeared to have DMDD, a community sample and a clinical sample from the same catchment area. On the basis of criteria obtained from interviews with parents, both samples were characterized by irritability and tantrums. However, 10.3% were captured by the CBCL profile in the community sample, whereas 32% were captured in the clinical sample (Carlson et al. 2016). We know immediately, then, that although both samples had individuals whose symptoms "met criteria," one appeared to have three times more individuals who were symptomatic. Scales like the CBCL are also somewhat sensitive to gender and age, unlike most criteria in categorical diagnoses. Data from the CBCL bipolar/dysregulation phenotype also suggest stability of the profile. Thus, youth with this profile are found to be significantly impaired and exhibit mood problems on follow-up (Althoff et al. 2010; Meyer et al. 2009).

At least three problems emerge with the dimensional approach, however. The first is deciding on a threshold. For instance, different studies have used different cut points for the dysregulation profile. Sometimes T scores for the three subscales are as low as 60, sometimes 67, sometimes 70 or higher. As Faraone et al. (2005) noted, "One can use various cut points on the CBCL-PBD to fit the purpose of the clinician or the investigator" (p. 522). That isn't reassuring. The second is that within any condition, the symptoms are also dimensional. With the CBCL phenotype, sometimes the sum of the scores is used, with ranges from a sum of 180 to 210, so that a child can have very high anxiety/depression and modest attention problems, or high aggression and attention problems and low anxiety/depression. This introduces considerable heterogeneity that may or may not be a part of the fundamental heterogeneity of the mood disorder. The final issue is what clinical condition the profiles reflect. The name "CBCL bipolar phenotype" has been changed to "CBCL dysregulation phenotype" because there was lack of consensus about whether the profile even described bipolar disorder, let alone was specific for it (Diler et al. 2009; Holtmann et al. 2007), although there is no disagreement that the profile describes seriously disturbed children.

Finally, the CBCL describes the child's current state (if used accurately), and unless one is specifically identifying current mania, it is unlikely that the CBCL could be used to diagnose a past manic episode. It thus may describe both who the child is (i.e., afflicted with chronic mood dysregulation) and what he or she has (which could include a manic episode).

Researchers in the field are actively trying to determine which measures are most likely to translate to meaningful clinical outcomes. Measurement issues provide important challenges to the field but should not invalidate the importance of objectively measuring how symptoms present over time and respond to treatment.

Comorbidity

As is well known, the conditions we diagnose and treat are not pure. This is not unique to psychiatry or to children. We have called co-occurring conditions "comorbidities." To some extent, the plethora of comorbidities with which we struggle emerged from the DSM-III "atheoretical" stance we described earlier: "If the criteria are met, then the individual has the disorder." Mood disorders co-occur with other mood disorders like anxiety, behavioral disorders, and developmental disorders. Do we truly think a child has six disorders that need treatment? Is one a complication of the other? Are the symptoms halo effects (e.g., having a headache is often a by-product of having a fever)? Many of us approach comorbidities like the Gordian knot. If you can figure out where to hit, you can solve the whole problem rather than trying to pick out each rope.

The relations of these comorbidities to one another in terms of when they occur (which is first, which is second, etc.) are rarely examined. Years ago, the faculty in Washington University's Department of Psychiatry characterized the relation between a mood disorder and its comorbid condition on the basis of which came first. If the depression or mania came first, it was called a "primary affective disorder." If another condition began first—for instance, an anxiety disorder or behavior disorder—the depression or mania was called a "secondary affective disorder" (Winokur 1979). There was some merit to this approach. For instance, patients with depressions secondary to psychiatric illnesses had an earlier age at onset, were more likely to have suicidal thoughts or to have made suicide attempts, were less likely to have memory problems, were less improved with treatment and more likely to relapse on follow-up, and had more alcoholism in their families than patients with depressions secondary to medical illnesses. Depressions secondary to medical illnesses seem to fit the category of reactive depression, and depressions secondary to psychiatric illnesses fit the definition of neurotic depression (Winokur et al. 1988).

Carlson and Cantwell (1980) used that approach to classify 28 children and adolescents who were given an affective disorder diagnosis on the basis of a structured interview and found that 12 (42.9%) had a primary affective disorder, and the rest (*n*=16, 57.1%) had another disorder first, and so had a secondary mood disorder. Only 11 of the 28 would have had their depression diagnosed with DSM-II. The authors concluded that the comorbid disorder "masked" the children's depressive disorder.

What we have realized with the passage of time is that neither comorbidity nor the mood disorder is necessarily fully expressed. A child can experience uncomplicated major depression (MDD), MDD with symptoms of one or more comorbidities (e.g., ADHD symptoms), MDD with full-criterion comorbidity (MDD and ADHD), or ADHD with depressive symptoms that may represent the unhappiness that occurs with constant failure, or possibly symptoms prodromal to future clinical depression. That eventuality makes the "primary/secondary" distinction difficult to operationalize. Many studies have required that criteria be met in order to say a disorder has begun, when, of course, that decision was made because it is difficult to really know when something truly started.

Longitudinal studies highlight another observation. In depressed youth, follow-up studies that have examined both the mood disorder and the comorbidity have found that the comorbid disorder continues to impair the subject, whereas the mood disorder relapses and remits (Kovacs et al. 2016). In bipolar disorder, increased severity of anxiety disorders and substance use disorders predicts longer time to recovery and less time to next depressive episode, as well as shorter time to next manic episode. Thus, worsening of comorbid conditions may constitute a precursor to mood episode recurrence or increase the duration of the mood disorder (Yen et al. 2016).

Cases

The following cases, in which the patients' identifying data and names have been altered, exemplify some of the issues raised above.

Issue: Diagnosing the Kind of Depression in the Face of Limited History and Determining Prognosis

Josh was 17 years old and starting his senior year of high school. He had long-standing, untreated ADHD and a significant learning disability. He was being educated in a self-contained class where teachers knew him well, described him as a respectful young man, and liked him. He was referred because of the "total change in his personality" that had occurred, in which he was irritable and agitated, went from crying to punching walls, walked out of class, and was seen as sad, anxious, withdrawn, illogical, and paranoid. He dropped the vocational program he had selected and shut down academically. Teachers felt he was terrified about graduating and that his depression was "reactive," meaning there was an obvious reason.

Although his parents observed that Josh had stopped hanging out with marijuana-using peers, was extremely irritable, and seemed more withdrawn, spacey, and paranoid, they did not recognize depression per se and had little to tell us about when it started. Josh himself was so depressed he mostly wept through his mental status exam. When he did speak, it was softly and with minimal output but with no overt thought disorder. He responded to everything verbally with "I'm not sure," but he scored in the severely depressed range (i.e., 44) on the Beck Depression Inventory (BDI; Beck et al. 1961). He acknowledged anxiety, suspiciousness, and possible hallucinations (he thought he heard critical voices but didn't know if they were "just my thoughts"), but no manic symptoms. Josh's parents were not knowledgeable about extended family history but denied psychiatric disorder in themselves. They had another child with severe cerebral palsy who consumed most of their time and energy.

Discussion

What is Josh's diagnosis? It could be a severe depression with psychosis, the first episode of an ultimate bipolar course, or developing schizophrenia. That differential is difficult in the best of circumstances, and his story highlights three important lessons. The first is that longitudinal history from good observers is critical but not always possible. In Joshua's case, his special education teachers and school psychologist gave the most useful information, and because they had known him for the past several years, they could document both when that change had taken place and the nature of the change. Psychiatric evaluations take detective work.

The second lesson is that it is crucial to determine the relevance of "precipitating events." Regardless of the causal contribution of such events, their utility is important in that stress elimination is helpful whether or not the stressor was the immediate cause of the problem. Josh was told that as a special education student he could remain in school for another year and complete the vocational program that he had dropped. That did nothing for his mood. He remained anxious about his future and was so depressed he could not think, let alone reason, about his occupational alternatives. Josh presents with features of both melancholic and reactive depression, so it is easy to see why classification has been so fraught with difficulty.

The final point is that we continue to struggle with what psychosis means in the context of depression and how it informs treatment. Is it a subtype (as the "binary" believers feel), a marker of severity (as the "unitary" believers feel), a harbinger of schizophrenia, or the first episode of bipolar disorder (although there was no obvious family history, parents' knowledge of their extended family was similar to their knowledge of their son)? The Suffolk County Mental Health Project, a study of first-episode psychosis (Bromet et al. 1992), reported that there were 80 participants with a baseline research diagnosis of MDD with psychosis. At 10-year follow-up (Ruggero et al. 2010), only 45% (*n*=36) of them retained their original diagnosis (although these were young adults, not children). Of those with an unstable diagnosis, 8.9% had their diagnosis switched to bipolar disorder, 16.7% had developed schizophrenia or schizoaffective disorder, and 37% had other diagnostic changes. Of the 36 who retained the MDD with psychosis diagnosis, 11 never had another episode, 12 had recurrent MDD with psychosis, and 13 had depressive episodes without psychosis. Kovacs has similar findings for her childhood depression cohort who are now adults (M. Kovacs, personal communication, May 3, 2018). Josh is old enough that these data are relevant for him. A first episode of severe depression is unstable diagnostically, so it is difficult to predict the outcome. Nevertheless, we have to treat what is in front of us while keeping an open mind diagnostically.

Josh's psychiatrist chose to treat his psychosis first to see the degree to which his mood would improve. His plan was to add an antidepressant. He planned to move aggressively with treatment. He also considered the possibility that Josh might need electroconvulsive therapy should he not respond to antidepressant treatment (Ghaziuddin et al. 2004).

Issue: "Characterological" Depression

Michelle is 15 years old and in regular tenth-grade classes. She has had problems with social anxiety, attention problems, and academic problems attributed to auditory processing since early elementary school. Full Scale IQ was 95, but receptive language scores were at the 15th percentile.

Michelle felt like she had always been bullied and victimized and remembered having been teased as far back as kindergarten. Her problems were exacerbated when the nude photograph of herself that her "boyfriend" talked her into sending to him was circulated at school. It is not clear when her current depression started, but it precipitated an overdose on fluoxetine. She also described panic attacks and felt that marijuana was the only thing that helped her calm down.

Michelle did not look depressed until she spoke about the photograph, at which point she became tearful and her spontaneous conversation was depressed and hopeless. She said, "I have negative thoughts; I'm OK with being made fun of; being bullied will happen forever."

Her score of 38 on the Children's Depression Inventory (CDI; Kovacs 1985) indicated severe depression. She said, "I get so down in the dumps I think I might never snap out of it." She was inconsistent about anger and irritability. On one occasion she said, "I never get angry," and on another she said, "I stay angry for a long time and I just don't SHOW my anger."

Michelle said she has had suicidal thoughts since fifth grade. She acted on her thoughts this time because "I was at a really low point." She let her mother know immediately, however, and said she stays alive because of her parents. She was able to list three positive things about herself.

Michelle also endorsed every single possible anxiety symptom (with the exception of obsessive-compulsive symptoms) on the Multidimensional Anxiety Scale for Children (MASC; March et al. 1997). On psychosis screening questions, she tended to over-endorse things, making herself look sicker than she is. For instance, she said "often" to "I have some beliefs that other people might find unusual or weird." When asked for examples, she said, "I think Donald Trump is a good president."

Family history was positive for learning disabilities and anxiety.

Discussion

Michelle illustrates the personality trait of neuroticism, one of the "big five" personality descriptors (see, e.g., Goldberg 1993). Depression is who she is rather than what she has. She evidences Aaron Beck's cognitive triad— that is, "automatic, spontaneous and seemingly uncontrollable negative thoughts" about the self, the environment, and the future (Beck et al. 1987). She feels worthless and ugly; she does not feel anyone cares about her; she is sure things will never change since they have always been that way. Not much was being accomplished in therapy. She said her therapist gave her some strategies to use on a piece of paper, but she did not read the paper and does not know where it is. She was prescribed a low dose of fluoxetine. She gets the usual monthly appointment. She clearly needs more vigorous treatment.

Michelle's case also illustrates how depression causes as well as results from stressful life events. Feeling depressed and unloved made her vulnerable to a predator who took advantage of her and got her to share a naked photograph, which, of course, was devastating and further reinforced her hopelessness.

Issues: Diagnostically Homeless, Poor Language Skills, Bipolar Sister

Trisha, age 12, was referred for refusing to go to school for 3 months. There were suggestions of an autism spectrum disorder because she had a significant language delay and social problems, but she did not have restricted and repetitive behaviors, and the diagnosis of autism was not made. She was irritable and had tantrums, and had been diagnosed with ADHD, however. Mom was not aware of any stressors or triggers for the school refusal.

Trisha often misinterpreted accidental behavior (like somebody bumping into her in the hallways) as an intentional harm. She had also become physically and verbally aggressive toward her mother to the point that her mother had to call the police to calm her down. She was quite remorseful about her rages. She said she felt "like a switch goes on" and afterward says, "I can't help it" and "I don't want to be this way."

Out of school, Trisha stayed in bed all day long and refused to take care of her hygiene (had not showered for over a month), and her mother also noted that "her room is a mess." Trisha's mood would switch quickly, and she would get easily upset about random things. Parent CBCL (Achenbach and Rescorla 2001) scores for Trisha were elevated for "thought problems" (T 70), attention problems (T 67), and withdrawn behavior (T 65), but not for anxiety or depression. The Child Mania Rating Scale (CMRS, Pavuluri et al. 2006) score was 14 (well below mania threshold). Teachers observed Trisha to be withdrawn (T 78) and anxious (T 70), and to have thought problems (T 83), social problems (T 70), attention problems (T 87), aggression (T 80), and conduct problems (T 75).

Trisha's Full Scale IQ was 87; there was no recent language testing. She was in a regular class with Resource Room, classified with "emotional disturbance." Her nurse practitioner had given her a "bipolar NOS [not otherwise specified]" diagnosis (assuming outbursts were evidence of pediatric bipolar disorder) and autism.

On mental status, Trisha was pretty but disheveled, and pleasant but spacey. It was difficult to get a linear narrative out of her. It was necessary to ask a specific question to get the next step in a sequence of events. She did not spontaneously provide much detail and had no sense of when things happened. She described what sounded like anxiety attacks (heart pounds, feels dizzy, has trouble breathing) "when I'm nervous," but couldn't say what made her nervous. In fact, she worried a lot about everything but never knew that what she was experiencing was anxiety. She also admitted to many ADHD symptoms.

On the CDI (Kovacs 1985), Trisha scored 35 (i.e., very depressed). She checked that she is sad many times, feels like crying all the time, does many things wrong, is bad many times, cannot concentrate, has to push to do schoolwork, is tired all the time, doesn't feel like eating, feels alone, never has fun, and is not sure if anyone even loves her. She said she feels weird and different from other children and is reminded of that fact by her peers. She understood the CDI items. It was expressive language where she suffered.

Trisha's parents were divorced. Her mother had been treated for depression; her father had been abusive, aggressive, and possibly depressed. Trisha's half sister carried a diagnosis of bipolar disorder, although no details were available about her symptoms.

Trisha was receiving counseling and medication management because of angry outbursts and difficulties focusing. Past medication trials included risperidone, aripiprazole, pindolol, haloperidol, valproate, low doses of OROS-methylphenidate, dexmethylphenidate, mixed amphetamine salts, atomoxetine, clonidine, and mirtazapine for sleep. It was clear from this regimen that the nurse practitioner was focusing on what she considered bipolar disorder, gingerly addressing ADHD.

Discussion

Trisha was chronically irritable with outbursts, but no one recognized her anxiety or depression. She did not understand what she was feeling, and her language skills further complicated her ability to volunteer this information. She could, however, respond to specific questions and to rating scales. In children with a history of language delay, it is often necessary to provide more structure to get at emotions, although it is also important to make sure the child understands the questions, because he or she might say yes or no to statements randomly and provide the wrong information.

Although Trisha appeared to have generalized anxiety, depression, and panic attacks, her clinical picture was quite different from Michelle's in the previous case. This is a point that Kendler (2016) has also made about the fact that our diagnoses do not give rise to homogeneous samples. However, even worse than that, Trisha has a comorbidity that does not even have a name. She does not quite have autism. She might have "social communication disorder," which was designed to address children with ADHD and social and language problems (both of which she has). Moreover, she had not received any language testing, so the level and quality of deficit had not been professionally documented. In our institution, we call children like Trisha "diagnostically homeless" (Weisbrot and Carlson 2004) because diagnostically they do not fit neatly anywhere but their symptoms have been recognized for years. We suspect many "diagnostically homeless" children are being diagnosed with autism spectrum disorder to get them services, and it is likely that Trisha needs more support than what she is getting in a regular class.

A review of Trisha's medications suggests that the ADHD was never treated adequately and that her clinician was afraid of appropriately medicating any anxiety or depression, had they been recognized. That is because of the assumption that Trisha's outbursts are "bipolar," or that having a "bipolar" half-sibling gives everyone else the diagnosis and antidepressants or adequate stimulants would make Trisha manic. Rates of bipolar disorder are certainly higher in family members of people with bipolar disorder than they are in family members of people without the disorder (Rasic et al. 2014). However, we do not know what kind of bipolar disorder Trisha's sister has because no one can describe symptoms for us. She may not even have bipolar disorder! She is also a half sister. Finally, even if her half sister has documented bipolar I disorder, that does not preclude treating Trisha's current problems. Although the odds compared with a nonbipolar family history are much higher in a person with a parent with mania, the likelihood of that person having a depressive disorder is still higher (see, e.g., Duffy et al. 2014; Mesman et al. 2013). In this case, we need to know more about the half sister, both her symptoms and whether she is responding to any particular treatment. The choice then is to have a discussion of risks versus benefits with the family. The other complication to keep in mind is that Trisha may be at higher risk for antidepressant-induced activation (not mania). This risk is higher in children with developmental disorders (Carlson and Mick 2003).

Finally, in addition to being treated for something she did not have, Trisha was not being treated adequately for her ADHD and language disorder. Thus, she was academically and socially overwhelmed and undertreated, and basically crawled into a hole emotionally and physically.

Issue: Adjustment Disorder or Major Depression and Social Anxiety Disorder

Jared is in third grade and was referred for "meltdowns," during which he says he wants to die and bites himself.

Unlike Trisha, who had something approximating autism but whose presentation did not meet the criteria, Jared has a history that is compatible with true high-functioning autism since age 2. He had extensive early intervention because of this and was successful with good special education support in an inclusion setting in kindergarten through second grade. He still had the social disconnect characteristic of autism but he was not picked on, apparently. His attendance was good, and there was no evidence of anxiety or depression in the past. He was successful enough academically that in third grade, he was placed in a regular classroom with Resource Room only. Jared was worried that there was no one for him to ask for extra help and feared that if he made mistakes he would get ridiculed. He could not tolerate being singled out and got embarrassed. If someone made fun of him or teased him, and he perceived it as a rejection (as happened the day his book bag was tossed in the air), Jared was devastated. His teachers were concerned about Jared's anxiety, emotion regulation, and negative beliefs (e.g., his feeling that "everyone hates me"). They noted that Jared has said he is sad and depressed and has even felt like killing himself (without a plan or history of attempts). Jared's mother felt his self-esteem had really suffered because of social problems, increased academic demands, and the absence of the support in the classroom that he had had in previous years. This was the first year in which he was anxious or depressed, so the onset was relatively recent.

On mental status, eye contact was poor and Jared spoke with a quiet voice. He could not answer open-ended questions. There was a huge latency of response during which he clearly struggled. However, on the CDI, which he read and seemed to understand, he scored 26. When asked about item endorsement, he could respond. Some of these comments, in brackets, were important: "I'm sad many times" ["When kids are mean; when I get bad grades"] (Jared said he gets 80s); "I'm not sure if things will work out" ["I think bad things will happen every day; I get yelled at by the teacher"]; "I have fun in some things" ["My friend has been to my house, but I've never been to his"]; "I'm sure that terrible things will happen to me" ["Kids being mean; I might get lost"]; "I hate myself" ["I do a lot of things wrong when I try my best; I'm only good at math and bad at everything else"]; "I think about killing myself, but I wouldn't do it ["It would be too painful; I wish I could die without pain"]. When asked if he thought his family would be sad, Jared said, "Dad wouldn't be sad ["He hates me; he acts like I'm a stranger"]; nobody really loves me" ["Only my mom; my sisters don't care; they'd just laugh if I broke my foot"].

Jared also endorsed many symptoms of social anxiety. On the MASC (March et al. 1997), for instance, he checked the following: "I worry about other people laughing at me; I'm afraid that other kids will make fun of me; I'm afraid other people will think I'm stupid; I worry about what other people think of me; I worry about doing something stupid or embarrassing; I get nervous if I have to perform in public; I have trouble asking other kids to play with me; I feel shy; and I worry about getting called on in class." He also had symptoms of separation and generalized anxiety.

Discussion

Jared is the third child to present with symptoms of depression and anxiety, and he is different again from the previous two children, although, like Trisha, he has difficulty volunteering symptoms verbally. Jared's depressive symptoms are relatively acute. They began, in fact, when he was removed from a supportive school placement to one where he had to function independently, which was difficult given his problematic language and executive function. Also, children were probably less tolerant of his quirkiness. Thus, Jared's residual autism symptoms are getting him into the most trouble. As with Trisha, his misunderstanding of social situations and his inability to think and talk quickly are contributing to his anxiety and depression. Unlike Trisha, he has functioned successfully in the past. His grades are acceptable at the moment, but keeping them up is coming at some cost—the meltdowns and emotional fragility at school. DSM specifies that if criteria for a major disorder are met, then a diagnosis of "adjustment disorder" cannot be given. However, Jared's history is better conceptualized as an adjustment disorder with mixed anxiety and depressed mood and autism spectrum disorder in partial remission. Treatmentwise, it makes more sense to give Jared back the academic support he needs rather than to prescribe medication for anxiety/depression. If symptoms persist after that intervention, the more serious diagnosis may be warranted.

Issue: Outburst Differential, Including DMDD and Reactive Depressive Symptoms

Six-year-old Bobby, who was taking immediate-release methylphenidate (MPH-IR) twice a day and guanfacine at night for his ADHD, was referred after he tried to set his house on fire with the purpose of burning it down and killing himself and his family. He was angry, which he often was, and said that his family only loved him when he was good, which he wasn't often. He had made numerous threats to get a gun so as to kill others and kill himself. His mother related that Bobby felt others were against him. He had become withdrawn, irritable, and depressed, and he did not enjoy much, and sometimes he talked about suicide. He had been that way since at least age 3. He was explosive (which Bobby admitted), silly, and hyperactive. On the Affect Reactivity Index (ARI; Stringaris et al. 2012), an index of irritability, he scored 16/16 (as high a score as can be gotten). Outbursts occurred daily at home and school, during which he whined, insulted, threatened, threw things, and destroyed property (the classroom had to be evacuated while he tore it apart), but he did not get aggressive toward people. On the CMRS (Pavuluri et al. 2006), he scored 25 by parent endorsement. On the CBCL (Achenbach and Rescorla 2001), T scores were elevated for aggression (T 83), delinquency (T 71), autism-like problems (T 71), withdrawn (68), anxious/depressed (T 67), and attention problems (T 67), and this fits the bipolar or dysregulation profile described earlier.

Bobby was also very irritable and oppositional in school. Teacher Report Form T scores indicated high aggressive behavior (T 75), attention problems (T 68), depression (T 69), odd behavior, and social problems (T 68).

Bobby reported feeling an anger level of 7/10, and he listed his sister hitting him, his father yelling at him, and his mom not buying him a toy as reasons he got angry. He identified his sadness as a 10/10. Reasons he gave included getting in trouble, people scolding him, and not being able to keep from "doing bad things." He also felt sad because he did not think his mom loved him. It was difficult to get anything out of Bobby regarding feeling happy. He had a dog who made him happy and that was it. Bobby reported that his level of being scared was a 4 out of 10. He reported worrying about teachers wanting him to do work, but he wanted to play with his friends instead. He worried that bad things would happen to his mom and dad, such as being kidnapped. When asked what would happen if they got kidnapped, he stated, "I would go nuts."

Bobby's IQ was 82, and his academic skills were somewhat better. He had been placed in a special education classroom both because of his outbursts and as a result of his difficulty paying attention.

Bobby's mother had ADHD. His father probably had learning disabilities, and he had dropped out of school in tenth grade and never gotten his GED.

We wondered if Bobby's ADHD would be better treated if his mood dysregulation were to improve. Thus, on one visit, we saw him unmedicated, then had him given a slightly higher dose of MPH-IR than he had been taking. Before the medication started to work, he was clearly hyperactive and distractible. Once the medication was working, about 45 minutes later, Bobby was more focused and somewhat less depressed and irritable, but with a constricted affect. His mother indicated that she did not like the "zombie" effect the medication was having on Bobby.

Discussion

Bobby presents the not uncommon problem of a child with ADHD who is in trouble all the time and wishes he were not. The question is whether he has the emotion dysregulation associated with ADHD (which is central to the disorder but was struck from the major DSM criteria in 1980 and put into the text as an associated feature; see Carlson and Klein 2014), whether he is appropriately unhappy because he is in trouble all the time, or whether he has a comorbid condition. The comorbid condition could be a major depression or DMDD.

Bobby is clearly unhappy. If we count criteria, his symptoms would probably meet MDD criteria (sad mood, irritability, withdrawal, suicidality, low self-esteem, relative anhedonia). His presentation also meets criteria for DMDD insofar as he is chronically irritable, he has frequent explosive outbursts, the problem has gone on for a year, and he is 6 years old. However, that diagnosis is not given if criteria are met for another condition we know how to treat, such as major depression.

The core issue is the degree to which Bobby's mood dysregulation is central to his ADHD versus to a primary mood disorder. Understanding developmental psychopathology is more than counting symptoms. Given this boy's age and level of ADHD severity, the most sensible strategy is to address the condition that can be most quickly treated. Although impairment is sometimes the way to decide treatment priority, it is difficult to judge what is causing the most impairment in this case. Fire setting and temper tantrums are what is causing the most immediate impairment, but neither of these are symptoms of ADHD or a mood disorder. The hope is that with improvement in behavior and decrease in impulsivity and tantrums, Bobby will be "good" more often and will experience an improvement in mood. Seeing the change in Bobby while taking his medication gave us the opportunity of explaining to his mother that her choice might have to be between a quieter child who was successful and one who was always in trouble and feeling terrible about it.

If improvement is not sufficient, we will have to address the depression directly. However, the approach is to treat the baseline condition thought to be explaining the outbursts/mood dysregulation. If that is only partially successful, the next step will be to address the remaining symptoms.

An algorithm I use to think through differential diagnosis of outbursts and whether they represent DMDD is illustrated in Figure 3–1. If the outbursts are rare, then DMDD is not considered. If they are frequent, then the question is whether they represent a change from usual self or are chronic. If they are of relatively new onset (or have a clear onset), the issues are somewhat different if the patient is a child or adolescent. If the condition is chronic, the question is whether the child is happy between outbursts or remains cranky. The most basic tenet for consideration, however, is whether there is something treatable behind the child's outbursts. DMDD has little treatment research. What little there is suggests that the child will need medications for mood, aggression, and attention; parents will need treatment for their own problems, as well as help in understanding their child's psychopathology and triggers. Both parents and child will need to develop anger management and self-control skills. Parent training will also be needed (Waxmonsky et al. 2016) (Figure 3–2). Given the severity of aggression that usually accompanies DMDD, the fact that ADHD is often co-occurring, and the chronicity of the problems, treatment will need to be ongoing.

Issue: Teen Says Mania and Parent Does Not See It

By her mother's history, Alicia had been a normal, somewhat reserved child and adolescent. Starting in ninth grade, she developed what sounds like both a severe depression with psychomotor retardation (was well as anhedonia, withdrawal, poor concentration, and self-esteem issues) and panic attacks. Alicia's grades would fall as she would procrastinate or be unmotivated about doing homework; however, with the end of the term or with a major project looming, Alicia seemed to pull herself together and get her grades up. She has an IQ of 140, so school was generally not a struggle. Mother also described "mood swings" in which Alicia went from being fine to being cranky and introverted, staying in her room. Mom couldn't say whether these spells lasted days or weeks. She never observed mania except for "giddy spells" in which Alicia would be extraordinarily silly with her younger siblings, but that lasted a few hours at most. Mom thought nothing of these periods, in fact, and mentioned them only when she was asked questions about mania/hypomania.

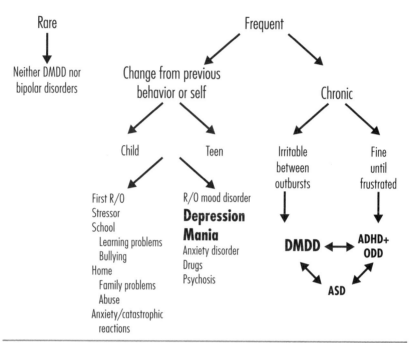

FIGURE 3–1. Differential diagnosis of explosive outbursts.
ASD = autism spectrum disorder; ADHD = attention-deficit/hyperactivity disorder;
DMDD = disruptive mood dysregulation disorder; ODD = oppositional defiant
disorder; R/O = rule out.

Alicia, now a high school senior, confirmed the depressive symptoms but
also clearly described periods of hypomania during which she talked and
laughed a lot, had "way too much energy," and did not feel tired. She
thought these periods could last a day, or as long as a week. Sleep was normal, and there were no psychotic symptoms or hypersexual behaviors. Alicia
said that the procrastination that her mother described was the result of her
depression (during which she was unmotivated to do much), and hypomanic
periods were when she became very productive and brought up her grades.

Although we initially got information from her mother and Alicia separately, we brought them together to try to reconcile the apparent disparity of information. Ultimately, Alicia's mother recognized the hypomanic
periods but had thought that Alicia was intentionally pulling herself together because of the impending term deadlines and the consequences of not
doing the projects or other assignments that were due. Alicia's mom also
thought the more productive periods indicated that Alicia was returning
to her premorbid self, when she was motivated and productive.

There was no family history of bipolar disorder. Alicia's father had untreated anxiety.

Alicia was in her senior year and had already been prescribed lithium
by her private psychiatrist. Although the mood fluctuations continued even

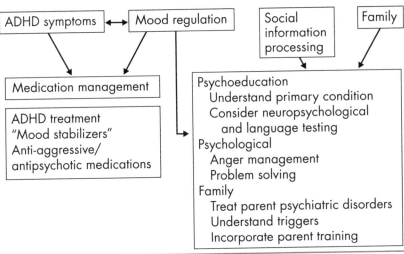

FIGURE 3–2.   Proposed management of explosive outbursts.

with the lithium, they were less extreme, and to Alicia's relief, the depression was much less of a problem. The reason Alicia and her mother sought consultation was to ask whether Alicia could stop lithium before going to college. Her mother did not want her to take medication, but Alicia was reluctant to stop because her depressions were too crippling.

Discussion

Alicia gives a fairly convincing history of bipolar II disorder. That is, her depressions have been much more impairing than her elevated mood, which her mother had barely even noticed. Indeed, when someone is depressed, it is sometimes difficult to distinguish a return to his or her normal euthymic state from a somewhat more elevated state. Alicia wanted her periodic depression treated and for that reason wanted to continue to take lithium. No one appeared troubled by her euthymic/hyperthymic periods. Had there been a question of full-blown mania, rather than hypomania, the information disparity would have been harder to reconcile. Mania is hard to miss, and if Alicia's mother missed it, we would need to understand why. We have had circumstances where the teen was dramatizing or over-reading moods, as well as times when the parent informant was oblivious for a variety of reasons. Access to other information sources and informants who can document the change in behavior and corroborate the type of behavior increases the certainty of the diagnosis of bipolar disorder.

Interestingly, as noted in Joshua's case, the original definition of "manic depression" included recurrent depression.

Regarding the advice Alicia and her mother were seeking, they were told that the summer before college is a bad time to stop medication and that they needed to wait for a time when she had a good support system in place. College was not that place. We recommended they find someone who was willing to follow and treat Alicia, in addition to Alicia's using the student counseling services. We also referred them to the Depression and Bipolar Support Alliance (www.dbsalliance.org).

Issue: Complex Comorbidities of Early-Onset Bipolar Disorder Versus Borderline Personality Disorder

Mariah, a high school senior, was convinced she had ADHD. She said she had had trouble thinking and concentrating since sixth grade (middle school). Her mother described her as a somewhat shy child who had done well academically. Her behavior in preschool and elementary school was completely unremarkable. Although her pediatrician was dubious about the diagnosis of ADHD, she prescribed OROS-methylphenidate (dose unknown), which "didn't help."

Mariah's mother is not sure when the drinking started, but she knows Mariah and her friends got drunk fairly regularly at "wild parties" by age 13. By age 15, Mariah not only was often drunk but also became promiscuous. Previously close to her mother, she became rude and irritable, more or less alienating her whole family.

Around the same time (the end of eighth grade), Mariah became obsessed with her weight and started vomiting to control it. Her room was described as disgusting and full of purged and half-eaten food. Even though she was having trouble completing homework, cutting classes, and missing tests, she demanded to be in honors classes and badgered the guidance counselor until her wishes were granted. Her quarterly secondary school grade point averages were interesting. In eighth grade they showed a steady decline from 92 to 81. In ninth grade they fluctuated from 81 to 67 to 84 to 71. In tenth they declined from 93 to 81 and in eleventh grade, they again fluctuated: 76, 90, 83, 64. Teacher comments indicated that it was incomplete work that was the problem when her grades were low.

Most recently, Mariah had become more withdrawn and depressed. Although the bingeing, purging, and dieting persisted, she stopped drinking, sneaking out at night, and being promiscuous. In fact, according to her mother, Mariah was mortified by her previous behavior. Mariah's mom described ADHD and oppositional defiant disorder symptoms, many anxiety symptoms, and depressive symptoms, but no mania.

On teacher ratings, Mariah was above grade level in her courses. There were mild ADHD symptoms ("sometimes" has difficulty with paying attention, following directions, being distracted, and being restless); the main symptoms exhibited in school were anxiety symptoms ("often" worries about her abilities in school, has difficulty controlling worries, is irritable, or acts restless). Depressive symptoms included "has little confidence," "difficulty concentrating," "overly tearful," and "can have an irritable unhappy mood." Interestingly, however, Mariah's guidance counselor reported that there were times when she was unusually cheerful, irritable, excessively active and talkative, or distractible; rapidly switched topics; and believed that she had the ability to do things that seemed unrealistic to an outside observer. The counselor also reported that Mariah could be reckless.

On mental status, Mariah stated that she had been depressed off and on since middle school. On the BDI (Beck et al. 1961) she scored a 31 (very depressed). During the interview Mariah was very tearful and apologized for each tissue she used.

Mariah also described "giddy and up" periods during which she drank excessively, engaged in indiscriminate sex, felt extremely energetic, and then got involved in many different things. These "up" periods evolved into a depressed mood so that for a time, she felt both energetic and depressed. Thus, she was drinking and hypersexual while still feeling depressed. She also described feeling very angry at times and irritable, and reported several instances in which she punched holes in the wall. She regretted her hypersexuality and drinking and stated that she felt like she lost control of herself during these times. She remembered these symptoms first occurring in middle school and lasting several months at a time.

Mariah first started drinking during middle school, with the onset possibly associated with a mood episode. She was shy, wanted to be popular, and felt less anxious when drinking. She drank several beers or hard liquor drinks two to four times per month and both passed out and blacked out. She ultimately stopped because she did not like how she felt afterward. However, she then felt more anxious and her mood worsened. Nevertheless, she made a decision to completely stop drinking. She denied current alcohol use and history of prior or current drug use. She had never been suicidal or self-injurious.

At the time she came in for consultation, Mariah had trouble thinking (which she attributed to ADHD), and indeed had difficulty on the cognitive tasks we asked her to do. (There was no psychoeducational testing available from school.) She had a bad reputation in school, and her relationship with her parents was poor. She was not enthusiastic about treatment because she feared medication would make her fat. She was in treatment, but with follow-up every 3 months.

There is a family history of depression, eating disorders, suicidality, alcohol abuse, and learning disabilities.

Discussion

The development of uncharacteristic, seemingly antisocial (e.g., sneaking out at night, getting drunk, promiscuity) and outlandish behaviors in a previously and seemingly well-adjusted person, and behaviors that clearly wax and wane over several years, strongly suggest a recurrent mood disorder. Her parents could not imagine what had come over their previously well-adjusted daughter. Mariah's mood descriptors, corroboration by her school counselor, and clear waxing and waning of grades strongly suggested bipolar I disorder and illustrate both how complicated and devastating adolescent-onset bipolar disorder can be.

For a young woman with a good premorbid history, adolescence brought with it not only bipolar I disorder, but alcohol abuse, an eating disorder (probably bulimia nervosa), and significant anxiety. The issue of comorbidities in general, and in bipolar disorder in particular, is complicated. Frequently comorbidities are an artifact of how we collect information. McElroy et al. (2011, 2016) have reported rates as high as 27% of bipolar patients (albeit adults) with a concomitant current DSM-5 eating disorder (mostly associated with bingeing), and compared with those without an eating disorder, these individuals were younger, were female, and had more suicidality, mood instability anxiety disorder, and substance use disorder. This constellation of problems sounds very much like behaviors associated with borderline personality disorder. Indeed, adults with borderline personality disorder and bipolar disorder have higher rates of these comorbidities than those without either of these disorders.

Distinguishing bipolar disorder, borderline personality disorder, and their combination is important in terms of treatment recommendations. Mariah did not have a history of tumultuous relationships. She did not fluctuate between overvaluing and undervaluing people in her life. Suicidality and self-injurious behavior were not part of her symptomatology. Medication is not a central component of borderline personality disorder, and it is very important in bipolar disorder. Mariah was not opposed to taking medication. Indeed, she was hoping medication for ADHD would help her. She did not want any medication that made her gain weight, however, and that added another layer of treatment difficulty.

Clinical Pearls

- Mood disorders in youth have many clinical presentations, only a few of which have been described in this chapter.

- Mood disorders are both homotypic and heterotypic in origins and outcomes. That is, they can be arrived at by a number of pathways (prior anxiety, family stress, temperament) and their outcomes are diverse (remission, recurrence, evolution into something else). Little is written in the child psychiatry literature about diagnostic stability (Carlson 2011). It stands to reason, however, that if diagnosis is unstable in adults, it should be even more so in children.

- Relying on one informant is fraught with inaccuracies, but there is no simple formula for combining information if it is discrepant. When there is doubt, informants should be asked about the discrepancy so that it can be clarified, and seeing parent and child together helps to develop a consensus.

- Multiple approaches may be necessary. In our clinic, we obtain rating scales from parents and teachers prior to doing the evaluation. For members of the American Academy of Child and Adolescent Psychiatry, there is a wonderful toolbox of forms and rating scales (https://www.aacap.org/AACAP/ Member_Resources/AACAP_Toolbox_for_Clinical_Practice_and_Outcomes/ Forms.aspx). DSM-5 has rating scales in the appendix and online. Rating scales allow the examiner to be thorough and to judge the severity of current symptoms, and provide a basis to measure improvement.

- If the child is presenting with outbursts, it will be necessary for the parent to keep track of their frequency, intensity, number, and duration. I have developed an irritability inventory (IRRI; Carlson et al. 2016) to help with that exercise.

- Clinical and systematic interviews of parent and child are the cornerstone of an evaluation. However, IQ, language testing, testing for learning disabilities, and urine screens for drugs are often relevant. Unfortunately, thorough evaluations are often not possible within the short time frame one has allotted by insurance reimbursement and clinic managers.

- Diagnostically, common things are common. In prepubertal children, attention-deficit/hyperactivity disorder with mood dysregulation will be much more common than mania.

- When there is uncertainty about the diagnosis (and sometimes a definitive diagnosis is really difficult to make because conditions are early in their course or information is inadequate), the clinician should discuss the issues with the family, pick a probable disorder to treat, and decide how it will be determined if the approach is a success or failure. Too often people give up too early and end up trying multiple things, and never make the trial long enough or strong enough to work.

- If two conditions are present and the clinician cannot decide which to pick, the child should be asked which he or she would most want to go away. Sometimes it is the comorbid disorder, and sometimes it is the mood disorder.

- Helping the child and family understand the phenomenology and course of mood disorders in general, and how the disorder is specifically affecting the child, is imperative, although clearly this approach is not unique to mood disorders.

References

Achenbach TM, Rescorla LA: Manual for the ASEBA School-Age Forms and Profiles. Burlington, University of Vermont, 2001

Althoff RR, Verhulst FC, Rettew DC, et al: Adult outcomes of childhood dysregulation: a 14-year follow-up study. J Am Acad Child Adolesc Psychiatry 49(11):1105–1116, 2010 20970698

Althoff RR, Ayer LA, Crehan ET, et al: Temperamental profiles of dysregulated children. Child Psychiatry Hum Dev 43(4):511–522, 2012 22271225

Altschule MD: The two kinds of depression according to St. Paul. Br J Psychiatry 113(500):779–780, 1967 4860435

American Psychiatric Association: Diagnostic and Statistical Manual of Mental Disorders, 3rd Edition. Washington, DC, American Psychiatric Association, 1980

Beck AT, Ward CH, Mendelson M, et al: An inventory for measuring depression. Arch Gen Psychiatry 4:561–571, 1961 13688369

Beck AT, Rush AJ, Shaw BF, et al: Cognitive Therapy of Depression. New York, Guilford, 1987

Biederman J, Wozniak J, Kiely K, et al: CBCL clinical scales discriminate prepubertal children with structured interview-derived diagnosis of mania from those with ADHD. J Am Acad Child Adolesc Psychiatry 34(4):464–471, 1995 7751260

Bromet EJ, Schwartz JE, Fennig S, et al: The epidemiology of psychosis: the Suffolk County Mental Health Project. Schizophr Bull 18(2):243–255, 1992 1621071

Burton R: The Anatomy of Melancholy (1621). New York, New York Review of Books, 2000

Cardoso de Almeida JR, Phillips ML: Distinguishing between unipolar depression and bipolar depression: current and future clinical and neuroimaging perspectives. Biol Psychiatry 73(2):111–118, 2013 22784485

Carlson GA: Diagnostic stability and bipolar disorder in youth. J Am Acad Child Adolesc Psychiatry 50(12):1202–1204, 2011 22115139

Carlson GA, Cantwell DP: Unmasking masked depression in children and adolescents. Am J Psychiatry 137(4):445–449, 1980 7361930

Carlson GA, Glovinsky I: The concept of bipolar disorder in children: a history of the bipolar controversy. Child Adolesc Psychiatr Clin N Am 18(2):257–271, vii, 2009 19264263

Carlson GA, Klein DN: How to understand divergent views on bipolar disorder in youth. Annu Rev Clin Psychol 10:529–551, 2014 24387237

Carlson GA, Klein DN: Commentary: frying pan to fire? Commentary on Stringaris et al. (2018). J Child Psychol Psychiatry 59(7):740–743, 2018 29924397

Carlson GA, Mick E: Drug-induced disinhibition in psychiatrically hospitalized children. J Child Adolesc Psychopharmacol 13(2):153–163, 2003 12880509

Carlson GA, Danzig AP, Dougherty LR, et al: Loss of temper and irritability: the relationship to tantrums in a community and clinical sample. J Child Adolesc Psychopharmacol 26(2):114–122, 2016 26783943

Casat CD, Powell K: The dexamethasone suppression test in children and adolescents with major depressive disorder: a review. J Clin Psychiatry 49(10):390–393, 1988 3049559

Casat CD, Arana GW, Powell K: The DST in children and adolescents with major depressive disorder. Am J Psychiatry 146(4):503–507, 1989 2648866

Diler RS, Birmaher B, Axelson D, et al: The Child Behavior Checklist (CBCL) and the CBCL-bipolar phenotype are not useful in diagnosing pediatric bipolar disorder. J Child Adolesc Psychopharmacol 19(1):23–30, 2009 19232020

Duffy A, Horrocks J, Doucette S, et al: The developmental trajectory of bipolar disorder. Br J Psychiatry 204(2):122–128, 2014 24262817

Dunner DL, Gershon ES, Goodwin FK: Heritable factors in the severity of affective illness. Biol Psychiatry 11(1):31–42, 1976 1260075

Faraone SV, Althoff RR, Hudziak JJ, et al: The CBCL predicts DSM bipolar disorder in children: a receiver operating characteristic curve analysis. Bipolar Disord 7(6):518–524, 2005 16403177

Fink M, Taylor MA: Electroconvulsive therapy: evidence and challenges. JAMA 298(3):330–332, 2007 17635894

Frommer EA: Treatment of childhood depression with antidepressant drugs. BMJ 1(5542):729–732, 1967 5335734

Ghaziuddin N, Kutcher SP, Knapp P, et al: Practice parameter for use of electroconvulsive therapy with adolescents. J Am Acad Child Adolesc Psychiatry 43(12):1521–1529, 2004 15564821

Goldberg LR: The structure of phenotypic personality traits. Am Psychol 48(1):26–34, 1993 8427480

Gurland BJ, Fleiss JL, Cooper JE, et al: Cross-national study of diagnosis of mental disorders: hospital diagnoses and hospital patients in New York and London. Compr Psychiatry 11(1):18–25, 1970 5411210

Holtmann M, Bölte S, Goth K, et al: Prevalence of the Child Behavior Checklist–pediatric bipolar disorder phenotype in a German general population sample. Bipolar Disord 9(8):895–900, 2007 18076540

Kendler KS: The phenomenology of major depression and the representativeness and nature of DSM criteria. Am J Psychiatry 173(8):771–780, 2016 27138588

Kovacs M: The Children's Depression Inventory (CDI). Psychopharmacol Bull 21(4):995–998, 1985 4089116

Kovacs M, Obrosky S, George C: The course of major depressive disorder from childhood to young adulthood: recovery and recurrence in a longitudinal observational study. J Affect Disord 203:374–381, 2016 27347807

Kraepelin E: Dementia Praecox and Paraphrenia. Leipzig, Barth, 1913

Kraepelin E: Die Erscheinungsformen des Irreseins. Z Gesamte Neurol Psychiatr 62:1–29, 1920

Lehmann HE: Psychiatric concepts of depression: nomenclature and classification. Can Psychiatr Assoc J 4(suppl):1–12, 1959 14415373

Leibenluft E, Charney DS, Towbin KE, et al: Defining clinical phenotypes of juvenile mania. Am J Psychiatry 160(3):430–437, 2003 12611821

Leonhard K: Aufteilung der endogenen Psychosen, 6 Auflage. Berlin, Akademie-Verlag, 1957

March JS, Parker JD, Sullivan K, et al: The Multidimensional Anxiety Scale for Children (MASC): factor structure, reliability, and validity. J Am Acad Child Adolesc Psychiatry 36(4):554–565, 1997 9100431

Margulies DM, Weintraub S, Basile J, et al: Will disruptive mood dysregulation disorder reduce false diagnosis of bipolar disorder in children? Bipolar Disord 14(5):488-496, 2012 22713098

McElroy SL, Frye MA, Hellemann G, et al: Prevalence and correlates of eating disorders in 875 patients with bipolar disorder. J Affect Disord 128(3):191–198, 2011 20674033

McElroy SL, Crow S, Blom TJ, et al: Prevalence and correlates of DSM-5 eating disorders in patients with bipolar disorder. J Affect Disord 191:216–221, 2016 26682490

Mesman E, Nolen WA, Reichart CG, et al: The Dutch bipolar offspring study: 12-year follow-up. Am J Psychiatry 170(5):542–549, 2013 23429906

Meyer SE, Carlson GA, Youngstrom E, et al: Long-term outcomes of youth who manifested the CBCL-Pediatric Bipolar Disorder phenotype during childhood and/or adolescence. J Affect Disord 113(3):227–235, 2009 18632161

National Institute of Mental Health: National Institute of Mental Health research roundtable on prepubertal bipolar disorder. J Am Acad Child Adolesc Psychiatry 40(8):871–878, 2001 11501685

Parker G, Fink M, Shorter E, et al: Issues for DSM-5: whither melancholia? The case for its classification as a distinct mood disorder. Am J Psychiatry 167(7):745–747, 2010 20595426

Pavuluri MN, Henry DB, Devineni B, et al: Child Mania Rating Scale: development, reliability, and validity. J Am Acad Child Adolesc Psychiatry 45(5):550–560, 2006 16601399

Rasic D, Hajek T, Alda M, et al: Risk of mental illness in offspring of parents with schizophrenia, bipolar disorder, and major depressive disorder: a meta-analysis of family high-risk studies. Schizophr Bull 40(1):28–38, 2014 23960245

Rie HE: Depression in childhood: a survey of some pertinent contributions. J Am Acad Child Psychiatry 5(4):653–685, 1966 5341688

Ruggero CJ, Carlson GA, Kotov R, Bromet EJ: Ten-year diagnostic consistency of bipolar disorder in a first-admission sample. Bipolar Disord 12(1):21–31, 2010 20148864

Rush AJ, Giles DE, Schlesser MA, et al: The dexamethasone suppression test in patients with mood disorders. J Clin Psychiatry 57(10):470–484, 1996 8909334

Stringaris A, Goodman R, Ferdinando S, et al: The Affective Reactivity Index: a concise irritability scale for clinical and research settings. J Child Psychol Psychiatry 53(11):1109–1117, 2012 22574736

Taylor MA, Fink M: Restoring melancholia in the classification of mood disorders. J Affect Disord 105(1–3):1–14, 2008 17659352

Waxmonsky JG, Waschbusch DA, Belin P, et al: A randomized clinical trial of an integrative group therapy for children with severe mood dysregulation. J Am Acad Child Adolesc Psychiatry 55(3):196–207, 2016 26903253

Weisbrot DW, Carlson GA: Diagnostically homeless: what to do if no diagnosis fits. Curr Psychiatr 4(2):25–41, 2004

Whalen DJ, Sylvester CM, Luby JL: Depression and anxiety in preschoolers: a review of the past 7 years. Child Adolesc Psychiatr Clin N Am 26(3):503–522, 2017 28577606

Winokur G: Unipolar depression: is it divisible into autonomous subtypes? Arch Gen Psychiatry 36(1):47–52, 1979 760696

Winokur G, Black DW, Nasrallah A: Depressions secondary to other psychiatric disorders and medical illnesses. Am J Psychiatry 145(2):233–237, 1988 3341468

Yen S, Stout R, Hower H, et al: The influence of comorbid disorders on the episodicity of bipolar disorder in youth. Acta Psychiatr Scand 133(4):324–334, 2016 26475572

4

Principles of Treatment of Mood Disorders Across Development

Isheeta Zalpuri, M.D.

Manpreet Kaur Singh, M.D., M.S.

Elaine is a 15-year-old girl with recent onset of depressed mood and reduced sleep since starting high school. Her parents recently moved from Chicago to New York. On initial evaluation, Elaine presented with depressed and irritable mood, 5-pound weight loss in the last month, anhedonia, and low energy. The family saw three therapists in the last year and stopped treatment after a few sessions every time Elaine showed some improvement in her symptoms. At one point in the last year, she also started citalopram, as prescribed by her pediatrician, but her parents did not notice much improvement after 8 weeks of taking 20 mg of citalopram daily. The family is now seeking treatment after Elaine expressed thoughts of wanting to die in the last week. On further evaluation, parents report that even as a young child, Elaine struggled with irritability following the birth of her younger sister. Irritability started around age 2, and symptoms worsened when she started attending day care 3 months later.

There is a strong family history of mental illness on the mother's side of the family. Elaine's mother herself suffered from postpartum depression when Elaine was born, and her father took over as the primary caregiver for Elaine at that time. Although her mother seemed to have benefited from a combination of therapy and citalopram, both she and Elaine's father are skeptical about starting another antidepressant for Elaine, given the lack of perceived efficacy with her last antidepressant trial and the black box warning of increased suicide risk in youth.

In this chapter, we provide an overview of the principles used for the treatment of mood disorders in youth, with a special focus on depression and bipolar disorders in children and adolescents across various stages of development.

Overview of Pharmacological Principles in Children and Adolescents: Pharmacodynamics and Pharmacokinetics

The Food and Drug Administration (FDA) guidelines for pediatric populations are subdivided into the following four groups: neonates (birth to 1 month), infants (1 month to 2 years), developing children (2 to 12 years), and adolescents (12 to 16 years) (U.S. Food and Drug Administration 1998). With regard to pharmacology, children are no longer considered "small adults," because youths and adults differ not only in body weight but also in physiology and biochemistry. Unfortunately, the long-term safety data for most drugs are lacking, and our knowledge of the benefits and risks of prolonged use of psychiatric medications is still emerging. Children have rapid growth within the first couple of years of life: body weight doubles in the first 6 months of life and triples during the first year. Body surface area also doubles during the first year of life. Studies have shown that even when normalized by body weight, pharmacokinetic parameters, including half-life, apparent volume of distribution, and total plasma clearance, vary among different age groups (Sumpter and Anderson 2009).

Differences in body composition and liver and kidney function account for pharmacokinetic differences between youth and adults. Importantly, liver metabolism and glomerular filtration, as measured by the glomerular filtration rate (GFR), are more efficient in children. GFR reaches adult rates by about 12 months of age. Renal function in newborns is immature, resulting in reduced renal clearance. GFR steadily rises in the first year, and adult values are reached by age 1. Nevertheless, liver and kidney function are so efficient that, in some instances, dosing adjustments of medications may need to be considered and balanced with other factors, such as drug absorption, distribution, and elimination, to optimize response.

Neurotransmitter levels also vary as a child's body develops. These levels increase concomitantly with synapse formation, with surges during perinatal periods, and subsequent leveling. Whereas serotonin levels stay relatively constant throughout life, norepinephrine levels increase with age. This likely explains the differential response in children and adults to tricyclic antidepressants. In contrast, dopamine receptor density decreases at age 3 and remains steady through the course of development (Herlenius and Lagercrantz 2004).

Drug absorption in neonates and infants is slower than in adolescents and adults, resulting in longer times to reach maximum plasma concentrations (Gibaldi 1984). Newborns also have a higher pH in their stomachs, so drugs that are weak acids are absorbed more slowly than those that are weak bases. Bioavailability of drugs in infants may also be higher because of reduced bacterial flora (Linday et al. 1987).

Children have a higher proportion of body fat compared with adults, which can result in a larger volume of distribution of lipid-soluble drugs. Furthermore, water-soluble drugs have a higher volume of distribution due to higher intracellular and extracellular water. Drug distribution is also higher in this age group because of increased free fraction secondary to lower albumin and α_1-acid glycoprotein concentrations. These drug distribution factors may play a role in the development of drug adverse effects.

Differences in enzyme and protein activity produce varied metabolic profiles and clearance in children when compared with adults. *Cytochrome P450 (CYP) system* refers to a group of enzymes called *monooxygenases*— critical for elimination of many drugs—that are expressed in every tissue, with the greatest expression in hepatic tissue. These enzymes catalyze the transformation of lipophilic drugs into more polar compounds that are then excreted by the kidneys. CYP-dependent medication metabolism is influenced by functional polymorphisms as well as development: CYP2D6 activity reaches adult range by 3–5 years of age. CYP3A4 activity reaches adult range by 6–12 months of age and increases relative to adult levels from 1 to 4 years of age, before declining to adult levels by the end of puberty. CYP2C19 activity reaches adult range by 6 months of age and peaks at 1.5–1.8 times adult values by 3–4 years of age, before decreasing by the end of puberty and returning to adult levels. And lastly, CYP1A2 activity reaches adult levels by 4 months of age and peaks at age 1–2 years, before declining to adult levels by end of puberty.

Given the potential of adverse effects, clinicians often prescribe psychotropic medications to children and adolescents at low doses and then titrate slowly. Although this may prevent the emergence of serious side effects at times, it also may delay improvement in symptomatology. Our field has made advancements in pharmacogenomic testing, which seems promising for predicting drug levels for some medications as well as side effects for some patients. Pharmacogenetic testing may help guide medication selection by leveraging variations in individual genes relevant to medication metabolism or predicting treatment response. Ideally, such testing would maximize the likelihood that a specific psychotropic medication produces the best therapeutic benefit while minimizing adverse effects (Wehry et al. 2018). It also has the potential to reduce treatment-emergent side effects and morbidity and enhance treatment response, as well as decrease inpatient admissions and readmissions due to lack of efficacy or side effects. However, we still need prospective studies to assess the benefit of medication selection and/or dose adjustments based on a patient's individual genotype prior to starting treatment. Also, most studies have been performed exclusively in adults, with results being extrapolated to the pediatric population. And whereas most studies have been performed on one gene at a time, it may take a combination of pharmacokinetic and pharmacodynamic genes to predict treatment response more accurately (Wehry et al. 2018).

Phases of Treatment

As in adults with mood disorders, the treatment of mood disorders in children can be divided into three phases: acute, continuation, and maintenance (Birmaher et al. 2007). A clinician's goal in the acute phase is to help the patient achieve an acute response to an intervention, with the broader goal of facilitating achievement of full symptomatic remission. In the context of treatment for mood disorders, *response* may clinically refer to either a lack of mood symptoms or a significant reduction in such symptoms for at least 2 weeks, whereas *remission* refers to a period of at least 2 weeks but less than 2 months with no or fewer mood symptoms. Clinical trials operationalize response and remission rates following standard definitions of response (≥50% measured symptom reduction from baseline) and remission (Young Mania Rating Scale ≤12 or Children's Depression Rating Scale—Revised ≤28). The goal in the continuation phase is to consolidate the response achieved in the acute phase and prevent *relapse,* which is defined as a period of mood symptoms during remission. The goal of the maintenance phase is to avoid *recurrence* of mood disorders, which is defined as the emergence of symptoms of depression during the period of recovery. *Recovery* refers to absence of significant symptoms of depression (e.g., no more than 1–2 symptoms) for ≥2 months (i.e., there is no new episode during this time period).

Each of these phases of treatment typically includes at minimum some psychoeducation for patients and their families, supportive psychotherapy, and collaboration with the patient's school. Psychoeducation involves providing patients and their parents/guardian, with information and knowledge about mood symptoms and associated conditions, and sharing resources that may be available to families in their local communities, in their treatment settings, and in carefully selected literature or bibliotherapy. Psychoeducation enables patients and their families to collaborate with the clinician in making informed treatment decisions. Successful treatments often involve working collaboratively with children, adolescents, and their caregivers to address questions raised about the risks, benefits, and alternatives to treatment. Psychoeducation has been well documented to improve adherence to treatment and reduce depressive symptoms (Brent et al. 1993; Renaud et al. 1998).

Supportive therapy has been found to be an important aspect of a patient's treatment. It includes face time with the patient and/or family, active listening and reflection, problem solving, and teaching basic coping skills in the face of stress or problems. Oftentimes pediatricians may not realize that they are providing this treatment modality in their day-to-day practice by suggesting lifestyle changes, sleep hygiene techniques, and screening for mood disorders, as well as providing psychoeducation to the families. All of these factors contribute to improve treatment adherence and facilitate remission of symptoms.

Apart from providing psychoeducation to the family, clinicians can engage the family in the treatment and ensure commitment to treatment not only from the patient but from the family as well. Often, parents are the only source for the child to be able to access the treatment that is needed. In most cases, parents also need to monitor their child's response, ensure adherence to the treatment, and provide a safety net in case the child experiences either symptom worsening or treatment-related side effects. Children and adolescents with mood disorders are at risk for self-harm/ suicide, and parents may need to closely monitor medication intake because of risk of overdose. It is possible that one or both parents or a sibling may benefit from treatment as well, or that the child's illness may benefit from some work focused around the parent-child relationship. Apart from this, if there is family dysfunction, marital conflict, or parent-child conflict, addressing it has been found to prevent interference with treatment progress.

School is such an important part of a child's life that mood symptoms could be secondary to problems in school, whether the problems are due to academic difficulties or interpersonal issues. A child's functioning in school might directly be impacted by a mood disorder or co-occurring condition. Thus, children and adolescents might need support from their schools, including specific accommodations to enable least restrictive learning before, during, or after a major mood episode. Developing these accommodations involves engaging the parents with school personnel, including counselors, student advocates, and teachers, who may all benefit from understanding how the symptoms manifest in a student and their impact on learning, and how treatment is conceptualized to help. Students may qualify for Emotional Disturbance disability and need a 504 or an Individualized Education Plan (IEP). Psychoeducation around the child's illness and treatment for school staff will be discussed further in Chapter 15 ("School-Based Interventions for Pediatric-Onset Mood Disorders").

Therapeutic Alliance and Leveraging the Placebo Response in Children

Therapeutic alliance refers to the collaborative relationships among the clinician, patient, family, and community when working with children and adolescents. Antidepressant trials in youth often fail because of treatment nonadherence (Woldu et al. 2011) or inadequate dosing or duration of medication. Strong and collaborative relationships among the treatment team have been found to have a positive impact on a child's mental health treatment. A strong therapeutic alliance leads to frequent parent participation in the treatment, whereas poor alliance can lead to treatment dropout. When seeing a clinician for the first time, families often have expectations and hopes that undergoing a consultation or having a better understanding of the illness may be enough and that they therefore may not need long-term ongoing treatment. Teens will also, at times, find improvement in symptoms if they can see a therapist in whom they can confide confidentially.

Randomized controlled trials (RCTs) have shown that 60% of children and adolescents with major depression respond to placebo. Placebo could be considered contact with a clinician in clinical settings, and placebo response has been found to be inversely associated with the severity of the illness. Although pharmacologically inert, placebo treatments are known to improve symptoms across various clinical conditions by virtue of patients' perceptions and beliefs about the treatment. Schafer et al.

(2018) suggest that placebo effects are part of a set of adaptive mechanisms for shaping nociceptive signaling based on its information value and anticipated optimal response in a given behavioral context. Also, Strawn et al. (2017) found that the degree of expectation of improvement in separation anxiety disorder raised the likelihood of a placebo-related decrease in anxiety symptoms, and this improvement occurred early in the course of treatment. There has been a large placebo response in trials of repetitive transcranial magnetic stimulation, which has been associated with depression improvement in the active treatment groups (Razza et al. 2018). The placebo effect also seems to be higher in younger patients than in older patients. This placebo response could be leveraged during treatment of this population, especially in those with milder forms of depression or subthreshold symptoms, and underscores the value of a supportive therapeutic approach.

Lessons Learned From TADS/TORDIA

Treatment for Adolescents with Depression Study (TADS) and Treatment of (SSRI) Resistant Depression in Adolescents (TORDIA) are two landmark, multicenter randomized clinical trials that were designed to evaluate the effectiveness of treatments for adolescents with major depressive disorder (MDD) and treatment-resistant depression, respectively.

Treatment for Adolescents with Depression Study

In TADS, a multisite clinical trial in which participants were recruited from 13 clinical sites, 439 adolescents ages 12–17 with a diagnosis of MDD were randomly assigned to one of four treatment groups: fluoxetine alone, cognitive-behavioral therapy (CBT) alone, combination of fluoxetine and CBT, and placebo (March et al. 2004). Participants were included if their symptoms met the DSM-IV criteria for MDD and they had a Children's Depression Rating Scale—Revised score > 45, had a Full Scale IQ > 80, and were antidepressant-free before consent. Concurrent psychostimulant medication was permitted. After 12 weeks, 71% of the participants responded to combination treatment, 61% responded to fluoxetine only, 43% to CBT only, and 35% to placebo only. It was found that a combination of fluoxetine and CBT was the best treatment approach for adolescents with depression compared with either of these interventions alone. By 12 weeks of treatment, 23% (102/439) of the youth had achieved remission (Kennard et al. 2006). The rate was significantly higher in the combination group (37%) as compared with the fluoxetine (23%), CBT (16%), and placebo (17%) groups, with odds ratios of 2.1 for combination versus fluoxetine, 3.3 for combination versus CBT, and 3.0 for combination versus placebo. Seventy-one percent of the youth no longer had symptoms that met criteria for major depression at the end of the acute treatment. Hence, it was concluded that during the acute phase, combination treatment was superior to monotherapy and placebo in terms of remission rates.

A majority of the samples had comorbid illness, which may have increased the probability of treatment seeking. The majority of the adolescents were from two-parent homes and families with higher-than-average annual incomes. Regardless, only one-third of the sample had sought treatment from a mental health specialist in the 3 months preceding study enrollment. The overall estimated remission rate for the 327 cases in the three active treatment arms was 27% at week 12, 40% at week 18, and 60% at week 36 (Curry et al. 2006). At 36 weeks, the remission rate was 60% in the combination treatment group, 55% in the fluoxetine-alone group, and 64% in the CBT-alone group. The recovery rate at week 36 was 65% for adolescents achieving remission during the acute phase (week 12) and 71% for adolescents achieving remission during the continuation phase (week 18), with no statistically significant difference in recovery rates. Most of the depressed sample had achieved remission by the end of 9 months of treatment.

This study highlights the importance of continuation- and maintenance-phase treatments, because symptoms improved with continuation of treatment and time. This could be one of the reasons why Elaine, whose case was mentioned at the beginning of this chapter, continued to have symptoms of depression despite seeing multiple providers. While the combination treatment arm and the fluoxetine arm achieved remission early in the course of treatment (week 6), combination treatment was superior to both the CBT-only and fluoxetine-only arms at weeks 12 and 18. However, all treatments converged in terms of rates of remission by week 24. These findings suggest that choosing a monotherapy treatment could lead to delay in remission rates for a considerable number of adolescents by 2–3 months. Hence, Elaine and her clinician may consider the relative value of combination treatment compared with either medication or therapy alone, given the superior remission rates demonstrated for combination treatment.

With regard to suicidal tendencies, at the beginning of the trial, 29% of the participants had clinically significant suicidal thoughts. The combination treatment evidenced the greatest reduction in suicidal thinking, although rates of suicidal thinking decreased among all treatment groups. Ten suicidal events occurred in the fluoxetine-alone arm (two attempts, eight ideation) versus six events in the combined arm (two attempts, three ideation, one self-harm), but this difference was not statistically significant at 12 weeks. However, TADS investigators reported significantly more suicidal events in the fluoxetine-alone arm at 36 weeks. Suicide-related events were twice as common among those participants who were treated with fluoxetine alone, and only the fluoxetine treatment arm was associated with more events than placebo (15% vs. 8% for combination and 6% for CBT). However, a causal relationship between fluoxetine and suicidal events was not established.

In conclusion, TADS found that the combination of fluoxetine and CBT was the most beneficial treatment for adolescents with MDD and the most effective treatment for reducing suicidal thinking. Remission rates were also higher in those adolescents receiving combination treatment.

Treatment of Resistant Depression in Adolescents

TORDIA was a multisite National Institute of Mental Health–funded study designed to address the fact that 40% of children and adolescents do not show adequate clinical response with medication, therapy, or combination treatment (Brent et al. 2008). In this 12-week study, adolescents who had not responded to a trial of an SSRI were randomly assigned to switch to an alternative SSRI (fluoxetine, citalopram, or paroxetine) or venlafaxine. The four treatment arms were an alternative SSRI, venlafaxine, SSRI with CBT, and venlafaxine with CBT. CBT and a switch to either medication regimen showed a higher response rate (54.8%; 95% confidence interval [CI]=47%, 62%) than a medication switch alone (40.5%; 95% CI=33%, 48%; $P=0.009$), but there was no difference in the response rate between venlafaxine and a second SSRI (48.2%; 95% CI=41%, 56% vs. 47.0%; 95% CI=40%, 55%; $P=0.83$). However, there was a greater increase in diastolic blood pressure and pulse and more frequent occurrence of skin problems during venlafaxine treatment than during SSRI treatment.

Nearly 40% of adolescents achieved remission after 6 months of treatment in this study. At week 12, those who had responded continued in their assigned treatment arm, and nonresponders received open treatment with medication and/or CBT for another 12 weeks, for a total of 24 weeks.

Of the 334 adolescents enrolled, 38.9% achieved remission by week 24. Initial treatment assignment did not affect remission rates. However, chances of remission were higher (61.6% vs. 18.3%) and time to remission was much quicker in those who demonstrated clinical response by week 12. Of those who responded by week 12, 19.6% had a relapse of depression by week 24. Lower depression scores; less hopelessness, anxiety, and family conflict; and absence of comorbid substance use also predicted remission. These findings also emphasized that ongoing treatment for treatment-resistant adolescents results in remission in about one-third of patients. Furthermore, earlier intervention among nonresponders may result in better outcomes. Augmentation with either a mood stabilizer or psychotherapy during the first 12 weeks resulted in eventual remission among nonresponders (Emslie et al. 2010).

Although there were no completed suicides, there were 58 suicide-related adverse events in 48 participants and 50 nonsuicidal adverse events in 31 participants (11 of these participants also had a suicidal adverse event). There was a significant reduction in suicidal ideation, but no differences were found between the different arms for suicidality or self-harm. However, a secondary analysis found that venlafaxine was associated with an increased risk of self-harm events when compared with SSRIs. In addition, those who received an antianxiety medication were more likely to engage in both suicidal and nonsuicidal self-injurious behaviors. In TORDIA, in contrast to TADS, there was no reported benefit from the addition of CBT on suicide-related events; this result could be related to increased severity of symptoms found in the TORDIA sample. Also, despite similar treatment length, the rate of remission in this sample at week 24 was lower than that in the TADS sample (Emslie et al. 2010).

This study showed that for adolescents who are not responding to an adequate trial of an SSRI, combination treatment with a switch to an SSRI or venlafaxine is equally efficacious. Chances of remission are also higher in those individuals who show a clinical response to treatment by the third month.

Use of Expert Guidelines

There are several clinical guidelines published to assist clinicians in the evaluation and treatment of mood disorders in youth. Two popular guidelines—the American Academy of Child and Adolescent Psychiatry [AACAP] practice parameters and Texas Children's Medication Algorithm Project (TMAP)—include expert opinions in the field from child and adolescent psychiatrists and allied mental health professionals. The

AACAP practice parameters (Birmaher et al. 2007) were developed following a review of the literature on the assessment and treatment of children and adolescents with depression and bipolar disorder. TMAP (Hughes et al. 2007), which is an update of the Texas Consensus Conference Panel on Medication Treatment of Childhood Major Depressive Disorder in 1999 (Hughes et al. 1999), was developed following a consensus conference that was held on January 13–14, 2005. This conference gathered together academic clinicians and researchers, practicing clinicians, administrators, consumers, and families to review, update, and incorporate the most current data to serve as a basis for recommendations of specific pharmacological approaches and clinical guidance on the treatment of MDD in children and adolescents.

These guidelines suggest that while working with pediatric populations, the clinician establishes a confidential relationship with the child or adolescent while maintaining a collaborative relationship with the parent or guardian, as well as other health and educational providers on the patient's treatment team. A comprehensive psychiatric assessment includes an evaluation of symptoms of depression as well as hypomania and mania, and also a thorough family psychiatric history. It is often helpful to keep a log of mood symptoms, including sleep onset and offset and the relationship of symptoms to stressors, diet, and medication changes. There are many mobile apps available for tracking mood and related symptoms. These can help patients and families understand the course of the illness, risk, and protective factors as well as aid clinicians in examining treatment response. Rating scales such as the Children's Depression Rating Scale—Revised and Young Mania Rating Scale can help the clinician assess and monitor the child's baseline symptoms as well as progress. Given the high prevalence of suicide risk in this population, the initial evaluation as well as every follow-up visit should always include a thorough safety assessment.

TMAP guidelines exist for treatment of depression in children and adolescents (Hughes et al. 2007). This expert panel emphasized the need for a thorough diagnostic evaluation in children prior to treatment initiation. Given the higher placebo response rate in trials in children compared with adults, the former may be particularly more responsive to supportive therapy and psychoeducation. For preadolescents, watchful waiting or active monitoring for a few weeks prior to medication initiation has been encouraged. Lifestyle management training and supportive management, psychoeducation, and family and school involvement are encouraged in each treatment phase. Suicide risk assessment is urged not only during initial assessment but also on an ongoing basis. Given that cognition and energy often improve prior to improvement in mood with the initiation of pharmacotherapy, suicide risk may be higher during the first few weeks. Hence, patients in this age group benefit from being seen frequently at the beginning of treatment.

For mild and uncomplicated depressive symptoms, supportive treatment is recommended as a first line of defense and may be the only treatment needed. The clinician should consider the family's cultural and religious preferences as part of the treatment plan. As noted above, it may be essential to work with the family on reducing conflicts and family dysfunction, as well as to facilitate referrals for either parent or siblings. Regular contact with a healthcare provider can at times result in improvement of symptoms. For mild symptoms, the patient can be observed for response after 4–6 weeks of supportive treatment (Birmaher et al. 2007). If symptoms do not remit, or for more severe or complicated forms of depression, the clinician should consider initiating psychotherapy. Psychotherapeutic approaches are typically tailored to the individual needs of the patient and may include modalities such as CBT, interpersonal psychotherapy (IPT), and dialectical behavior therapy (DBT). Selection of type of therapy is based on both the symptomatology and the type of psychotherapy available. CBT and IPT have been demonstrated to be effective treatments for mild to moderate depression. For example, Curry et al. (2006) found that CBT considerably reduces depressive symptoms in prepubertal children.

For moderate to severe symptoms, the clinician should consider psychotherapy from the start. At times, depending on the family's and clinician's decision, the clinician can also consider a trial of psychotropic medication or combination (therapy and medication) treatment as the initial step. The decision depends on various factors, including the severity of symptoms, suicidality, and how family members have responded to psychotropic medications. It is usually recommended that psychotropic medication management be associated with supportive therapy or another therapeutic modality.

In children and adolescents, SSRI monotherapy is indicated as a first-line pharmacological intervention (according to the TMAP guideline) for depression. If this is not effective, a trial of another SSRI is indicated. Currently, fluoxetine (8–18 years old) and escitalopram (12–18 years old) are the only FDA-approved agents for the treatment of depression in this population. Sertraline (Wagner et al. 2003) and citalopram (Wagner et al. 2004) have had positive results in randomized trials in this age group and can be tried as an alternative. These results, however, have not been replicated. SSRIs should be started at a low dose, with careful titration and reduction in dose if side effects emerge. It is important to continue treatment for 6–12 months in order to consolidate response to acute treatment and to avoid relapses. Studies have found a high risk of relapse within 4 months of symptomatic improvement.

For children and adolescents who do not respond to the medications used above, an alternative SSRI is recommended. Whereas paroxetine is included in this stage, it is usually better to avoid it in this group because of the potential for side effects, increased hostility, and agitation as compared with other SSRIs (Hughes et al. 2007). For partial responders in Stage 1, augmentation of the current SSRI is recommended. However, there are a limited number of studies that prove the efficacy of these agents, and recommendations are based on adult studies. These agents include mirtazapine and sustained-release bupropion.

If the child experiences two failed SSRI monotherapy trials, it is important to reassess the diagnosis and comorbid disorders. It is also important to consider psychotherapy if the child and the family are not already participating in it, or to consider another psychotherapeutic modality. If symptoms still persist, an alternative antidepressant monotherapy, with either bupropion, venlafaxine, duloxetine, or mirtazapine, can be initiated. Again, this recommendation is based on adult data, although there is one RCT that produced positive results for venlafaxine used for treatment of depression in adolescents (Brent et al. 2008). Although aripiprazole has been found to be efficacious as an adjunctive therapy in MDD in adults, there are no RCTs of this medication in adolescents. There is some evidence that quetiapine, when added as an adjunct to SSRIs, can reduce aggression, irritability, and depressive symptoms in children and adolescents (Podobnik et al. 2012). On the basis of adult data, one may try lithium and thyroid as adjunct agents too. Given that children and adolescents are more vulnerable to side effects than adults, and also that there is still a paucity of research on combination treatments, one may want to consider augmentation of antidepressants with lithium, quetiapine, aripiprazole, or thyroid replacement, but only if the child or adolescent has failed adequate monotherapy as well as psychotherapy trials. There are emerging data for the potential benefit of transcranial magnetic stimulation or electroconvulsive therapy in pediatric populations. These will be covered in detail in a later chapter (see Chapter 16, "Preventative and Emerging Pharmacological and Nonpharmacological Treatments").

When considering a diagnosis of bipolar disorder, clinicians must carefully assess preschool children presenting with mood and behavioral concerns for other factors, including developmental disorders, psychosocial stressors, parent-child conflicts, and temperamental difficulties (McClellan et al. 2007). Given the complexity of the illness, it is helpful to consider a comprehensive treatment plan. Often this includes providing psychoeducation to the family, psychotherapeutic interventions, and medications. Psychotherapeutic interventions that have been found to be effective include family-focused therapy and interpersonal and social rhythm therapy. These modalities help address the functional and developmental impairments, while providing skill building, problem-solving techniques, and support to the family. As with depression treatments, these help with rapport building and enhancing treatment compliance to prevent relapses. The choice of medication depends on the phase of the illness, presence of confounding symptoms (rapid cycling, psychotic symptoms), safety profile, patient's history of medication response, family history, and patient/family's preference of medication. Lithium (approved for patients 12 years and older), and antipsychotic medications such as aripiprazole (12 years and older), asenapine (10 years and older), risperidone (10 years and older), quetiapine (10 years and older), and olanzapine (13 years and older), are the primary treatment for acute mania. Lithium is also approved for maintenance therapy. Lurasidone was recently approved for the treatment of bipolar depression in children and adolescents ages 10–17 years (DelBello et al. 2017). Most children and adolescents with bipolar I disorder require ongoing medication therapy to prevent relapse, and some may even need lifelong treatment (McClellan et al. 2007). Given the potential for adverse effects, baseline labs such as complete blood cell counts, liver function tests, serum creatinine, pregnancy test, hemoglobin A_{1C}, and fasting lipid panel, followed by regular labs (every 3–6 months), are often indicated when these medications are being used. For those with severe symptoms in this population, if medication is not effective and/or tolerated because of side effects, ECT may be used in adolescents.

Recommendations for Prevention in At-Risk Populations

Youth who have parents with depression or bipolar disorder are at increased risk for developing depression and other mental health disorders. A 20-year follow-up study of offspring of depressed and nondepressed parents showed that the risk of developing depression in the former group was three times higher, and social impairment was also greater in this group. The highest incidence of MDD was between ages 15 to 20 years, with females largely affected (Weissman et al. 2006). Offspring of parents with bipolar disorder also have relatively more impaired psychosocial functioning, require more psychiatric treatment, have higher rates of placement in special education classes (Henin et al. 2005), display fewer social skills, and exhibit poorer peer social networks, including attachment difficulties in infancy. Early age at onset is a poor prognostic factor for the severity and duration of depressive episodes in adulthood, and the clinical picture is further complicated by serious morbidity, comorbidity, and suicidality throughout the entire course of the illness. Most adults with recurrent depression have their first depressive episode as a teen (Pine et al. 1998), implying that adolescence is a crucial developmental period in which to identify cases and to intervene. Given the potential for high morbidity, early identification and prevention in this population are important. An RCT conducted to prevent depressive episodes in at-risk offspring (ages 13–18 years) of depressed parents showed that a brief group cognitive therapy prevention program reduced the risk of depression in this group (Clarke et al. 2001). The intervention consisted of 15 one-hour sessions for groups of 6–10 adolescents, led by a therapist, where the adolescents were taught cognitive restructuring techniques to identify negative thoughts, with a special focus on beliefs related to having a depressed parent. Two other manual- and family-based preventive intervention programs targeted at preventing depression in healthy children, ages 8–15 years, found that these programs had long-standing positive effects on problem solving in the families around parental illness (Beardslee et al. 2003). Enhancing the children's knowledge of parental mood disorder promoted resilience-related qualities in them. Parents were also provided with psychoeducation about their illness as well as taught positive steps that they could take to promote healthy lifestyle and functioning in their children.

As in the case of Elaine, those adolescents with a prior history of extreme irritability in childhood, prior depressive episode, or other psychiatric illness are also at high risk for developing a depressive episode in adolescence or adult life. This emphasizes the importance of prevention, early detection, and intervention as well as appropriate treatment when needed, along with treatment compliance. Youth with a history of depression are at high risk for self-injurious or suicidal behaviors. The estimated lifetime prevalence of suicidal ideation, suicide plans, and suicide attempts in adolescents ages 13–18 years is 12.1%, 4.0%, and 4.1%, respectively (Nock et al. 2013). In the National Comorbidity Survey Replication, MDD and dysthymia were found to be the most prevalent lifetime disorders in adolescents (Merikangas et al. 2010). Given that suicidal behavior is more common in those with an underlying psychiatric illness, it is important to recognize the signs and symptoms to take preventive measures, and to treat the underlying disorder. This is where collaboration with the patient's family, other providers, and school personnel is crucial. Youth with a prior history of suicide attempt or a family history of attempts or completed suicide are at higher risk for suicide themselves. Apart from regular check-ins and psychotherapeutic modalities, including DBT, mentalization-based treatment for adolescents (MBT-A) and mindfulness-based cognitive therapy (MBCT) are effective for suicide-related symptoms and self-harm behaviors.

To date, there has been a lack of a strong evidence base for pharmacological approaches to treating suicidal behavior. No pharmacological intervention has been found to conclusively decrease self-harm in an RCT in children and adolescents (Hawton et al. 2015). However, medication can address underlying symptoms of mood disorders. Since pharmacological treatments may increase short-term suicide risk in some patients, close monitoring of certain medications may be needed because of overdose risk. Moreover, it is ideal for parents/guardians to be in charge of the medication and ensure compliance. Hence, it is important to start medications at a low dose and titrate slowly, with careful monitoring of suicide risk. Clinicians must weigh the risks of increased suicidality from exposure to certain pharmacological agents against the risks of increased suicidality from leaving suicidal symptoms untreated.

As noted earlier, another at-risk population is the offspring of parents with bipolar disorder. The risk of developing bipolar disorder is amplified if both parents have a diagnosis of bipolar disorder. In children and adolescents who are at high risk of developing a bipolar disorder, an initial approach may aim at promoting resilience as well as lifestyle changes, including regular physical activity or exercise, good sleep hygiene, and proper nutrition. Offspring of parents with bipolar disorder often have increased sleep disturbance symptoms, including excessive daytime sleepiness, headaches after awakening, and nightmares, compared with youth offspring of parents without bipolar disorder (Sebela et al. 2017). Because shortened sleep duration can have a negative impact on ventral striatum-insula brain connectivity during reward processing (Soehner et al. 2016), high-risk youth with poor sleeping habits are more likely to develop bipolar disorder when compared with good or variable sleepers (Levenson et al. 2017). Sleep interventions in youth with anxiety or ADHD have been found to show benefit and must be considered for this population as well.

Omega-3 fatty acids have neuroprotective and neurotrophic properties and have been found in an RCT to be efficacious, compared with placebo, in combination with psychoeducational psychotherapy in these youth (Fristad et al. 2015).

If these modalities are ineffective or the illness is more severe, the clinician should consider social rhythm, family-based, and individual or group psychotherapeutic interventions. With regard to psychotherapeutic interventions, family-focused therapy, psychoeducational psychotherapy, and child- and family-focused CBT have been known to be particularly effective in reducing mood symptoms in offspring of parents with bipolar disorder (Miklowitz et al. 2011, 2013). These treatments focus on the entire family and include problem solving as well as emotion regulation. MBCT for children (MBCT-C) has also been found to be efficacious for this group for anxiety (Cotton et al. 2016). MBCT-C is a manualized group psychotherapeutic intervention that incorporates cognitive-behavioral principles and mindfulness exercises to enhance attention regulation and nonjudgmental acceptance of thoughts and emotions in the moment. Interpersonal and social rhythm therapy focuses on stabilizing daily rhythms and interpersonal relationships and may be beneficial for these youth; however, there is a need for controlled trials with longitudinal follow-up to assess whether this intervention can help prevent or delay onset of disorder in high-risk adolescents (Goldstein et al. 2014). Many of these trials are limited by small sample size, and there is still limited evidence supporting the treatment of these high-risk youth to prevent psychiatric symptoms from progressing to threshold bipolar disorder (Zalpuri and Singh 2017).

Pharmacological interventions can either be next in line or be used in combination with psychotherapy, depending of the symptoms, availability of treatment, and joint decision made by the patient, family, and the clinician. However, very few studies have evaluated the efficacy of pharmacological interventions for the treatment of symptoms in high-risk adolescents, and the literature is currently mixed. When considering antidepressant medications as an option for the treatment of depression or anxiety in this population, the clinician must start at a low dose and titrate as needed, with careful attention to any treatment-emergent adverse events in order to prevent a switch to a hypomanic or manic episode. In situations in which antidepressants are not effective or lead to adverse events, mood stabilizers such as lithium or lamotrigine, or newly emerging atypical antipsychotic medications that have favorable risk-benefit profiles such as lurasidone, may be reasonable alternatives.

Although it is important to intervene early and prevent a manic episode, not all youth at risk for bipolar disorder will develop mania. Similarly, not all youth with a depressive episode will have recurrence of depression in adulthood. Primary, secondary, and tertiary prevention strategies are carefully contextualized and matched to symptom presentation and functional impairment. Hence, although prevention is crucial to reduce illness burden, clinicians treating adolescents may want to balance the ethical principles of beneficence and nonmaleficence, given that psychotropic medications also have adverse effects, especially on the developing brains of youth.

Clinical Pearls

- Psychotherapy is often the first line of treatment of mood disorders in children and adolescents.

- Because of ongoing developmental changes in their brains as well as lack of enough research and evidence, when managing pharmacology in children and adolescents, clinicians should follow these primary principles: 1) start low and go slow and 2) schedule regular follow-ups.

- Offspring of depressed and bipolar disorder parents are at high risk for developing mood disorders. Prevention and early intervention are key in addressing emerging mood disorders in this group.

Strategies for treating initial and refractory depressions

- Current guidelines are informed by large clinical trials but high placebo response.

- Novel antidepressants approved by the U.S. Food and Drug Administration for use in adults are being tested in youth.

- Combined medication and psychotherapy may yield better results than either alone.

Safety of current evidence-based treatments

- Suicide risk and mania assessment should be conducted on all youth treated for mood disorders.

- Youth with a familial risk of bipolar disorder may be at higher risk for side effects from antidepressants compared with the general population.

Preventative and emerging treatments

- Sleep- and exercise-based interventions may be useful for primary prevention.

- Clinicians should balance the risks and benefits of novel pharmacological, digital, and nonpharmacological (e.g., transcranial magnetic stimulation) treatments.

Strategies for treating pediatric mania and side effects

- Current guidelines are informed by large clinical trials.

- Weight gain and sedation are the most common and problematic adverse effects for atypical antipsychotics.

- Youth with a familial risk of bipolar disorder may be at higher risk for side effects from antidepressants compared with the general population.

Application of evidence-based treatments

- There is a strong evidence base for antidepressants and atypical antipsychotics from large randomized controlled trials.

- Combined medication and psychotherapy is optimal.

- Atypical antipsychotics and lithium are effective to treat pediatric mania.

- Psychotherapy, aripiprazole, lithium, lamotrigine, and lurasidone may be effective for bipolar depression; potential for maintenance and high-risk cohorts.

References

Beardslee WR, Gladstone TR, Wright EJ, et al: A family-based approach to the prevention of depressive symptoms in children at risk: evidence of parental and child change. Pediatrics 112(2):e119–e131, 2003 12897317

Birmaher B, Brent D, Bernet W, et al; AACAP Work Group on Quality Issues: Practice parameter for the assessment and treatment of children and adolescents with depressive disorders. J Am Acad Child Adolesc Psychiatry 46(11):1503–1526, 2007 18049300

Brent DA, Poling K, McKain B, et al: A psychoeducational program for families of affectively ill children and adolescents. J Am Acad Child Adolesc Psychiatry 32(4):770–774, 1993 8340297

Brent D, Emslie G, Clarke G, et al: Switching to another SSRI or to venlafaxine with or without cognitive behavioral therapy for adolescents with SSRI-resistant depression: the TORDIA randomized controlled trial. JAMA 299(8):901–913, 2008 18314433

Clarke GN, Hornbrook M, Lynch F, et al: A randomized trial of a group cognitive intervention for preventing depression in adolescent offspring of depressed parents. Arch Gen Psychiatry 58(12):1127–1134, 2001 11735841

Cotton S, Luberto CM, Sears RW, et al: Mindfulness-based cognitive therapy for youth with anxiety disorders at risk for bipolar disorder: a pilot trial. Early Interv Psychiatry 10(5):426–434, 2016 25582800

Curry J, Rohde P, Simons A, et al; TADS Team: Predictors and moderators of acute outcome in the Treatment for Adolescents with Depression Study (TADS). J Am Acad Child Adolesc Psychiatry 45(12):1427–1439, 2006 17135988

DelBello MP, Goldman R, Phillips D, et al: Efficacy and safety of lurasidone in children and adolescents with bipolar I depression: a double-blind, placebo-controlled study. J Am Acad Child Adolesc Psychiatry 56(12):1015–1025, 2017 29173735

Emslie GJ, Mayes T, Porta G, et al: Treatment of Resistant Depression in Adolescents (TORDIA): week 24 outcomes. Am J Psychiatry 167(7):782–791, 2010 20478877

Fristad MA, Young AS, Vesco AT, et al: A randomized controlled trial of individual family psychoeducational psychotherapy and omega-3 fatty acids in youth with subsyndromal bipolar disorder. J Child Adolesc Psychopharmacol 25(10):764–774, 2015 26682997

Gibaldi M: Gastrointestinal absorption: physicochemical considerations, in Biopharmaceutics and Clinical Pharmacokinetics, 3rd Edition. Philadelphia, PA, Lea & Febiger, 1984, pp 44–63

Goldstein TR, Fersch-Podrat R, Axelson DA, et al: Early intervention for adolescents at high risk for the development of bipolar disorder: pilot study of interpersonal and social rhythm therapy (IPSRT). Psychotherapy (Chic) 51(1):180–189, 2014 24377402

Hawton K, Witt KG, Taylor Salisbury TL, et al: Interventions for self-harm in children and adolescents. Cochrane Database Syst Rev (12):CD012013, 2015 26688129

Henin A, Biederman J, Mick E, et al: Psychopathology in the offspring of parents with bipolar disorder: a controlled study. Biol Psychiatry 58(7):554–561, 2005 16112654

Herlenius E, Lagercrantz H: Development of neurotransmitter systems during critical periods. Exp Neurol 190 (suppl 1):S8–S21, 2004 15498537

Hughes CW, Emslie GJ, Crismon ML, et al: The Texas Children's Medication Algorithm Project: report of the Texas Consensus Conference Panel on Medication Treatment of Childhood Major Depressive Disorder. J Am Acad Child Adolesc Psychiatry 38(11):1442–1454, 1999 10560232

Hughes CW, Emslie GJ, Crismon ML, et al; Texas Consensus Conference Panel on Medication Treatment of Childhood Major Depressive Disorder: Texas Children's Medication Algorithm Project: update from Texas Consensus Conference Panel on Medication Treatment of Childhood Major Depressive Disorder. J Am Acad Child Adolesc Psychiatry 46(6):667–686, 2007 17513980

Kennard B, Silva S, Vitiello B, et al; TADS Team: Remission and residual symptoms after short-term treatment in the Treatment of Adolescents with Depression Study (TADS). J Am Acad Child Adolesc Psychiatry 45(12):1404–1411, 2006 17135985

Levenson JC, Soehner A, Rooks B, et al: Longitudinal sleep phenotypes among offspring of bipolar parents and community controls. J Affect Disord 215:30–36, 2017 28315578

Linday L, Dobkin JF, Wang TC, et al: Digoxin inactivation by the gut flora in infancy and childhood. Pediatrics 79(4):544–548, 1987 3822671

March J, Silva S, Petrycki S, et al; Treatment for Adolescents with Depression Study (TADS) Team: Fluoxetine, cognitive-behavioral therapy, and their combination for adolescents with depression: Treatment for Adolescents with Depression Study (TADS) randomized controlled trial. JAMA 292(7):807–820, 2004 15315995

McClellan J, Kowatch R, Findling RL; Work Group on Quality Issues: Practice parameter for the assessment and treatment of children and adolescents with bipolar disorder. J Am Acad Child Adolesc Psychiatry 46(1):107–125, 2007 17195735

Merikangas KR, He JP, Burstein M, et al: Lifetime prevalence of mental disorders in U.S. adolescents: results from the National Comorbidity Survey Replication—Adolescent Supplement (NCS-A). J Am Acad Child Adolesc Psychiatry 49(10):980–989, 2010 20855043

Miklowitz DJ, Chang KD, Taylor DO, et al: Early psychosocial intervention for youth at risk for bipolar I or II disorder: a one-year treatment development trial. Bipolar Disord 13(1):67–75, 2011 21320254

Miklowitz DJ, Schneck CD, Singh MK, et al: Early intervention for symptomatic youth at risk for bipolar disorder: a randomized trial of family focused therapy. J Am Acad Child Adolesc Psychiatry 52(2):121–131, 2013 23357439

Nock MK, Green JG, Hwang I, et al: Prevalence, correlates, and treatment of lifetime suicidal behavior among adolescents: results from the National Comorbidity Survey Replication Adolescent Supplement. JAMA Psychiatry 70(3):300–310, 2013 23303463

Pine DS, Cohen P, Gurley D, et al: The risk for early adulthood anxiety and depressive disorders in adolescents with anxiety and depressive disorders. Arch Gen Psychiatry 55(1):56–64, 1998 9435761

Podobnik J, Foller Podobnik I, Grgic N, et al: The effect of add-on treatment with quetiapine on measures of depression, aggression, irritability and suicidal tendencies in children and adolescents. Psychopharmacology (Berl) 220(3):639–641, 2012

Razza LB, Moffa AH, Moreno ML, et al: A systematic review and meta-analysis on placebo response to repetitive transcranial magnetic stimulation for depression trials. Prog Neuropsychopharmacol Biol Psychiatry 81:105–113, 2018 29111404

Renaud J, Brent DA, Baugher M, et al: Rapid response to psychosocial treatment for adolescent depression: a two-year follow-up. J Am Acad Child Adolesc Psychiatry 37(11):1184–1190, 1998 9808930

Schafer SM, Geuter S, Wager TD: Mechanisms of placebo analgesia: a dual-process model informed by insights from cross-species comparisons. Prog Neurobiol 160:101–122, 2018 29108801

Sebela A, Novak T, Kemlink D, Goetz M: Sleep characteristics in child and adolescent offspring of parents with bipolar disorder: a case control study. BMC Psychiatry 17(1):199, 2017 28549429

Soehner AM, Bertocci MA, Manelis A, et al: Preliminary investigation of the relationships between sleep duration, reward circuitry function, and mood dysregulation in youth offspring of parents with bipolar disorder. J Affect Disord 205:144–153, 2016 27442458

Strawn JR, Dobson ET, Mills JA, et al: Placebo response in pediatric anxiety disorders: results from the Child/Adolescent Anxiety Multimodal Study. J Child Adolesc Psychopharmacol 27(6):501–508, 2017 28384010

Sumpter A, Anderson BJ: Pediatric pharmacology in the first year of life. Curr Opin Anaesthesiol 22(4):469–475, 2009 19593898

U.S. Food and Drug Administration: Guidance for industry: general considerations for pediatric pharmacokinetic studies for drugs and biological products. Rockville, MD, U.S. Department of Health and Human Services, November 1998

Wagner KD, Ambrosini P, Rynn M, et al; Sertraline Pediatric Depression Study Group: Efficacy of sertraline in the treatment of children and adolescents with major depressive disorder: two randomized controlled trials. JAMA 290(8):1033–1041, 2003 12941675

Wagner KD, Robb AS, Findling RL, et al: A randomized, placebo-controlled trial of citalopram for the treatment of major depression in children and adolescents. Am J Psychiatry 161(6):1079–1083, 2004 15169696

Wehry AM, Ramsey L, Dulemba SE, et al: Pharmacogenomic testing in child and adolescent psychiatry: an evidence-based review. Curr Probl Pediatr Adolesc Health Care 48(2):40–49, 2018 29325731

Weissman MM, Wickramaratne P, Nomura Y, et al: Offspring of depressed parents: 20 years later. Am J Psychiatry 163(6):1001–1008, 2006 16741200

Woldu H, Porta G, Goldstein T, et al: Pharmacokinetically and clinician-determined adherence to an antidepressant regimen and clinical outcome in the TORDIA trial. J Am Acad Child Adolesc Psychiatry 50(5):490–498, 2011 21515198

Zalpuri I, Singh MK: Treatment of psychiatric symptoms among offspring of parents with bipolar disorder. Curr Treat Options Psychiatry 4(4):341–356, 2017 29503793

5

Neuroscience of Early-Onset Depression

Uma Rao, M.D.

Tiffany Lei, B.S.

The aim of this chapter is to describe recent findings on the neuroscience of early-onset depression. Specifically, we focus on the evolving understanding of the developmental neuroscience of emotion regulation, cognitive function, and social behavior as it applies to the risk, pathophysiology, treatment, and clinical course of early-onset depression. The implications of these findings for the diagnosis and treatment of early-onset depression as well as directions for future research also are discussed.

This work was supported, in part, by grants from the National Institutes of Health (R01DA040966, R01MD010757, R01MH108155, and UL1TR001414).

Developmental Influences on Vulnerability to Depression

The risk for depression increases markedly during the transition from childhood to adolescence (Avenevoli et al. 2015; Kessler et al. 2001). Almost two-thirds of the adult cases of depression have onset in adolescence (Johnson et al. 2018; Klein et al. 2013). The increased risk for depression in adolescence parallels neurodevelopmental changes in brain function that occur during this period. Adolescence is a crucial developmental stage marked by a confluence of physical, biological, psychological, and social changes. The elevated levels of gonadal steroid hormones with the onset of puberty sculpt and reorganize neural circuits (Sisk and Zehr 2005). The changes in neural circuits are associated with cognitive advances, such as the ability for abstract thinking, generalizations across situations, organization, planning, and decision-making skills (Crone and Elzinga 2015; Luna et al. 2010). The adolescent brain also gains a better perspective of a variety of emotional and social cues (Baird et al. 1999; Herba and Phillips 2004), leading to better self-awareness and social understanding (Crone and Dahl 2012; Kilford et al. 2016). These social-cognitive developments in conjunction with interpersonal transitions (e.g., changes in social roles in family and peer relationships) and social-contextual changes (e.g., school transitions) culminate in maturational changes that occur in neural circuits responding to rewards, danger, and stress (Fuhrmann et al. 2015; Guyer et al. 2016; Somerville et al. 2010).

The maturational transitions described above offer tremendous opportunities for youth to promote emotion regulation, social learning, and affiliation as well as to set long-term goals and aspirations (Crone and Dahl 2012; Guyer et al. 2016; Kilford et al. 2016). Because the developing brain regions underlying emotional, cognitive, and behavioral systems mature at different rates (Casey et al. 2016; Ernst 2014), and since these systems are under the control of both integrative and independent biological processes (Blakemore et al. 2010; Brenhouse and Andersen 2011; Sisk and Zehr 2005), this developmental period is also marked by heightened vulnerability (Lamblin et al. 2017; Paus et al. 2008; Somerville et al. 2010). The normative developmental transitions associated with adolescence might serve as sensitive periods for the activation of specific processes involved in the onset, persistence, and recurrence of depressive episodes (Andersen and Teicher 2008; Avenevoli et al. 2015; Davey et al. 2008; Guyer et al. 2016; Kessler et al. 2001).

Developmental Changes in the Brain

Except for infancy, adolescence is perhaps the greatest time of neural change and maturation (Gogtay et al. 2004; Lebel and Deoni 2018; Khundrakpam et al. 2016). Although there is a minimal increase in brain size beyond toddlerhood, remodeling of gray and white matter occurs throughout adolescence and into early adulthood (Giorgio et al. 2010; Wilke et al. 2007). In the gray matter, these changes are nonlinear and region specific. The gray-matter changes occur in the form of increased myelination of different cortical connections or synaptic pruning or both, with a net reduction in cortical thickness and gray-matter volume (Giorgio et al. 2010; Gogtay et al. 2004; Khundrakpam et al. 2016; Sowell et al. 2004; Wilke et al. 2007).

Simultaneously, there is a linear increase in white-matter density during adolescence, associated with increases in the diameter and myelination of axons forming the fiber tracts along with increased neural size and proliferation of glia (Giorgio et al. 2010; Lebel and Deoni 2018; Paus 2010). Myelination increases the speed of neural transmission (Paus 2010). Synaptic pruning is the process by which excess connections (synapses) between the neurons are removed, thereby increasing the efficiency of cognitive processing through the creation of dedicated structural neural networks (Durston and Casey 2006; Durston et al. 2006; Khundrakpam et al. 2013; Luna et al. 2010; Mimura et al. 2003). Disturbances in these developmental patterns can adversely affect emotion and behavioral regulation (Disner et al. 2011; Weir et al. 2012).

Brain Regions and Networks Involved in Social-Emotional Processing

The neural systems associated with emotion processing can be conceptualized not only as systems involved in emotions and motivation but also, more broadly, as a network of *valuing* systems that are involved in learning about rewards and threats and in regulating *approach* and *avoidance* behaviors accordingly (Ernst 2014). During adolescence, the most salient types of rewards and threats are typically in the social domain (e.g., being admired, being accepted or rejected by peers, having early romantic and sexual experiences). Therefore, it is important to recognize the inherent overlap between emotion and social processing during the adolescent development (Crone and Dahl 2012; Guyer et al. 2016; Kilford et al. 2016).

The conceptual frameworks of adolescent neurodevelopment (Blakemore et al. 2010; Casey et al. 2016; Crone and Dahl 2012; Davey et al. 2008; Ernst 2014; Guyer et al. 2016; Kilford et al. 2016; Nelson et al. 2005; Somerville et al. 2010), as well as empirical work in animal (Andersen and Teicher 2008; Brenhouse and Andersen 2011) and adult human (Hamilton et al. 2013; Mayberg 2003; Panksepp 2010; Phillips et al. 2003; Price and Drevets 2010; Wager et al. 2008) samples, have guided neuroimaging studies on brain regions and networks involved in social-emotional processing in adolescents (Burnett et al. 2011; Crone and Dahl 2012; Crone and Elzinga 2015). These investigations have focused on the amygdala, striatum, insula, anterior cingulate cortex (ACC), and a number of regions within the prefrontal cortex (PFC). These regions work together to assign salience, promote learning, monitor conflict, compute relative valence of social stimuli, and integrate this information to generate and guide emotionally laden behaviors toward wider goals and within the contexts in which they occur.

The initial functional magnetic resonance imaging (fMRI) studies emphasized localized patterns of activation within specific brain regions (Miller et al. 2015), but there has been a recent trend to delineate patterns of functional connectivity between these regions and brain areas that subserve different functional processes (Ernst et al. 2015; Khundrakpam et al. 2016). Although social-emotional processing also includes motivational components and learning about rewards and threats, empirical research in emotional and motivational-reward aspects has taken a parallel approach rather than an integrated approach in studying these two aspects. Moreover, most studies on motivational-reward processing have focused on monetary (rather than social) rewards to examine how the ventral striatum, a subcortical brain region that becomes active when an individual receives or expects a reward (Haber and Knutson 2010; Telzer 2016), responds to risks and rewards in adolescents compared with adults.

Although some neuroscientists describe emotion and cognition as separable processes subserved by different regions of the brain, such as the amygdala for emotion and the PFC for cognition, functional interactions between the amygdala and PFC mediate emotional influences on cognitive processes, and vice versa. For example, emotion regulation is broadly defined as the monitoring, evaluation, and modifying of emotional reactions in order to accomplish goals, thereby requiring cognitive control of the emotional experience and expression (Thompson 1994). Hence, these two mental processes are inextricably linked and are represented in dynamic neural networks composed of interconnected prefrontal and limbic brain structures (Ahmed et al. 2015; Gyurak et al. 2012; Hariri et al.

2000; Heyder et al. 2004). The following subsections focus on developmental changes in the neural circuits/networks involved in cognitive-emotional and motivational-reward processes because circuits/networks play a crucial role in the key features of unipolar major depressive disorder (namely, negative mood and anhedonia).

Developmental Changes in Neural Circuits Involved in Emotion Regulation

Connections between the limbic structures and PFC make up the core neural circuitry involved in emotion generation and regulation (Lee et al. 2012; Morawetz et al. 2017; Phan et al. 2004). The primary structures within the limbic system include the amygdala, hippocampus, thalamus, hypothalamus, basal ganglia, and cingulate gyrus. The amygdala is the emotion center of the brain (Bellani et al. 2011; Hare et al. 2005; Hariri et al. 2000), whereas the hippocampus plays an essential role in the formation of new memories about past experiences (Campbell and Macqueen 2004; Panksepp 2010). Moreover, the hippocampus is highly sensitive to stress, particularly during the early developmental period, and depression is recognized as a stress-sensitive illness (McEwen 1999; Sapolsky 2003; Spinelli et al. 2009).

The PFC plays an important role in emotion regulation (Conson et al. 2015; Iordan and Dolcos 2017), and it also mediates higher cognitive capacities, including reasoning, planning, and behavioral control (Burgess and Stuss 2017; Crone and Elzinga 2015; Fuster 2002; Luna et al. 2010). The ventral part of the ACC is connected to the other limbic structures, and it is involved in assessing the salience of emotion and motivation (Allman et al. 2001; Bush et al. 2000; Hamani et al. 2011). In contrast, the dorsal part of the ACC is connected with the PFC and parietal cortex and serves as a central station for processing top-down and bottom-up stimuli (Allman et al. 2001; Bush et al. 2000).

The limbic structures and PFC continue to develop after birth. Specifically, volumetric changes in the amygdala and hippocampus continue during childhood and adolescence (Giedd et al. 1996; Uematsu et al. 2012). Some of these volumetric changes correspond to pubertal development (Goddings et al. 2014). Neuroimaging studies using growth mapping techniques suggest that the PFC matures more slowly than the other brain regions (Gogtay et al. 2004), and its development parallels the observed improvements in emotion regulation, cognitive control, and behavioral inhibition that emerge during the adolescent transition into adulthood (Crone and Elzinga 2015; Gyurak et al. 2012; Khundrakpam et al. 2013;

Luna et al. 2010; Sowell et al. 2004). Longitudinal fMRI studies show that activations in some brain regions, such as the prefrontal, temporal, and parietal cortex, are relatively stable over time and can be used as predictors for cognitive functions, whereas activations in other brain regions, such as the amygdala and ventral striatum, are more variable over time (Crone and Elzinga 2015). This variability in activations in limbic regions has implications for emotion generation and regulation.

Connections between limbic regions and the PFC are essential for effective emotion regulation (Ahmed et al. 2015; Casey et al. 2016; Crone and Elzinga 2015; Gyurak et al. 2012; Wager et al. 2008), and they are slow to develop. Adolescence is a period of remarkable changes in both structural and functional connections between the amygdala and PFC, at which time they begin to exhibit adultlike patterns of regulatory function (Casey et al. 2016; Dougherty et al. 2015; Gabard-Durnam et al. 2014; Gee et al. 2013; Perlman and Pelphrey 2011; Scherf et al. 2013; Swartz et al. 2014; Vink et al. 2014). These strengthening connections are developing at the same time that high amygdala reactivity to emotional stimuli (e.g., faces) is observed (Guyer et al. 2008; Hare et al. 2008; Somerville et al. 2011). Even though these maturational changes allow for the continued development of the limbic-cortical circuitry during adolescence, the instability (plasticity) of this system when the PFC responsivity is not yet fully developed (Hare et al. 2008; Monk et al. 2003) increases vulnerability to environmental stress (Lupien et al. 2009; Moriceau et al. 2004; Tottenham and Galván 2016) and unregulated emotion generation.

Developmental Changes in Neural Circuits Involved in Motivational-Reward Processes

The mesostriatal and mesocorticolimbic dopamine pathways are involved in processing natural rewards and reward-directed behavior (Schultz 2010; Telzer 2016). The mesostriatal-mesocorticolimbic dopamine system includes reciprocal dopamine projections from the ventral tegmental area in the midbrain into the ventral striatum, the limbic structures (amygdala in particular), and the orbitofrontal cortex (OFC). In fact, the ability to regulate emotion relies heavily on the dynamic interactions among the amygdala, PFC, and ventral striatum (Ernst 2014; Hare et al. 2005; Somerville et al. 2010; Tottenham and Galván 2016). Both the amygdala and ventral striatum are involved in emotional associative learning; they exhibit responsivity to both positive (appetitive) and negative (aversive) stimuli (Paton et al. 2006; Telzer 2016). However, differences in their roles also have been described. For instance, the amygdala is typically implicated in identifying highly salient emotional stimuli and serving as an attentional gate for associative learning (Ernst 2014; Li et al. 2011; Pearce and Hall 1980). In contrast, the ventral striatum is more likely to be implicated in reward-based learning, which involves computing a prediction error based on anticipated outcomes (Li et al. 2011; Schultz 2010).

Models of emotion-laden behavior suggest that the organization among PFC, amygdala, and ventral striatum allows for the dynamic coordination of emotional learning and responding through Pavlovian and instrumental processes that link emotion to action. The PFC is an association area that coordinates and regulates information throughout the brain. The amygdala has strong bidirectional projections with the PFC (Barbas et al. 2003; Morawetz et al. 2017), whereas the ventral striatum receives unidirectional projections from the amygdala and PFC, including excitatory projections that facilitate reward learning (Stuber et al. 2011), and it sends indirect projections back to the PFC (Cardinal et al. 2002; Casey et al. 2016; Cho et al. 2013). A developmental resting-state fMRI study in humans has indicated that the connectivity from the amygdala to the ventral striatum is present starting in early childhood (Fareri et al. 2015). However, the functional significance of these amygdala–ventral striatum connections has not been evaluated carefully in humans, and much of the developmental work has approached the function of these two regions in parallel rather than in coordination.

The dopamine system undergoes significant reorganization during adolescence (Telzer 2016). Increases in dopamine signaling peak during adolescence (Chambers et al. 2003; Wahlstrom et al. 2010). In rodents, adolescent-specific peaks were observed in the density of dopamine receptors in the ventral striatum (Andersen et al. 1997; Philpot et al. 2009; Tarazi et al. 1999). Also, dopamine concentrations and the density of dopamine fibers projecting to the PFC increase during adolescence (Brenhouse et al. 2008). A human postmortem study has reported similar peaks in dopamine expression during adolescence (Haycock et al. 2003). In addition, fMRI studies have shown that the ventral striatum is significantly more active in adolescents when compared with children and adults while receiving primary rewards (Galván and McGlennen 2013), secondary rewards (Ernst et al. 2005; Galván et al. 2006; Van Leijenhorst et al. 2010), or social rewards (Chein et al. 2011; Guyer et al. 2009), as well as in the presence of appetitive social cues (Somerville et al. 2011). In contrast to these findings, a few studies reported blunted ventral striatal activation in adolescents compared with adults during anticipation of rewards (Bjork et al. 2010). Hypoactivation of the ventral striatum has been interpreted to mean that adolescents may attain less positive feelings from rewarding stimuli, which drives them to seek out greater reward-inducing experiences that increase activity in dopamine-related circuitry (Spear 2000).

Theoretical Models of Neural Responses to Motivational-Reward Processing During Adolescent Development

The prevailing view regarding the literature on adolescent brain development is that heightened activity in the mesolimbic dopamine system serves as a liability, orienting adolescents toward risky behaviors, increasing their sensitivity to social evaluation and loss, and resulting in compromised well-being (Chambers et al. 2003; Schneider et al. 2012; Somerville et al. 2011; Wahlstrom et al. 2010). An alternative view proposed is that heightened dopaminergic sensitivity increases risk-taking behaviors that may be adaptive for promoting survival and skill acquisition (Spear 2000). The tendency to approach, explore, and take risks during adolescence may serve an adaptive purpose that affords a unique opportunity for adolescents to attain new experiences at a time when youth are primed to learn from their environments and leave the safety of their caregivers (Crone and Dahl 2012; Spear 2000). This conceptualization suggests that risk-taking itself is a normative and adaptive behavior. Heightened ventral striatum reactivity may therefore be an adaptive response as long as the system is not in overdrive and adolescents only engage in moderate levels of risk taking (Crone and Dahl 2012; Spear 2011).

Some scientists have conceptualized an adaptive role of reward sensitivity such that striatal reactivity can actually lead adolescents away from risks and psychopathology (Pfeifer and Allen 2012; Telzer 2016). Recent evidence suggests that increased dopamine neural signaling and heightened striatal reactivity may actually motivate adolescents to engage in more prosocial behaviors, facilitating improved cognition, and ultimately protect them from developing depression or engaging in health-compromising risky behaviors (Pfeifer et al. 2011; Telzer et al. 2013, 2014). For example, adolescents participated in a simulated driving session during which they could make decisions to engage in safe or risky behavior (Cascio et al. 2015). The participants completed the task in the presence of either a high- or low-risk peer. Behaviorally, adolescents made significantly fewer risky choices (i.e., drove through intersections with red lights) in the presence of low-risk peers compared with high-risk peers. At the neural level, youth who displayed greater activation in the ventral striatum engaged in fewer risky behaviors in the presence of cautious peers. In contrast, ventral striatal activation was not associated with being influenced by risky peers or with driving behavior when alone.

In a longitudinal investigation, adolescents completed a prosocial task at baseline in which they could choose to donate earnings to their family or keep monetary rewards for themselves (Telzer et al. 2010, 2011). The participants also completed a risk-taking task (the BART; Lejuez et al. 2002), during which they could inflate a virtual balloon that gave them increasing monetary rewards with each pump but could explode at any point and result in a loss of all earnings attained for that balloon. Participants who showed heightened ventral striatal activation during prosocial decisions toward their family experienced longitudinal declines in depressive symptoms over the following year (Telzer et al. 2014). In contrast, those who showed heightened ventral striatal activation when keeping earnings for themselves on the prosocial task (i.e., selfish decisions), or who showed heightened ventral striatal activation during the risk-taking (BART) task, experienced increases in depressive symptoms over the following year (Telzer et al. 2014). In a separate study, adolescents who manifested increased striatal activation in response to prosocial decisions also showed longitudinal declines in risky behaviors (Telzer et al. 2013).

These findings highlight the importance of considering the context in which the ventral striatal activation occurs. Heightened dopamine signaling may therefore be a neurobiological marker for approach-related behaviors, regardless of the perceived outcome (i.e., adaptive or maladaptive). On the one hand, it may be channeled toward motivated behaviors that are highly adaptive, such as orientation toward motivationally positive behaviors (e.g., striving for academic success, engaging in goal-oriented or prosocial behaviors). Alternatively, dopamine signaling may be directed toward motivated behaviors that can be highly maladaptive depending on the motivational context (e.g., dangerous driving behaviors, risky sexual behaviors).

Other research has shown that the ventral striatum is involved in emotion regulation. In a longitudinal study of youth followed during the adolescent transition, participants were scanned twice to examine how neural responses to emotional facial expressions changed over time (Pfeifer et al. 2011). Longitudinal increases in ventral striatal reactivity were associated with decreases in risky behavior and declines in susceptibility to peer influence over time. The ventral striatum was functionally coupled with the amygdala in the negative direction during processing of emotional faces, suggesting that the ventral striatum may regulate and dampen heightened amygdala response to emotionally arousing stimuli (Pfeifer et al. 2011).

Others have reported ventral striatal activation during cognitive reappraisal of negative emotions in adolescents (McRae et al. 2012), further highlighting its role in emotion regulation. Masten et al. (2009) found that heightened ventral striatal activation during social exclusion was associated with dampened self-reported emotional distress and less activation in brain regions involved in "social pain" processing, confirming that the ventral striatum is crucial for regulating negative emotion in adolescents. Given its role in reward processing, the ventral striatum may aid in the reappraisal of negative experiences into positive interpretations (Masten et al. 2009; McRae et al. 2012; Wager et al. 2008), serving a protective role against psychopathology.

Sex Differences in Depression and Neural Circuitry

Epidemiological studies have consistently demonstrated that females are two to three times more likely than males to develop depression (Avenevoli et al. 2015; Kessler et al. 2001). A developmental trend is observed for sex differences in the prevalence of depression. Prior to adolescence, the rate of depressive disorders is about equal in boys and girls (Hankin et al. 1998; Kessler et al. 2001; Wade et al. 2002). During early to middle adolescence, the rate of depressive symptoms and disorders in girls rises by two to three times that of boys (Hankin et al. 1998; Kessler et al. 2001; Wade et al. 2002), a trend that continues into adulthood (Hankin et al. 1998). Sex differences in brain structure and function also have been reported (Andersen et al. 1997; Giedd et al. 2006; Giorgio et al. 2010; Goddings et al. 2014; Kaczkurkin et al. 2018; Lebel and Deoni 2018; Sowell et al. 2004; Yurgelun-Todd et al. 2002). However, whether the neural developmental patterns associated with depressive symptoms differ between males and females is less clear (Kaczkurkin et al. 2018). Few studies have focused on this question.

In a longitudinal study of adolescents at high risk for depression (Whittle et al. 2014), divergent patterns of brain development between male and female subjects were associated with risk for depression onset; depression was associated with greater amygdala growth in female subjects but attenuated growth in male subjects. Moreover, the development of depressive disorder was associated with smaller nucleus accumbens volume over time in female subjects but not in male subjects. In a study of neural responses to an emotional face-processing task in depressed adolescents, sex differences were observed in the supramarginal gyrus, posterior cingulate cortex, and cerebellum in response to sad relative to neutral distractors (Chuang et al. 2017). In healthy volunteers, greater ventromedial PFC activation during the receipt of reward at baseline predicted a greater increase in depressive symptoms at follow-up in males but not females (Hanson et al. 2015), whereas reduced OFC activation during loss at baseline predicted greater depressive symptoms at follow-up in females but not males (Jin et al. 2017). The clinical significance of these sex differences is not clear. More work is needed to identify the effects of sex on brain development and depression.

Explanatory Models of Early-Onset Depression

Incorporating developmental and neuroscience frameworks, several theoretical models have been proposed to explain the increased vulnerability to depression and other psychopathology during adolescence (Casey et al. 2008, 2016; Crone and Dahl 2012; Ernst 2014; Forbes and Dahl 2005, 2012; Nelson et al. 2005, 2016). A summary of these theoretical frameworks is provided in Table 5–1.

An integration of the earlier iterations of the various models indicates that the increased vulnerability to depression and other psychiatric disorders during adolescence may be due to an imbalance between the relative structural and functional maturity of brain systems critical to emotional and incentive-based behavior (subcortical regions such as the amygdala and ventral striatum) compared with the brain systems mediating cognitive and impulse control (e.g., PFC), suggesting that the PFC exerts less regulatory control over subcortical regions in adolescents relative to adults (Casey et al. 2008, 2016; Ernst 2014; Nelson et al. 2005; Somerville et al. 2010). This framework provides a heuristic model for explaining the neurodevelopmental basis for the emotional and behavioral changes observed in adolescence.

In conceptualizing the ways in which the development of regulatory mechanisms lags behind the development of emotional brain systems, this imbalance model seems particularly appropriate for explaining the increased rates of dysregulated behaviors, especially risky behaviors, which emerge during adolescence but decline when regulatory brain systems reach adult levels of maturity (Moffitt 1993; Rutter et al. 2006). However, this model cannot explain the high rates of depression that start in adolescence but persist through adulthood (Rao and Chen 2009), by which time, presumably, the regulatory mechanisms whose delayed development puta-

TABLE 5–1.   Models of developmental changes contributing to risk for depression

Proposed model	Theoretical framework
Imbalance model (Casey et al. 2008, 2016)	1. Divergent developmental courses of two brain systems: the subcortical socioemotional system matures earlier than the cortical cognitive-control system, leading to dysregulated emotion/behavior (Casey et al. 2008). 2. Integrated circuit-based perspective: the development and functioning of components of these two neural systems are inextricably linked in their influence over emotion and behavior (Casey et al. 2016).
Flexible frontal cortical engagement (Crone and Dahl 2012)	Pubertal changes induce increased social-affective influences on goals and behavior that, in turn, interact with changes in cognitive control and social-cognitive development contributing to flexibility in the engagement of frontal cortical systems, depending on the motivational salience of the context. These changes can result in positive or negative growth trajectories.
Triadic model (Ernst 2014)	Neural circuitry is composed of reward/approach, avoidance, and regulatory components. Depression is associated with changes in two of the triadic model's arms—decreased approach and increased avoidance—and this mismatch cannot be corrected by the still immature regulatory component.
Dysregulated positive affect model (Forbes and Dahl 2005, 2012)	Reward system undergoes developmental changes across the life span. Depression results from a reduction in positive affectivity (a factor that indexes active engagement with the environment). Differences between depressed and nondepressed groups are most evident during adolescence, when levels of reward function are particularly high in the nondepressed group.
Social information processing model (Nelson et al. 2005, 2016)	Brain processes governing social behavior comprise three broad functional nodes: the perceptual node, the affective node, and the cognitive-regulatory node. During adolescence, the *affective node* (equivalent to the subcortical limbic system) outpaces maturation of the cortically based *cognitive-regulatory node*. The mismatch creates a vulnerability in which strong emotional responses to social stimuli are not tempered by the yet-to-mature regulatory mechanisms.

tively gave rise to emotional dysregulation have matured (Gogtay et al. 2004). This theory also appears to hold that emotional and motivational systems are composed primarily of subcortical structures, whereas the regulatory systems are cortical. More recently, the very concept that emotion and emotion regulation (or emotion and cognition) exist as separable processes has been questioned (Ahmed et al. 2015; Wager et al. 2008).

The imbalance model was further refined to account for the complexity of brain and behavioral changes across adolescence. These dynamic integrated circuit-based models stress 1) the importance of studying brain connectivity within/between limbic, emotional-motivational, and cognitive-control brain circuits (Casey et al. 2016); 2) the influence of social context and affiliation on observed neural sensitivities (Kilford et al. 2016; Nelson et al. 2016); and 3) the importance of pubertal changes and cortical-subcortical flexible interactions (Crone and Dahl 2012).

In contrast to the models described above, Davey and colleagues (2008) proposed that the maturation of the PFC itself might be responsible for the development and maintenance of depression. According to this prefrontal-development model, there is a cost to the ability of the PFC to make decisions in complex social environments that take into account the consequences of decisions into the future, resulting in a heightened vulnerability to depression when anticipated future rewards are not attained. As described earlier, there is substantial remodeling and maturation of the dopaminergic reward system and PFC during adolescence, which coincides with the adolescent entering the complex world of adult peer and romantic relationships, in which the rewards that can be obtained (e.g., group affiliation, romantic love, social status) are abstract and temporally distant from the proximal context. Development of the PFC makes it possible to pursue such complex and distal rewards, which are, however, tenuous and more readily frustrated than the more immediate rewards. Davey et al. (2008) hypothesized that when these distant rewards are unattainable, they suppress the reward system. When the suppression of the reward system is extensive and occurs for an extended period of time, it manifests as depressive disorder.

The functional significance of the dopaminergic system's more extensive integration with the PFC during adolescence is that the nature of the represented rewards becomes more sophisticated. The net result is the ability of adolescents to be motivated by, and to respond to, rewards that are more distal and complex (Schultz 2010). For example, serotonin interacts with the dopamine system to further shape reward function (Benloucif and Galloway 1991; Di Mascio et al. 1998), possibly by reducing impulsive overresponding to proximal emotional stimuli in favor of maintaining emotional engagement with the long-term goals (Katz 1999; Spoont 1992). Davey et al. (2008) proposed that the initial episodes of clinical depression during adolescence often result from the frustration, or the omission, of highly anticipated social reward(s). Abstract social rewards have a greater salience and are associated with an active state of arousal (Bechara and Damasio 2005; Panksepp 2010). When an anticipated reward is omitted, it has the effect of transiently suppressing the neural reward system (Schultz 2010). Omission of rewards that are extended in their representation into the more distant future will cause a correspondingly prolonged suppression of the reward system, resulting in depression.

Neural System Approaches to Early-Onset Depression

To capture the complex phenomenology of depression, we may need to adopt a multimodal/network approach. Consistent with this framework, recent investigations of early-onset depression have moved beyond localized changes in specific regions to a neural systems approach (Khundrakpam et al. 2013, 2016). Additionally, studies of adult depression indicate that combined structural and functional techniques offer complementary information on pathophysiology and treatment prediction (de Kwaasteniet et al. 2013). Accordingly, multimodal approaches have gained momentum. In addition to the fronto-limbic and fronto-striatal systems that have been implicated in depression, neural system studies in adult samples have focused on the intrinsic functional organization of the brain, wherein functionally homogeneous neural regions appear to show correlated activity even when they have not been actively prompted (Hamilton et al. 2013). A brief overview of the identified neural networks, including the default mode, executive, and salience networks, is provided below.

Default Mode Network

The default mode network (DMN) has been implicated in depressive symptoms experienced across the lifespan. The DMN is composed of the posterior cingulate cortex (PCC), bilateral parietal cortex, medial PFC (mPFC), and medial temporal lobe (MTL) (Raichle et al. 2001). In healthy individuals, this network of structures shows metabolic activity at rest but a corresponding reduction in activity during an active task. To corroborate the network pattern of activity in the DMN, Greicius et al. (2009) simultaneously examined structural and functional connectivity. Using an independent probabilistic component analysis approach, they identified white-matter tracts that directly connected the PCC to mPFC and PCC to MTL, but not to structures outside the DMN. These results indicate that the temporal correlation of activity in these regions at rest is likely due, at least partly, to tracts that link DMN regions directly.

The DMN is primarily involved in self-referential processes such as rumination. Failure to deactivate DMN areas during tasks requiring cognitive engagement is thought to reflect an "inability" to disengage from self-related thought processes. Because maladaptive ruminative thinking manifests frequently in depression, increased activity of the DMN at rest (due to spontaneous rumination) is strongly implicated in depression. Consistent with this hypothesis, increased activity/functional connectivity in the DMN at rest has been linked to increased rumination of negative thoughts in adult patients with depression (Hamilton et al. 2013; Li et al. 2018), and anomalous gray-matter structural networks support this formulation of depression (Singh et al. 2013). Some studies also found that individuals with depression did not demonstrate the typical pattern of deactivation in several components of the DMN during presumably self-relevant active and passive processing of negative stimuli (Hamilton et al. 2013). The restoration of connectivity of this network and corresponding symptom improvement following treatment serve as additional evidence for the crucial role of the DMN in the pathophysiology of depression (Li et al. 2018).

Executive Network

In contrast to the DMN, which is more active at rest than during task performance, the executive network (EN), comprising the dorsolateral PFC (DLPFC) and lateral parietal cortex, has nodes that become selectively activated with executive task performance (Seeley et al. 2007). Cognitive theories of depression posit a cyclical relationship between negative affective responding and depressed mood, in which negative affective biases promote depressed mood that, in turn, exacerbates negative emotional responding, which further increases negative biases. Consistent with this theory, studies with depressed patients found decreased activation of the DLPFC at rest and in response to negative stimuli, but not to positive stimuli (Hamilton et al. 2013; Li et al. 2018). Even though the DLPFC is underactive both at rest and in response to negative stimuli in depression, it appears there is little overlap in the two states. Both regions fell within the boundaries of the EN (Seeley et al. 2007), but the part of DLPFC that showed reliable under-responding to negative stimuli was contralateral and posterior relative to the part of the DLPFC that was underactivated at rest in depression (Hamilton et al. 2013). These findings suggest that tonic (resting-state) and phasic (affective-response) neural functional anomalies in depression are undergirded by separate components of a functionally coherent network.

Salience Network

The salience network (SN), which also becomes more active during task performance, includes the anterior insula, the amygdala, and the dorsal ACC (Seeley et al. 2007). The SN is primarily involved in guiding behavior in response to both external and internal salient stimuli, and it was shown to correlate with state anxiety (Seeley et al. 2007). The SN has been linked to emotional overreactivity in depression, and heightened response in the SN nodes has been documented in depression across a wide range of negative conditions, but not to positive stimuli (Hamilton et al. 2013; Li et al. 2018).

An important difference between dysfunction in the SN and dysfunction in the DMN and EN in depression is that whereas all primary nodes of the SN are affected, some components of the EN and DMN (primarily the parietal components) have not been found to exhibit aberrant activation in depression (Hamilton et al. 2013). Despite these differences, all three intrinsic networks appear to be affected in depression (Hamilton et al. 2013; Li et al. 2018; Wang et al. 2016). Wang et al. (2016) proposed that the dynamic alteration and imbalance among these intrinsic networks, both in the resting-state and rest-task transition stages, contribute to cognitive vulnerability in depression. Under conditions of negative stimuli during the rest-to-task transition, Wang et al. identified three types of aberrant network interactions as facilitators of vulnerability to depression and dysphoric mood, each through a different cognitive mechanism: DMN dominance over the EN, an impaired SN-mediated switching between the DMN and EN, and ineffective EN modulation of the DMN. The interrelated networks and brain-activity changes between rest and task states provide a neural system perspective on cognitive vulnerability and resilience to depression, and may potentially guide the development of new intervention strategies for this disabling illness.

Structural Brain Changes Associated With Depression

Major findings from structural MRI (sMRI) and diffusion tensor imaging (DTI) studies in youth with early-onset depression will be summarized.

The sMRI technique provides regional volumetric and cortical thickness information. DTI can provide additional information on axonal integrity and bundle coherence of white-matter tracts, which can be used to estimate the structural efficiency of neural pathways. Additionally, data from studies in youth at risk for depression will be reviewed.

Volumetric and Cortical Changes Associated With Early-Onset Depression

Neuroimaging studies in early-onset unipolar depression began with volumetric studies of isolated brain regions that served to identify key nodes of the frontal-limbic circuitry. A brief summary of these studies is presented (for reviews, see Hulvershorn et al. 2011; Weir et al. 2012). Similar to the observations in adults (Price and Drevets 2010; Schmaal et al. 2017), many studies in pediatric depression identified structural alterations in frontal regions, including the PFC, OFC, and ACC (Hulvershorn et al. 2011; Schmaal et al. 2017; Weir et al. 2012). However, in contrast to the adult findings, which indicated reduced volume in these regions, some pediatric studies of depression found increased volume. It has been argued that the discrepancy between pediatric and adult studies may be accounted for by severity and protracted duration of the illness, resulting in neural loss in adult samples.

Regarding the subcortical structures, inconsistent findings have been reported in amygdala volume changes in adult depression, but a reduction in hippocampal volume has been replicated in many studies, particularly in early-onset and recurrent cases (Campbell and Macqueen 2004; Price and Drevets 2010; Schmaal et al. 2017). In the pediatric samples, amygdala and hippocampal volumes appeared, overall, to be smaller in depressed individuals compared with healthy control subjects (Hulvershorn et al. 2011; Weir et al. 2012). The smaller volumes were associated with early life adversity, family history of depression, onset during adolescence, and comorbid anxiety disorders (Hulvershorn et al. 2011). A few studies examined gray-matter changes in the striatum in pediatric depression, in which smaller striatal and caudate volumes were observed, and the volume changes may be inversely correlated with depression severity (Hulvershorn et al. 2011; Schmaal et al. 2017; Weir et al. 2012).

Volumetric abnormalities were observed in key brain regions of the frontal-limbic network in early-onset depression. Several moderating variables have been identified, including age, sex, age at onset and duration of illness, symptom severity, medication exposure, family history, comorbidity, and early life adversity (reviewed in Hulvershorn et al. 2011; Schmaal et al. 2017; Weir et al. 2012). Most of the studies were limited by modest sample sizes, precluding the ability to systematically address the effect of these moderating variables.

More recently, studies have focused on cortical thickness and surface area differences in early-onset depression from healthy controls (Hulvershorn et al. 2011; Schmaal et al. 2017). Studies in adult depression generally reported cortical thinning, but adolescent studies reported both cortical thinning and thickening, or no differences, in certain regions (Schmaal et al. 2017). The differences in findings between adolescent and adult depression may be due to the ongoing maturational changes as cortical thickness decreases linearly during adolescence owing to synaptic pruning, myelination, and other remodeling effects. These processes cause a delay in maturation (i.e., delayed thinning) of the cortex in adolescent depression, resulting in greater cortical thickness during various stages of brain maturation but a thinner cortex eventually. Consistent with this hypothesis, depressive and anxiety symptoms were associated with greater cortical thickness in some studies of adolescent depression (Schmaal et al. 2017). In contrast to greater cortical thickness, a bilateral reduction in total surface area has been observed in adolescent depression (Schmaal et al. 2017), reflecting a diffuse pattern of local surface area deficits. Surface area deficits have been seen in the medial OFC and superior frontal gyrus as well as in the visual, somatosensory, and motor areas (Schmaal et al. 2017). These deficits have been found in youth with recurrent episodes, suggesting a negative effect of multiple episodes on the cortex.

Development of cortical thickness and development of surface area occur independently (Winkler et al. 2010) and result from different neurobiological processes, representing distinct features of cortical maturation at various stages of development (Anderson 2011). In the ENIGMA Major Depressive Disorder Working Group study (consisting of 20 cohorts worldwide), with data obtained from 10,105 adolescent and adult subjects, cortical surface area differences were not detected in adult patients with early-onset depression compared with their healthy control counterparts (Schmaal et al. 2017), suggesting that the smaller cortical surface area in adolescent depression indicates delayed cortical maturation (i.e., delayed expansion). Some regions with observed surface area abnormalities in adolescent depression, including the lingual gyrus, medial OFC, and superior frontal gyrus (Schmaal et al. 2017), undergo a more protracted maturational process (Wierenga et al. 2014) and may be especially prone to delayed maturation in adolescent depression. Delayed maturation may alter functional connections with other regions through decreased growth and branching of dendritic trees and the number of synapses associated with gray-matter volume (Anderson 2011), and such alterations may persist into adulthood even if the surface area measures normalize when the transition into adulthood takes place. The absence of cortical surface area abnormalities in adult depressed patients with an early age at onset (Schmaal et al. 2017) could indicate such normalization.

Volumetric and Cortical Changes Associated With Vulnerability to Depression

Data on volumetric changes in at-risk samples are emerging (for review, see Jones et al. 2017). In a longitudinal study, we examined hippocampal changes in depressed adolescents, healthy adolescents with familial risk for depression, and healthy low-risk controls (Rao et al. 2010). We found that the depressed and high-risk groups had smaller bilateral hippocampal volumes compared with controls. In particular, early life adversity was associated with smaller hippocampal volumes, and smaller hippocampal volumes partially mediated the effect of early life adversity on the onset of depression during follow-up (Rao et al. 2010). In a longitudinal study of at-risk youth based on affective temperament who had no prior history of depressive disorders, reduced growth of the hippocampus and attenuated reduction in putamen volume over time (between early and middle adolescence) were associated with the onset of depression. Sex moderated the association between amygdala growth and depression; exaggerated growth of the amygdala was associated with depression onset in female subjects, whereas attenuated growth of the amygdala was associated with depression in male subjects. A smaller nucleus accumbens volume across time was associated with depression in female subjects only (Whittle et al. 2014). Other studies examined the association between gray-matter volume in subcortical structures at baseline and increases in depressive symptoms over time in pediatric samples (reviewed in Jones et al. 2017).

A recent study, using machine learning in a sample of 10- to 15-year-old female subjects (with and without familial risk), found that adolescents who later developed depression had thicker gray matter of the left insula and thinner gray matter of the right medial OFC prior to symptom onset (Foland-Ross et al. 2015). These findings suggest that alterations in the developmental trajectories of cortical and subcortical gray matter during adolescence may represent a neurobiological vulnerability for development of depression during this critical period, and therefore might provide clues for etiological mechanisms of this disorder. Furthermore, sex differences in the association between gray-matter volume in subcortical structures and risk for depression (Whittle et al. 2014) further support the idea that male and female youth are likely to be at different points in non-linear growth trajectories during adolescence (Kaczkurkin et al. 2018).

White-Matter Tract Changes Associated With Early-Onset Depression

Fractional anisotropy (FA) is the most common DTI-based index of white-matter microstructure, with higher values indicative of greater structural integrity and improved organization, cohesion, and compactness of the fiber tracts. Other metrics also can be calculated, including mean diffusivity (MD), which estimates the overall magnitude of diffusion; axial diffusivity (AD), which measures diffusion along the primary direction of diffusion; and radial diffusivity (RD), which reflects the amount of diffusion perpendicular to the primary diffusion direction. Although the precise cellular mechanisms of change in each diffusion metric remain unclear, higher FA and AD, coupled with lower RD and MD, are generally considered to reflect better structural integrity, increased myelination, and greater cohesion of white-matter pathways (Cascio et al. 2007; Lebel and Deoni 2018; Paus 2010). A large number of DTI studies in healthy volunteers showed a general increase in FA and decrease in MD with normal maturation in childhood, adolescence, and early adulthood (Cascio et al. 2007; Lebel and Deoni 2018).

DTI has been used extensively to study adult depression, and a recent meta-analysis of first-episode, drug-naïve patients with major depression found robust evidence of white-matter deficits in the interhemispheric connections and frontal-subcortical neural circuits (Chen et al. 2017). In the first documented DTI study in early-onset depression (Cullen et al. 2010), connectivity between the subgenual ACC and amygdala was examined. Adolescent patients with depression had lower FA values on the right side compared with healthy controls. Additionally, lower FA values were observed in several white-matter tracts in depressed youth, including the left and right uncinate fasciculi, left and right inferior fronto-occipital fasciculi, left anterior cingulum, and left superior longitudinal fasciculus. Subsequent studies confirmed reduced FA values in the white-matter tracts connecting frontal-limbic regions (Bessette et al. 2014; Henderson et al. 2013; LeWinn et al. 2014), the thalamus (Bessette et al. 2014; Henderson et al. 2013), the genu of the corpus callosum, internal and external capsule tracts, and the midbrain (Bessette et al. 2014). Furthermore, lower FA values in the cingulum were linked to greater depression severity, whereas poorer integrity of the anterior thalamus radiations was associated with more severe anhedonia (Henderson et al. 2013).

Although the number of studies assessing white-matter connectivity is limited and the sample sizes in these studies are modest, there is evidence that connectivity-based disruptions are associated with early-onset depression. In particular, white-matter integrity of the cingulum and anterior thalamic radiation may have an impact on symptom presentation and illness severity. Hypotheses regarding the developmental course of these abnormal brain networks should be addressed in future longitudinal studies, with adequate power to assess the effects of covariates such as age at onset and duration of illness, treatment history, comorbidity, and family history.

White-Matter Tract Changes Associated With Vulnerability to Depression

In a study of healthy adolescents at familial risk for depression, we observed lower FA values in the left cingulum, splenium of the corpus callosum, superior longitudinal fasciculus, uncinate fasciculus, and inferior fronto-occipital fasciculus (Huang et al. 2011). Moreover, reduced FA values in the cingulum, superior longitudinal fasciculus, and/or uncinate fasciculus were associated with the onset of depression at longitudinal follow-up (U. Rao and H. Huang, unpublished data, 2012). In a separate sample of adolescents exposed to childhood maltreatment, without a prior history of psychopathology, we found that lower FA values in the superior longitudinal fasciculi and right cingulum–hippocampus projection at baseline were associated with increased risk for depression at longitudinal follow-up (Huang et al. 2012). Collectively, these preliminary findings suggest that deficits in white-matter tracts connecting the limbic and frontal regions may serve as neurobiological risk markers for the development of unipolar depression during adolescence.

Functional Brain Changes Associated With Depression

In the following subsections, we summarize both resting-state and task-based fMRI findings in individuals with early-onset depression and in those at risk for depression. The fMRI techniques indirectly quantify neural activity during rest (spontaneous fluctuations) or while an individual is completing a task by measuring the blood oxygen level–dependent (BOLD) signal. Compared with task-based fMRI, resting-state functional connectivity (RSFC) offers an attractive framework for studying pediatric samples because of its practical benefits, including minimal demands on compliance and short acquisition times. Also, the highly replicable nature of resting-state fMRI measurements, within and across subjects, makes RSFC findings potentially more universally comparable.

Intrinsic Neural Functional Connectivity in Early-Onset Depression

Intrinsic functional connectivity alterations in the major neural networks associated with adult depression were studied extensively, and the findings were summarized earlier in this chapter (see section "Neural System Approaches to Early-Onset Depression"). Empirical data on RSFC in early-onset depression are emerging (for reviews, see Hulvershorn et al. 2011; Kerestes et al. 2013). These studies used a range of methods to measure RSFC, including seed-based correlations, graph theory, and independent component analysis. They consistently found increased connectivity in the mPFC areas, including the pregenual ACC (most consistently BA32) and subgenual ACC (BA25) as well as dorsomedial (BA8) and ventromedial (BA10) divisions of the PFC, in adolescent depression. Of note, these mPFC areas are components of the DMN; they mediate emotion processing and also correlate with distinct symptom profiles such as rumination and illness severity (Kerestes et al. 2013). In contrast to the increased RSFC within the mPFC regions, reduced RSFC was observed between frontal and limbic regions (Connolly et al. 2017; Cullen et al. 2014; Geng et al. 2016). In unmedicated adolescents with depression, reduced RSFC between the amygdala and insula at baseline predicted greater increases in depressive symptoms 3 months later (Connolly et al. 2017). In another investigation, alterations in DMN, EN, and SN connectivity predicted suicidal behaviors in depressed adolescents (Ordaz et al. 2018).

Emerging findings on RSFC in early-onset depression emphasize the importance of medial neural network (DMN) disturbances in contributing to the clinical manifestation of self-referential processes, including negative rumination. Given the consistent evidence of alterations in the subgenual ACC in depression, and the clinical importance of the subgenual ACC as a target site for deep brain stimulation (Chau et al. 2017; Mayberg 2003; Price and Drevets 2010), studies examining the treatment implications of this region in pediatric samples hold promise.

Intrinsic Functional Connectivity Changes Associated With Vulnerability to Depression

In a longitudinal investigation of adolescents who had no evidence of psychopathology at baseline, Scheuer et al. (2017) found that adolescents who reported a significant increase in depressive symptoms over a 4-year follow-up period manifested reduced amygdala-frontal connectivity at baseline compared with those who showed no change in depressive symptoms during the corresponding period. In a longitudinal study with repeated resting-state fMRI scans (average interval 2 years), youth who showed decreased functional connectivity between the subgenual ACC and other cortical regions over time had more severe depressive symptoms at follow-up (Strikwerda-Brown et al. 2015). Finally, increased left ventral striatum node strength (a measure of reward-related RSFC) at baseline in 6- to 12-year-olds predicted elevated risk for depressive disorder during longitudinal follow-up (Pan et al. 2017). These findings suggest that functional connectivity alterations within limbic or striatal subcortical regions or their connectivity with the frontal regions, as well as weakening of the connectivity of these regions across time, may serve as vulnerability markers for adolescent depression.

Provoked Functional Connectivity Changes Associated With Early-Onset Depression

In a recent review of functional connectivity studies in adult depression, Li et al. (2018) identified alterations in four primary neural networks: increased connectivity of a ventral limbic affective network may be associated with excessive negative mood (dysphoria); decreased connectivity of a frontal-striatal reward network accounts for loss of interest, motivation, and pleasure (anhedonia); enhanced DMN connectivity may underlie depressive rumination; and diminished connectivity of a dorsal cognitive-control network is associated with cognitive deficits, especially ineffective top-down control of negative thoughts and emotions.

Task-based fMRI investigations in early-onset depression focused on these domains as well; earlier studies examined only regional changes, whereas more recent studies have taken a network-based approach (for reviews, see Hulvershorn et al. 2011; Kerestes et al. 2013; Miller et al. 2015). In an earlier comprehensive review of task-based fMRI studies of depression in adolescents and young adults, Kerestes et al. (2013) identified four primary domains: emotion processing, cognitive control, affective cognition, and reward processing. Elevated activity was observed in the ACC, ventromedial PFC, OFC, and amygdala across these domains. In a recent meta-analysis comparing voxelwise activation patterns during a variety of affective-processing and executive functioning tasks in 246 adolescents with major depression and 274 age-matched healthy controls, depressed youth showed reliable patterns of both general and task-specific effects in the following regions: hyperactivation in subgenual ACC and ventrolateral PFC and hypoactivation in the caudate across aggregated tasks; hyperactivation in the thalamus and parahippocampal gyrus during affective-processing tasks; hypoactivation in the cuneus, dorsal cingulate cortex, and dorsal anterior insula during executive functioning tasks; hypoactivity in the posterior insula during positive-valence tasks; and hyperactivity in the DLPFC and superior temporal cortex during negative-valence tasks (Miller et al. 2015). The authors have suggested that the altered activations in several distributed brain networks help explain the seemingly disparate symptoms of depression in youth, similar to those observed in adult depression (Li et al. 2018). Adolescent depression also is characterized by aberrant functional cross-talk of the PFC with the striatum (Forbes and Dahl 2012; Keren et al. 2018; Luking et al. 2016).

The findings from task-based fMRI studies in early-onset depression converge on hypo- and hyperactivation deficits in the frontal, limbic, and striatal regions implicated in the various aspects of emotion processing and regulation as well as reward-processing deficits (Figure 5–1). It is hypothesized that reduced frontal-limbic connectivity specifically reflects ineffective recruitment of the PFC to manage amygdala activity, whereas increased connectivity reflects prolonged and persistent experience of negative emotion. Considered together, the identified neural correlates of early-onset depression are analogous to the findings in adults. Preliminary evidence suggests that some deficits may be present even during remission (Burkhouse et al. 2017) and may serve as risk factors for recurrent episodes.

Provoked Functional Connectivity Changes Associated With Vulnerability to Depression

Monk et al. (2008) studied children and adolescents at high and low familial risk for depression and examined face processing during passive viewing of emotion faces and also during constrained viewing (i.e., asked to rate specific aspects of the face during viewing). High-risk youth showed greater amygdala and nucleus accumbens activity during passive fear-face processing and reduced nucleus accumbens activation during passive happy-face processing. In exploratory analysis, constraining the attention was associated with higher mPFC activation in the high-risk group, consistent with amygdala dampening. In a study of adolescents at familial risk for depression, Mannie et al. (2008) reported that high-risk youth failed to mount the expected activation in pregenual ACC to both positive and negative words during the emotional Stroop task. It is not

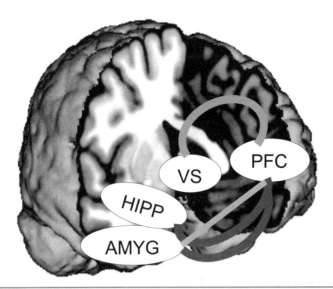

FIGURE 5–1.   A hypothesized model of fronto-limbic and fronto-striatal connectivity deficits in early-onset depression. (*see color plate 1*)
Red denotes increased connectivity, and *blue* denotes reduced connectivity.
AMYG=amygdala; HIPP=hippocampus; PFC=prefrontal cortex; VS=ventral striatum.

clear if these alterations in frontal and subcortical regions increase the risk for depression. In another study of healthy adolescents at baseline, greater subgenual ACC activation during peer exclusion was associated with greater increases in parent-reported depressive symptoms during the following year (Masten et al. 2011).

Various reward-based decision-making paradigms have been employed to demonstrate that reduced ventral striatal activation in healthy youth is predictive of later escalation in depressive symptoms or a clinical diagnosis (for a review, see Jones et al. 2017). For example, lower baseline ventral striatal activation during eudaimonic decisions (decisions involving self-sacrifice) compared with hedonic (reward-based) decisions (Telzer et al. 2014), or during reward anticipation (Morgan et al. 2013), was predictive of greater increases in depressive symptoms over time in adolescents. Additionally, a greater reduction in ventral striatal activation during reward processing over 2 years was associated with more depressive symptoms at follow-up (Hanson et al. 2015), and lower ventral striatal activation during reward anticipation at baseline predicted transition to subthreshold/clinical depression in previously asymptomatic adolescents (Stringaris et al. 2015). Prefrontal activation during reward- and loss-based decision making also may be predictive of future depressive symptom severity in a sex-dependent manner (Hanson et al. 2015; Jin et al. 2017).

Neural Correlates of Treatment Response in Pediatric Depression

Several studies investigated potential neural markers for successful treatment outcomes in adult depression (for reviews, see Chakrabarty et al. 2016; Chau et al. 2017; Gudayol-Ferré et al. 2015; Li et al. 2018). Extension of these findings to adolescents has been limited to a few studies with modest sample sizes. In depressed adolescents, reduced subgenual ACC activation in response to rewards versus losses (Straub et al. 2015), and decreased RSFC between the amygdala and DLPFC and insula (Straub et al. 2017), prior to treatment, predicted poorer response (i.e., less reduction in depressive symptoms) following cognitive-behavioral therapy (CBT). Additionally, lower RSFC of the amygdala with left supplementary motor area and with right precentral gyrus but greater connectivity with right central opercular cortex and Heschl's gyrus predicted a favorable response to treatment with selective serotonin reuptake inhibitors in depressed adolescents (Klimes-Dougan et al. 2018). In the same study, greater activation of the ACC and left medial frontal gyrus in response to an emotion processing task predicted better treatment response.

In a longitudinal study, researchers acquired fMRI scans in depressed adolescents while viewing facial expressions at baseline and 8 weeks later following open-label treatment with fluoxetine (Tao et al. 2012). Before treatment, depressed youth showed exaggerated brain activation in multiple regions, including the frontal, temporal, and limbic cortices, compared with healthy controls. Fluoxetine treatment normalized the activation in most regions, including the amygdala, OFC, and subgenual ACC. Cullen et al. (2016) examined functional connectivity changes before and after treatment with a selective serotonin reuptake inhibitor for 8 weeks. Favorable response to treatment was associated with increased RSFC of the amygdala with the right frontal cortex, but decreased RSFC with right precuneus and right PCC, from baseline to posttreatment. Also, clinical improvement was associated with decreased activation in rostral and subgenual ACC in response to a negative emotion task but increased activation in the insula and other regions. Chattopadhyay et al. (2017) examined changes in RSFC of the emotional ("hot") and cognitive-control ("cold") neural networks in response to CBT in depressed adolescents. Successful treatment with CBT ameliorated the observed baseline-heightened connectivity in the emotional-processing network, but there were no changes in the cognitive-control network. In another study of depressed adolescents, CBT induced increased regional cerebral blood flow (measured via arterial spin labeling) in the right DLPFC, right caudate nucleus, and left inferior parietal lobe (Sosic-Vasic et al. 2017).

Functional connectivity within/between frontal-limbic structures serves as an indicator for which groups of individuals might benefit most from certain types of treatment. More importantly, these findings are in line with the literature, suggesting that reduced connectivity within the limbic and fronto-limbic systems and reduced reward-related limbic activations are predictive of greater symptom severity and depression onset (Jones et al. 2017); treatment appears to ameliorate these deficits.

Clinical Implications and Future Directions for Research

A growing body of research in early-onset depression has identified certain structural and functional brain changes, some at the regional level and others at a systems level. Certain alterations are evident before the clinical manifestation of depressive symptoms in at-risk youth and seem to predict the onset of illness. Preliminary evidence that treatment may restore some functional connectivity deficits with corresponding symptom improvement serves as additional support for the crucial role of these networks in the pathophysiology of early-onset depression. Even though there is some consistency in the structural and functional brain changes between early-onset and adult-onset illness, some findings have differed, possibly reflecting ongoing neuroplastic changes and the impact that chronic illness may have on neural connectivity.

Despite enormous technological advances in neuroimaging in the past two decades, our knowledge of the neural mechanisms of early-onset depression lags significantly behind that of adult depression. Many studies in pediatric samples consist of modest sample sizes with cross-sectional designs. Hence, it is not clear how the maturational changes across child, adolescent, and adult development relate to the vulnerability and maintenance of depression. More information is needed on which neural changes are specific to depression and how family history, severity of illness, symptom patterns, and comorbid conditions influence the findings. It is not clear which neural changes are preexisting and increase vulnerability to the disorder or which are sequelae of the illness. Furthermore, it is not known with any certainty if the observed brain changes are temporary, state-like conditions that resolve without any sequelae, are temporary but still place an individual on a delayed trajectory toward normal development, or whether any disruption to the normal maturational process during this period permanently and deleteriously affects the neural systems. The effect of disease course on the neurobiological substrate also has not been studied. The utility of neural markers in the diagnosis, treatment, and prognosis of the disorder, as well as the neural changes in response to treatment, should be established. Tragically, early-onset depression is associated with frequent recurrence, but unique opportunities possibly exist for neural recovery, highlighting the need for early, effective intervention.

Perhaps the most obvious implication from this review is the need for more prospective research in youngsters. Efforts should build on the recent findings in high-risk youth to better understand neural markers of disease susceptibility, their stability, and their ability to predict treatment response and illness course. Studies of depressed children and adolescents have a number of advantages compared with studies of adults: confounding factors such as repeated episodes, long duration of illness, multiple medications, and co-occurring medical problems are minimized. Given that adolescence is a high-risk period for the onset of depression, in a relatively short follow-up period, it is possible to identify both preexisting and "scar" markers of depression. Since early-onset depression recurs and persists into adulthood, comprehensive research in pediatric samples also holds promise for preventing adverse adult outcomes.

Scientists should identify clear structure/function hypotheses that implement, but go beyond, the current diagnostic system to translate clinical neuroscience findings into a new classification system based on pathophysiology and etiological processes. Such models also can explain the heterogeneity and high rates of comorbidity in depression in youth. Adding genetic information to neuroimaging will likely provide knowledge on the contributions of genes to network-level functioning. It is important to obtain neural measures before and after behavioral, pharmacological, or somatic treatment. Such studies will shed light on the mechanisms through which treatments work and can provide new targets for treatment development. It is also critical to identify baseline predictors of treatment outcome (i.e., moderators) to help move the field toward more personalized care.

Clinical Pearls

- The markedly increased risk for depression during adolescence may be associated with simultaneous maturational changes in neural networks involved in social-emotional and reward processing during this developmental period.

- Developmental trends in sex differences in the prevalence of depression and maturational brain changes also have been observed. However, more work is needed to identify the effects of sex on brain development and depression during the adolescent transition.

- To capture the complex phenomenology of depression, we need to adopt a multimodal/network approach to studying brain changes associated with depression.

- Certain neural alterations are evident before the clinical manifestation of depressive symptoms in at-risk youth and seem to predict the onset of illness, suggesting their clinical significance for targeted prevention efforts.

- Even though there is some consistency in the structural and functional brain changes between early-onset and adult-onset depression, some findings have differed, possibly reflecting ongoing neuroplastic changes and the impact that chronic illness may have on neural connectivity.

- Scientists should identify clear brain structure/function hypotheses that go beyond the current diagnostic system to translate clinical neuroscience findings into a new classification system based on pathophysiology and etiological processes.

References

Ahmed SP, Bittencourt-Hewitt A, Sebastian CL: Neurocognitive bases of emotion regulation development in adolescence. Dev Cogn Neurosci 15:11–25, 2015 26340451

Allman JM, Hakeem A, Erwin JM, et al: The anterior cingulate cortex: the evolution of an interface between emotion and cognition. Ann N Y Acad Sci 935(1):107–117, 2001 11411161

Andersen SL, Teicher MH: Stress, sensitive periods and maturational events in adolescent depression. Trends Neurosci 31(4):183–191, 2008 18329735

Andersen SL, Rutstein M, Benzo JM, et al: Sex differences in dopamine receptor overproduction and elimination. Neuroreport 8(6):1495–1498, 1997 9172161

Anderson BJ: Plasticity of gray matter volume: the cellular and synaptic plasticity that underlies volumetric change. Dev Psychobiol 53(5):456–465, 2011 21678393

Avenevoli S, Swendsen J, He JP, et al: Major depression in the National Comorbidity Survey—Adolescent Supplement: prevalence, correlates, and treatment. J Am Acad Child Adolesc Psychiatry 54(1):37.e2–44.e2, 2015 25524788

Baird AA, Gruber SA, Fein DA, et al: Functional magnetic resonance imaging of facial affect recognition in children and adolescents. J Am Acad Child Adolesc Psychiatry 38(2):195–199, 1999 9951219

Barbas H, Saha S, Rempel-Clower N et al: Serial pathways from primate prefrontal cortex to autonomic areas may influence emotional expression. BMC Neurosci 4:25, 2003 14536022

Bechara A, Damasio AR: The somatic marker hypothesis: a neural theory of economic decision. Games Econ Behav 52:336–372, 2005

Bellani M, Baiano M, Brambilla P: Brain anatomy of major depression, II: focus on amygdala. Epidemiol Psychiatr Sci 20(1):33–36, 2011 21657113

Benloucif S, Galloway MP: Facilitation of dopamine release in vivo by serotonin agonists: studies with microdialysis. Eur J Pharmacol 200(1):1–8, 1991 1769366

Bessette KL, Nave AM, Caprihan A, et al: White matter abnormalities in adolescents with major depressive disorder. Brain Imaging Behav 8(4):531–541, 2014 24242685

Bjork JM, Smith AR, Chen G, et al: Adolescents, adults and rewards: comparing motivational neurocircuitry recruitment using fMRI. PLoS One 5(7):e11440, 2010 20625430

Blakemore SJ, Burnett S, Dahl RE: The role of puberty in the developing adolescent brain. Hum Brain Mapp 31(6):926–933, 2010 20496383

Brenhouse HC, Andersen SL: Developmental trajectories during adolescence in males and females: a cross-species understanding of underlying brain changes. Neurosci Biobehav Rev 35(8):1687–1703, 2011 21600919

Brenhouse HC, Sonntag KC, Andersen SL: Transient D1 dopamine receptor expression on prefrontal cortex projection neurons: relationship to enhanced motivational salience of drug cues in adolescence. J Neurosci 28(10):2375–2382, 2008 18322084

Burgess PW, Stuss DT: Fifty years of prefrontal cortex research: impact on assessment. J Int Neuropsychol Soc 23(9–10):755–767, 2017 29198274

Burkhouse KL, Jacobs RH, Peters AT, et al: Neural correlates of rumination in adolescents with remitted major depressive disorder and healthy controls. Cogn Affect Behav Neurosci 17(2):394–405, 2017 27921216

Burnett S, Sebastian C, Cohen Kadosh K, et al: The social brain in adolescence: evidence from functional magnetic resonance imaging and behavioural studies. Neurosci Biobehav Rev 35(8):1654–1664, 2011 21036192

Bush G, Luu P, Posner MI: Cognitive and emotional influences in anterior cingulate cortex. Trends Cogn Sci 4(6):215–222, 2000 10827444

Campbell S, Macqueen G: The role of the hippocampus in the pathophysiology of major depression. J Psychiatry Neurosci 29(6):417–426, 2004 15644983

Cardinal RN, Parkinson JA, Hall J, et al: Emotion and motivation: the role of the amygdala, ventral striatum, and prefrontal cortex. Neurosci Biobehav Rev 26(3):321–352, 2002 12034134

Cascio CJ, Gerig G, Piven J: Diffusion tensor imaging: application to the study of the developing brain. J Am Acad Child Adolesc Psychiatry 46(2):213–223, 2007 17242625

Cascio CN, Carp J, O'Donnell MB, et al: Buffering social influence: neural correlates of response inhibition predict driving safety in the presence of a peer. J Cogn Neurosci 27(1):83–95, 2015 25100217

Casey BJ, Getz S, Galvan A: The adolescent brain. Dev Rev 28(1):62–77, 2008 18688292

Casey BJ, Galván A, Somerville LH: Beyond simple models of adolescence to an integrated circuit-based account: a commentary. Dev Cogn Neurosci 17:128–130, 2016 26739434

Chakrabarty T, Ogrodniczuk J, Hadjipavlou G: Predictive neuroimaging markers of psychotherapy response: a systematic review. Harv Rev Psychiatry 24(6):396–405, 2016 27824635

Chambers RA, Taylor JR, Potenza MN: Developmental neurocircuitry of motivation in adolescence: a critical period of addiction vulnerability. Am J Psychiatry 160(6):1041–1052, 2003 12777258

Chattopadhyay S, Tait R, Simas T, et al: Cognitive behavioral therapy lowers elevated functional connectivity in depressed adolescents. EBioMedicine 17:216–222, 2017 28258922

Chau DT, Fogelman P, Nordanskog P, et al: Distinct neural-functional effects of treatments with selective serotonin reuptake inhibitors, electroconvulsive therapy, and transcranial magnetic stimulation and their relations to regional brain function in major depression: a meta-analysis. Biol Psychiatry Cogn Neurosci Neuroimaging 2(4):318–326, 2017 29560920

Chein J, Albert D, O'Brien L, et al: Peers increase adolescent risk taking by enhancing activity in the brain's reward circuitry. Dev Sci 14(2):F1–F10, 2011 21499511

Chen G, Guo Y, Zhu H, et al: Intrinsic disruption of white matter microarchitecture in first-episode, drug-naive major depressive disorder: a voxel-based meta-analysis of diffusion tensor imaging. Prog Neuropsychopharmacol Biol Psychiatry 76:179–187, 2017 28336497

Cho YT, Ernst M, Fudge JL: Cortico-amygdala-striatal circuits are organized as hierarchical subsystems through the primate amygdala. J Neurosci 33(35):14017–14030, 2013 23986238

Chuang J-Y, Hagan CC, Murray GK, et al: Adolescent major depressive disorder: neuroimaging evidence of sex difference during an affective go/no-go task. Front Psychiatry 8:119, 2017

Connolly CG, Ho TC, Blom EH, et al: Resting-state functional connectivity of the amygdala and longitudinal changes in depression severity in adolescent depression. J Affect Disord 207:86–94, 2017 27716542

Conson M, Errico D, Mazzarella E, et al: Transcranial electrical stimulation over dorsolateral prefrontal cortex modulates processing of social, cognitive and affective information. PLoS One 10(5):e0126448, 2015 25951227

Crone EA, Dahl RE: Understanding adolescence as a period of social-affective engagement and goal flexibility. Nat Rev Neurosci 13(9):636–650, 2012 22903221

Crone EA, Elzinga BM: Changing brains: how longitudinal functional magnetic resonance imaging studies can inform us about cognitive and social-affective growth trajectories. Wiley Interdiscip Rev Cogn Sci 6(1):53–63, 2015 26262928

Cullen KR, Klimes-Dougan B, Muetzel R, et al: Altered white matter microstructure in adolescents with major depression: a preliminary study. J Am Acad Child Adolesc Psychiatry 49(2):173–183.e1, 2010 20215939

Cullen KR, Westlund MK, Klimes-Dougan B, et al: Abnormal amygdala resting-state functional connectivity in adolescent depression. JAMA Psychiatry 71(10):1138–1147, 2014 25133665

Cullen KR, Klimes-Dougan B, Vu DP, et al: Neural correlates of antidepressant treatment response in adolescents with major depressive disorder. J Child Adolesc Psychopharmacol 26(8):705–712, 2016 27159204

Davey CG, Yücel M, Allen NB: The emergence of depression in adolescence: development of the prefrontal cortex and the representation of reward. Neurosci Biobehav Rev 32(1):1–19, 2008 17570526

de Kwaasteniet B, Ruhe E, Caan M, et al: Relation between structural and functional connectivity in major depressive disorder. Biol Psychiatry 74(1):40–47, 2013 23399372

Di Mascio M, Di Giovanni G, Di Matteo V, et al: Selective serotonin reuptake inhibitors reduce the spontaneous activity of dopaminergic neurons in the ventral tegmental area. Brain Res Bull 46(6):547–554, 1998 9744293

Disner SG, Beevers CG, Haigh EA, et al: Neural mechanisms of the cognitive model of depression. Nat Rev Neurosci 12(8):467–477, 2011 21731066

Dougherty LR, Blankenship SL, Spechler PA, et al: An fMRI pilot study of cognitive reappraisal in children: divergent effects on brain and behavior. J Psychopathol Behav Assess 37(4):634–644, 2015 26692636

Durston S, Casey BJ: What have we learned about cognitive development from neuroimaging? Neuropsychologia 44(11):2149–2157, 2006 16303150

Durston S, Davidson MC, Tottenham N, et al: A shift from diffuse to focal cortical activity with development. Dev Sci 9(1):1–8, 2006 16445387

Ernst M: The triadic model perspective for the study of adolescent motivated behavior. Brain Cogn 89:104–111, 2014 24556507

Ernst M, Nelson EE, Jazbec S, et al: Amygdala and nucleus accumbens in responses to receipt and omission of gains in adults and adolescents. Neuroimage 25(4):1279–1291, 2005 15850746

Ernst M, Torrisi S, Balderston N, et al: fMRI functional connectivity applied to adolescent neurodevelopment. Annu Rev Clin Psychol 11:361–377, 2015 25581237

Fareri DS, Gabard-Durnam L, Goff B, et al: Normative development of ventral striatal resting state connectivity in humans. Neuroimage 118:422–437, 2015 26087377

Foland-Ross LC, Sacchet MD, Prasad G, et al: Cortical thickness predicts the first onset of major depression in adolescence. Int J Dev Neurosci 46:125–131, 2015 26315399

Forbes EE, Dahl RE: Neural systems of positive affect: relevance to understanding child and adolescent depression? Dev Psychopathol 17(3):827–850, 2005 16262994

Forbes EE, Dahl RE: Research Review: altered reward function in adolescent depression: what, when and how? J Child Psychol Psychiatry 53(1):3–15, 2012 22117893

Fuhrmann D, Knoll LJ, Blakemore SJ: Adolescence as a sensitive period of brain development. Trends Cogn Sci 19(10):558–566, 2015 26419496

Fuster JM: Frontal lobe and cognitive development. J Neurocytol 31(3–5):373–385, 2002 12815254

Gabard-Durnam LJ, Flannery J, Goff B, et al: The development of human amygdala functional connectivity at rest from 4 to 23 years: a cross-sectional study. Neuroimage 95:193–207, 2014 24662579

Galván A, McGlennen KM: Enhanced striatal sensitivity to aversive reinforcement in adolescents versus adults. J Cogn Neurosci 25(2):284–296, 2013 23163417

Galván A, Hare TA, Parra CE, et al: Earlier development of the accumbens relative to orbitofrontal cortex might underlie risk-taking behavior in adolescents. J Neurosci 26(25):6885–6892, 2006 16793895

Gee DG, Humphreys KL, Flannery J, et al: A developmental shift from positive to negative connectivity in human amygdala-prefrontal circuitry. J Neurosci 33(10):4584–4593, 2013 23467374

Geng H, Wu F, Kong L, et al: Disrupted structural and functional connectivity in prefrontal-hippocampus circuitry in first-episode medication-naive adolescent depression. PLoS One 11(2):e0148345, 2016 26863301

Giedd JN, Vaituzis AC, Hamburger SD, et al: Quantitative MRI of the temporal lobe, amygdala, and hippocampus in normal human development: ages 4–18 years. J Comp Neurol 366(2):223–230, 1996 8698883

Giedd JN, Clasen LS, Lenroot R, et al: Puberty-related influences on brain development. Mol Cell Endocrinol 254–255:154–162, 2006 16765510

Giorgio A, Watkins KE, Chadwick M, et al: Longitudinal changes in grey and white matter during adolescence. Neuroimage 49(1):94–103, 2010 19679191

Goddings AL, Mills KL, Clasen LS, et al: The influence of puberty on subcortical brain development. Neuroimage 88:242–251, 2014 24121203

Gogtay N, Giedd JN, Lusk L, et al: Dynamic mapping of human cortical development during childhood through early adulthood. Proc Natl Acad Sci USA 101(21):8174–8179, 2004 15148381

Greicius MD, Supekar K, Menon V, et al: Resting-state functional connectivity reflects structural connectivity in the default mode network. Cereb Cortex 19(1):72–78, 2009 18403396

Gudayol-Ferré E, Peró-Cebollero M, González-Garrido AA, et al: Changes in brain connectivity related to the treatment of depression measured through fMRI: a systematic review. Front Hum Neurosci 9:582, 2015 26578927

Guyer AE, Monk CS, McClure-Tone EB, et al: A developmental examination of amygdala response to facial expressions. J Cogn Neurosci 20(9):1565–1582, 2008 18345988

Guyer AE, McClure-Tone EB, Shiffrin ND, et al: Probing the neural correlates of anticipated peer evaluation in adolescence. Child Dev 80(4):1000–1015, 2009 19630890

Guyer AE, Silk JS, Nelson EE: The neurobiology of the emotional adolescent: from the inside out. Neurosci Biobehav Rev 70:74–85, 2016 27506384

Gyurak A, Goodkind MS, Kramer JH, et al: Executive functions and the down-regulation and up-regulation of emotion. Cogn Emotion 26(1):103–118, 2012 21432634

Haber SN, Knutson B: The reward circuit: linking primate anatomy and human imaging. Neuropsychopharmacology 35(1):4–26, 2010 19812543

Hamani C, Mayberg H, Stone S, et al: The subcallosal cingulate gyrus in the context of major depression. Biol Psychiatry 69(4):301–308, 2011 21145043

Hamilton JP, Chen MC, Gotlib IH: Neural systems approaches to understanding major depressive disorder: an intrinsic functional organization perspective. Neurobiol Dis 52:4–11, 2013 23477309

Hankin BL, Abramson LY, Moffitt TE, et al: Development of depression from preadolescence to young adulthood: emerging gender differences in a 10-year longitudinal study. J Abnorm Psychol 107(1):128–140, 1998 9505045

Hanson JL, Hariri AR, Williamson DE: Blunted ventral striatum development in adolescence reflects emotional neglect and predicts depressive symptoms. Biol Psychiatry 78(9):598–605, 2015 26092778

Hare TA, Tottenham N, Davidson MC, et al: Contributions of amygdala and striatal activity in emotion regulation. Biol Psychiatry 57(6):624–632, 2005 15780849

Hare TA, Tottenham N, Galvan A, et al: Biological substrates of emotional reactivity and regulation in adolescence during an emotional go-nogo task. Biol Psychiatry 63(10):927–934, 2008 18452757

Hariri AR, Bookheimer SY, Mazziotta JC: Modulating emotional responses: effects of a neocortical network on the limbic system. Neuroreport 11(1):43–48, 2000 10683827

Haycock JW, Becker L, Ang L, et al: Marked disparity between age-related changes in dopamine and other presynaptic dopaminergic markers in human striatum. J Neurochem 87(3):574–585, 2003 14535941

Henderson SE, Johnson AR, Vallejo AI, et al: A preliminary study of white matter in adolescent depression: relationships with illness severity, anhedonia, and irritability. Front Psychiatry 4:152, 2013 24324445

Herba C, Phillips M: Annotation: development of facial expression recognition from childhood to adolescence: behavioural and neurological perspectives. J Child Psychol Psychiatry 45(7):1185–1198, 2004 15335339

Heyder K, Suchan B, Daum I: Cortico-subcortical contributions to executive control. Acta Psychol (Amst) 15(2–3):271–289, 2004 14962404

Huang H, Fan X, Williamson DE, Rao U: White matter changes in healthy adolescents at familial risk for unipolar depression: a diffusion tensor imaging study. Neuropsychopharmacology 36(3):684–691, 2011 21085111

Huang H, Gundapuneedi T, Rao U: White matter disruptions in adolescents exposed to childhood maltreatment and vulnerability to psychopathology. Neuropsychopharmacology 37(12):2693–2701, 2012 22850736

Hulvershorn LA, Cullen K, Anand A: Toward dysfunctional connectivity: a review of neuroimaging findings in pediatric major depressive disorder. Brain Imaging Behav 5(4):307–328, 2011 21901425

Iordan AD, Dolcos F: Brain activity and network interactions linked to valence-related differences in the impact of emotional distraction. Cereb Cortex 27(1):731–749, 2017 26543041

Jin J, Narayanan A, Perlman G, et al: Orbitofrontal cortex activity and connectivity predict future depression symptoms in adolescence. Biol Psychiatry Cogn Neurosci Neuroimaging 2(7):610–618, 2017 29226267

Johnson D, Dupuis G, Piche J, et al: Adult mental health outcomes of adolescent depression: a systematic review. Depress Anxiety 35(8):700–716, 2018 29878410

Jones SA, Morales AM, Lavine JB, et al: Convergent neurobiological predictors of emergent psychopathology during adolescence. Birth Defects Res 109(20):1613–1622, 2017 29251844

Kaczkurkin AN, Raznahan A, Satterthwaite TD: Sex differences in the developing brain: insights from multimodal neuroimaging. Neuropsychopharmacology June 6, 2018 [Epub ahead of print] 29930385

Katz LD: Dopamine and serotonin: integrating current affective engagement with longer-term goals. Behav Brain Sci 22(3):527, 1999

Keren H, O'Callaghan G, Vidal-Ribas P, et al: Reward processing in depression: a conceptual and meta-analytic review across fMRI and EEG studies. Am J Psychiatry June 20, 2018 [Epub ahead of print] 29921146

Kerestes R, Davey CG, Stephanou K, et al: Functional brain imaging studies of youth depression: a systematic review. Neuroimage Clin 4:209–231, 2013 24455472

Kessler RC, Avenevoli S, Ries Merikangas K: Mood disorders in children and adolescents: an epidemiologic perspective. Biol Psychiatry 49(12):1002–1014, 2001 11430842

Khundrakpam BS, Reid A, Brauer J, et al; Brain Development Cooperative Group: Developmental changes in organization of structural brain networks. Cereb Cortex 23(9):2072–2085, 2013 22784607

Khundrakpam BS, Lewis JD, Zhao L, et al: Brain connectivity in normally developing children and adolescents. Neuroimage 134:192–203, 2016 27054487

Kilford EJ, Garrett E, Blakemore SJ: The development of social cognition in adolescence: an integrated perspective. Neurosci Biobehav Rev 70:106–120, 2016 27545755

Klein DN, Glenn CR, Kosty DB, et al: Predictors of first lifetime onset of major depressive disorder in young adulthood. J Abnorm Psychol 122(1):1–6, 2013 22889243

Klimes-Dougan B, Westlund Schreiner M, Thai M, et al: Neural and neuroendocrine predictors of pharmacological treatment response in adolescents with depression: a preliminary study. Prog Neuropsychopharmacol Biol Psychiatry 81:194–202, 2018 29100972

Lamblin M, Murawski C, Whittle S, et al: Social connectedness, mental health and the adolescent brain. Neurosci Biobehav Rev 80:57–68, 2017 28506925

Lebel C, Deoni S: The development of brain white matter microstructure. Neuroimage January 3, 2018 [Epub ahead of print] 29305910

Lee H, Heller AS, van Reekum CM, et al: Amygdala-prefrontal coupling underlies individual differences in emotion regulation. Neuroimage 62(3):1575–1581, 2012 22634856

Lejuez CW, Read JP, Kahler CW, et al: Evaluation of a behavioral measure of risk taking: the Balloon Analogue Risk Task (BART). J Exp Psychol Appl 8(2):75–84, 2002 12075692

LeWinn KZ, Connolly CG, Wu J, et al: White matter correlates of adolescent depression: structural evidence for frontolimbic disconnectivity. J Am Acad Child Adolesc Psychiatry 53(8):899–909, 909.e1–909.e7, 2014 25062597

Li BJ, Friston K, Mody M, et al: A brain network model for depression: from symptom understanding to disease intervention. CNS Neurosci Ther June 21, 2018 [Epub ahead of print] 29931740

Li J, Schiller D, Schoenbaum G, et al: Differential roles of human striatum and amygdala in associative learning. Nat Neurosci 14(10):1250–1252, 2011 21909088

Luking KR, Pagliaccio D, Luby JL, et al: Reward processing and risk for depression across development. Trends Cogn Sci 20(6):456–468, 2016 27131776

Luna B, Padmanabhan A, O'Hearn K: What has fMRI told us about the development of cognitive control through adolescence? Brain Cogn 72(1):101–113, 2010 19765880

Lupien SJ, McEwen BS, Gunnar MR, et al: Effects of stress throughout the lifespan on the brain, behaviour and cognition. Nat Rev Neurosci 10(6):434–445, 2009 19401723

Mannie ZN, Norbury R, Murphy SE, et al: Affective modulation of anterior cingulate cortex in young people at increased familial risk of depression. Br J Psychiatry 192(5):356–361, 2008 18450659

Masten CL, Eisenberger NI, Borofsky LA, et al: Neural correlates of social exclusion during adolescence: understanding the distress of peer rejection. Soc Cogn Affect Neurosci 4(2):143–157, 2009 19470528

Masten CL, Eisenberger NI, Borofsky LA, et al: Subgenual anterior cingulate responses to peer rejection: a marker of adolescents' risk for depression. Dev Psychopathol 23(1):283–292, 2011 21262054

Mayberg HS: Modulating dysfunctional limbic-cortical circuits in depression: towards development of brain-based algorithms for diagnosis and optimised treatment. Br Med Bull 65:193–207, 2003 12697626

McEwen BS: Stress and hippocampal plasticity. Annu Rev Neurosci 22:105–122, 1999 10202533

McRae K, Gross JJ, Weber J, et al: The development of emotion regulation: an fMRI study of cognitive reappraisal in children, adolescents and young adults. Soc Cogn Affect Neurosci 7(1):11–22, 2012 22228751

Miller CH, Hamilton JP, Sacchet MD, et al: Meta-analysis of functional neuroimaging of major depressive disorder in youth. JAMA Psychiatry 72(10):1045–1053, 2015 26332700

Mimura K, Kimoto T, Okada M: Synapse efficiency diverges due to synaptic pruning following overgrowth. Phys Rev E Stat Nonlin Soft Matter Phys 68(3 Pt 1):031910, 2003 14524806

Moffitt TE: Adolescence-limited and life-course-persistent antisocial behavior: a developmental taxonomy. Psychol Rev 100(4):674–701, 1993 8255953

Monk CS, McClure EB, Nelson EE, et al: Adolescent immaturity in attention-related brain engagement to emotional facial expressions. Neuroimage 20(1):420–428, 2003 14527602

Monk CS, Klein RG, Telzer EH, et al: Amygdala and nucleus accumbens activation to emotional facial expressions in children and adolescents at risk for major depression. Am J Psychiatry 165(1):90–98, 2008 17986682

Morawetz C, Bode S, Baudewig J, et al: Effective amygdala-prefrontal connectivity predicts individual differences in successful emotion regulation. Soc Cogn Affect Neurosci 12(4):569–585, 2017 27998996

Morgan JK, Olino TM, McMakin DL, et al: Neural response to reward as a predictor of increases in depressive symptoms in adolescence. Neurobiol Dis 52:66–74, 2013 22521464

Moriceau S, Roth TL, Okotoghaide T, et al: Corticosterone controls the developmental emergence of fear and amygdala function to predator odors in infant rat pups. Int J Dev Neurosci 22(5–6):415–422, 2004 15380840

Nelson EE, Leibenluft E, McClure EB, et al: The social re-orientation of adolescence: a neuroscience perspective on the process and its relation to psychopathology. Psychol Med 35(2):163–174, 2005 15841674

Nelson EE, Jarcho JM, Guyer AE: Social re-orientation and brain development: an expanded and updated view. Dev Cogn Neurosci 17:118–127, 2016 26777136

Ordaz SJ, Goyer MS, Ho TC, et al: Network basis of suicidal ideation in depressed adolescents. J Affect Disord 226:92–99, 2018 28968564

Pan PM, Sato JR, Salum GA, et al: Ventral striatum functional connectivity as a predictor of adolescent depressive disorder in a longitudinal community-based sample. Am J Psychiatry 174(11):1112–1119, 2017 28946760

Panksepp J: Affective neuroscience of the emotional BrainMind: evolutionary perspectives and implications for understanding depression. Dialogues Clin Neurosci 12(4):533–545, 2010 21319497

Paton JJ, Belova MA, Morrison SE, et al: The primate amygdala represents the positive and negative value of visual stimuli during learning. Nature 439(7078):865–870, 2006 16482160

Paus T: Growth of white matter in the adolescent brain: myelin or axon? Brain Cogn 72(1):26–35, 2010 19595493

Paus T, Keshavan M, Giedd JN: Why do many psychiatric disorders emerge during adolescence? Nat Rev Neurosci 9(12):947–957, 2008 19002191

Pearce JM, Hall G: A model for Pavlovian learning: variations in the effectiveness of conditioned but not of unconditioned stimuli. Psychol Rev 87(6):532–552, 1980 7443916

Perlman SB, Pelphrey KA: Developing connections for affective regulation: age-related changes in emotional brain connectivity. J Exp Child Psychol 108(3):607–620, 2011 20971474

Pfeifer JH, Allen NB: Arrested development? Reconsidering dual-systems models of brain function in adolescence and disorders. Trends Cogn Sci 16(6):322–329, 2012 22613872

Pfeifer JH, Masten CL, Moore WE III, et al: Entering adolescence: resistance to peer influence, risky behavior, and neural changes in emotion reactivity. Neuron 69(5):1029–1036, 2011 21382560

Phan KL, Wager TD, Taylor SF, et al: Functional neuroimaging studies of human emotions. CNS Spectr 9(4):258–266, 2004 15048050

Phillips ML, Drevets WC, Rauch SL, et al: Neurobiology of emotion perception, I: the neural basis of normal emotion perception. Biol Psychiatry 54(5):504–514, 2003 12946879

Philpot RM, Wecker L, Kirstein CL: Repeated ethanol exposure during adolescence alters the developmental trajectory of dopaminergic output from the nucleus accumbens septi. Int J Dev Neurosci 27(8):805–815, 2009 19712739

Price JL, Drevets WC: Neurocircuitry of mood disorders. Neuropsychopharmacology 35(1):192–216, 2010 19693001

Raichle ME, MacLeod AM, Snyder AZ, et al: A default mode of brain function. Proc Natl Acad Sci USA 98(2):676–682, 2001 11209064

Rao U, Chen LA: Characteristics, correlates, and outcomes of childhood and adolescent depressive disorders. Dialogues Clin Neurosci 11(1):45–62, 2009 19432387

Rao U, Chen LA, Bidesi AS, et al: Hippocampal changes associated with early life adversity and vulnerability to depression. Biol Psychiatry 67(4):357–364, 2010 20015483

Rutter M, Kim-Cohen J, Maughan B: Continuities and discontinuities in psychopathology between childhood and adult life. J Child Psychol Psychiatry 47(3–4):276–295, 2006 16492260

Sapolsky RM: Stress and plasticity in the limbic system. Neurochem Res 28(11):1735–1742, 2003 14584827

Scherf KS, Smyth JM, Delgado MR: The amygdala: an agent of change in adolescent neural networks. Horm Behav 64(2):298–313, 2013 23756154

Scheuer H, Alarcón G, Demeter DV, et al: Reduced fronto-amygdalar connectivity in adolescence is associated with increased depression symptoms over time. Psychiatry Res Neuroimaging 266:35–41, 2017 28577433

Schmaal L, Hibar DP, Sämann PG, et al: Cortical abnormalities in adults and adolescents with major depression based on brain scans from 20 cohorts worldwide in the ENIGMA Major Depressive Disorder Working Group. Mol Psychiatry 22(6):900–909, 2017 27137745

Schneider S, Peters J, Bromberg U, et al; IMAGEN Consortium: Risk taking and the adolescent reward system: a potential common link to substance abuse. Am J Psychiatry 169(1):39–46, 2012 21955931

Schultz W: Dopamine signals for reward value and risk: basic and recent data. Behav Brain Funct 6:24, 2010 20416052

Seeley WW, Menon V, Schatzberg AF, et al: Dissociable intrinsic connectivity networks for salience processing and executive control. J Neurosci 27(9):2349–2356, 2007 17329432

Singh MK, Kesler SR, Hadi Hosseini SM, et al: Anomalous gray matter structural networks in major depressive disorder. Biol Psychiatry 74(10):777–785, 2013 23601854

Sisk CL, Zehr JL: Pubertal hormones organize the adolescent brain and behavior. Front Neuroendocrinol 26(3–4):163–174, 2005 16309736

Somerville LH, Jones RM, Casey BJ: A time of change: behavioral and neural correlates of adolescent sensitivity to appetitive and aversive environmental cues. Brain Cogn 72(1):124–133, 2010 19695759

Somerville LH, Fani N, McClure-Tone EB: Behavioral and neural representation of emotional facial expressions across the lifespan. Dev Neuropsychol 36(4):408–428, 2011 21516541

Sosic-Vasic Z, Abler B, Grön G, et al: Effects of a brief cognitive behavioural therapy group intervention on baseline brain perfusion in adolescents with major depressive disorder. Neuroreport 28(6):348–353, 2017 28328739

Sowell ER, Thompson PM, Leonard CM, et al: Longitudinal mapping of cortical thickness and brain growth in normal children. J Neurosci 24(38):8223–8231, 2004 15385605

Spear LP: The adolescent brain and age-related behavioral manifestations. Neurosci Biobehav Rev 24(4):417–463, 2000 10817843

Spear LP: Rewards, aversions and affect in adolescence: emerging convergences across laboratory animal and human data. Dev Cogn Neurosci 1(4):392–400, 2011 21918675

Spinelli S, Chefer S, Suomi SJ, et al: Early life stress induces long-term morphologic changes in primate brain. Arch Gen Psychiatry 66(6):658–665, 2009 19487631

Spoont MR: Modulatory role of serotonin in neural information processing: implications for human psychopathology. Psychol Bull 112(2):330–350, 1992 1454898

Straub J, Plener PL, Sproeber N, et al: Neural correlates of successful psychotherapy of depression in adolescents. J Affect Disord 183:239–246, 2015 26025370

Straub J, Metzger CD, Plener PL, et al: Successful group psychotherapy of depression in adolescents alters fronto-limbic resting-state connectivity. J Affect Disord 209:135–139, 2017 27912160

Strikwerda-Brown C, Davey CG, Whittle S, et al: Mapping the relationship between subgenual cingulate cortex functional connectivity and depressive symptoms across adolescence. Soc Cogn Affect Neurosci 10(7):961–968, 2015 25416726

Stringaris A, Vidal-Ribas Belil P, Artiges E, et al; IMAGEN Consortium: The brain's response to reward anticipation and depression in adolescence: dimensionality, specificity, and longitudinal predictions in a community-based sample. Am J Psychiatry 172(12):1215–1223, 2015 26085042

Stuber GD, Sparta DR, Stamatakis AM, et al: Excitatory transmission from the amygdala to nucleus accumbens facilitates reward seeking. Nature 475(7356):377–380, 2011 21716290

Swartz JR, Carrasco M, Wiggins JL, et al: Age-related changes in the structure and function of prefrontal cortex-amygdala circuitry in children and adolescents: a multi-modal imaging approach. Neuroimage 86:212–220, 2014 23959199

Tao R, Calley CS, Hart J, et al: Brain activity in adolescent major depressive disorder before and after fluoxetine treatment. Am J Psychiatry 169(4):381–388, 2012 22267183

Tarazi FI, Tomasini EC, Baldessarini RJ: Postnatal development of dopamine D1-like receptors in rat cortical and striatolimbic brain regions: an autoradiographic study. Dev Neurosci 21(1):43–49, 1999 10077701

Telzer EH: Dopaminergic reward sensitivity can promote adolescent health: a new perspective on the mechanism of ventral striatum activation. Dev Cogn Neurosci 17:57–67, 2016 26708774

Telzer EH, Masten CL, Berkman ET, et al: Gaining while giving: an fMRI study of the rewards of family assistance among white and Latino youth. Soc Neurosci 5(5–6):508–518, 2010 20401808

Telzer EH, Masten CL, Berkman ET, et al: Neural regions associated with self control and mentalizing are recruited during prosocial behaviors towards the family. Neuroimage 58(1):242–249, 2011 21703352

Telzer EH, Fuligni AJ, Lieberman MD, et al: Ventral striatum activation to prosocial rewards predicts longitudinal declines in adolescent risk taking. Dev Cogn Neurosci 3:45–52, 2013 23245219

Telzer EH, Fuligni AJ, Lieberman MD, et al: Neural sensitivity to eudaimonic and hedonic rewards differentially predict adolescent depressive symptoms over time. Proc Natl Acad Sci USA 111(18):6600–6605, 2014 24753574

Thompson RA: Emotion regulation: a theme in search of definition. Monogr Soc Res Child Dev 59(2–3):25–52, 1994 7984164

Tottenham N, Galván A: Stress and the adolescent brain: amygdala-prefrontal cortex circuitry and ventral striatum as developmental targets. Neurosci Biobehav Rev 70:217–227, 2016 27473936

Uematsu A, Matsui M, Tanaka C, et al: Developmental trajectories of amygdala and hippocampus from infancy to early adulthood in healthy individuals. PLoS One 7(10):e46970, 2012 23056545

Van Leijenhorst L, Gunther Moor B, Op de Macks ZA, et al: Adolescent risky decision-making: neurocognitive development of reward and control regions. Neuroimage 51(1):345–355, 2010 20188198

Vink M, Derks JM, Hoogendam JM, et al: Functional differences in emotion processing during adolescence and early adulthood. Neuroimage 91:70–76, 2014 24468408

Wade TJ, Cairney J, Pevalin DJ: Emergence of gender differences in depression during adolescence: national panel results from three countries. J Am Acad Child Adolesc Psychiatry 41(2):190–198, 2002 11837409

Wager TD, Davidson ML, Hughes BL, et al: Prefrontal-subcortical pathways mediating successful emotion regulation. Neuron 59(6):1037–1050, 2008 18817740

Wahlstrom D, White T, Luciana M: Neurobehavioral evidence for changes in dopamine system activity during adolescence. Neurosci Biobehav Rev 34(5):631–648, 2010 20026110

Wang X, Öngür D, Auerbach RP, et al: Cognitive vulnerability to major depression: view from the intrinsic network and cross-network interactions. Harv Rev Psychiatry 24(3):188–201, 2016 27148911

Weir JM, Zakama A, Rao U: Developmental risk I: depression and the developing brain. Child Adolesc Psychiatr Clin N Am 21(2):237–259, vii, 2012 22537725

Whittle S, Lichter R, Dennison M, et al: Structural brain development and depression onset during adolescence: a prospective longitudinal study. Am J Psychiatry 171(5):564–571, 2014 24577365

Wierenga LM, Langen M, Oranje B, et al: Unique developmental trajectories of cortical thickness and surface area. Neuroimage 87:120–126, 2014 24246495

Wilke M, Krägeloh-Mann I, Holland SK: Global and local development of gray and white matter volume in normal children and adolescents. Exp Brain Res 178(3):296–307, 2007 17051378

Winkler AM, Kochunov P, Blangero J, et al: Cortical thickness or grey matter volume? The importance of selecting the phenotype for imaging genetics studies. Neuroimage 53(3):1135–1146, 2010 20006715

Yurgelun-Todd DA, Killgore WD, Young AD: Sex differences in cerebral tissue volume and cognitive performance during adolescence. Psychol Rep 91(3 Pt 1):743–757, 2002 12530718

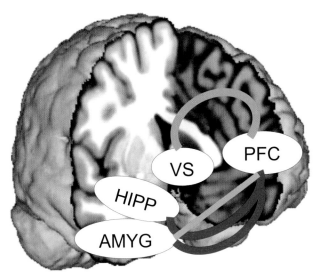

PLATE 1. *(Figure 5–1)* **A hypothesized model of fronto-limbic and fronto-striatal connectivity deficits in early-onset depression.**

Red denotes increased connectivity, and *blue* denotes reduced connectivity. AMYG=amygdala; HIPP=hippocampus; PFC=prefrontal cortex; VS=ventral striatum.

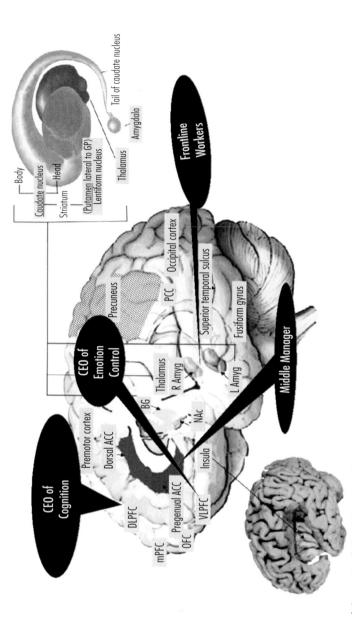

PLATE 2. (*Figure 6–1*) **Key functional regions deployed in pediatric bipolar disorder (PBD).**

ACC==anterior cingulate cortex; BG==basal ganglia; GP==globus pallidus; DLPFC=dorsolateral prefrontal cortex; MPFC=medial prefrontal cortex; NAc=nucleus accumbens; OFC=orbitofrontal cortex; PCC=posterior cingulate cortex; VLFPC=ventrolateral prefrontal cortex.

Source. Adapted from Pavuluri 2015a.

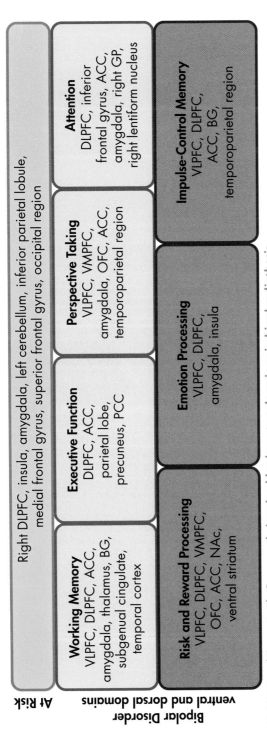

At Risk

Right DLPFC, insula, amygdala, left cerebellum, inferior parietal lobule, medial frontal gyrus, superior frontal gyrus, occipital region

Bipolar Disorder
ventral and dorsal domains

Working Memory
VLPFC, DLPFC, ACC, amygdala, thalamus, BG, subgenual cingulate, temporal cortex

Executive Function
DLPFC, ACC, parietal lobe, precuneus, PCC

Perspective Taking
VLPFC, VMPFC, amygdala, OFC, ACC, temporoparietal region

Attention
DLPFC, inferior frontal gyrus, ACC, amygdala, right GP, right lentiform nucleus

Risk and Reward Processing
VLPFC, DLPFC, VMPFC, OFC, ACC, NAc, ventral striatum

Emotion Processing
VLPFC, DLPFC, amygdala, insula

Impulse-Control Memory
VLPFC, DLPFC, ACC, BG, temporoparietal region

PLATE 3. *(Figure 6–2)* **Commonly involved brain network regions in bipolar diathesis.**

Brain function in various regions overlaps across individuals at risk for BD (HR group) and those with pediatric bipolar disorder (PBD), as well as across all the domains in PBD. *Blue* indicates predominantly dorsal domains, engaged in cognitive processes and highly interconnected across the brain in PBD. *Pink* indicates predominantly ventral domains, emotionally charged and highly interconnected across the brain in PBD.

ACC=anterior cingulate cortex; BG=basal ganglia; DLPFC=dorsolateral prefrontal cortex; GP=globus pallidus; NAc=nucleus accumbens; OFC=orbitofrontal cortex; PCC=posterior cingulate cortex; VLPFC=ventrolateral prefrontal cortex; VMPFC=ventromedial PFC.

All findings are noted as "relative to healthy volunteers."

Effort, comparison group, and type of task engagement determine the level of activation in brain regions. Therefore, increases and decreases in functional activity are not specified.

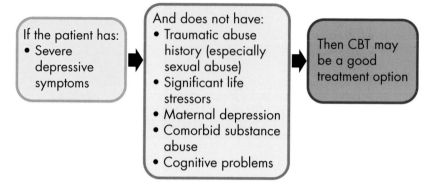

PLATE 4. *(Figure 7–1)* Treatment decision making: cognitive-behavioral therapy.

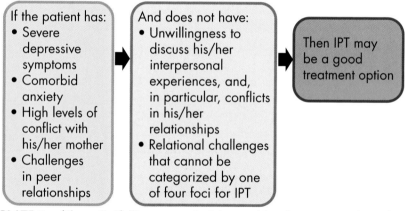

PLATE 5. *(Figure 7–2)* Treatment decision making: interpersonal psycho-therapy.

6

Neuroscience of Childhood-Onset Bipolar Disorder

TRANSLATION OF SCIENCE TO SERVICE

Amber C. May, M.D.

Sally M. Weinstein, Ph.D.

Julie Carbray, Ph.D.

Mani N. Pavuluri, M.D., Ph.D.

Jake is an 11-year-old boy who was brought to the clinic for a follow-up treatment session by his parents and older siblings. In the office, he plays video games on his iPad until his parents ask him to stop and engage in the interview. The iPad has a protective cover, in case he throws it across the room because of poor impulse control and judgment during his manic state. He demonstrates poor mood regulation, shouting loudly and incessantly without eye contact. He is frustrated by everyone who impedes his virtual play, demonstrating cognitive inflexibility. His parents desperately try to calm him, eventually promising a reward of his favorite double chocolate ice cream after the visit. They complain that Jake is perpetually reward seeking and that rewards are the only way to get him to cooperate. He is overweight because of excessive, uncontrolled eating habits further complicated by antipsychotic medication that increases his appetite. He is inattentive, unable to sit still or focus on any question asked during the interview. Jake begins pacing around the room, agitated with mixed dysphoria and excitement, along with hyperarousal and poor reasoning, while anticipating the ice cream treat. Jake has a poor working memory and has challenges keeping information "online." Since he was diagnosed with attention-deficit/hyperactivity disorder (ADHD), the school implemented an individualized education plan (IEP). His accommodations include a one-on-one aide who helps him overcome poor executive function including challenges with problem solving, forward planning, and organization. Genetic history includes his mother carrying a diagnosis of bipolar disorder (BD), a sister with disruptive mood dysregulation disorder (DMDD), and a brother with ADHD.

The presentation described above is complicated, yet not uncommon in a patient with childhood-onset BD or pediatric bipolar disorder (PBD) with complex comorbid diagnoses. Such a case challenges the clinician to conceptualize the illness features and dysfunction across multiple brain domains. Jake is a child at genetic risk for BD who developed the illness on longitudinal clinical follow-up.

Upon early recognition, there are two key clinical tasks. First, the family must be educated about the complexity of BD, and the diagnosis must be explained as a brain disorder in understandable terms. Second, the treatment goals must be prioritized to address the symptoms of illness and the domains of dysfunction. In this chapter we present an overview of the emerging evidence of brain abnormalities in individuals at risk for and in youth diagnosed with BD.

There are two caveats to consider at the outset. First, although the research spans over the past two decades, the diagnostic criteria changed in 2013 (American Psychiatric Association 2013). Thus, patients now labeled with DMDD per DSM-5 (American Psychiatric Association 2013) may have been included under BD not otherwise specified according to DSM-IV-TR criteria (American Psychiatric Association 2000) in the studies that were launched prior to 2013. Severe mood dysregulation (SMD) is a definition originally developed for research encompassing significantly impairing irritability and hyperarousal symptoms akin to mania, but without discrete episodes (Leibenluft 2011). SMD was used as the basis for the DSM-5 diagnostic criteria for DMDD with the exclusion of the hypomanic symptoms and hyperarousal (Sparks et al. 2014). Mood dys-regulation is a common feature in BD and DMDD. Moreover, DMDD may precede the onset of PBD.

Second, it is challenging to be precise and definitive in interpreting study findings in which subjects have illness features that are inherently complex and display heterogeneity in severity, episode type, or medication status. Furthermore, the majority of studies of children at risk for developing BD are evaluated cross-sectionally with heterogeneous features and do not include subjects with prodromal symptoms but without a family history of PBD (Garrett et al. 2015; Roybal et al. 2015; Singh et al. 2013b; Tseng et al. 2015; Wiggins et al. 2017). In some longitudinal studies (e.g., the Longitudinal Assessment of Manic Symptoms [LAMS] study), the concept of mood dysregulation as a domain is introduced without partiality to the episodic nature of bipolar illness (Bertocci et al. 2016; Versace et al. 2017).

Brain regions and circuits that support this complex presentation of symptoms require an orientation. Structural brain changes compared with healthy volunteers, including enlargement or reduction inconsistent with typical development, are interpreted as pathological or compensatory.

The key brain regions discussed in this chapter in relation to their operative function in imaging studies are as follows (Figure 6–1):

1. The prefrontal cortex (PFC) has several regions of higher cognitive, emotional, and social functions.

    a. The dorsolateral PFC (DLPFC; middle frontal gyrus; Brodmann area [BA] 9 and BA 46) is referred to as the "CEO of cognition" because of its key role as a cognitive region primarily responsible for managing decision making, working memory, planning, and cognitive flexibility (Barbey et al. 2013; Goldman-Rakic 1995).

    b. The ventrolateral PFC (VLPFC; inferior frontal gyrus; BA 45 and BA 47) is referred to as the "CEO of emotion control" because of its critical function in emotion regulation along with the DLPFC by virtue of its strong cortico-cortical connection (Wager et al. 2008). In addition, the VLPFC has multiple roles in exerting motor inhibition (Levy and Wagner 2011) and performance monitoring (Fuster 2008) with its connectivity to the basal ganglia and the anterior cingulate and amygdala, respectively.

    c. The medial PFC (MPFC; medial portions of BA 10–12 and BA 25) is implicated in emotion processing (via the amygdala), memory (via the hippocampus), and higher-order sensory regions (via the insula). The PFC's fundamental role is in social cognitive abilities such as self-reflection, interpersonal perception, and theory of mind/mentalizing (Amodio and Frith 2006; Grossmann 2013).

    d. The orbitofrontal cortex (OFC; BA 10 and BA 11) is involved in decision making and expectation and in estimating the affective value of rewards (Kringelbach 2005). Therefore, the OFC is key in comparing expected versus actual delivery of reward/punishment, facilitating adaptive learning.

2. The insula is anteriorly contiguous with the VLPFC and closely linked to the MPFC and the amygdala. The insula plays a central role in experiencing somatic sensations such as physiological arousal (Pavuluri and May 2015).

3. The anterior cingulate cortex (ACC) is an intermediary cortex with the role of a "middle manager" or central station that connects top-down and bottom-up pathways of the PFC executive regions and the subcortical regions.

    a. The dorsal ACC moderates performance errors.

    b. The ventral or pregenual ACC (BA 24) is key to emotion processing and reward learning. The ACC takes on a compensatory role in the case of PFC dysfunction.

    c. The subgenual ACC (BA 25) is a key serotonin transporter region implicated in processing negative emotion (e.g., sadness) (Mayberg et al. 1999) and memory formation along with the hippocampus (Nieuwenhuis and Takashima 2011).

4. The posterior cingulate cortex (PCC) is involved in cognitive introspection and concentration (Leech and Sharp 2014).

5. The amygdala's functions include emotion processing and generating a reaction to positive or negative perceptions. As a "frontline worker," the amygdala is responsible for primal emotions, emotion regulation (with the VLPFC), emotional memory formation (with the hippocampus), emotionally driven attention (with the DLPFC), and reward seeking (with the nucleus accumbens) (Phelps and LeDoux 2005).

6. The basal ganglia has multiple regions involved in the psychopathology of bipolar diathesis (Robinson et al. 2012). Subregions include the dorsal (caudate and putamen) and ventral striatum (nucleus accumbens and the olfactory tubercle), globus pallidus, ventral pallidum, substantia nigra, and subthalamic nuclei.

    a. The caudate and putamen are other "frontline workers" involved in trial-and-error–based learning of repetitive behavior, task switching (with the DLPFC), and impulse control (with the VLPFC).

b. Working memory (Schroll and Hamker 2013) is facilitated with the basal ganglia acting as a gateway, whereas the DLPFC holds information online (i.e., remembering while thinking and operating a task) in short bursts. The globus pallidus is involved in movement and activity.

c. The nucleus accumbens moderates reward seeking and aversion through dopamine supplied by the ventral tegmental area and ventral pallidum, and glutamate from the amygdala, hippocampus, and OFC (Pavuluri et al. 2017).

Brain Structure in Youth With Bipolar Disorder

Structural Abnormalities in Youth With Bipolar Disorder

Abnormal structural gray-matter findings in patients with PBD include increased volume in the basal ganglia and decreased volume in the ACC, DLPFC, VLPFC, amygdala, and left hippocampus (Adler et al. 2006; Chiu et al. 2008; DelBello et al. 2004; Dickstein et al. 2005; Frazier et al. 2005; Gao et al. 2013; Gold et al. 2016; Wilke et al. 2004). Decreased gray-matter volume in the DLPFC was observed both in BD patients and more recently in DMDD patients relative to healthy volunteers. The decreased DLPFC volume in BD patients was also observed in direct comparisons with anxiety disorder patients who had increased gray matter (Gold et al. 2016). On longitudinal follow-up, greater bilateral cingulum length predicted fewer manic symptoms (Bertocci et al. 2016); this attests to the crucial role of the ACC.

Altered white-matter integrity with lower fractional anisotropy has also been reported using diffusion tensor imaging studies capturing the U fibers of the frontolimbic system (Weathers et al. 2012), the anterior and posterior corona radiata, and the corpus callosum (Barnea-Goraly et al. 2009; Frazier et al. 2007; Gao et al. 2013; Kafantaris et al. 2009; Pavuluri et al. 2009c).

Structural Abnormalities in Youth at Risk for Bipolar Disorder

Early intervention is a commonly overlooked aspect of treatment for PBD. Preventive intervention could lessen the suffering of affected individuals and

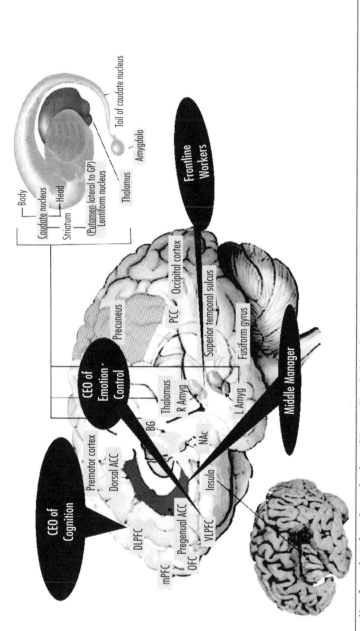

FIGURE 6–1. Key functional regions deployed in pediatric bipolar disorder (PBD). *(see color plate 2)*

ACC=anterior cingulate cortex; Amyg=amygdala; BG=basal ganglia; DLPFC=dorsolateral prefrontal cortex; GP==globus pallidus; L=left; MPFC=medial prefrontal cortex; NAc=nucleus accumbens; OFC=orbitofrontal cortex; PCC=posterior cingulate cortex; R=right; VLPFC=ventrolateral prefrontal cortex.

Source. Adapted from Pavuluri 2015a.

families by decreasing severity as well as reducing associated economic loss (Bechdolf et al. 2010). Identifying intergenerational characteristics and behavioral patterns of psychopathology is the key. Genetic loading leads to high-risk (HR) status for developing BD, with increased risk for developing affective disorders, and specifically BD by 10-fold compared with the general population (Kim et al. 2017; Whalley et al. 2013). By studying the population at risk for PBD, researchers may identify early biomarkers of brain dysfunction that can be utilized as screening measures. Decoding a biosignature can aid in identifying vulnerability prior to disease manifestation (Bechdolf et al. 2012; Chang et al. 2004; Fusar-Poli et al. 2012; Kim et al. 2017; Lee et al. 2014; Phillips and Kupfer 2013; Singh et al. 2008a).

Thus far, published studies of HR patients have had seemingly contradictory results as to whether structural differences exist. Often, these studies are limited by sample size or to a comparison with BD patients or healthy volunteers (Barbey et al. 2013; Bechdolf et al. 2010; Dunlop et al. 2015; Ladouceur et al. 2013; Lee et al. 2014; Thermenos et al. 2011). Significant studies have not found structural differences in asymptomatic offspring of bipolar parents (Hajek et al. 2008, 2009; Singh et al. 2008a).

However, other studies do report structural changes in HR patients with active symptoms or disease progression. HR youth may not manifest structural abnormalities until the emergence of clinical symptoms (Fusar-Poli et al. 2012; Kim et al. 2017; Lim et al. 2013). In a meta-analysis of neuroimaging studies, the HR group had larger intracerebral gray-matter volumes compared with BD patients (Fusar-Poli et al. 2012). A cross-sectional MRI study noted decreased insula and amygdala volumes compared with healthy volunteers in symptomatic, functionally impaired HR patients who developed PBD within a year (Bechdolf et al. 2012). Another study found that prior to clinical symptoms of BD, symptomatic HR youth displayed inhibited temperaments associated with decreased right hippocampal volumes (Kim et al. 2017). These results add to the literature showing that decreased right hippocampal volumes may be a risk factor for mood disorders (Chen et al. 2010; Frazier et al. 2005; Inal-Emiroglu et al. 2015; Pfeifer et al. 2008; Röttig et al. 2007).

Further longitudinal studies can determine if the findings of decreased gray-matter volume, decreased insula and amygdala volumes, and a correlation between inhibited temperament and hippocampal volume could be utilized as screening tools for BD (Bechdolf et al. 2012; Chang et al. 2004; Fusar-Poli et al. 2012; Kim et al. 2017; Singh et al. 2008a). These findings may only be detectable after symptoms and psychopathology have reached a certain threshold or level of functional impairment (Fusar-Poli et al. 2012; Kim et al. 2017; Lim et al. 2013).

Brain Function in
Youth With Bipolar Disorder

Functional Abnormalities in Youth With Bipolar Disorder: Targets for Intervention

Education for families with BD spectrum emphasizes how a single diagnostic label of BD does not do justice to the patient's experience. The complex clinical problems are best understood through the lens of multidomain dysfunction. This section outlines the research findings on these domains as a window into understanding how the brain functions in the context of BD. Note that all study findings generated are based on group data, so the deficits reported are not necessarily present in every single patient with BD. However, the gestalt of emerging literature informs and trains the clinical eye. Neuropsychological testing may attest to these deficits, in addition to astute clinical observation. Currently, there is not yet an established neuroimaging test to conduct at an individual and clinical level to make a diagnosis of BD.

Impaired Emotion Processing

> He demonstrates poor mood regulation, shouting loudly and incessantly without eye contact.

Excessive reactivity to negative emotions, impaired facial emotion recognition, and missed social cues are common problems in BD.

Findings from computer-based testing

Even while in a stabilized mood, BD patients had difficulty detecting subtle emotions. This signifies a trait deficit regardless of illness state (McClure et al. 2005). Furthermore, patients with BD interpreted hostility in neutral faces (Rich et al. 2005) or underestimated very intense happy and sad emotions (Schenkel et al. 2007). If patients had been acutely ill or very young at symptom onset, they had more problems differentiating emotions (Schenkel et al. 2012).

Clinician's role.   Translation of these findings for families fosters understanding about their children's emotions and behaviors. Educating the family about cognitive control and its role in delayed gratification and impulsive behaviors can lead to "coaching" moments in which parents can help with impulsivity and reactivity in real time. Patients may miss subtle emotional cues or misinterpret intense emotions, and this could result in hostile attributions with emotionally driven parental responses. Subsequent mood dysregulation or rapid cycling leads to familial stress. Clinicians can teach parents how to recognize and manage environmental triggers, perceived or real, often by distraction through engagement in cognitive tasks (Pavuluri 2015a).

Findings from fMRI studies

Negative stimuli (e.g., angry faces or hurtful words) have a greater impact compared with positive stimuli in eliciting impaired affective circuitry in BD. The VLPFC exerts emotional control along with the DLPFC. Together, they modulate the overactive amygdala, which receives and processes both internal and external emotional cues and feeling states. Research shows that the right VLPFC is overactive while exerting effortful control during less severe mood episodes. Interestingly, brain activity is absent in this region during severe mania. The research is inconclusive about whether the abnormalities are primarily cortical (VLPFC/DLPFC) or subcortical (amygdala). Rather, it is likely that cortical and subcortical networks interact, resulting in brainwide system-level dysfunction (Chang et al. 2004; Kim et al. 2012; Pavuluri et al. 2006b). Posterior to the VLPFC, the insula engages in processing negative emotions and sensorimotor information (Pavuluri and May 2015).

Clinician's role.   As noted earlier, several studies demonstrated that BD patients respond to negative emotion with underactivity in the right VLPFC and the DLPFC along with overactivity in the amygdala. This finding indicates that children with BD are highly sensitive to negative stimuli. Environmental intervention can be crucial, particularly in finding "the right fit" for a child's school, classroom setup, and teachers. Clinicians can partner with parents in educating other caretakers and teachers about the value of demonstrating compassion, particularly for children with mood dysregulation.

In addition, the amygdala showed less activity when directly labeling facial emotion versus when attending to a cognitive task (e.g., estimating the age of an emotional face) (Pavuluri et al. 2009a). Focusing on recognizing facial emotions may improve the affective circuitry function in PBD. This can be practiced by focusing one's full attention to emotion reading versus working on task completion simultaneously.

Executive Dysfunction

His accommodations include a one-on-one aide who helps him overcome poor executive function, including challenges with problem solving, forward planning, and organization.

Impaired executive function manifests as poor verbal elocution, disorganization, and inflexibility.

Findings from computer-based testing

Executive dysfunction progresses with age (Pavuluri et al. 2009b), persists regardless of mood stabilization (Pavuluri et al. 2006b, 2009b, 2010b), and manifests irrespective of co-occurring ADHD (Dickstein et al. 2004; Pavuluri et al. 2006b). Patients with BD have impaired functionality in the following areas: cognitive flexibility, adaptation to changing risks and rewards, frustration tolerance to negative consequences (Rich et al. 2005, 2010), error monitoring with feedback (Patino et al. 2013; Rich et al. 2010), forward planning with changing rules (Gorrindo et al. 2005), and processing speed (Doyle et al. 2005). A meta-analysis of the aforementioned studies highlighted deficits in planning, inhibition, flexibility, intelligence, and academic functioning (Joseph et al. 2008). Furthermore, negative emotional material has been shown to interfere with the executive function of language, including encoding, recall, and detailed narration (Jacobs et al. 2011). The degree of depressive symptoms appeared to adversely impact recall of less significant details, but not the essence of the story.

Clinician's role.   Parents often report challenges that relate to executive dysfunction when presented with the following situations: adapting to dynamic environmental demands, transitioning between activities, planning tasks, and completing multi-step tasks. To mitigate these difficulties, an IEP may allow provisions such as tutors aiding in multistepped learning, increased test-taking duration, and reduced homework requirements. These interventions decrease cognitive burden and increase motivation through the generation of successful experiences. Clinicians can encourage communication and storytelling, which improves recall and allows for processing negative experiences, thereby decreasing frustration.

Findings from fMRI studies on cognitive/mental flexibility

Mental flexibility, a subdomain of executive function, is the ability to shift from one task to another without rigidity or frustration. Patients with BD showed increased DLPFC-ACC-parietal activity, recruiting regions responsible for cognitive control and visuospatial strategies (Dickstein et al. 2010). This maladaptive activity is greater in response to failed reversal trials paired with punishment, as illustrated by increased activity in the precuneus and PCC. BD and SMD patients may show no differences in the decreased level of caudate activity, which is considered responsible for switching and learning new rules.

Clinician's role.   The consequent functional impairment that ensues from the above-described maladaptive function can lead to diagnostic confusion that can only be clarified by a comprehensive diagnostic interview. It is important to underscore that conducting a diagnostic assessment and understanding domain dysfunction are interlinked but not interchangeable concepts. In educating families, we help them understand how, for example, BD coexists with poor attention or cognitive inflexibility. The decision-making regions (e.g., DLPFC), attentional regions (e.g., the ACC and PCC), and learning and adaptation regions (e.g., the caudate) are affected in both BD and SMD. Inflexibility or decreased capacity to adapt is a deficit often noted in youth with BD. Thus, a clinician can work with these patients on skill building toward flexibility (PFC support), focus (ACC support), and adaptation/ability to switch tasks (caudate effort).

Impulsivity

> The iPad has a protective cover, in case he throws it across the room because of poor impulse control and judgment during his manic state.

Studies show impaired ability to control and accurately time impulsive responses, both emotionally explosive verbal expressions and physical outbursts.

Findings from computer-based testing

Impulse control has been examined with various versions of the stop-signal task, which tests for the ability to inhibit a motor act preparing to be executed. Findings consistently indicate that BD patients have decreased accuracy and increased intrasubject variability in response times. Poor attention to performance monitoring and inability to delay gratification may also contribute to premature reactivity or impulsivity. Impulsivity commonly manifests in both ADHD and BD and may arise from differential engagement of affective and cognitive systems in these disorders (Pavuluri and May 2014). Negative stimuli during interpersonal interactions can hinder optimal functioning. Additionally, comorbid internalizing emotional states (depression or anxiety) may lead to selection bias.

The clinical features of impulsivity were not correlated with the response inhibition measures: behavioral findings indicate poor inhibition in halting action midway when cues were given to stop.

Clinician's role.   Treatment strategies entail helping the patient develop insight into exercising cognitive control with mindful decision making. Educating the family about cognitive control and its role in delayed gratification and impulsive behaviors can lead to "coaching" moments during which parents can help with impulsivity and reactivity in real time.

Findings from fMRI studies

Across the entire bipolar spectrum, fMRI studies of various tasks probing response inhibition have illustrated highly consistent findings implicating dysfunction in the ACC and VLPFC. The VLPFC's dual role in exerting emotional and motor control and the ACC's dual role of emotion processing and cognitive error correction may explain the involvement of these regions in modulating both emotions and response inhibition.

Two contiguous pathophysiological processes implicate PFC regions in cognitive control and temporal-parietal regions in scanning with attention. Whereas patients with ADHD demonstrate cognitively driven impulsivity, patients with BD suffer from both cognitive and emotional impulsivity that involves frontostriatal (Deveney et al. 2012; Leibenluft et al. 2007; Weathers et al. 2012) and frontolimbic (Cerullo et al. 2009; Passarotti et al. 2011) circuitry (Pavuluri 2015a, 2015b).

Clinician's role.   Studies revealed that frontostriatal regions show increased activity with effort and decreased activity with failed inhibition. The act of paying attention is associated with underfunctioning frontal regions such as the VLPFC and DLPFC. The posterior cortical regions (e.g., the temporal and parietal regions) and subcortical regions (e.g., the basal ganglia) appear to compensate for frontal deficits. Treatment interventions for improved brain function may target mood regulation, error checking, and cognitive control.

Reward and Risk Processing

> They complain that Jake is perpetually reward seeking and that rewards are the only way to get him to cooperate.

Major areas of brain dysfunction in BD include hyperexcitability with rewards, inability to tolerate delayed gratification, and excessive frustration with loss during behavioral reward tasks.

Findings from computer-based tasks

Studies show that the pathophysiology of BD involves a lack of response to reinforcement and anticipated outcome. There is a shift away from the correct responses, whether reward or unexpected loss. Additionally, feedback sensitivity drops significantly with frustration induced by rigged feedback (Rich et al. 2005, 2010) or distraction by non-reward-related stimuli (Patino et al. 2013).

Clinician's role.   Children with BD have excessive reactions to negative stimuli, low frustration tolerance, inflexibility in attention-shifting tasks, and difficulty adapting to a dynamic environment. Additionally, patients with BD are more strongly motivated by immediate reward and gratification. These reward- and risk-modulated responses can be understood through interrelated multidomain dysfunctions in affect regulation, attention, and cognitive flexibility. These brain domains should be the targets for intervention.

Reward processing examined through fMRI studies

Reward processing involves a complex system encompassing emotional evaluation, decision making, and motivation. Dysfunctional reward networks in a child with PBD are hypothesized to occur at the interface of the *reward-centric* ventromedial PFC (VMPFC)– or OFC—ventral striatal circuitry (May et al. 2004) and the *emotion-centric* DLPFC-VLPFC-ACC-limbic circuitry. In addition to the studies in PBD, normative studies illustrate greater activation in the VMPFC, amygdala, and nucleus accumbens during winning compared with losing in behavioral reward tasks. For adolescents and adults, the degree of activation is proportional to reward (Bjork and Hommer 2007; May et al. 2004). Striatal regions show reduced activation during reward anticipation in adolescents relative to adults (Bjork and Hommer 2007). Patients with BD may show altered evaluation and appraisal of reward contingencies with impaired task completion. This results in excessive excitability or frustration, and reduced motivation (Singh et al. 2013a, 2014).

Clinician's role.   Motivation/reward circuitry and emotion regulation circuitry are closely linked in the ventral portion of the brain. Hyperarousal, poorly timed responses, intense reward seeking, and excessive excitation associated with reward and risk are explained by deficits in fronto-temporo-parieto-subcortical circuits (Passarotti et al. 2011). The increased incidence in PBD of substance use is related to dysfunction in closely connected subcortical regions—that is, the nucleus accumbens and the amygdala (Pavuluri et al. 2017). An increased risk for obesity and cardiovascular disease in BD may similarly be rooted in aberrant engagement of reward networks (e.g., food cravings), with or without exposure to atypical antipsychotic medications (Goldstein et al. 2015). Educating families to intervene in the cycle of intense reward seeking through biological explanation, increasing the repertoire of positive channels of motivation (constructive rewards), and providing assistance with deliberation of pros and cons during decision making (recruiting PFC) may help shape the underlying traits. Adaptive reward responses may be amenable to change through modification of existing preventive psychological interventions such as behavior modification strategies and parent training of effective reward contingencies.

Inattention

> He is inattentive, unable to sit still or focus on any question asked during the interview.

The construct of attention includes alertness, selectivity, focus, sustained attention, divided attention, and inhibition from distraction.

Findings from computer-based testing

Attention problems in BD include perseverance, low vigilance, false-responding with target insensitivity, and variable intraindividual response timing (Dickstein et al. 2004; Doyle et al. 2005; Pavuluri et al. 2006b, 2009b; Strakowski et al. 2010). These patients demonstrate selective attentional bias to negative stimuli such as angry faces (Pavuluri et al. 2007) and negative words (Whitney et al. 2012). PBD patients struggle with impaired problem solving when exposed to negative words (Pavuluri et al. 2008) and matching emotional words (Passarotti et al. 2013). Selective attentional bias has been demonstrated across domains of executive function and in the context of internalizing symptoms of depression and anxiety. Since BD is a disorder of emotion, selection bias appears impaired when the target is emotionally laden. Impairment in selection bias is more severe if the emotion is negative (Passarotti et al. 2013) versus when the target is emotionally neutral (Rich et al. 2006, 2010).

Findings from fMRI studies

A recent meta-analysis has shown that when patients with PBD relative to healthy volunteers engaged in attentional tasks, there was increased activation seen in the inferior frontal gyrus versus decreased activation in the amygdala. Differential patterns of underactivity were also noted in the dorsal attentional system—that is, the frontostriatal circuit (DLPFC, ACC, right lentiform nucleus, and right globus pallidus)—in patients with PBD relative to the healthy volunteers.

Clinician's role.   Given that BD is an emotional disorder, clinicians should be cognizant of sensitivity to negative stimuli that impacts focused attention. Clinicians may also observe patients with PBD to have negative biases to relatively neutral information. Finally, clinicians should recognize and treat comorbid internalizing disorders; thereby inattention problems may be ameliorated, which could improve school performance.

Working Memory Deficits

> Since he was diagnosed with attention-deficit/hyperactivity disorder (ADHD), the school implemented an Individual Education Plan (IEP).

Commonly, PBD patients have difficulty remembering numbers or words, especially if complex or multistep learning is involved. These deficits directly impact academic achievement (Pavuluri et al. 2006a, 2006b).

Findings from computer-based testing

Working memory is the ability to hold information online for short periods of time while accomplishing a task. This domain is critical for learning and day-to-day operations. Impaired verbal working memory in BD is associated with poor reading and reduced vigilance with math challenges (Pavuluri et al. 2006b). A longitudinal follow-up after 3 years showed persistent difficulties in working memory, including verbal memory (Pavuluri et al. 2006b, 2009b).

Findings from fMRI studies

Working memory deficits in BD are associated with impaired DLPFC-ACC-thalamic–basal ganglia circuitry (Adler et al. 2006; Chang et al. 2004). In BD relative to ADHD patients, tasks involving working memory under emotional challenge engaged the emotional circuitry regions within the ventral PFC and subgenual cingulate (Passarotti et al. 2010a). In contrast, patients with ADHD had only the dorsal cognitive, fronto-striatal, and fronto-parietal circuits engaged during these tasks. Interestingly, when patients with BD or ADHD are compared with healthy volunteers, both the cognitive and emotional regions are underactive. Additionally, the cognitive and affective regions underactive in BD patients with angry/negative emotions are overactive with happy emotions. In BD relative to healthy volunteer studies, negative stimuli consistently have greater impact on prefrontal regions and may decrease activation, whereas positive stimuli can engage the PFC regions with increased activity.

A study of brain network connectivity showed that for patients with BD, regions involved in the affective network circuitry (VLPFC-amygdala) and the facial emotion processing circuitry (fronto-temporo-amygdala) are not firing in synchrony with the rest of the corresponding brain network regions during a working memory task (Passarotti et al. 2010a, 2010b). Simultaneously, working memory circuitry is overengaged or hyperconnected (Passarotti et al. 2012). This pattern of differences illustrates interlinked, potentially compensatory processes at the interface of emotional and cognitive networks in BD.

Clinician's role. Working or verbal memory may not be completely rectified with medication. Brain functional studies show that working memory and affective circuitries are both dysfunctional in BD and ADHD, although affective circuits are malfunctioning to a greater degree in BD. Negative stimuli impair the ability of PFC regions to function effectively. To optimize academic productivity, patients should be provided a tranquil working environment and have reduced demands on working memory. Findings from functional neuroimaging studies delineate how ADHD and BD have shared dysfunction in affective and cognitive circuits relative to healthy volunteers. This explains the co-occurrence of emotional and cognitive problems in both disorders.

Perspective-Taking Deficits

> Shouting loudly and incessantly without eye contact.

Perspective taking, a dimension of theory of mind (ToM), is the ability to understand the point of view of others (Schenkel et al. 2008, 2014). Inability to grasp others' social cues or perspectives, especially in the context of stressful negative events, leads to social difficulties.

Findings from computer-based and fMRI studies

Individuals with SMD and those with BD have shared involvement of the amygdala, VLPFC, and emotion processing circuits. In fact, subjects with SMD show deficits across social reciprocity tasks involving social awareness, social cognition, social communication, and social motivation (Whitney et al. 2013).

Research shows that the same neural circuitry may be involved for PBD and ToM deficits. ToM domain dysfunction encompasses the following regions: MPFC (deployed in self-referential thinking), ACC (involved in error monitoring), amygdala (engaged in processing emotions), and OFC (involved in decision making and evaluation of rewards). Similar and interlinked regions affected in BD are the amygdala, ACC, OFC, MPFC, and other PFC regions such as the DLPFC and VLPFC (Altshuler et al. 2005; Blumberg et al. 1999; Chang et al. 2004; Kronhaus et al. 2006; Krüger et al. 2006; Pavuluri et al. 2005, 2007; Yurgelun-Todd et al. 2000). Other studies have suggested that neural correlates of perspective taking include the MPFC and temporoparietal junction (Hynes et al. 2006; Völlm et al. 2006).

One study revealed that the true intentions behind subtle hints during a negatively valenced affective story task were poorly recognized by BD patients (Schenkel et al. 2008). A later study showed poor performance on perspective taking and peer relations in BD type I patients relative to healthy volunteers; this was not the case for BD type II (Schenkel et al. 2014).

Clinician's role.   First, it is important to differentiate BD from autism spectrum disorder given the shared abnormalities in executive function, cognitive inflexibility, and perspective-taking deficits. Second, helping youth to practice thinking in terms of "walking in others' shoes" expands the repertoire of subtleties in interpersonal communication. This may be especially useful for improving parent-child interactions.

Impaired Function at the Interface of Emotion and Cognition

> Jake begins pacing around the room, agitated with mixed dysphoria and excitement, along with hyperarousal and poor reasoning, while anticipating the ice cream treat.

Findings from fMRI studies

In youth with BD, any excessive emotional stimuli will offset the ability to problem-solve because of mood dysregulation that destabilizes cognitive capacities. Negative emotions trigger amygdala activation along with the pregenual ACC in BD. The VLPFC is more affected in BD than in ADHD during a working memory task (Passarotti et al. 2010a, 2010b).

Clinician's role.   Understanding the impact on emotional dysfunction in the VLPFC, DLPFC, and amygdala illustrates that negative consequences may result in poor functioning of cortical cognitive and emotion control regions. This dysfunction may originate from abnormalities in either the amygdala, the PFC, or both. Psychotherapy principles should eliminate utilization of negative consequences and instead advocate for appropriate timing, tone of voice, and modulated use of language with corrective feedback. This employs a major shift away from the practice of using negative consequences in youth with mood dysregulation. Child- and family-focused cognitive-behavioral therapy was developed and tested in BD youth on the basis of these principles (West et al. 2014).

Functional Abnormalities in Youth at Risk for BD

A 2014 meta-analysis eloquently summarized the relevant fMRI studies comparing brain function in PBD, HR individuals, and healthy volunteers (Lee et al. 2014). The right DLPFC, insula, inferior parietal lobule, and left cerebellum regions demonstrated significantly greater activation in the HR group compared with the healthy volunteer group. There was also more activity found in the right DLPFC, right insula, and left cerebellum in the HR individuals compared with patients with PBD. This difference was hypothesized to be due to HR individuals using compensatory mechanisms in their cognition and emotional-processing regions. The meta-analysis facilitated a group comparison of fMRIs studies that showed that in the HR population, compared with PBD patients, the DLPFC and dorsal circuitry hub (e.g., insula, parietal lobe) are more involved. Although some studies found that HR individuals had increased amygdala activity (Bechdolf et al. 2012), the meta-analysis did not corroborate this finding (Lee et al. 2014). Another meta-analysis of neuroimaging studies demonstrated increased activity regardless of task in the left superior frontal gyrus, medial frontal gyrus, and left insula of HR youth compared with healthy volunteers (Fusar-Poli et al. 2012).

Brain regions and networks involved in affect processing have been investigated for dysfunction in HR individuals because this is a known impairment in patients with BD. Scientists have been searching for risk endophenotypes: specific biomarkers associated with bipolar illness that are genetically linked and state independent (Hasler et al. 2006; Wiggins et al. 2017). Facial emotion processing studies of HR youth for BD reveal dysfunction across the PFC, amygdala, dorsolateral, and occipital regions, which may be potential risk endophenotypes (Breakspear et al. 2015; Ladouceur et al. 2013; Manelis et al. 2015; Mourão-Miranda et al. 2012; Olsavsky et al. 2012; Singh et al. 2014; Tseng et al. 2015; Wiggins et al. 2017).

Neural Correlates of Treatment Response in Youth With Bipolar Disorder

Neural Correlates of Pharmacotherapy Response

When families are uncertain about the impact of medications, clinicians can provide education on the evidence of pharmacotherapy's reparative effect on emotional and cognitive systems due to brain plasticity. The first series of fMRI studies in pediatric mania examined the effects of lamotrigine, risperidone, and divalproex sodium individually as well as through a pharmacotherapy algorithm. The impact of medications was examined through the changes in the brain regions recruited while subjects were engaged in emotion processing, response inhibition, and executive function. The common biomarker of pharmacotherapy response appeared to be an increase in VLPFC activity in BD patients relative to healthy volunteers (Pavuluri 2014). Later, this finding was replicated in the LAMS study, in which medicated youth with BD were compared with two groups: unmedicated youth with BD and medicated youth without BD (Horwitz et al. 2010). Medicated youth with BD showed attenuation of abnormal deactivation in the VLPFC during emotion processing of angry faces (Hafeman et al. 2014).

The impact of lamotrigine was examined during probing of the impulse-control domain. Findings showed increased activity in the MPFC and pregenual, subgenual, and posterior cingulate cortices in BD versus increased striatal activity in healthy volunteers (Pavuluri et al. 2010b). Similarly, lamotrigine was proven to reduce bipolar depression with increased activity in the MPFC, DLPFC, striatum, and PCC relative to activity in these regions in healthy volunteers during an affective task of rating emotions (Chang et al. 2008). In a double-blind randomized study that compared the effects of divalproex versus risperidone, divalproex treatment for mania increased the connectivity of the subgenual cortex within the frontostriatal circuitry during response inhibition (Pavuluri et al. 2010a). Thus, the subgenual cingulate cortex is recruited during mood stabilization through probing the impulse-control domain with the antiepileptic agents divalproex and lamotrigine. In contrast, the insula is recruited during mood stabilization while probing the impulse-control domain with the second-generation antipsychotic risperidone (Pavuluri et al. 2010a).

The impact of mood-stabilizing medications was also tested during probing of the interface between working memory (cognitive) and emotion processing domains. Specifically, when patients were challenged with recalling angry faces, the VLPFC-MPFC and medial temporal regions showed increased activity with the antiepileptic agents lamotrigine and divalproex posttreatment (Pavuluri et al. 2011). In the same context, in response to risperidone, the subgenual cingulate and ventral striatum showed greater activation posttreatment (Pavuluri et al. 2011).

While probing the interface between executive function and emotion processing domains, negative word matching powerfully elicited medication effects. Indeed, evaluative brain regions (i.e., MPFC and ACC) showed increased activity with risperidone, divalproex, and lamotrigine (Pavuluri et al. 2012a, 2012b). However, under a negative emotional challenge, the cognitive DLPFC activation response was reduced with lamotrigine and risperidone. This provides a rationale for the suggestion that cognitive enhancers may be needed post–mood stabilization, based on medications used or for improvement of the residual attention difficulties intrinsic to BD (Pavuluri et al. 2009b). Furthermore, prognostic markers of clinical outcome have begun to emerge, with greater amygdala activity at baseline as a marker for poor outcome in the case of risperidone (possibly involving greater effort to subdue the amygdala). In contrast, MPFC activity was a marker for a good outcome (a sign of greater deployment of higher cortical regions) in the case of divalproex on direct comparison of these medication groups.

Overall, these results indicate three key ideas. First, negative or angry stimuli are more successful in eliciting drug-related activity than happy or neutral faces in probing group differences. Second, medications differentially engage the brain circuitry based on neurochemistry and tasks. Third, an appreciation of state-versus-trait effects on the brain has emerged. With all medications, the amygdala showed reduced activity from baseline along with recovery from a manic state but remained active relative to that of healthy volunteers (trait marker), whereas the PFC regions were normalized with mood stabilization (state marker) (Passarotti et al. 2011). However, long-term treatment for at least 4 months with a standardized algorithm led to increased amygdala connectivity (Wegbreit et al. 2011) in the affective circuitry and normalized subcortical activity (Yang et al. 2013).

In conclusion, these discoveries give rise to the concept that antiepileptics and antipsychotics complement each other by virtue of their variability in action by reversing the brain dysfunction across domains.

Neural Correlates of Psychotherapy Response

An emerging area of literature utilizes neuroimaging to explore changes at the brain level in response to psychotherapy for BD in youth. In a small preliminary study of depressed adolescents with BD, Diler et al. (2013) examined neural activity in response to an implicit emotional-processing task at baseline and after 6 weeks of open psychotherapy as usual plus medication management. Across treatment, youth demonstrated decreased neural activity in the left occipital cortex in response to intense fearful stimuli, and increased left insula, left cerebellum, and right VLPFC in response to intense happy stimuli. Findings suggest improved emotion processing—namely, attention away from negative emotions and attention to positive emotions—in response to treatment for depression in BD youth. Additionally, a recent study examined youth at high risk for BD (as defined by familial risk in concert with current mood symptoms) before and 4 months after family-focused treatment for BD or treatment as usual (Garrett et al. 2015). Results indicated improved DLPFC activation and reduced amygdala activation across psychotherapy, and with family-focused treatment in particular. Moreover, improvement in DLPFC activation corresponded to improvement in mania symptoms across treatment, thus highlighting the DLPFC as a possible neural mechanism of clinical improvement in response to psychotherapy. Continued research in this area is critical to refine and tailor psychosocial interventions to specifically target the neurobiological dysfunction inherent in BD in youth.

Conclusion

In patients with PBD, it is the rule rather than the exception that multiple brain domains are affected (as summarized in Figure 6–2) with impairment of daily function. What is not addressed by the literature in any group data of studies is the invariable complexity encumbered by multidomain involvement at an individual level.

Empirical findings led to the development of RAINBOW therapy[1] and problem-solving pharmacotherapy for addressing symptoms of BD and potential comorbidities (West et al. 2014, 2018). Just as not all symptoms need be present to diagnose BD, not all domains need be affected in any single individual patient. Clinical strategies to overcome cognitive issues include setting up tutoring for multistepped learning, reducing homework to decrease cognitive burden, increasing motivation through positive reinforcement, lengthening test-taking duration, allowing appropriate time

---

[1]Cognitive-behavioral therapy that includes Routine; Affect regulation; I can do it; No negative thoughts; Be a good friend and balanced lifestyle; Oh, how can we solve the problems; and Ways to get support.

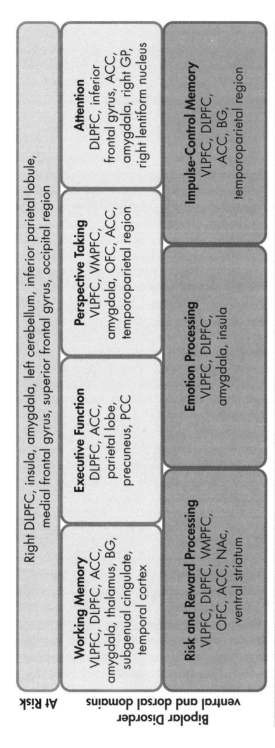

FIGURE 6–2.   Commonly involved brain network regions in bipolar diathesis. (*see color plate 3*)

Brain function in various regions overlaps across individuals at risk for bipolar disorder (high-risk group) and those with pediatric bipolar disorder (PBD), as well as across all the domains in PBD. *Blue* indicates predominantly dorsal domains, engaged in cognitive processes and highly interconnected across the brain in PBD. *Pink* indicates predominantly ventral domains, emotionally charged and highly interconnected across the brain in PBD.

ACC=anterior cingulate cortex; BG=basal ganglia; DLPFC=dorsolateral prefrontal cortex; GP=globus pallidus; NAc=nucleus accumbens; OFC=orbitofrontal cortex; PCC=posterior cingulate cortex; VLPFC=ventrolateral prefrontal cortex; VMPFC=ventromedial prefrontal cortex.

All findings are noted as "relative to healthy volunteers." Effort, comparison group, and type of task engagement determine the level of activation in brain regions. Therefore, increases and decreases in functional activity are not specified.

to accomplish tasks, developing cues for transition, and assisting with problem solving through preparation and planning.

When the critical dysfunction at the interface of emotional and cognitive systems is considered, there is abundant evidence that negative emotions impair cognitive function. Addressing this impairment demands not only the above-mentioned strategies but also environmental manipulation to provide compassionate care. An array of options, summarized above, tailored to the individual patient and his or her unique system of caretakers, is key for a personalized approach. Accurate assessment, educating families with comprehensible language on the complex neurobiology of the brain and behavioral dysfunction that underlies emotional and cognitive problems, and chemical intervention paired with dynamic psychosocial interventions lead to precision in addressing individual and family needs. Understanding all elements facilitates appreciation of the complexity of interlinked brain domain functions as well as the environmental impact at an individual level when striving toward precision care.

Clinical Pearls

- Clinicians can delineate dysfunction across two tiers: abnormal behavior aligned with various dimensions of brain function and clinical symptoms of bipolar diatheses (BD).

- Emotion processing can involve negative emotional stimuli triggering emotional outbursts, explained by hyperactivity in the amygdala and hypoactivity in the dorsolateral prefrontal cortex (DLPFC) and the ventrolateral prefrontal cortex (VLPFC). These findings support the need for providing compassionate care at home and school as well as for designing psychotherapeutic models such as *child and family focused cognitive-behavior therapy* (CFF-CBT a.k.a. RAINBOW therapy). Conversely, incorporating negative consequences is not part of CFF-CBT.

- Recognizing and tuning into facial emotions, negative or positive, can decrease activity in the amygdala. Conversely, participating in cognitive tasks without attention to decoding emotions may lead to being hijacked by the overreactive amygdala.

- The DLPFC–anterior cingulate cortex (ACC)–parietal regions may be affected in BD, leading to mental inflexibility and inability to switch between activities.

- High comorbidity with attention-deficit/hyperactivity disorder (ADHD) explains the shared clinical features of impulsivity. The VLPFC has a dual role in exerting emotional control and motor control. Similarly, the ACC has a dual role in emotion processing and error correction. Inattention and working memory deficits are common in BD and involve the DLPFC, ACC, and basal ganglia. Both diagnoses of BD and ADHD, either present together or alone, have these shared dimensional deficits with common affected brain regions.

- Preliminary findings on pharmacotherapy and psychotherapy show promising results in reversing the impairment across the interconnected emotional and cognitive brain networks.

References

Adler CM, DelBello MP, Strakowski SM: Brain network dysfunction in bipolar disorder. CNS Spectr 11(4):312–320, quiz 323–324, 2006 16641836

Altshuler L, Bookheimer S, Proenza MA, et al: Increased amygdala activation during mania: a functional magnetic resonance imaging study. Am J Psychiatry 162(6):1211–1213, 2005 15930074

American Psychiatric Association: Diagnostic and Statistical Manual of Mental Disorders, 4th Edition, Text Revision. Washington, DC, American Psychiatric Association, 2000

American Psychiatric Association: Diagnostic and Statistical Manual of Mental Disorders, 5th Edition. Arlington, VA, American Psychiatric Association, 2013

Amodio DM, Frith CD: Meeting of minds: the medial frontal cortex and social cognition. Nat Rev Neurosci 7(4):268–277, 2006 16552413

Barbey AK, Koenigs M, Grafman J: Dorsolateral prefrontal contributions to human working memory. Cortex 49(5):1195–1205, 2013 22789779

Barnea-Goraly N, Chang KD, Karchemskiy A, et al: Limbic and corpus callosum aberrations in adolescents with bipolar disorder: a tract-based spatial statistics analysis. Biol Psychiatry 66(3):238–244, 2009 19389661

Bechdolf A, Nelson B, Cotton SM, et al: A preliminary evaluation of the validity of at-risk criteria for bipolar disorders in help-seeking adolescents and young adults. J Affect Disord 127(1–3):316–320, 2010 20619465

Bechdolf A, Wood SJ, Nelson B, et al: Amygdala and insula volumes prior to illness onset in bipolar disorder: a magnetic resonance imaging study. Psychiatry Res 201(1):34–39, 2012 22281200

Bertocci MA, Bebko G, Versace A, et al: Predicting clinical outcome from reward circuitry function and white matter structure in behaviorally and emotionally dysregulated youth. Mol Psychiatry 21(9):1194–1201, 2016 26903272

Bjork JM, Hommer DW: Anticipating instrumentally obtained and passively received rewards: a factorial fMRI investigation. Behav Brain Res 177(1):165–170, 2007 17140674

Blumberg HP, Stern E, Ricketts S, et al: Rostral and orbital prefrontal cortex dysfunction in the manic state of bipolar disorder. Am J Psychiatry 156(12):1986–1988, 1999 10588416

Breakspear M, Roberts G, Green MJ, et al: Network dysfunction of emotional and cognitive processes in those at genetic risk of bipolar disorder. Brain 138 (Pt 11):3427–3439, 2015 26373604

Cerullo MA, Adler CM, Lamy M, et al: Differential brain activation during response inhibition in bipolar and attention-deficit hyperactivity disorders. Early Interv Psychiatry 3(3):189–197, 2009 22640382

Chang K, Adleman NE, Dienes K, et al: Anomalous prefrontal-subcortical activation in familial pediatric bipolar disorder: a functional magnetic resonance imaging investigation. Arch Gen Psychiatry 61(8):781–792, 2004 15289277

Chang KD, Wagner C, Garrett A, et al: A preliminary functional magnetic resonance imaging study of prefrontal-amygdalar activation changes in adolescents with bipolar depression treated with lamotrigine. Bipolar Disord 10(3):426–431, 2008 18402630

Chen MC, Hamilton JP, Gotlib IH: Decreased hippocampal volume in healthy girls at risk of depression. Arch Gen Psychiatry 67(3):270–276, 2010 20194827

Chiu S, Widjaja F, Bates ME, et al: Anterior cingulate volume in pediatric bipolar disorder and autism. J Affect Disord 105(1–3):93–99, 2008 17568686

DelBello MP, Zimmerman ME, Mills NP, et al: Magnetic resonance imaging analysis of amygdala and other subcortical brain regions in adolescents with bipolar disorder. Bipolar Disord 6(1):43–52, 2004 14996140

Deveney CM, Connolly ME, Jenkins SE, et al: Neural recruitment during failed motor inhibition differentiates youths with bipolar disorder and severe mood dysregulation. Biol Psychol 89(1):148–155, 2012 22008364

Dickstein DP, Treland JE, Snow J, et al: Neuropsychological performance in pediatric bipolar disorder. Biol Psychiatry 55(1):32–39, 2004 14706422

Dickstein DP, Milham MP, Nugent AC, et al: Frontotemporal alterations in pediatric bipolar disorder: results of a voxel-based morphometry study. Arch Gen Psychiatry 62(7):734–741, 2005 15997014

Dickstein DP, Gorrostieta C, Ombao H, et al: Fronto-temporal spontaneous resting state functional connectivity in pediatric bipolar disorder. Biol Psychiatry 68(9):839–846, 2010 20739018

Diler RS, Segreti AM, Ladouceur CD, et al: Neural correlates of treatment in adolescents with bipolar depression during response inhibition. J Child Adolesc Psychopharmacol 23(3):214–221, 2013 23607410

Doyle AE, Wilens TE, Kwon A, et al: Neuropsychological functioning in youth with bipolar disorder. Biol Psychiatry 58(7):540–548, 2005 16199011

Dunlop BW, Kelley ME, McGrath CL, et al: Preliminary findings supporting insula metabolic activity as a predictor of outcome to psychotherapy and medication treatments for depression. J Neuropsychiatry Clin Neurosci 27(3):237–239, 2015 26067435

Frazier JA, Chiu S, Breeze JL, et al: Structural brain magnetic resonance imaging of limbic and thalamic volumes in pediatric bipolar disorder. Am J Psychiatry 162(7):1256–1265, 2005 15994707

Frazier TW, Demeter CA, Youngstrom EA, et al: Evaluation and comparison of psychometric instruments for pediatric bipolar spectrum disorders in four age groups. J Child Adolesc Psychopharmacol 17(6):853–866, 2007 18315456

Fusar-Poli P, Howes O, Bechdolf A, et al: Mapping vulnerability to bipolar disorder: a systematic review and meta-analysis of neuroimaging studies. J Psychiatry Neurosci 37(3):170–184, 2012 22297067

Fuster JM: The Prefrontal Cortex. London, Elsevier, 2008

Gao W, Jiao Q, Qi R, et al: Combined analyses of gray matter voxel-based morphometry and white matter tract-based spatial statistics in pediatric bipolar mania. J Affect Disord 150(1):70–76, 2013 23477846

Garrett AS, Miklowitz DJ, Howe ME, et al: Changes in brain activation following psychotherapy for youth with mood dysregulation at familial risk for bipolar disorder. Prog Neuropsychopharmacol Biol Psychiatry 56:215–220, 2015 25283342

Gold AL, Brotman MA, Adleman NE, et al: Comparing brain morphometry across multiple childhood psychiatric disorders. J Am Acad Child Adolesc Psychiatry 55(12):1027.e3–1037.e3, 2016 27871637

Goldman-Rakic PS: Architecture of the prefrontal cortex and the central executive. Ann N Y Acad Sci 769:71–83, 1995 8595045

Goldstein BI, Carnethon MR, Matthews KA, et al; American Heart Association Atherosclerosis; Hypertension and Obesity in Youth Committee of the Council on Cardiovascular Disease in the Young: Major depressive disorder and bipolar disorder predispose youth to accelerated atherosclerosis and early cardiovascular disease: a scientific statement from the American Heart Association. Circulation 132(10):965–986, 2015 26260736

Gorrindo T, Blair RJ, Budhani S, et al: Deficits on a probabilistic response-reversal task in patients with pediatric bipolar disorder. Am J Psychiatry 162(10):1975–1977, 2005 16199850

Grossmann T: The role of medial prefrontal cortex in early social cognition. Front Hum Neurosci 7:340, 2013 23847509

Hafeman DM, Bebko G, Bertocci MA, et al: Abnormal deactivation of the inferior frontal gyrus during implicit emotion processing in youth with bipolar disorder: attenuated by medication. J Psychiatr Res 58:129–136, 2014 25151338

Hajek T, Bernier D, Slaney C, et al: A comparison of affected and unaffected relatives of patients with bipolar disorder using proton magnetic resonance spectroscopy. J Psychiatry Neurosci 33(6):531–540, 2008 18982176

Hajek T, Gunde E, Slaney C, et al: Striatal volumes in affected and unaffected relatives of bipolar patients—high-risk study. J Psychiatr Res 43(7):724–729, 2009 19046588

Hasler G, Drevets WC, Gould TD, et al: Toward constructing an endophenotype strategy for bipolar disorders. Biol Psychiatry 60(2):93–105, 2006 16406007

Horwitz SM, Demeter CA, Pagano ME, et al: Longitudinal Assessment of Manic Symptoms (LAMS) study: background, design, and initial screening results. J Clin Psychiatry 71(11):1511–1517, 2010 21034684

Hynes CA, Baird AA, Grafton ST: Differential role of the orbital frontal lobe in emotional versus cognitive perspective-taking. Neuropsychologia 44(3):374–383, 2006 16112148

Inal-Emiroglu FN, Resmi H, Karabay N, et al: Decreased right hippocampal volumes and neuroprogression markers in adolescents with bipolar disorder. Neuropsychobiology 71(3):140–148, 2015 25925781

Jacobs RH, Pavuluri MN, Schenkel LS, et al: Negative emotion impacts memory for verbal discourse in pediatric bipolar disorder. Bipolar Disord 13(3):287–293, 2011 21676131

Joseph MF, Frazier TW, Youngstrom EA, et al: A quantitative and qualitative review of neurocognitive performance in pediatric bipolar disorder. J Child Adolesc Psychopharmacol 18(6):595–605, 2008 19108664

Kafantaris V, Kingsley P, Ardekani B, et al: Lower orbital frontal white matter integrity in adolescents with bipolar I disorder. J Am Acad Child Adolesc Psychiatry 48(1):79–86, 2009 19050654

Kim E, Garrett A, Boucher S, et al: Inhibited temperament and hippocampal volume in offspring of parents with bipolar disorder. J Child Adolesc Psychopharmacol 27(3):258–265, 2017 27768380

Kim P, Thomas LA, Rosen BH, et al: Differing amygdala responses to facial expressions in children and adults with bipolar disorder. Am J Psychiatry 169(6):642–649, 2012 22535257

Kringelbach ML: The human orbitofrontal cortex: linking reward to hedonic experience. Nat Rev Neurosci 6(9):691–702, 2005 16136173

Kronhaus DM, Lawrence NS, Williams AM, et al: Stroop performance in bipolar disorder: further evidence for abnormalities in the ventral prefrontal cortex. Bipolar Disord 8(1):28–39, 2006 16411978

Krüger S, Alda M, Young LT, et al: Risk and resilience markers in bipolar disorder: brain responses to emotional challenge in bipolar patients and their healthy siblings. Am J Psychiatry 163(2):257–264, 2006 16449479

Ladouceur CD, Diwadkar VA, White R, et al: Fronto-limbic function in unaffected offspring at familial risk for bipolar disorder during an emotional working memory paradigm. Dev Cogn Neurosci 5:185–196, 2013 23590840

Lee MS, Anumagalla P, Talluri P, et al: Meta-analyses of developing brain function in high-risk and emerged bipolar disorder. Front Psychiatry 5:141, 2014 25404919

Leech R, Sharp DJ: The role of the posterior cingulate cortex in cognition and disease. Brain 137 (Pt 1):12–32, 2014 23869106

Leibenluft E: Severe mood dysregulation, irritability, and the diagnostic boundaries of bipolar disorder in youths. Am J Psychiatry 168(2):129–142, 2011 21123313

Leibenluft E, Rich BA, Vinton DT, et al: Neural circuitry engaged during unsuccessful motor inhibition in pediatric bipolar disorder. Am J Psychiatry 164(1):52–60, 2007 17202544

Levy BJ, Wagner AD: Cognitive control and right ventrolateral prefrontal cortex: reflexive reorienting, motor inhibition, and action updating. Ann N Y Acad Sci 1224(1):40–62, 2011 21486295

Lim CS, Baldessarini RJ, Vieta E, et al: Longitudinal neuroimaging and neuropsychological changes in bipolar disorder patients: review of the evidence. Neurosci Biobehav Rev 37(3):418–435, 2013 23318228

Manelis A, Ladouceur CD, Graur S, et al: Altered amygdala-prefrontal response to facial emotion in offspring of parents with bipolar disorder. Brain 138 (Pt 9):2777–2790, 2015 26112339

May JC, Delgado MR, Dahl RE, et al: Event-related functional magnetic resonance imaging of reward-related brain circuitry in children and adolescents. Biol Psychiatry 55(4):359–366, 2004 14960288

Mayberg HS, Liotti M, Brannan SK, et al: Reciprocal limbic-cortical function and negative mood: converging PET findings in depression and normal sadness. Am J Psychiatry 156(5):675–682, 1999 10327898

McClure EB, Treland JE, Snow J, et al: Deficits in social cognition and response flexibility in pediatric bipolar disorder. Am J Psychiatry 162(9):1644–1651, 2005 16135623

Mourão-Miranda J, Almeida JR, Hassel S, et al: Pattern recognition analyses of brain activation elicited by happy and neutral faces in unipolar and bipolar depression. Bipolar Disord 14(4):451–460, 2012 22631624

Nieuwenhuis IL, Takashima A: The role of the ventromedial prefrontal cortex in memory consolidation. Behav Brain Res 218(2):325–334, 2011 21147169

Olsavsky AK, Brotman MA, Rutenberg JG, et al: Amygdala hyperactivation during face emotion processing in unaffected youth at risk for bipolar disorder. J Am Acad Child Adolesc Psychiatry 51(3):294–303, 2012 22365465

Passarotti AM, Sweeney JA, Pavuluri MN: Emotion processing influences working memory circuits in pediatric bipolar disorder and attention-deficit/hyperactivity disorder. J Am Acad Child Adolesc Psychiatry 49(10):1064–1080, 2010a

Passarotti AM, Sweeney JA, Pavuluri MN: Neural correlates of response inhibition in pediatric bipolar disorder and attention deficit hyperactivity disorder. Psychiatry Res 181(1):36–43, 2010b 19926457

Passarotti AM, Sweeney JA, Pavuluri MN: Fronto-limbic dysfunction in mania pretreatment and persistent amygdala over-activity post-treatment in pediatric bipolar disorder. Psychopharmacology (Berl) 216(4):485–499, 2011 21390505

Passarotti AM, Ellis J, Wegbreit E, et al: Reduced functional connectivity of prefrontal regions and amygdala within affect and working memory networks in pediatric bipolar disorder. Brain Connect 2(6):320–334, 2012 23035965

Passarotti AM, Fitzgerald JM, Sweeney JA, et al: Negative emotion interference during a synonym matching task in pediatric bipolar disorder with and without attention deficit hyperactivity disorder. J Int Neuropsychol Soc 19(5):601–612, 2013 23398984

Patino LR, Adler CM, Mills NP, et al: Conflict monitoring and adaptation in individuals at familial risk for developing bipolar disorder. Bipolar Disord 15(3):264–271, 2013 23528067

Pavuluri MN: Neurobiology of bipolar disorder in youth: brain domain dysfunction is translated to decode the pathophysiology and understand the nuances of the clinical manifestation. Front Psychiatry 5:141, 2014

Pavuluri MN: Neurobiology of bipolar disorder in youth: brain domain dysfunction is translated to decode the pathophysiology and understand the nuances of the clinical manifestation, in Bipolar Disorder in Youth: Presentation, Treatment, and Neurobiology. Edited by Strakowski SM, DelBello MP, Adler CM. New York, Oxford University Press, 2015a, pp 282–304

Pavuluri MN: Neuroscience-based formulation and treatment for early onset bipolar disorder: a paradigm shift. Curr Treat Options Psychiatry 2(3):229–251, 2015b

Pavuluri MN, May A: Differential treatment of pediatric bipolar disorder and attention-deficit/hyperactivity disorder. Psychiatr Ann 44(10):471–480, 2014

Pavuluri MN, May A: I feel, therefore, I am: the insula and its role in human emotion, cognition, and the sensory-motor system. AIMS Neuroscience 2(1):18–27, 2015

Pavuluri MN, Herbener ES, Sweeney JA: Affect regulation: a systems neuroscience perspective. Neuropsychiatr Dis Treat 1(1):9–15, 2005 18568120

Pavuluri MN, O'Connor MM, Harral EM, et al: Impact of neurocognitive function on academic difficulties in pediatric bipolar disorder: a clinical translation. Biol Psychiatry 60(9):951–956, 2006a 16730333

Pavuluri MN, Schenkel LS, Aryal S, et al: Neurocognitive function in unmedicated manic and medicated euthymic pediatric bipolar patients. Am J Psychiatry 163(2):286–293, 2006b 16449483

Pavuluri MN, O'Connor MM, Harral E, et al: Affective neural circuitry during facial emotion processing in pediatric bipolar disorder. Biol Psychiatry 62(2):158–167, 2007 17097071

Pavuluri MN, O'Connor MM, Harral EM, et al: An fMRI study of the interface between affective and cognitive neural circuitry in pediatric bipolar disorder. Psychiatry Res 162(3):244–255, 2008 18294820

Pavuluri MN, Passarotti AM, Harral EM, et al: An fMRI study of the neural correlates of incidental versus directed emotion processing in pediatric bipolar disorder. J Am Acad Child Adolesc Psychiatry 48(3):308–319, 2009a 19242292

Pavuluri MN, West A, Hill SK, et al: Neurocognitive function in pediatric bipolar disorder: 3-year follow-up shows cognitive development lagging behind healthy youths. J Am Acad Child Adolesc Psychiatry 48(3):299–307, 2009b 19182689

Pavuluri MN, Yang S, Kamineni K, et al: Diffusion tensor imaging study of white matter fiber tracts in pediatric bipolar disorder and attention-deficit/hyperactivity disorder. Biol Psychiatry 65(7):586–593, 2009c 19027102

Pavuluri MN, Henry DB, Findling RL, et al: Double-blind randomized trial of risperidone versus divalproex in pediatric bipolar disorder. Bipolar Disord 12(6):593–605, 2010a 20868458

Pavuluri MN, Passarotti AM, Mohammed T, et al: Enhanced working and verbal memory after lamotrigine treatment in pediatric bipolar disorder. Bipolar Disord 12(2):213–220, 2010b 20402714

Pavuluri MN, Passarotti AM, Lu LH, et al: Double-blind randomized trial of risperidone versus divalproex in pediatric bipolar disorder: fMRI outcomes. Psychiatry Res 193(1):28–37, 2011 21592741

Pavuluri MN, Ellis JA, Wegbreit E, et al: Pharmacotherapy impacts functional connectivity among affective circuits during response inhibition in pediatric mania. Behav Brain Res 226(2):493–503, 2012a 22004983

Pavuluri MN, Passarotti AM, Fitzgerald JM, et al: Risperidone and divalproex differentially engage the fronto-striato-temporal circuitry in pediatric mania: a pharmacological functional magnetic resonance imaging study. J Am Acad Child Adolesc Psychiatry 51(2):157.e5–170.e5, 2012b 22265362

Pavuluri MN, Volpe K, Yuen A: Nucleus accumbens and its role in reward and emotional circuitry: a potential hot mess in substance use and emotional disorders. AIMS Neuroscience 4(1):52–70, 2017

Pfeifer JC, Welge J, Strakowski SM, et al: Meta-analysis of amygdala volumes in children and adolescents with bipolar disorder. J Am Acad Child Adolesc Psychiatry 47(11):1289–1298, 2008 18827720

Phelps EA, LeDoux JE: Contributions of the amygdala to emotion processing: from animal models to human behavior. Neuron 48(2):175–187, 2005 16242399

Phillips ML, Kupfer DJ: Bipolar disorder diagnosis: challenges and future directions. Lancet 381(9878):1663–1671, 2013 23663952

Rich BA, Schmajuk M, Perez-Edgar KE, et al: The impact of reward, punishment, and frustration on attention in pediatric bipolar disorder. Biol Psychiatry 58(7):532–539, 2005 15953589

Rich BA, Vinton DT, Roberson-Nay R, et al: Limbic hyperactivation during processing of neutral facial expressions in children with bipolar disorder. Proc Natl Acad Sci USA 103(23):8900–8905, 2006 16735472

Rich BA, Holroyd T, Carver FW, et al: A preliminary study of the neural mechanisms of frustration in pediatric bipolar disorder using magnetoencephalography. Depress Anxiety 27(3):276–286, 2010 20037920

Robinson JL, Laird AR, Glahn DC, et al: The functional connectivity of the human caudate: an application of meta-analytic connectivity modeling with behavioral filtering. Neuroimage 60(1):117–129, 2012 22197743

Röttig D, Röttig S, Brieger P, et al: Temperament and personality in bipolar I patients with and without mixed episodes. J Affect Disord 104(1–3):97–102, 2007 17428544

Roybal DJ, Barnea-Goraly N, Kelley R, et al: Widespread white matter tract aberrations in youth with familial risk for bipolar disorder. Psychiatry Res 232(2):184–192, 2015 25779034

Schenkel LS, Pavuluri MN, Herbener ES, et al: Facial emotion processing in acutely ill and euthymic patients with pediatric bipolar disorder. J Am Acad Child Adolesc Psychiatry 46(8):1070–1079, 2007 17667485

Schenkel LS, Marlow-O'Connor M, Moss M, et al: Theory of mind and social inference in children and adolescents with bipolar disorder. Psychol Med 38(6):791–800, 2008 18208632

Schenkel LS, West AE, Jacobs R, et al: Cognitive dysfunction is worse among pediatric patients with bipolar disorder Type I than Type II. J Child Psychol Psychiatry 53(7):775–781, 2012 22339488

Schenkel LS, Chamberlain TF, Towne TL: Impaired theory of mind and psychosocial functioning among pediatric patients with Type I versus Type II bipolar disorder. Psychiatry Res 215(3):740–746, 2014 24461271

Schroll H, Hamker FH: Computational models of basal-ganglia pathway functions: focus on functional neuroanatomy. Front Syst Neurosci 7:122, 2013 24416002

Singh MK, DelBello MP, Adler CM, et al: Neuroanatomical characterization of child offspring of bipolar parents. J Am Acad Child Adolesc Psychiatry 47(5):526–531, 2008a 18356766

Singh MK, DelBello MP, Strakowski SM: Temperament in child offspring of parents with bipolar disorder. J Child Adolesc Psychopharmacol 18(6):589–593, 2008b 19108663

Singh MK, Chang KD, Kelley RG, et al: Reward processing in adolescents with bipolar I disorder. J Am Acad Child Adolesc Psychiatry 52(1):68–83, 2013a 23265635

Singh MK, Jo B, Adleman NE, et al: Prospective neurochemical characterization of child offspring of parents with bipolar disorder. Psychiatry Res 214(2):153–160, 2013b 24028795

Singh MK, Kelley RG, Howe ME, et al: Reward processing in healthy offspring of parents with bipolar disorder. JAMA Psychiatry 71(10):1148–1156, 2014 25142103

Sparks GM, Axelson DA, Yu H, et al: Disruptive mood dysregulation disorder and chronic irritability in youth at familial risk for bipolar disorder. J Am Acad Child Adolesc Psychiatry 53(4):408–416, 2014 24655650

Strakowski SM, Fleck DE, DelBello MP, et al: Impulsivity across the course of bipolar disorder. Bipolar Disord 12(3):285–297, 2010 20565435

Thermenos HW, Makris N, Whitfield-Gabrieli S, et al: A functional MRI study of working memory in adolescents and young adults at genetic risk for bipolar disorder: preliminary findings. Bipolar Disord 13(3):272–286, 2011 21676130

Tseng WL, Bones BL, Kayser RR, et al: An fMRI study of emotional face encoding in youth at risk for bipolar disorder. Eur Psychiatry 30(1):94–98, 2015 25172156

Versace A, Sharma V, Bertocci MA, et al: Using machine learning and surface reconstruction to accurately differentiate different trajectories of mood and energy dysregulation in youth. PLoS One 12(7):e0180221, 2017 28683115

Völlm BA, Taylor AN, Richardson P, et al: Neuronal correlates of theory of mind and empathy: a functional magnetic resonance imaging study in a nonverbal task. Neuroimage 29(1):90–98, 2006 16122944

Wager TD, Davidson ML, Hughes BL, et al: Prefrontal-subcortical pathways mediating successful emotion regulation. Neuron 59(6):1037–1050, 2008 18817740

Weathers JD, Stringaris A, Deveney CM, et al: A developmental study of the neural circuitry mediating motor inhibition in bipolar disorder. Am J Psychiatry 169(6):633–641, 2012 22581312

Wegbreit E, Ellis JA, Nandam A, et al: Amygdala functional connectivity predicts pharmacotherapy outcome in pediatric bipolar disorder. Brain Connect 1(5):411–422, 2011 22432455

West AE, Weinstein SM, Peters AT, et al: Child- and family focused cognitive-behavioral therapy for pediatric bipolar disorder: a randomized clinical trial. J Am Acad Child Adolesc Psychiatry 53(11):1168–1178, 2014 25440307

West AE, Weinstein SM, Pavuluri MN: Rainbow: A Child- and Family-Focused Cognitive-Behavioral Treatment for Pediatric Bipolar Disorder: Clinician Guide. New York, Oxford University Press, 2018

Whalley HC, Sussmann JE, Romaniuk L, et al: Prediction of depression in individuals at high familial risk of mood disorders using functional magnetic resonance imaging. PLoS One 8(3):e57357, 2013 23483904

Whitney J, Joormann J, Gotlib IH, et al: Information processing in adolescents with bipolar I disorder. J Child Psychol Psychiatry 53(9):937–945, 2012 22390273

Whitney J, Howe M, Shoemaker V, et al: Socio-emotional processing and functioning of youth at high risk for bipolar disorder. J Affect Disord 148(1):112–117, 2013 23123133

Wiggins JL, Brotman MA, Adleman NE, et al: Neural markers in pediatric bipolar disorder and familial risk for bipolar disorder. J Am Acad Child Adolesc Psychiatry 56(1):67–78, 2017 27993231

Wilke M, Kowatch RA, DelBello MP, et al: Voxel-based morphometry in adolescents with bipolar disorder: first results. Psychiatry Res 131(1):57–69, 2004 15246455

Yang H, Lu LH, Wu M, et al: Time course of recovery showing initial prefrontal cortex changes at 16 weeks, extending to subcortical changes by 3 years in pediatric bipolar disorder. J Affect Disord 150(2):571–577, 2013 23517886

Yurgelun-Todd DA, Gruber SA, Kanayama G, et al: fMRI during affect discrimination in bipolar affective disorder. Bipolar Disord 2(3 Pt 2):237–248, 2000 11249801

Part 2
TREATMENT

7

Evidence-Based Psychotherapies for Pediatric Depressive Disorders

Pilar Santamarina, Ph.D.

M. Melissa Packer, M.A.

Peter, a 10-year-old, was recently brought to a child mental health clinic by his parents because of concerns about irritability, somatic complaints, negativity, frequent crying, and a drop in school performance. Peter's parents first noticed these behaviors at the beginning of the school year, and the behaviors progressively increased over the last 6 months in intensity and frequency to the point of creating a lot of family conflict. Peter attends fifth grade at a public elementary school.

Peter lives with his parents and has no siblings. His family relocated from Boston to San Diego a year ago because of his father's job. The family adjusted well to the move, and both parents continue to work full time. Aside from the move, another source of stress for the family was the fact that Peter's maternal grandfather, who has chronic major depressive disorder, was recently hospitalized after trying to end his life. Peter's parents described their son as a smart boy with more interest in chess and intellectual pursuits than in sports activities compared with his peers. Although Peter is shy, he has never had problems making and keeping friends. In the past few months, his parents have noted a lack of interest in playing chess or other activities that were previously enjoyable for Peter.

When Peter went to the clinic, the clinician evaluating him noticed that he avoided eye contact and spoke very little. During the first few psychotherapy sessions, the clinician focused on strengthening the therapeutic alliance with Peter. After several sessions, Peter felt more comfortable talking about his feelings. He reported that at the beginning of the school year, he was glad to go to school because he made some friends and joined their group of friends. However, after noticing how smart he was in class, this peer group labeled him as a nerd and began excluding him. Peter felt alone but did not say anything in order to avoid concerning his parents. However, when he gave up his extracurricular activities and his school absences increased, his parents inevitably became concerned.

On the basis of a comprehensive clinical evaluation, the clinician determined that Peter's symptoms met the criteria for a depressive disorder. Peter's treatment began with psychoeducation sessions about depression for him and his parents. Then, to increase activation, the clinician engaged Peter with activity selection strategies to identify specific positive activities from which he could derive pleasure. Peter also received relaxation sessions to manage his social anxiety. With sufficient mastery over his anxiety, Peter was gradually able to improve his school attendance. In therapy, Peter rehearsed social skills to improve interpersonal functioning and practiced cognitive techniques to alter negative interpretations of social situations. Peter's parents also learned how to enhance their ability to effectively parent Peter during these stressful situations.

Evidence-Based Psychotherapies for Pediatric Depression

As we can see in other chapters of this book, depression in youth is a common, chronic, and recurrent condition (Brent and Weersing 2010) associated with negative consequences, including occupational and educational impairments, social difficulties and poor peer relationships, increased rate of smoking and substance abuse, lower life satisfaction, and reduced global functioning (Lewinsohn et al. 1998; Thapar et al. 2012; Verboom et al. 2014). Consequently, there is a need to find effective interventions to treat depression in this age group. The objective of this chapter is to review evidence-based psychosocial interventions for pediatric depression that are commonly used as first-line treatments of symptoms.

This chapter began with a case that represents the typical initial symptoms observed in depressed youth. Children and adolescents are more likely than adults to display an irritable rather than a sad mood; thus, psychosocial treatments in youth are tailored to accommodate this important developmental difference. Over the last three decades, evidence for the effectiveness of psychosocial treatments for depression in children and adolescents has grown (Qin et al. 2015). Currently, many different types of psychotherapy are being used in clinical practice to treat depression in children and adolescents. These may include therapies such as cognitive-behavioral therapy (CBT), interpersonal psychotherapy (IPT), family therapy, play therapy, relaxation techniques, motivational interviewing, and psychodynamic psychotherapies. The two most commonly studied psychotherapies in the treatment of pediatric depression are CBT and IPT.

CBT is based on the premise that depression comes from maladaptive information processing strategies and is sustained by dysfunctional behavioral responses to aberrant cognitions (Beck et al. 1979). The therapy concentrates on identifying and modifying the utility, content, and structure of cognitions that accompany negative affect. The intervention also teaches patients other methods of behaving or thinking (Lemmens et al. 2015) to improve their mood and functioning. It is well established that CBT is efficacious in the treatment of adult depression (Cuijpers et al. 2013). Some of the interventions based on the CBT model include social skills, self-control therapy (which teaches self-management skills), cognitive restructuring, and problem-solving strategies.

IPT is a manualized, typically time-limited psychotherapeutic approach that was designed for the treatment of acute major depressive episodes but has been adapted for other psychological disorders (Klerman 1984; Weissman et al. 2007). It is less structured than CBT. The focus of IPT is on present psychosocial and interpersonal events and problem areas associated with depression and affect (Markowitz 2010; Schramm et al. 2011). The therapeutic relationship is described as helpful and supportive. Components include addressing grief, role transitions, interpersonal role conflicts, and interpersonal deficits (Mufson et al. 2004). Mechanisms of change in IPT include 1) augmenting social support, 2) reducing interpersonal stress, 3) aiding emotional processing, and 4) cultivating interpersonal skills (Lipsitz and Markowitz 2013). IPT has shown efficacy in treating major depressive disorder in many studies in adults (Markowitz 2010).

There are several versions of psychotherapy available for depressed youth. These formats vary widely depending on the theoretical orientation used and the nature of the patient's problems. Individual psychotherapy involves one-on-one interaction with a therapist and, as such, does not focus as much on the live, dynamic relational interactions that occur in therapy sessions as a group or family format would. The areas of focus in individual therapy, however, can still comprise improving relationships and social skills. Group psychotherapy can take the form of a prevention program, a psychoeducation program, or a process-oriented approach in which individuals in the group speak about their experiences while commenting on or relating to the experiences of others in the group. The family format of psychotherapy can encompass a blend of characteristics from the individual and group therapy formats in that relational issues and dynamics are navigated in session, and individual skill-building can be taught and practiced in sessions but applied, at least in part, to family dynamics.

In this chapter, we review findings from randomized controlled trials (RCTs) in order to present the current evidence base for psychosocial treatments in youth depression. We discuss main results obtained from the most current reviews published to date that synthesize the extant literature.

Evidence was categorized following an adaptation of the Task Force on Promotion and Dissemination of Psychological Procedures criteria (Southam-Gerow and Prinstein 2014). Within this classification system, treatments are assessed based on five methods criteria and then categorized into five levels of efficacy. An intervention study is considered of good quality if it 1) involves a randomized controlled trial (RCT) design; 2) uses treatment manuals; 3) clearly defines its target population and inclusion criteria; 4) uses reliable and valid outcome measures to assess the intervention targets; and 5) utilizes appropriate statistical analyses and a sample size large enough to detect possible intervention effects.

On the basis of this classification, evidence was categorized into level 1, or "well-established treatments" when at least two studies demonstrated that a treatment was more effective than placebo or an alternative intervention or was as effective as a well-established treatment and were carried out by two different research teams. An intervention was deemed level 2, or "probably efficacious," if at least two studies showed the treatment to be superior to a wait-list condition but independent replication by different research teams was lacking. Level 3, or "possibly efficacious treatments," was used as a classification for a treatment if at least one RCT showed that the treatment was superior to a no-treatment control group and met all five methods criteria, or if at least two clinical trials were in favor of the treatment and met at least two methods criteria of the last four. "Experimental criteria," or level 4, was utilized for treatments that have not been tested in an RCT or if their efficacy has been shown in at least one study not meeting level 3 criteria. For "treatments of questionable efficacy," or level 5, the results showed that the treatment was not superior to another treatment or a type of control group. Criteria for evidence-based psychotherapies are summarized in Table 7–1.

In line with previous reviews, the next two subsections are organized according to studies conducted with children and those conducted with adolescents (Table 7–2).

TABLE 7–1. Criteria for evidence-based psychotherapies

Methods criteria

M1	Group design: a randomized controlled design
M2	Treatment manuals
M3	Population clarified
M4	Reliable and valid outcome assessment measures
M5	Appropriate data analysis

Evidence criteria

Level 1: Well-established treatments	At least two studies demonstrated that the treatment was more efficacious than pill or psychological placebo or an alternative intervention, or was as effective as a well-established treatment; were carried out by two independent research teams; and used all five methods criteria
Level 2: Probably efficacious treatments	Treatments must meet all five methods criteria and be shown to be superior to a wait list in at least two studies or meet well-established criteria in at least one study (Level 2 will not involve independent research groups)
Level 3: Possibly efficacious treatments	At least one good randomized controlled trial (RCT) showed that the treatment was more effective than wait-list group and the trial used all five methods criteria; or at least two clinical studies meeting at least two of criteria 2, 3, 4, or 5
Level 4: Experimental treatments	Not yet tested in an RCT; efficacy demonstrated in at least one study but not sufficient to meet level 3 criteria
Level 5: Treatments of questionable efficacy	Treatment has not been found to be superior to another treatment or a type of control group

---

Evidence-Based Psychotherapies for Children

Depression in children younger than 12 years is less common than among adolescents. Thus, the evidence on the effectiveness of psychotherapy in children compared with adolescents is more limited. In 1998, Kaslow and Thompson carried out one of the first comprehensive reviews of psychosocial interventions for children with depression. The authors assessed specific manualized protocols rather than theoretical orientations (e.g., CBT or IPT). Kaslow and Thompson analyzed seven studies that had enrolled children under age 12 years. Most studies included interventions that were based on a

TABLE 7–2. Randomized clinical trials and reviews of psychosocial treatments for depression in children and adolescents

Trial	Design	Sample	Treatment	Measures	Results
Asarnow et al. 2005	RCT	N=418 Ages: 13–21 Depressive symptoms	CBT vs. usual care	CES-D, MCS-12, and a scale to assess satisfaction with mental health care	CBT group had more improvement in depressive symptoms and quality of life, and greater satisfaction with mental health care, compared with usual care
Brent et al. 1997	RCT	N=107 Ages: 13–18 Depressive disorder	Individual CBT, family therapy, or individual supportive therapy	K-SADS, BDI	CBT was more effective than the other conditions
Brent et al. 2008 (TORDIA)	RCT	N=334 Ages: 12–18 Fluoxetine-resistant depressive disorder	4 conditions, switching to a different SSRI, a different SSRI+CBT, venlafaxine, or venlafaxine+CBT	CDRS-R, CGI, K-SADS	CBT+either medication condition had greater improvements compared with medication alone Venlafaxine showed fewer adverse effects

TABLE 7–2. Randomized clinical trials and reviews of psychosocial treatments for depression in children and adolescents *(continued)*

Trial	Design	Sample	Treatment	Measures	Results
Clarke et al. 1999	RCT	N=123 Ages: 14–18 Major depression or dysthymia	Adolescent group CBT; adolescent-parent group CBT or wait-list control	K-SADS, LIFE	CBT was superior to wait list in reducing depressive symptoms
Clarke et al. 2001	RCT	N=49 Ages: 13–18 Adolescent offspring of depressed parents	Usual care vs. usual care+group CBT	K-SADS, CBCL, HAM-D, GAF, CES-D	Group CBT may reduce the risk for depression in the adolescent offspring of parents with depression
Clarke et al. 2002	RCT	N=47 Ages: 13–18 Depressed adolescent offspring of depressed parents	Group CBT vs. usual care	K-SADS, CBCL, HAM-D, GAF, CES-D	Group CBT did not appear to be incrementally beneficial for depressed offspring of depressed parents
Clarke et al. 2005	RCT	N=152 Ages: 12–18 Depressive disorder	Antidepressant vs. antidepressant+ CBT	K-SADS, CES-D, YSR, CGAS, SAS-SR, SF-12	CBT had only a weak effect on reducing depressive symptoms

TABLE 7–2.   Randomized clinical trials and reviews of psychosocial treatments for depression in children and adolescents (*continued*)

Trial	Design	Sample	Treatment	Measures	Results
Cook and Gorraiz 2016	Meta-analysis	12 studies Adolescents Symptoms related to borderline personality disorder	DBT		DBT was effective in reducing NSSI and depression; the effect size was large for NSSI and small for depression
David-Ferdon and Kaslow 2008	Review	24 studies Children and adolescents Depressive disorders or elevated depressive symptoms	CBT, IPT-A, nondirected support, and family systems		CBT for children and CBT and IPT for adolescents appear to be the most promising interventions
De Cuyper et al. 2004	RCT	N=20 Ages: 10–12 Elevated depressive symptoms	CBT vs. wait-list condition	CDI, SPPC, STAIC, CBCL	CBT was superior to control group at posttreatment; results had not been steadily maintained at 12-month follow-up
Diamond et al. 2002	RCT	N=32 Ages: 13–17 Major depressive disorder	ABFT vs. wait-list condition	K-SADS, BDI, CBCL, SRFF, BHS, SIQ, YSR	ABFT was superior in reducing depression and anxiety compared with wait list

TABLE 7–2. Randomized clinical trials and reviews of psychosocial treatments for depression in children and adolescents (*continued*)

Trial	Design	Sample	Treatment	Measures	Results
Diamond et al. 2010	RCT	N=66 Ages: 12–17 Elevated depressive symptoms and suicidality	ABFT (family intervention) vs. usual care	SIQ, BDI, SSI	ABFT was more efficacious than usual care in reducing suicidal ideation and depressive symptoms
Dobson et al. 2010	RCT	N=46 Ages: 13–18 Elevated depressive symptoms	Group CBT (CWS) vs. supportive therapy	CES-D, CDI, BAI, MASQ, CBCL-YSR, SES	Both treatments were effective; CBT was not superior to supportive therapy
Forti-Buratti et al. 2016	Review	7 RCTs Children (≤12 years old) Depressive disorders	CBT, family therapy, and father-child interaction		Review did not find any evidence in favor of CBT; not enough studies for other therapies
Gillham et al. 2006	RCT	N=271 Ages: 11–12 Elevated depressive symptoms	PRP vs. usual care	CASQ, CDI, DICA-R, D-SADS	PRP prevented depression and anxiety symptoms, and adjustment disorders
Goodyer et al. 2007	RCT	N=208 Ages: 11–17 Depressive disorder	SSRI medication vs. SSRI+CBT	K-SADS, CDRS-R, CGAS, CGI	Combination of CBT+SSRI did not improve depressive symptoms

TABLE 7–2. Randomized clinical trials and reviews of psychosocial treatments for depression in children and adolescents (*continued*)

Trial	Design	Sample	Treatment	Measures	Results
Kahn et al. 1990	RCT	$N=68$ Ages: 11–13	CBT vs. wait-list condition	Measures of depression and self-esteem	All treatment conditions, relative to wait-list-control group, evidenced significant decrease in depression and increase in self-esteem
Kaslow and Thompson 1998	Review	14 studies included (children and adolescents)	CBT, IPT-A, family therapy, and supportive therapy		No treatments met criteria for well established; two programs (self-control therapy and CWD-A) were probably efficacious
Kerfoot et al. 2004	RCT	$N=52$ Age mean: 13.9 Elevated depressive symptoms	CBT or TAU delivered by social workers	K-SADS; MFQ; HoNOSCA, SDQ	No differences between groups were found; training social workers in CBT is not effective in improving depression
Lewinsohn et al. 1990	RCT	$N=59$ Ages: 14–18 Depressive disorders	CWD for adolescents and parents, CWD only adolescents, or wait-list condition	K-SADS; BDI, SAQ, SPQ, CES-D, PBI, DAS, IC, CBCL, PES	Treatments improved in the depression measures compared with wait-list group; adolescent-and-parent group was more effective compared with only adolescent group

TABLE 7–2. Randomized clinical trials and reviews of psychosocial treatments for depression in children and adolescents (*continued*)

Trial	Design	Sample	Treatment	Measures	Results
Liddle and Spence 1990	RCT	*N*=21 Ages: 7–11 Depressive disorder	CBT (social competence training), attention placebo control, or no treatment	CDI, CDRS-R	Depressive symptoms decreased at posttreatment in all conditions; results remained steady at 2-month follow-up
Luby et al. 2012	RCT	*N*=54 Ages: 3–7 Depressive disorder	PCIT-ED vs. psychoeducation	PAPA, PFC-S, HBQ, KIDSEDF, ERC, BRIEF, BDI-II, PSI	Both groups improved in several domains; PCIT-ED showed a greater number of domains
March et al. 2004	RCT	*N*=439 Ages: 12–17 Major depressive disorder	Fluoxetine alone, CBT alone, or CBT with fluoxetine or placebo	K-SADS, CDRS-R, CGI, RADS, SIQ	Combination of fluoxetine with CBT offered the most favorable results
Melvin et al. 2006	RCT	*N*=73 Ages: 12–18 Depressive disorder	CBT, antidepressant alone, or CBT + antidepressant	K-SADS, RADS, RCMAS, SIQ	All treatments improved depression; the advantages of a combined approach were not evident
Mufson et al. 1999	RCT	*N*=48 Ages: 12–18 Depressive disorder	IPT-A vs. clinical monitoring	HAMD, K-SADS, DISC, BDI, CGAS, CGI, SAS-SR	IPT-A showed improvement in depressive symptoms, social functioning, and problem-solving skills

TABLE 7–2. Randomized clinical trials and reviews of psychosocial treatments for depression in children and adolescents (*continued*)

Trial	Design	Sample	Treatment	Measures	Results
Mufson et al. 2004	RCT	N=63 Ages: 12–18 Depressive disorder	IPT-A vs. TAU	K-SADS, HAMD, C-GAS, BDI, CGI, SAS-SR	IPT-A showed greater symptom reduction and improvement in overall functioning compared with TAU
Nelson et al. 2003	RCT	N=28 Ages: 8–14 Depressive disorder	Face-to-face CBT vs. videoconferencing CBT	K-SADS, CDI	Both conditions were effective
Richardson et al. 2014	RCT	N=101 Ages: 13–17 Depressive disorder	CBT vs. TAU	K-SADS, CDRS-R, CIS, PHQ-9	CBT improved depressive symptoms compared with TAU
Roberts et al. 2003	RCT	N=189 Ages: 11–13 Elevated depressive symptoms	PRP vs. usual care	CDI, CASQ, RCMAS, CBCL	No intervention effects were found for depression; less anxiety was reported in intervention group compared with control group at 6-month follow-up
Rohde et al. 2004	RCT	N=93 Ages: 13–17 Major depressive disorder and conduct disorder	CWD-A vs. tutoring control condition	BDI-II, HAMD, CBCL, CGAS, SAS-SR	CWD-A was superior to tutoring in reducing depression and improving social functioning posttreatment

TABLE 7–2. Randomized clinical trials and reviews of psychosocial treatments for depression in children and adolescents (*continued*)

Trial	Design	Sample	Treatment	Measures	Results
Rohde et al. 2014	RCT	*N*=170 Ages: 13–18 Major depressive disorder and substance use disorder	CBT after FFT, FFT after CBT, or FFT+CBT	K-SADS, CDRS-R, TLFB	All three conditions reduced depressive symptoms at post-treatment, 6- and 12-month follow-up; FFT followed by CBT improved substance use
Rosselló and Bernal 1999	RCT	*N*=71 Ages: 13–18 Depressive disorder	CBT, IPT, or wait list	CDI, PHCSCS, SAS, FEICS, CBCL	Both CBT and IPT were more effective than wait list
Rosselló et al. 2008	RCT	*N*=112 Ages: 12–18 Depressive disorder	Individual CBT, group CBT, individual IPT, or group IPT	CDI, PHCSCS, CBCL, SAS, DISC	CBT and IPT were effective in both group and individual formats; CBT showed greater decreases in depressive symptoms and improved self-concept than IPT
Sanford et al. 2006	RCT	*N*=41 Ages: 13–18 Depressive disorder	Usual care vs. usual care+family psychoeducation	K-SADS, RADS, SSAI, FAD, ACL, CGAS	Family therapy showed greater improvement in social functioning and adolescent-parent relationships
Shirk et al. 2014	RCT	*N*=43 Ages: 13–17 Depression+trauma	Mindfulness+CBT vs. TAU	Pre-post K-SADS, BDI-II, TESI-C; CBCL; PHCSCS	No differences between groups were found

TABLE 7–2. Randomized clinical trials and reviews of psychosocial treatments for depression in children and adolescents (*continued*)

Trial	Design	Sample	Treatment	Measures	Results
Stallard et al. 2012	RCT	$N=1,064$ Ages: 12–16 Elevated depressive symptoms	CBT, attention control, or usual school provision	MFQ, CATS, SES, RCADS, SDEC	No differences were found between conditions; no improvement in depressive symptoms was noted
Stark et al. 1987	RCT	$N=29$ Ages: 9–12 Elevated depressive symptoms	Self-control, problem-solving, or wait list	CDI, CDS, CDRS-R, CBCL, CSEI, RCMAS	Both experimental groups were superior to wait list in improving depressive symptoms; effects remained steady at 8-week follow-up
Stark et al. 1991	RCT	$N=24$ Ages: 9–13 Elevated depressive symptoms	CBT *vs.* counseling group	K-SADS-P, CDI, ATQ, CSEI, HSC	Both groups improved in depression; improvement in CBT was superior to that in counseling; effects remained steady at 7-month follow-up
Stice et al. 2008	RCT	$N=341$ Ages: 14–19 Elevated depressive symptoms	Group CBT, supportive therapy CBT bibliography, or assessment control	K-SADS, BDI, SAS-SR, substance use, EDDI	CBT was superior to the other conditions for improving depression at posttreatment and 6-month follow-up

TABLE 7–2. Randomized clinical trials and reviews of psychosocial treatments for depression in children and adolescents (*continued*)

Trial	Design	Sample	Treatment	Measures	Results
Szigethy et al. 2014	RCT	N=217 Ages: 9–17 Depressive disorder and inflammatory bowel disease	CBT (PASCET) vs. supportive therapy	CDI; K-SADS; CDRS-R; CGAS	Both treatments were effective; no between-group differences were noted
Trowell et al. 2007	RCT	N=72 Ages: 9–15 Depressive disorder	Individual psycho-dynamic therapy vs. family therapy	K-SADS, CDI, MFQ, CGAS	Both interventions were effective in improving depressive symptoms
Vostanis et al. 1996	RCT	N=57 Ages: 8–17 Depressive disorder	CBT vs. nonfocused control intervention	K-SADS, MFQ, RCMAS, SEI, AS	Both groups improved in depressive and anxiety symptoms, self-esteem, and social functioning
Weersing et al. 2017	Review	42 RCTs Children and adolescents Depressive disorders	CBT, IPT-A, family therapy, and psychodynamic therapy		Evidence for child treatments is weaker than for adolescent interventions; CBT for children appears to be possibly efficacious; CBT and IPT-A are well-established interventions for adolescents

TABLE 7–2. Randomized clinical trials and reviews of psychosocial treatments for depression in children and adolescents (*continued*)

Trial	Design	Sample	Treatment	Measures	Results
Weisz et al. 2009	RCT	N=57 Ages: 8–17 Depressive disorder	CBT (PASCET program) vs. usual care	Diagnostic Interview Schedule for Children (DISC-C and DISC-P), CDI, CBCL, ETOS	No group differences in depression were found; CBT was superior for parent engagement, medication use and dosage, cost, and speed of improvement
Wood et al. 1996	RCT	N=48 Ages: 9–17 Depressive disorder	CBT vs. relaxation	MFQ, RCMAS, SES, ABS	CBT was superior to relaxation in depressive symptoms at posttreatment follow-up; no differences in measures of anxiety were found
Young et al. 2006	RCT	N=41 Ages: 13–17 Elevated depressive symptoms	IPT-A vs. school counseling (SC)	CES-D, K-SADS, CGAS	IPT group had fewer depression symptoms and better overall functioning postintervention and at 6-month follow-up
Young et al. 2010	RCT	N=57 Ages: 13–17 Elevated depressive symptoms	IPT-A vs. school counseling	K-SADS, CGAS, CES-D, CDRS-R	IPT-A improved depressive symptoms after 6 months; no differences after 18 months—patients with IPT stabilized and school counseling continue improving

TABLE 7–2. Randomized clinical trials and reviews of psychosocial treatments for depression in children and adolescents (*continued*)

Trial	Design	Sample	Treatment	Measures	Results

Note. ABFT=attachment-based family therapy; ABS=Antisocial Behavior Scale; ACL=Adjective Check List; AS=Aggression Scale; ATQ=Automatic Thoughts Questionnaire; BAI=Beck Anxiety Inventory; BDI-II=Beck Depression Inventory–II; BHS=Beck Hopelessness Scale; BRIEF=Behavior Rating Inventory of Executive Function—Preschool Version; CASQ=Children's Attributional Style Questionnaire; CATS=Children's Automatic Thoughts Scale; CBCL=Child Behavior Checklist; CBT=cognitive-behavioral therapy; CDI=Children's Depression Inventory; CDRS-R=Children's Depression Rating Scale—Revised; CDS=Children's Depression Scale; CES-D=Center for Epidemiologic Studies—Depression Scale; CGAS=Children's Global Assessment Scale; CGI=Clinical Global Impression; CIS=Columbia Impairment Scale; CSEI=Coopersmith Self-Esteem Inventory; CWD-A=Adolescent Coping With Depression Course; DAS=Dysfunctional Attitudes Scale; DBT=dialectical behavior therapy; DICA-R=Diagnostic Interview for Children and Adolescents—Revised; DISC=Diagnostic Interview Schedule for Children; EDDI=Eating Disorder Diagnostic Interview; ERC=Emotion Regulation Checklist; ETOS=Expectations of Therapy Outcome Scale; FAD=Family Assessment Device; FEICS=Family Emotional Involvement and Criticism Scale; FFT=functional family therapy; GAF=Global Assessment of Functioning Scale; HAMD=Hamilton Depression Rating Scale; HBQ=Health and Behavior Questionnaire; HoNOSCA=Health of the Nation Outcome Scale for Children and Adolescents; HSC=Hopelessness Scale for Children; IC=Issues Checklist; IPT-A=interpersonal therapy for adolescents; KIDSEDF=Penn Emotion Differentiation Test; K-SADS=Schedule for Affective Disorders and Schizophrenia for School-Age Children; LIFE=Longitudinal Inventory Follow-up Evaluation; MASQ=Mood and Anxiety Symptom Questionnaire; MCS-12=Mental Health Summary Score; MFQ=Mood and Feelings Questionnaire; NSSI=nonsuicidal self-injury; PAPA=Preschool Age Psychiatric Assessment; PASCET=Primary and Secondary Control Enhancement Training; PBI=Personality Behavior Inventory; PCIT-ED=Parent-Child Interaction Therapy Emotion Development; PES=Pleasant Events Schedule; PFC-S=Preschool Feelings Checklist—Scale Version; PHCSCS=Piers-Harris Children's Self-Concept Scale; PHQ-9=Patient Health Questionnaire–9; PRP=Penn Resiliency Program; PSI=Parenting Stress Index; RADS=Reynolds Adolescent Depression Scale; RCADS=Revised Child Anxiety and Depression Scale; RCMAS=Revised Children's Manifest Anxiety Scale; RCT=randomized controlled trial; SAS-SR=Social Adjustment Scale—Self-Report; SAQ=State Anxiety Questionnaire; SDEC=Scale Developments and Educational Correlates; SDQ=Strengths and Difficulties Questionnaire; SES=Self-Esteem Scale; SIQ=Suicidal Ideation Questionnaire; SPPC=Self-Perception Profile for Children; SPQ=Schizotypal Personality Questionnaire; SF-12=Short Form-12; SRFF=Self-Report of Family Functioning; SSAI=Structured Social Adjustment Interview; SSRI=selective serotonin reuptake inhibitor; STAIC=State-Trait Anxiety Inventory for Children; TAU=treatment as usual; TESI-C=Trauma Experiences Screening Interview; TORDIA=Treatment of (SSRI) Resistant Depression in Adolescents; TLFB=Timeline Followback Interview (drugs used daily); YSR=Youth Self-Report.

cognitive-behavioral model, including modules such as social skills training, self-control therapy, cognitive restructuring, or problem-solving strategies. All of the interventions presented were conducted in a school setting with a group format. The review concluded that no treatments showed well-established evidence for treating childhood depression, and the one therapy that was considered only "probably effective" was self-control therapy for children with elevated depressive symptoms (Stark et al. 1987). Self-control therapy was tested in 29 children ages 9–12 years with depressive symptoms assessed with the Children's Depression Inventory (CDI; Kovacs 1996). Youth were assigned to three different groups: self-control treatment focused on teaching self-management skills, problem-solving therapy in order to improve social behavior and self-management of unpleasant events, and a wait-list control condition. Subjects following both active treatments improved in depressive symptomatology compared with the wait-list group. These results were replicated several years later, including with only self-control therapy (Stark et al. 1991). Importantly, these studies involved treatment of youth with depressive symptoms rather than youth with an established diagnosis of a depressive disorder based on DSM-III-R (American Psychiatric Association 1987). Thus, the evidence is limited to youth who may have nonspecific depressive symptoms that may or may not be related to a depressive disorder. For young children, this limitation may not be too problematic, given that symptoms of depression can remain sub-threshold or ill-defined for many years before meeting threshold diagnostic criteria but yet may cause sufficient impairment to warrant intervention.

Psychotherapy for childhood depression was reviewed again 20 years later by David-Ferdon and Kaslow (2008). In contrast to Kaslow's previous review, the review included both youth who met diagnostic criteria for a depressive disorder from clinical settings and youth who showed elevated depressive symptom scores from school settings. David-Ferdon and Kaslow analyzed 10 additional RCTs conducted with child samples published since 1998. Most studies used interventions based on CBT that involved teaching skills to monitor mood symptoms, regulate emotions, schedule pleasant activities, restructure cognitive thoughts, improve communication, and achieve problem resolution. Some studies focused on other theoretical orientations, such as psychodynamic therapy, family therapy, and a combination of psychoeducation and support therapy. David-Ferdon and Kaslow (2008) also included individual, group, and child and parent dyadic formats, and studies whose primary endpoint was to reduce depressive symptoms.

In general, David-Ferdon and Kaslow observed that many interventions were effective in improving depressive symptoms in school and clinical settings compared with control conditions (e.g., wait-list, community services). However, none of the psychosocial treatments reviewed was deemed to be a well-established intervention in depressive children. Regarding follow-up studies, the results varied. Some of them showed improvement of depressive symptoms at 3 and 6 months' follow-up, whereas others did not show any improvement at follow-up. David-Ferdon and Kaslow concluded that further studies were needed to evaluate the long-term benefits of psychosocial interventions for depression in children. None of the studies showed high methodological quality because of small sample size, unclear inclusion and exclusion criteria, and problems with diagnostic information and with the randomization protocol. For the second part of the review, David-Ferdon and Kaslow organized the evidence in support of specific programs, modalities of intervention, and theoretical orientations. On the basis of the Task Force on the Promotion and Dissemination of Psychological Procedures guidelines, the review authors found that there were no specific programs deemed to be well-established interventions. Two programs met criteria for "probably efficacious" interventions for depressive children: self-control therapy (Stark et al. 1987, 1991), consistent with the previous review (Kaslow and Thompson 1998), and the Penn Prevention Program (Gillham et al. 2006; Roberts et al. 2003). The Penn Prevention Program developed a manual for group therapy with 10- to 14-year-old youth based on cognitive-behavioral theories. During the sessions, the therapists taught skills on identifying the links between thoughts and feelings of depression and anxiety and then generating alternative thoughts.

Regarding modality classification schemata, two modalities were considered well established: group CBT for children and group CBT for children and parents. These modalities were more effective in reducing depressive symptoms than control or other treatments, and studies were replicated by two independent research teams.

Finally, when theoretical orientations were analyzed using a broad approach, the review concluded that CBT met criteria for a well-established intervention and behavior therapy met criteria for a probably effective intervention.

A recent review evaluated RCTs published between 2008 and 2014 and reevaluated previously reviewed evidence (Weersing et al. 2017). This review only included subjects whose symptoms met diagnostic criteria for depressive disorders and also analyzed well-designed RCTs with null or negative findings. This review considered some of the studies included in the previous review but excluded others that did not meet the methods criteria. Finally, they included seven RCTs for the children sample, only one of which had been published since the last review (Weisz et al. 2009). In this pool of seven studies, one showed positive findings in favor of CBT compared with the wait-list condition (Kahn et al. 1990). Four studies showed confusing findings on CBT because of the range of comparison conditions used (De Cuyper et al. 2004; Nelson et al. 2003; Stark et al. 1987; Weisz et al. 2009). Two studies did not find significant findings between CBT and control conditions (Liddle and Spence 1990; Vostanis et al. 1996). The review concluded that there were no well-established psychological treatments for child depression. The most effective treatments in this age group were group CBT, technology-assisted CBT, and behavior therapy, all of which were classified as "possibly efficacious." Thus, CBT as a broader theoretical orientation did not meet criteria to be considered a probably efficacious or a well-established intervention, as suggested by the David-Ferdon and Kaslow (2008) review, because the Weersing review included studies with null results and excluded subsyndromal symptoms. Other types of therapies, such as individual CBT, psychodynamic therapy, and family-based intervention, did not show enough evidence because of the paucity of studies, so they were considered "experimental" for child depression.

A systematic review and meta-analysis published in 2016 focused on assessing the efficacy of psychological treatments for depressive children up to 12 years of age (Forti-Buratti et al. 2016). The authors of this review searched for all relevant RCTs (published and unpublished) in the main databases and included seven studies. Five out of seven studies used CBT in either individual or group format (Brent et al. 2008; Liddle and Spence 1990; March et al. 2004; Stallard et al. 2012; Stark et al. 1987), one study used family therapy (Luby et al. 2012), and another one tested the efficacy between family therapy and psychodynamic psychotherapy (Trowell et al. 2007). The authors suggested that combined results from the studies are not enough to confirm that CBT is better than no treatment. The evidence base was even more limited for family therapy and psychodynamic therapy.

In conclusion, there is no clear preponderance of evidence on which psychological treatment is the most effective for children with depression, in part because of the paucity of studies researching depression interventions in this young age group. In general, there is relatively more evidence in favor of the CBT paradigm than with other orientations, but the evidence level is still limited. Additional evidence is needed to confirm the effectiveness and the comparative effectiveness of the aforementioned interventions in children.

Evidence-Based Psychotherapies for Adolescents

On the basis of the prevalence and age at onset of depression, there are expectedly more studies conducted in adolescents with depression than in children. In the review by Kaslow and Thompson (1998), seven studies with adolescents were assessed. The subjects showed elevated depression symptoms or had symptoms that met diagnostic criteria for major depressive disorder or dysthymia. The authors determined that there were no treatments meeting criteria for well-established interventions, but one treatment program was probably efficacious in adolescents: the Adolescent Coping With Depression (CWD-A) treatment developed by Lewinsohn et al. (1990). This treatment uses a manual for a cognitive-behavioral group intervention in order to teach skills for increasing pleasant activities, relaxation, restructuring depressive thoughts, and improving social skills.

In the next review, published in 2008, David-Ferdon and Kaslow included 18 studies that used samples of adolescents between 12 and 18 years of age. Twelve studies enrolled adolescents with symptoms that met DSM-III-R or DSM-IV (American Psychiatric Association 1987, 1994) criteria for depressive disorders , and six studies included adolescents at high risk for developing a depressive disorder based on elevated depressive symptoms. Compared with the child studies reviewed, there were more studies with adolescents that included participants with clinical depressive disorders rather than some level of depressive symptoms. Interventions could be facilitated in individual, group, and adolescent-parent formats, as in studies presenting interventions for children. Most interventions were based on the CBT model (Asarnow et al. 2005; Clarke et al. 1999; March et al. 2004; Rohde et al. 2004). There were studies that included IPT for adolescents that consisted of helping adolescents recognize their feelings and think about how interpersonal events might affect their mood, improving communication and problem-solving skills, enhancing social functioning, and decreasing depressive symptoms (Mufson et al. 1999, 2004; Young et al. 2006). Another one used a family intervention following an attachment-based model to guide the process of repairing conflict-ridden relationships (Diamond et al. 2002). All of these interventions (CBT, IPT, and family intervention) proved to be superior to their respective control groups in reducing depressive symptoms. There was more evidence in favor of CBT and IPT than there was in favor of family interventions. However, no psychosocial intervention has been clearly established as the superior treatment for depressed adolescents. Regarding follow-up studies with periods between 1 and 24 months postintervention, evidence remains inconclusive. Some results found that improvement in depressive symptoms was maintained over time, whereas other studies showed no differences in depression between treatment group and control group at follow-up.

On the basis of the Task Force on Promotion and Dissemination of Psychological Procedures, David-Ferdon and Kaslow (2008) classified interventions by their specific program, modality, and theoretical orientation.

They concluded that no specific psychosocial intervention for depressive adolescents had been classified as well established since 1998. Consistent with the previous review by Kaslow and Thompson (1998), CWD-A was deemed to be probably efficacious (Lewinsohn et al. 1990; Rohde et al. 2004). IPT was also considered a probably efficacious intervention (Mufson et al. 1999, 2004).

With regard to modality classification, CBT group treatment with adolescents (Clarke et al. 1999; Lewinsohn et al. 1990) and individual IPT were considered well-established interventions (Mufson et al. 1999, 2004). Other modalities under CBT, such as adolescent group therapy with parent component, individual therapy, and adolescent group plus parent/family component, were considered probably efficacious. Studies that focused on bibliotherapy, primary care services enhanced with CBT, and group IPT were considered experimental.

Finally, the authors tested evidence for adolescent depression from a broad theoretical perspective. On the basis of the number of studies published, both CBT and IPT were deemed to be well-established orientations in this population. Other approaches, such as supportive therapy, family-based intervention, and behavior therapy, were considered to be experimental because there were not enough studies in favor of their efficacy.

The recent review by Weersing et al. (2017) added 13 new RCTs with adolescent samples, published from 2008 to 2014, and reevaluated studies previously reviewed. The authors included both treatment and prevention programs. As in previous reviews, CBT, IPT, and family-based intervention were included. In total, 27 trials under the CBT orientation were tested in this review. The recent review included 14 RCTs that used individual CBT, six trials from the previous reviews (Asarnow et al. 2005; Brent et al. 1997; March et al. 2004; Melvin et al. 2006; Rosselló and Bernal 1999; Wood et al. 1996), four new RCTs published after 2007 (Brent et al. 2008; Richardson et al. 2014; Shirk et al. 2014; Szigethy et al. 2014), and three trials published prior to 2008 but excluded in the previous reviews (Clarke et al. 2005; Goodyer et al. 2007; Kerfoot et al. 2004). Seven out of 14 studies found positive results in favor of CBT compared with the control condition. The rest of the RCTs failed to find statistically significant differences from comparison conditions. Twelve studies in which CBT for adolescents was implemented using group format met criteria for inclusion in this review (Clarke et al. 1999, 2001, 2002, 2005; Dobson et al. 2010; Lewinsohn et al. 1990; Rohde et al. 2004, 2014; Rosselló et al. 2008; Stallard et al. 2012; Stice et al. 2008; Wijnhoven et al. 2014). Among all RCTs using group CBT for adolescents, seven showed positive effects in favor of CBT, and five studies found null results.

Given the obtained findings, Weersing et al., in their review, concluded that individual CBT, group CBT, and CBT overall met the criteria for well-established treatments. However, there were not enough studies for bibliotherapy-assisted CBT, which was deemed possibly efficacious, or for technology-assisted CBT, which was considered to be experimental. IPT also met criteria for a well-established treatment. Six trials were conducted in adolescent samples, and five of them had positive findings. Individual format under the IPT approach showed efficacy in several studies, being considered as well established (Mufson et al. 1999, 2004; Rosselló and Bernal 1999; Rosselló et al. 2008). Three RCTs using group IPT were included (Rosselló et al. 2008; Young et al. 2006, 2010). Only in two trials did group IPT show efficacy, so it was deemed probably efficacious.

Five studies analyzed family-based interventions (Brent et al. 1997; Diamond et al. 2002, 2010; Rohde et al. 2014; Sanford et al. 2006). Whereas some of them found positive results supporting family-based therapy, others failed to find a superior effect associated with the family component compared with a control condition. Thus, family therapy was classified as possibly efficacious.

Regarding durability of effects of interventions over follow-up, most of the studies included in the review by Weersing et al. (2017) followed up with participants 1 or 2 years after the end of the treatment. Differences between CBT or IPT and control groups were greater in follow-ups conducted closer to the end of treatment than for follow-ups conducted as late as 24 months after treatment. This narrowed gap between treatment and control conditions on follow-up could be explained by the possibility that patients assigned to the control groups improved in depressive symptoms over follow-up in congruence with the hypothesis of symptomatic remission and course of nontreated depression (Kovacs 1996).

Psychosocial interventions have also been compared with medication conditions over time. One of these studies is a trial conducted by the Treatment for Adolescents with Depression Study Team (March et al. 2004), which was previously cited in this chapter. The team enrolled 439 adolescents ages 12–17 years with a diagnosis of major depressive disorder of at least moderate severity. The researchers compared the effects of fluoxetine alone, CBT alone, CBT with fluoxetine, and placebo. The combination of fluoxetine with CBT, compared with the other conditions, resulted in the most relative benefit for adolescents with moderate to severe depression. Interestingly, about 60% of adolescents with major depressive disorder will respond to either an antidepressant medication or an empirically validated psychotherapy, and a similar proportion of depressed adolescents will show symptomatic remission after 6 months of treatment

(Weisz et al. 2006). However, at least 40% of adolescents with depression do not show clinical response to any of these interventions.

Another trial designed to compare psychosocial interventions with medication conditions in adolescents with treatment-resistant depression is the Treatment of (SSRI) Resistant Depression in Adolescents (TORDIA) trial (Brent et al. 2008). The study enrolled 334 adolescents between 12 and 18 years old with severe and chronic depression resistant to SSRI antidepressants. The effect of CBT and another antidepressant combined resulted in improvement of clinical symptoms compared with a switch to another medication without CBT, underscoring the importance of psychotherapy in treatment-resistant depression.

Another type of therapy that is spurring interest in the field of depressive disorders is dialectical behavior therapy (DBT). DBT belongs to the third wave of CBT interventions. This therapy, developed by Marsha Linehan as a treatment for adults with borderline personality disorder (BPD) (Linehan 1993), combines individual and group sessions in order to enhance skills to regulate emotions. Evidence has shown that DBT is associated with greater reductions in symptoms related to BPD in adults (Kliem et al. 2010; Stoffers et al. 2012). Recently, DBT has been adapted for youth with difficulties in regulating emotions and who may engage in self-injurious behavior (Miller et al. 2006). A recent meta-analysis about the effectiveness of DBT showed that DBT was effective in reducing nonsuicidal self-injury (NSSI) and depression, but the effect size was large for NSSI and small for depression (Cook and Gorraiz 2016). The authors suggested that further research on DBT interventions to treat adolescent depression is needed (see Chapter 13, "Management of Suicidal Youth," for more details on DBT).

In conclusion, data from systematic reviews suggest that CBT and IPT should be considered the main options for treating depression in adolescents (Zhou et al. 2015). Other psychotherapies have been understudied in adolescence. In addition, the combination of antidepressant and CBT should be considered mainly in moderately severe depression.

Comparative Effectiveness of Psychotherapies in Treating Youth With Depression

There is a shortage of comparative effectiveness studies for psychotherapeutic interventions among youth. However, according to a systematic review of the literature, the level of evidence in children with depression suggests that CBT is the most effective among all psychosocial interventions, classified as only possibly efficacious in young children (Weersing et al. 2017). CBT interventions that were considered possibly efficacious among children included group CBT, technology-assisted CBT, and behavior therapy. Unfortunately, there is no clear evidence in support of a superior psychosocial treatment that is effective in depressed children because of the dearth of studies researching depression interventions in this age group. In general, there is more evidence in favor of the CBT paradigm than with other orientations, but the extant evidence level remains low.

Among adolescents with depression, arguably the most rigorous review of the literature suggests that CBT and IPT have the most evidence. Specifically, individual CBT, group CBT, CBT overall, and individual IPT are considered well-established treatments, and group IPT is classified as probably efficacious. Although CBT and IPT for depression in adults have been demonstrated to be comparably effective over several decades of research, comparative effectiveness for these treatments is unknown in children or adolescents because of a dearth of RCTs in this area and a relative overrepresentation of CBT trials in the extant pediatric literature. Thus, the effectiveness of these treatments is an important future direction for research in the optimization and personalization of treatment in children. Clearly, knowing whether one therapy is significantly more effective for treating youth depression than all others would be important for the treatment outcomes of symptom remission and improved well-being, and would mitigate societal costs of this ubiquitous public health concern. For many reasons, however, it is difficult to find a panacea for youth depression given the lack of rigorously designed RCTs, the overrepresentation of CBT in RCTs, and variability in presentations of depression that might render different psychotherapies more effective for some presentations but not for others. Another inconsistency in psychotherapy research that complicates the endeavor to determine the most effective treatment is the different constructs used for treatment effectiveness (e.g., variety of outcome measures used, whether benefits are followed long term and found to be maintained over time).

Another reason for the importance of comparative psychotherapy studies for youth depression is that not starting with the right therapy could have adverse effects on clinical course. This could come in the form of deterioration of a patient's condition or a lack of improvement in a patient's condition. The latter could adversely affect the patient's clinical course by holding back that patient's progress or creating distress and hopelessness if and when the patient perceives a lack of treatment response. Although more research has been devoted to harm that can come from psychotherapy not

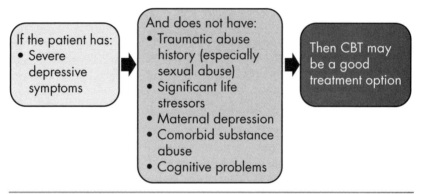

FIGURE 7–1.   Treatment decision making: cognitive-behavioral therapy (CBT). (*see color plate 4*)

delivered well (e.g., lack of competency or compassion on the part of the therapist), there is some evidence that certain treatment modalities may be ineffective or harmful to certain patients (Dimidjian and Hollon 2010; Lilienfeld 2007). For example, there is evidence that relaxation training can give rise to panic attacks among a small group of patients (Adler et al. 1987). Therefore, although relaxation has largely been helpful for most patients, it may be detrimental for a few. Research on treatment modalities that can be harmful, whether for small patient groups with certain characteristics or more broadly, is needed. Notwithstanding these challenges, the field has made efforts to better understand treatment personalization, which can increase treatment effectiveness in its own right for specific individuals or groups of people with important similarities by examining treatment predictors, moderators, and mediators.

How to Match a Patient With a Therapeutic Approach: Treatment Recommendations

Given that CBT holds the most evidence to date for treatment of depression in children and that both CBT and IPT are considered to be the most efficacious interventions for adolescent depression, this section will focus primarily on those forms of psychotherapy (Figures 7–1 and 7–2).

Research is limited on which components of psychotherapy, whether included in CBT, IPT, or other psychotherapies, are most effective for treating youth depression. Relatedly, to date there has been limited evidence for particular treatment mechanisms (i.e., underlying psychologi-

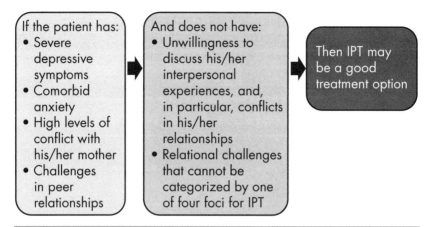

FIGURE 7–2. Treatment decision making: interpersonal psychotherapy (IPT). (*see color plate* 5)

cal, social, and neurophysiological processes by which therapeutic change occurs) proposed for each therapy, such as cognitive alterations for CBT and resolution of interpersonal difficulties for IPT (Lipsitz and Markowitz 2013; Longmore and Worrell 2007). However, some recommendations can be found in the literature for matching youth on the basis of their symptoms, presentation, and/or life and family circumstances to appropriate treatments or for identifying youth for whom certain treatments may not be effective.

The aforementioned Weersing et al. (2017) review, in addition to investigating youth depression RCT outcomes, examined the mechanisms and limitations of treatment response in the form of predictors, moderators, and mediators. Predictors were coded as baseline features of youth and families that were linked to poor treatment response regardless of condition, according to a system devised by Kraemer et al. (2002). In treatment planning, these predictors can help a provider decide which treatment strategies *not* to use with a particular patient or family affected by youth depression. In the review, moderators were recognized as baseline variables that related to differential responses to an intervention. Moderators hold utility in making clinical judgments about who should receive a particular intervention. Moderators may also be beneficial in treatment development, because they aid in ascertaining areas of limitation in the mechanisms of action in certain interventions. Mediation analyses test the causal theories undergirding treatment models (e.g., alteration in negative cognitive style leads to modification in depressive symptoms according to CBT), and findings from these analyses may help inform providers toward refining and fortifying interventions. Of note, as in the broader pediatric depression treatment literature, substantiation of predictors, moderators, and mediators of youth depression treatment comes mostly from depressed adolescent samples and CBT trials.

Predictor analyses in such trials have determined that demographic factors do not appear to play a considerable predictive role in treatment response (Weersing et al. 2017). However, this may be attributed to the fact that age has been tested solely within an adolescent sample rather than across the broader age span from childhood through adolescence. Moreover, treatment effects decrease as adolescents get older (Curry et al. 2006). The Weersing review found that low global functioning, higher levels of depression symptoms, high levels of suicidality, cognitive distortions, comorbid anxiety, family conflict, and hopelessness most dependably predicted poor response in both treatment and control conditions for youth depression.

Weersing et al. (2017) found that no child depression trial conducted any moderator analyses. Demographic factors were not significant moderators of CBT effects among adolescents, perhaps because of restriction of age range. A few studies suggested that CBT effects were heightened in participants with more severe depressive symptoms (Asarnow et al. 2009; Curry et al. 2006). In addition, CBT may separate more from a control condition if there are co-occurring psychiatric disorders other than substance abuse. Notably, although comorbid anxiety predicted poor response across conditions, CBT appears to be less affected by the co-occurrence of anxiety than control interventions. On the other hand, the authors found CBT to be less robust in the face of significant life stress. In one important moderator analysis, maternal depression occurring temporally with treatment participation in youth removed the relative advantage of CBT over other psychotherapies (Brent et al. 1998). CBT is more likely to have positive effects in youth *without* traumatic abuse histories (Asarnow et al. 2009; Barbe et al. 2004; Shamseddeen et al. 2011; Shirk et al. 2014). Sexual abuse seems to be most consistently linked to poor CBT outcome and failure of CBT to outdo control conditions (Lewis et al. 2010; Shamseddeen et al. 2011).

Few moderators of IPT effects have been reported. Comorbid anxiety and depression severity have been examined as clinical moderators, but the results are mixed across studies (Weersing et al. 2017). Nevertheless, IPT effects were most favorable for depressed adolescents with higher levels of conflict with their mothers and more challenges in relationships with their peers at baseline (Gunlicks-Stoessel et al. 2010). In contrast, studies of other family-based interventions have not found evidence for distinct efficacy due to moderating variables.

The term *mediator* is used to signify a source or mechanism of change in therapeutic outcomes and psychological research in general (Kazdin and Nock 2003). There are seven criteria for inferring a causal relation in research: strong association, specificity, experiment, temporality, gradient, consistency, and plausibility/coherence. The first four are the minimum criteria, but the rest are ideal and if met strengthen the case for certain mediators found. In the context of psychotherapeutic outcomes research, *strong association* refers to showing a strong relation between the psychotherapeutic intervention and the supposed mechanism of change (i.e., the mediator). *Specificity* pertains to demonstrating the specificity of the associations between the psychotherapeutic intervention, hypothesized mechanism, and outcome. *Experiment criterion* refers to using an experiment to show that manipulating the hypothesized causal force is related to change in the outcome examined. Effectively designed experiments can eliminate other possible explanations for the seen effects apart from the condition(s) engineered by the experimentalist. *Temporal precedence criterion* refers to the demonstration that the incident of or alteration in the hypothesized mechanism preceded change in the outcome in question. *Gradient criterion* means that an increased manifestation of the mediator is related to greater change in the outcome being examined. *Consistency* is a criterion to be met as well via the replication of a result, which is not unique to substantiating psychotherapeutic mechanisms of change but is important for all scientific research. Finally, one must determine whether the mediator is *plausible and coherent*—meaning whether a credible explanation can be clearly articulated—and whether the finding is integrative within the more general scientific literature (Kazdin and Nock 2003).

The Weersing review selected studies for this section by reviewing their already existing pool for pertinent analyses and searching for secondary articles from the same data sets, considering only empirical examinations of posttreatment data in which treatment and control conditions were considered separately rather than pooled for analysis, and results were given for primary depression outcomes. Six CBT trials met entry criteria for mediation analysis (Weersing et al. 2017), yielding inconclusive results. Specifically, cognitive and behavioral adjustment may relate to change in depressive symptoms, but these outcomes are inconsistent across studies and/or measures of processes. A cognitive bibliotherapy trial for adolescents with mild depression seen in primary care (Ackerson et al. 1998) showed that adjustment of dysfunctional attitudes, but not negative automatic thoughts as assessed by the Automatic Thoughts Questionnaire (ATQ; Hollon and Kendall 1980), was a significant mediator of the intervention's effects on self-reported depression symptoms only. In contrast, another trial of CBT adapted for depressed adolescents with comorbid conduct disorder (Kaufman et al. 2005) found nonsignificant results for dysfunctional attitudes yet small significant effects on negative automatic thoughts in improving depressive symptoms. In a trial comparing a CBT prevention program with supportive therapy and bibliotherapy control conditions (Stice et al. 2010), reduction in depression symptoms scores in the CBT prevention group was mediated by a reduction in depressogenic thinking using the ATQ and augmented involvement in pleasant activities. However, on closer examination, it looked like changes in depressive symptoms temporally preceded change in the mediators, so this finding should be interpreted with caution. In TADS, cognitive style mediated higher effects of combination treatment above CBT with placebo intervention on interviewer-rated depressive symptoms (Jacobs et al. 2009). However, this finding was also undermined by a lack of clear evidence of sequential precedence presenting cognitive change prior to symptom outcome as well as the generally weak effects of CBT alone in this trial on both the mediator and the outcomes. Another mediator analysis with the TADS data set examining motivational factors ran into the same issue of temporal change (Lewis et al. 2009). Kolko et al.'s (2000) reanalysis of a comparative trial of cognitive, family, and supportive therapy (Brent et al. 1997) aiming to examine mediation through a different measure of cognitive attitudes (Children's Negative Cognitive Errors Questionnaire; Leitenberg et al. 1986) rendered inconclusive findings due in part to missing data that compromised power.

A review conducted by Cheung et al. (2013) based its examination of treatment recommendations on the Guidelines for Adolescent Depression in Primary Care (GLAD-PC), an initiative in North America to foster guidelines for the treatment of adolescent depression. Although these guidelines were explained in the context of primary care, they can be useful for mental health providers as well. The review dealt primarily with the treatment of depression in adolescents, given the higher prevalence of the disorder in and wider body of research for that group. Treatment of depression in children was touched on briefly.

For mild adolescent depression, a period of hands-on support and monitoring for 6–8 weeks combined with assessment using brief validated scales may be helpful before proposing treatment with antidepressants or psychotherapy (Cheung et al. 2007). RCTs have shown that up to 20% of depressed youth improve from regular symptom monitoring, nondirective supportive therapy, and/or regular specialist care (Cheung et al. 2007; Goodyer et al. 2008). Monitoring and active support can involve arranging frequent follow-up visits, having youth engage in preferred extracurricular and school activities and connect to a peer support group, establishing self-management goals with depressed youth and families, and sharing educational resources (Cheung et al. 2007). This kind of approach not only is helpful for mild depression but also may be helpful when adolescents decline active treatment.

For moderate to severe adolescent depression, CBT or IPT is recommended. CBT is a viable option as monotherapy for adolescent depression, although a potential contraindication is the presence of cognitive problems such as learning disabilities that would make the discussions and homework assignments in CBT difficult. Considerations regarding the suitability of a depressed adolescent for IPT include whether the patient would be willing to discuss his or her interpersonal experiences, and conflicts in particular in his or her relationships, as well as whether relational challenges can be categorized by one of four foci for IPT: grief, interpersonal role transitions, interpersonal role disputes, or interpersonal deficits (Cheung et al. 2013).

Depression in children younger than 12 years is less ubiquitous than amid adolescents; nonetheless, it can be dependably diagnosed in children as early as 3 years of age (Bufferd et al. 2012). Because there is significantly less evidence for treatment of depression in children than for their adolescent counterparts, there are no definitive psychotherapy recommendations in the very young child except for meta-analytic (Weisz et al. 2006) and RCT data, which indicate that both psychoeducation and a parenting intervention reduced severity of depression in 3- to 7-year-olds (Luby et al. 2012). Interestingly, the latter trial found that the parenting intervention, in addition to reducing depression severity, also showed benefit for emotion recognition skills and executive functioning.

Children of parents with depression are at increased risk for developing depression themselves. In fact, by the age of 20, offspring of depressed parents have a 40% chance of having a major depressive episode, after which age the rate increases (Beardslee et al. 1993). There is a dearth of research on effective treatments for children of depressed parents, particularly *currently depressed* children of parents with current or remitted depression. A review (Boyd and Gillham 2009) on aspects of this topic distinguished multiple interventions that can be used for depressed parents and their children. Most important is to treat the parents' depression, an approach that has been shown to lead to parallel improvement in the parental depression alongside improvement in the children's behavioral and emotional symptoms (Gunlicks and Weissman 2008). It can be beneficial to the parents' treatment to include a focus on their parenting experiences and to teach behavioral parenting techniques, which also may improve children's functioning. Psychoeducation on parental depression and its impact on children can be fruitful, as can interventions with the intent to improve relationships, communication, and empathy between parents and their children (Boyd and Gillham 2009). Interventions that instruct about coping skills directly to children may be particularly helpful in preventing and reducing depression in children of depressed parents (Clarke et al. 2001, 2002).

Notwithstanding the need for additional evidence and clarity in the literature regarding psychotherapeutic treatments for youth depression, there is exciting and unique progress being made in this field that may expand options and accessibility for youth depression through the use of advancing technology. For example, accessibility to various Web-based CBT apps and other mental health-related apps has increased. Given youth's engagement and comfort level with technology and social media, which is sometimes beyond their potential engagement and comfort level in speaking with an adult therapist about their struggles, these options may be advantageous. However, live conversation may be crucial to improving symptoms. Web-based CBT apps have shown efficacy but are marked by poor adherence. Some researchers see promise in conversational agents in offering a convenient yet more engaging way of getting timely support. A recent study found this to be the case in decreasing symptoms of depression and anxiety in young adults who had access for 2 weeks to a fully automated conversational agent (Woebot) that conversed using self-help content based on CBT principles (Fitzpatrick et al. 2017).

Considering the results extracted from RCTs, the following clinical guidelines provide some general recommendations for treating depression in youth (National Institute for Health and Care Excellence 2005): 1) for mild depression, it is recommended that clinicians use a psychological intervention that has shown some favorable evidence for being effective for children and adolescents in general (CBT, IPT, family therapy, or supportive therapy); and 2) for moderate to severe depression, it is recommended to offer the psychological treatments that have been shown to be more effective in controlled studies. For children, CBT is the most recommendable intervention. For adolescents, CBT monotherapy is recommended in the absence of cognitive problems, and IPT is recommended as long as the patient is willing to discuss his or her interpersonal experiences and the patient's relational conflicts fit within the foci of IPT. If depression is resistant to psychological treatment after four to six sessions, considering combined therapy (antidepressant and psychological therapy) is recommended. There are no clear-cut psychotherapy recommendations for very young children, but there are data suggesting that psychoeducation and parenting interventions could be helpful. CBT effects may be amplified in participants with more severe depressive symptoms and can be helpful in the face of co-occurring psychiatric disorders except for substance abuse. CBT may be less robust in the face of significant life stress and/or maternal depression. CBT is more likely to be fruitful for youth *without* traumatic abuse histories, especially sexual abuse. IPT may be especially favorable for depressed adolescents with high levels of conflict with their mothers and peer relationship challenges.

Conclusion

In general, the available scientific evidence for the psychotherapeutic treatment of depressive disorders in youth is insufficient, of low quality, and inconclusive. Although there is some evidence in reducing depressive symptoms by using certain therapies, treatments are especially limited in the case of children under 12 years old and at follow-up. In the studies analyzed, CBT, particularly in group format, and IPT in adolescents individually seem to show a beneficial effect, mainly in reducing depressive symptoms at posttreatment. RCTs focused on comparing only CBT with IPT would be helpful, since it is unclear which of these two treatments is most effective for treatment of adolescent or child depression. Along with this clarity, there is a need to elucidate the moderators and mechanisms of change in these treatments, specifically in youth depression and then by age group (i.e., adolescent versus child), so that mental health providers are better poised to match specific presentations of depression and circumstances to appropriate interventions. In addition, few controlled studies evaluating family, psychodynamic, or other psychological interventions were found, and data supporting their efficacy are limited. Further research is needed to establish more evidence for psychotherapies that address youth depression and to better pair treatments, treatment modalities (group versus individual treatment format), and treatment components to different presentations of depression in youth.

Clinical Pearls

- Cognitive-behavioral therapy (CBT) appears to be the most promising intervention for children with depression, while CBT and interpersonal psychotherapy (IPT) are considered the most effective treatments for adolescents, with well-established evidence.

- There is some evidence in favor of the effectiveness of family therapy for adolescents, although more research is needed.

- The combination of an antidepressant with CBT is more effective than an antidepressant alone for adolescents with moderate to severe depression or in treatment-resistant depression.

- CBT may be conducive for youth with severe depressive symptoms and without a traumatic abuse history (especially sexual abuse), significant life stressors, maternal depression, comorbid substance abuse, and cognitive problems.

- IPT may be conducive for youth with severe depressive symptoms, comorbid anxiety, high levels of conflict with their mothers, and challenges in peer relationships.

References

Ackerson J, Scogin F, McKendree-Smith N, et al: Cognitive bibliotherapy for mild and moderate adolescent depressive symptomatology. J Consult Clin Psychol 66(4):685–690, 1998 9735587

Adler CM, Craske MG, Barlow DH: Relaxation-induced panic (RIP): when resting isn't peaceful. Integr Psychiatry 5(2):94–100, 1987

American Psychiatric Association: Diagnostic and Statistical Manual of Mental Disorders, 3rd Edition, Revised. Washington, DC, American Psychiatric Association, 1987

American Psychiatric Association: Diagnostic and Statistical Manual of Mental Disorders, 4th Edition. Washington, DC, American Psychiatric Association, 1994

Asarnow JR, Jaycox LH, Duan N, et al: Effectiveness of a quality improvement intervention for adolescent depression in primary care clinics: a randomized controlled trial. JAMA 293(3):311–319, 2005 15657324

Asarnow JR, Emslie G, Clarke G, et al: Treatment of selective serotonin reuptake inhibitor–resistant depression in adolescents: predictors and moderators of treatment response. J Am Acad Child Adolesc Psychiatry 48(3):330–339, 2009 19182688

Barbe RP, Bridge JA, Birmaher B, et al: Lifetime history of sexual abuse, clinical presentation, and outcome in a clinical trial for adolescent depression. J Clin Psychiatry 65(1):77–83, 2004 14744173

Beardslee WR, Keller MB, Lavori PW, et al: The impact of parental affective disorder on depression in offspring: a longitudinal follow-up in a nonreferred sample. J Am Acad Child Adolesc Psychiatry 32(4):723–730, 1993 8340291

Beck AT, Rush A, Shaw B, et al: Cognitive Therapy of Depression. New York, Guilford, 1979

Boyd RC, Gillham JE: Review of interventions for parental depression from toddlerhood to adolescence. Curr Psychiatry Rev 5(4):226–235, 2009 20824114

Brent D, Weersing VR: Depressive disorders in childhood and adolescence, in Rutter's Child and Adolescent Psychiatry, 5th Edition. Edited by Rutter MJ, Bishop D, Pine D, et al. New York, Wiley-Blackwell, 2010, pp 587–612

Brent DA, Holder D, Kolko D, et al: A clinical psychotherapy trial for adolescent depression comparing cognitive, family, and supportive therapy. Arch Gen Psychiatry 54(9):877–885, 1997 9294380

Brent DA, Kolko DJ, Birmaher B, et al: Predictors of treatment efficacy in a clinical trial of three psychosocial treatments for adolescent depression. J Am Acad Child Adolesc Psychiatry 37(9):906–914, 1998 9735610

Brent D, Emslie G, Clarke G, et al: Switching to another SSRI or to venlafaxine with or without cognitive behavioral therapy for adolescents with SSRI-resistant depression: the TORDIA randomized controlled trial. JAMA 299(8):901–913, 2008 18314433

Bufferd SJ, Dougherty LR, Carlson GA, et al: Psychiatric disorders in preschoolers: continuity from ages 3 to 6. Am J Psychiatry 169(11):1157–1164, 2012 23128922

Cheung AH, Zuckerbrot RA, Jensen PS, et al; GLAD-PC Steering Group: Guidelines for Adolescent Depression in Primary Care (GLAD-PC), II: treatment and ongoing management. Pediatrics 120(5):e1313–e1326, 2007 17974724

Cheung AH, Kozloff N, Sacks D: Pediatric depression: an evidence-based update on treatment interventions. Curr Psychiatry Rep 15(8):381, 2013 23881712

Clarke GN, Rohde P, Lewinsohn PM, et al: Cognitive-behavioral treatment of adolescent depression: efficacy of acute group treatment and booster sessions. J Am Acad Child Adolesc Psychiatry 38(3):272–279, 1999 10087688

Clarke GN, Hornbrook M, Lynch F, et al: A randomized trial of a group cognitive intervention for preventing depression in adolescent offspring of depressed parents. Arch Gen Psychiatry 58(12):1127–1134, 2001 11735841

Clarke GN, Hornbrook M, Lynch F, et al: Group cognitive-behavioral treatment for depressed adolescent offspring of depressed parents in a health maintenance organization. J Am Acad Child Adolesc Psychiatry 41(3):305–313, 2002 11886025

Clarke GN, Debar L, Lynch F, et al: A randomized effectiveness trial of brief cognitive-behavioral therapy for depressed adolescents receiving antidepressant medication. J Am Acad Child Adolesc Psychiatry 44(9):888–898, 2005 16113617

Cook NE, Gorraiz M: Dialectical behavior therapy for nonsuicidal self-injury and depression among adolescents: preliminary meta-analytic evidence. Child Adolesc Ment Health 21(2):81–89, 2016

Cuijpers P, Hollon SD, van Straten A, et al: Does cognitive behaviour therapy have an enduring effect that is superior to keeping patients on continuation pharmacotherapy? A meta-analysis. BMJ Open 3(4):e002542, 2013 23624992

Curry J, Rohde P, Simons A, et al; TADS Team: Predictors and moderators of acute outcome in the Treatment for Adolescents with Depression Study (TADS). J Am Acad Child Adolesc Psychiatry 45(12):1427–1439, 2006 17135988

David-Ferdon C, Kaslow NJ: Evidence-based psychosocial treatments for child and adolescent depression. J Clin Child Adolesc Psychol 37(1):62–104, 2008 18444054

De Cuyper S, Timbremont B, Braet C, et al: Treating depressive symptoms in schoolchildren: a pilot study. Eur Child Adolesc Psychiatry 13(2):105–114, 2004 15103536

Diamond GS, Reis BF, Diamond GM, et al: Attachment-based family therapy for depressed adolescents: a treatment development study. J Am Acad Child Adolesc Psychiatry 41(10):1190–1196, 2002 12364840

Diamond GS, Wintersteen MB, Brown GK, et al: Attachment-based family therapy for adolescents with suicidal ideation: a randomized controlled trial. J Am Acad Child Adolesc Psychiatry 49(2):122–131, 2010 20215934

Dimidjian S, Hollon SD: How would we know if psychotherapy were harmful? Am Psychol 65(1):21–33, 2010 20063907

Dobson KS, Ahnberg Hopkins J, Fata L, et al: The prevention of depression and anxiety in a sample of high-risk adolescents: a randomized controlled trial. Can J Sch Psychol 25(4):291–310, 2010

Fitzpatrick KK, Darcy A, Vierhile M: Delivering cognitive behavior therapy to young adults with symptoms of depression and anxiety using a fully automated conversational agent (Woebot): a randomized controlled trial. JMIR Ment Health 4(2):e19, 2017 28588005

Forti-Buratti MA, Saikia R, Wilkinson EL, et al: Psychological treatments for depression in pre-adolescent children (12 years and younger): systematic review and meta-analysis of randomised controlled trials. Eur Child Adolesc Psychiatry 25(10):1045–1054, 2016 26969618

Gillham JE, Hamilton J, Freres DR, et al: Preventing depression among early adolescents in the primary care setting: a randomized controlled study of the Penn Resiliency Program. J Abnorm Child Psychol 34(2):203–219, 2006 16741684

Goodyer I, Dubicka B, Wilkinson P, et al: Selective serotonin reuptake inhibitors (SSRIs) and routine specialist care with and without cognitive behaviour therapy in adolescents with major depression: randomised controlled trial. BMJ 335(7611):142–146, 2007 17556431

Goodyer IM, Dubicka B, Wilkinson P, et al: A randomised controlled trial of cognitive behaviour therapy in adolescents with major depression treated by selective serotonin reuptake inhibitors: the ADAPT trial. Health Technol Assess 12(14):iii–iv, ix–60, 2008 18462573

Gunlicks ML, Weissman MM: Change in child psychopathology with improvement in parental depression: a systematic review. J Am Acad Child Adolesc Psychiatry 47(4):379–389, 2008 18388766

Gunlicks-Stoessel M, Mufson L, Jekal A, et al: The impact of perceived interpersonal functioning on treatment for adolescent depression: IPT-A versus treatment as usual in school-based health clinics. J Consult Clin Psychol 78(2):260–267, 2010 20350036

Hollon SD, Kendall PC: Cognitive self-statements in depression: development of an automatic thoughts questionnaire. Cognit Ther Res 4(4):383–395, 1980

Jacobs RH, Silva SG, Reinecke MA, et al: Dysfunctional Attitudes Scale perfectionism: a predictor and partial mediator of acute treatment outcome among clinically depressed adolescents. J Clin Child Adolesc Psychol 38(6):803–813, 2009 20183664

Kahn JS, Kehle TJ, Jenson WR, et al: Comparison of cognitive-behavioral, relaxation, and self-modeling interventions for depression among middle-school students. School Psych Rev 19:196–211, 1990

Kaslow NJ, Thompson MP: Applying the criteria for empirically supported treatments to studies of psychosocial interventions for child and adolescent depression. J Clin Child Psychol 27(2):146–155, 1998 9648032

Kaufman NK, Rohde P, Seeley JR, et al: Potential mediators of cognitive-behavioral therapy for adolescents with comorbid major depression and conduct disorder. J Consult Clin Psychol 73(1):38–46, 2005 15709830

Kazdin AE, Nock MK: Delineating mechanisms of change in child and adolescent therapy: methodological issues and research recommendations. J Child Psychol Psychiatry 44(8):1116–1129, 2003 14626454

Kerfoot M, Harrington R, Harrington V, et al: A step too far? Randomized trial of cognitive-behaviour therapy delivered by social workers to depressed adolescents. Eur Child Adolesc Psychiatry 13(2):92–99, 2004 15103534

Klerman GL (ed): Interpersonal Psychotherapy of Depression. New York, Basic Books, 1984

Kliem S, Kröger C, Kosfelder J: Dialectical behavior therapy for borderline personality disorder: a meta-analysis using mixed-effects modeling. J Consult Clin Psychol 78(6):936–951, 2010 21114345

Kolko DJ, Brent DA, Baugher M, et al: Cognitive and family therapies for adolescent depression: treatment specificity, mediation, and moderation. J Consult Clin Psychol 68(4):603–614, 2000 10965636

Kovacs M: Presentation and course of major depressive disorder during childhood and later years of the life span. J Am Acad Child Adolesc Psychiatry 35(6):705–715, 1996 8682751

Kraemer HC, Wilson GT, Fairburn CG, et al: Mediators and moderators of treatment effects in randomized clinical trials. Arch Gen Psychiatry 59(10):877–883, 2002 12365874

Leitenberg H, Yost LW, Carroll-Wilson M: Negative cognitive errors in children: questionnaire development, normative data, and comparisons between children with and without self-reported symptoms of depression, low self-esteem, and evaluation anxiety. J Consult Clin Psychol 54(4):528–536, 1986 3745607

Lemmens LHJM, Arntz A, Peeters F, et al: Clinical effectiveness of cognitive therapy v. interpersonal psychotherapy for depression: results of a randomized controlled trial. Psychol Med 45(10):2095–2110, 2015 25640151

Lewinsohn PM, Clarke GN, Hops H, et al: Cognitive-behavioral treatment for depressed adolescents. Behav Ther 21(4):385–401, 1990

Lewinsohn PM, Rohde P, Seeley JR: Major depressive disorder in older adolescents: prevalence, risk factors, and clinical implications. Clin Psychol Rev 18(7):765–794, 1998 9827321

Lewis CC, Simons AD, Silva SG, et al: The role of readiness to change in response to treatment of adolescent depression. J Consult Clin Psychol 77(3):422–428, 2009 19485584

Lewis CC, Simons AD, Nguyen LJ, et al: Impact of childhood trauma on treatment outcome in the Treatment for Adolescents with Depression Study (TADS). J Am Acad Child Adolesc Psychiatry 49(2):132–140, 2010 20215935

Liddle B, Spence SH: Cognitive-behaviour therapy with depressed primary school children: a cautionary note. Behav Cogn Psychother 18:85–102, 1990

Lilienfeld SO: Psychological treatments that cause harm. Perspect Psychol Sci 2(1):53–70, 2007 26151919

Linehan M: Cognitive Behavioral Treatment of Borderline Personality Disorder. New York, Guilford, 1993

Lipsitz JD, Markowitz JC: Mechanisms of change in interpersonal therapy (IPT). Clin Psychol Rev 33(8):1134–1147, 2013 24100081

Longmore RJ, Worrell M: Do we need to challenge thoughts in cognitive behavior therapy? Clin Psychol Rev 27(2):173–187, 2007 17157970

Luby J, Lenze S, Tillman R: A novel early intervention for preschool depression: findings from a pilot randomized controlled trial. J Child Psychol Psychiatry 53(3):313–322, 2012 22040016

March J, Silva S, Petrycki S, et al: Fluoxetine, cognitive-behavioral therapy, and their combination for adolescents with depression. JAMA 292(7):807–820, 2004, 15315995

Markowitz JC: IPT and PTSD. Depress Anxiety 27(10):879–881, 2010 20886608

Melvin GA, Tonge BJ, King NJ, et al: A comparison of cognitive-behavioral therapy, sertraline, and their combination for adolescent depression. J Am Acad Child Adolesc Psychiatry 45(10):1151–1161, 2006 17003660

Miller AL, Rathus JH, Linehan MM: Dialectical Behavior Therapy With Suicidal Adolescents. New York, Guilford, 2006

Mufson L, Weissman MM, Moreau D, et al: Efficacy of interpersonal psychotherapy for depressed adolescents. Arch Gen Psychiatry 56(6):573–579, 1999 10359475

Mufson L, Dorta KP, Wickramaratne P, et al: A randomized effectiveness trial of interpersonal psychotherapy for depressed adolescents. Arch Gen Psychiatry 61(6):577–584, 2004 15184237

National Institute for Health and Care Excellence: Depression in children and young people: identification and management. NICE Guidelines, September 2005. Available at: https://www.nice.org.uk/guidance/cg28. Accessed September 14, 2018.

Nelson E-L, Barnard M, Cain S: Treating childhood depression over videoconferencing. Telemed J E Health 9(1):49–55, 2003 12699607

Qin B, Zhou X, Michael KD, et al: Psychotherapy for depression in children and adolescents: study protocol for a systematic review and network meta-analysis. BMJ Open 5(2):e005918, 2015 25681311

Richardson LP, Ludman E, McCauley E, et al: Collaborative care for adolescents with depression in primary care: a randomized clinical trial. JAMA 312(8):809–816, 2014 25157724

Roberts C, Kane R, Thomson H, et al: The prevention of depressive symptoms in rural school children: a randomized controlled trial. J Consult Clin Psychol 71(3):622–628, 2003 12795585

Rohde P, Clarke GN, Mace DE, et al: An efficacy/effectiveness study of cognitive-behavioral treatment for adolescents with comorbid major depression and conduct disorder. J Am Acad Child Adolesc Psychiatry 43(6):660–668, 2004 15167082

Rohde P, Waldron HB, Turner CW, et al: Sequenced versus coordinated treatment for adolescents with comorbid depressive and substance use disorders. J Consult Clin Psychol 82(2):342–348, 2014 24491069

Rosselló J, Bernal G: The efficacy of cognitive-behavioral and interpersonal treatments for depression in Puerto Rican adolescents. J Consult Clin Psychol 67(5):734–745, 1999 10535240

Rosselló J, Bernal G, Rivera-Medina C: Individual and group CBT and IPT for Puerto Rican adolescents with depressive symptoms. Cultur Divers Ethnic Minor Psychol 14(3):234–245, 2008 18624588

Sanford M, Boyle M, McCleary L, et al: A pilot study of adjunctive family psychoeducation in adolescent major depression: feasibility and treatment effect. J Am Acad Child Adolesc Psychiatry 45(4):386–495, 2006 16601642

Schramm E, Zobel I, Dykierek P, et al: Cognitive behavioral analysis system of psychotherapy versus interpersonal psychotherapy for early onset chronic depression: a randomized pilot study. J Affect Disord 129(1–3):109–116, 2011 20822814

Shamseddeen W, Asarnow JR, Clarke G, et al: Impact of physical and sexual abuse on treatment response in the Treatment of Resistant Depression in Adolescent Study (TORDIA). J Am Acad Child Adolesc Psychiatry 50(3):293–301, 2011 21334569

Shirk SR, Deprince AP, Crisostomo PS, et al: Cognitive behavioral therapy for depressed adolescents exposed to interpersonal trauma: an initial effectiveness trial. Psychotherapy (Chic) 51(1):167–179, 2014 24377410

Southam-Gerow MA, Prinstein MJ: Evidence base updates: the evolution of the evaluation of psychological treatments for children and adolescents. J Clin Child Adolesc Psychol 43(1):1–6, 2014 24294989

Stallard P, Sayal K, Phillips R, et al: Classroom based cognitive behavioural therapy in reducing symptoms of depression in high risk adolescents: pragmatic cluster randomised controlled trial. BMJ 345:e6058, 2012, 23043090

Stark KD, Reynolds WM, Kaslow NJ: A comparison of the relative efficacy of self-control therapy and a behavioral problem-solving therapy for depression in children. J Abnorm Child Psychol 15(1):91–113, 1987 3571741

Stark KD, Rouse LW, Livingston R: Treatment of depression during childhood and adolescence: cognitive-behavioral procedures for the individual and family, in Child and Adolescent Therapy: Cognitive-Behavioral Procedures. Edited by Kendall PC. New York, Guilford, 1991, pp 165–206

Stice E, Rohde P, Seeley JR, et al: Brief cognitive-behavioral depression prevention program for high-risk adolescents outperforms two alternative interventions: a randomized efficacy trial. J Consult Clin Psychol 76(4):595–606, 2008 18665688

Stice E, Rohde P, Seeley JR, et al: Testing mediators of intervention effects in randomized controlled trials: an evaluation of three depression prevention programs. J Consult Clin Psychol 78(2):273–280, 2010 20350038

Stoffers JM, Völlm BA, Rücker G, et al: Psychological therapies for people with borderline personality disorder. Cochrane Database Syst Rev 8(8):CD005652, 2012 22895952

Szigethy E, Bujoreanu SI, Youk AO, et al: Randomized efficacy trial of two psychotherapies for depression in youth with inflammatory bowel disease. J Am Acad Child Adolesc Psychiatry 53(7):726–735, 2014 24954822

Thapar A, Collishaw S, Pine DS, et al: Depression in adolescence. Lancet 379(9820):1056–1067, 2012 22305766

Trowell J, Joffe I, Campbell J, et al: Childhood depression: a place for psychotherapy: an outcome study comparing individual psychodynamic psychotherapy and family therapy. Eur Child Adolesc Psychiatry 16(3):157–167, 2007 17200793

Verboom CE, Sijtsema JJ, Verhulst FC, et al: Longitudinal associations between depressive problems, academic performance, and social functioning in adolescent boys and girls. Dev Psychol 50(1):247–257, 2014 23566082

Vostanis P, Feehan C, Grattan E, et al: A randomised controlled out-patient trial of cognitive-behavioural treatment for children and adolescents with depression: 9-month follow-up. J Affect Disord 40:105–116, 1996 8882920

Weersing VR, Jeffreys M, Do MT, et al: Evidence base update of psychosocial treatments for child and adolescent depression. J Clin Child Adolesc Psychol 46(1):11–43, 2017 27870579

Weissman MM, Markowitz JC, Klerman GL: Clinician's Quick Guide to Interpersonal Psychotherapy. New York, Oxford University Press, 2007

Weisz JR, McCarty CA, Valeri SM: Effects of psychotherapy for depression in children and adolescents: a meta-analysis. Psychol Bull 132(1):132–149, 2006 16435960

Weisz JR, Southam-Gerow MA, Gordis EB, et al: Cognitive-behavioral therapy versus usual clinical care for youth depression: an initial test of transportability to community clinics and clinicians. J Consult Clin Psychol 77(3):383–396, 2009 19485581

Wijnhoven LAMW, Creemers DHM, Vermulst AA, et al: Randomized controlled trial testing the effectiveness of a depression prevention program ("Op Volle Kracht") among adolescent girls with elevated depressive symptoms. J Abnorm Child Psychol 42(2):217–228, 2014 23893066

Wood A, Harrington R, Moore A: Controlled trial of a brief cognitive-behavioural intervention in adolescent patients with depressive disorders. J Child Psychol Psychiatry 37(6):737–746, 1996 8894955

Young JF, Mufson L, Davies M: Efficacy of interpersonal psychotherapy—adolescent skills training: an indicated preventive intervention for depression. J Child Psychol Psychiatry 47(12):1254–1262, 2006 17176380

Young JF, Mufson L, Gallop R: Preventing depression: a randomized trial of interpersonal psychotherapy–adolescent skills training. Depress Anxiety 27(5):426–433, 2010 20112246

Zhou X, Hetrick SE, Cuijpers P, et al: Comparative efficacy and acceptability of psychotherapies for depression in children and adolescents: a systematic review and network meta-analysis. World Psychiatry 14(2):207–222, 2015 26043339

Evidence-Based Psychotherapies for Pediatric Bipolar Disorders

David J. Miklowitz, Ph.D.

Ethan, a 13-year-old with depression, who had both a sister and a grandparent with bipolar disorder (BD), was evaluated at a child outpatient service. Following a diagnostic interview, he was diagnosed with major depressive disorder (current and past), although the evaluator noted the presence of transient hypomanic symptoms. His presentation also met criteria for attention-deficit/hyperactivity disorder (ADHD) and oppositional defiant disorder. His parents reported that Ethan was performing poorly in school despite an above-average IQ. He had been in a string of schools for kids with "severe mental illness" or "emotional and cognitive disorders," most of whom had autism or psychosis. The family was middle class and lived in a rural area. His mother was a real estate agent, and his father owned an import/export business. He had a 21-year-old sister who had a developmental disability and had been diagnosed with BD at age 13. His sister lived in the home but in her parents' estimation was not stable enough to attend family sessions. Ethan received 12 family-focused therapy

(FFT) sessions with his mother and father, conducted by a trained family clinician.

During the first family session, Ethan's father began by listing all of the things Ethan had done in the past several months to "destroy the family atmosphere." These included inconsistent school performance; staying up too late playing video games; being irritable, especially when asked to interrupt his game-playing; being grumpy at the dinner table; getting into altercations with kids at school in situations when he felt insulted or left out; and, more generally, "poisoning the atmosphere wherever he goes." Ethan responded to his father's tirade by intermittently crying and cursing. When Ethan calmed down, the clinician asked him to describe his most recent episode of depression. Ethan was articulate in describing his symptoms but felt that his parents were unaware of his degree of suffering and generally ignored him when he was down.

Ethan showed some insight into his problems. He complained bitterly that his father "is always after me to do better....He never tells me I'm doing good enough." He spoke about feeling stigmatized by attending a school for emotionally disturbed kids. His conflicts with his mother centered on her apparent inability to help him obtain accommodations at his school, such as getting extensions on his homework due dates. He expressed anger at her unwillingness to have him moved to another school.

His mother reported that Ethan became quite angry when denied things at home (e.g., access to a particular video game that involved interacting with his few friends). His father complained that Ethan was pushing everyone around and holding the other family members "hostage" with his mood swings and irritability. Ethan's mother defended him by saying that her husband was unable to hold a conversation with Ethan without attaching a criticism in some way. She noted a recent example: His father asked him how his school day went, and Ethan said, simply, "Fine." His father countered with "Maybe you'd be doing better if you talked to me about it once in a while."

Ethan's father had his own history of major depression, and his grandmother had an undiagnosed BD. Both parents agreed that Ethan tended to act out externally or express suicidal thoughts after negative family exchanges involving criticism or judgment. Given her protective feelings toward Ethan, Ethan's mother occasionally interfered with her husband's efforts to talk to Ethan when he expressed suicidal thoughts.

Treatment Goals

The clinician offered Ethan and his family a 12-session course of FFT for youth at high risk for BD (FFT-HR; Miklowitz et al. 2013). Disordered communication was notable as a target, as was a lack of acknowledgment of Ethan's mood disorder in his parents' formulation of his problems. The FFT-HR program consisted of four sessions of family psychoeducation (recognition and early intervention with prodromal signs of mood episodes; recognizing and attempting to reduce the impact of stressors), four sessions of communication enhancement training (directed exercises to practice effective dyadic communication strategies), and four sessions of problem-solving skills training. Ethan also met with a psychiatrist, who prescribed risperidone, lamotrigine, and the central nervous system stimulant Vyvanse (lisdexamfetamine dimesylate) for ADHD.

The family clinician worked with the family on the following objectives: 1) encourage the parents to recognize the underlying biological bases of Ethan's disorder, and the degree to which his aversive behaviors might not be fully under his control; 2) encourage parents to recognize Ethan's hypersensitivity to critical comments, and to work toward decreasing the frequency of negative communication; 3) increase the frequency of positive communication from both parents toward the child and the child toward parents; 4) assist the father in framing his positive feedback in ways that didn't put pressure on Ethan; and 5) help Ethan to recognize and label his emotional reactions when his parents or peers said or did things that made him feel rejected, and to try to distinguish his reactions from their intentions.

Course of Treatment

The family psychoeducation sessions were used to encourage an open discussion between Ethan and his parents about what "depression" meant to each of them (they had each experienced it in themselves) and, similarly, what stimuli in the family environment were associated with Ethan's irritable "meltdowns." His parents and Ethan listed his early warning signs of depression and irritability (e.g., withdrawal from family interaction) and discussed how best to help him when his mood worsened. He asked his parents to "Ask me what's wrong," "Talk to me," or "Take me out somewhere." He also highlighted the importance of staying away from judgmental statements that, he felt, made him feel worse. In turn, his father requested that he be more open to talking about what was bothering him.

Communication training had a more direct impact on the family's interactions, especially between Ethan and his father. Ethan learned the steps of *active listening* and *positive requests for change* very quickly. He responded especially well to the exercises involving *expressing positive feelings about specific behaviors*. Not only did he appreciate his parents' acknowledgment regarding his attempts to be a good student, but the exercises allowed him to express appreciation toward his mother, who he recognized had been working hard to find him the right school (despite his frustrations). Notably, his father practiced giving Ethan specific positive feedback (e.g., "I appreciate how hard you're working on your math assignments") without adding a "tail" at the end (e.g., "especially when you think of how much money we spent on tutoring last summer").

Problem solving mainly focused on his school situation and what kinds of changes needed to be made, either in his individualized education plan within the existing school or in another school. The clinician encouraged Ethan's mother to reconsider her "helicopter parenting" (her husband's words) style in relation to his schooling (e.g., calling his teachers constantly), which, Ethan reported, was contributing to his anxiety. Finally, the clinician encouraged the father and son to spend more time together after school and on weekends so that they could begin to see each other in a more positive light.

Outcome

Ethan benefited from learning to label his emotions. Instead of the pervasive "good" or "bad" emotions he described at the beginning, he was increasingly able to identify more nuanced states such as anxiety, threat, guilt, anger, sadness, or, on the upside, feeling "super excited," or "amped up." Use of these terms in skill-training exercises was of considerable help when he tried to explain to either parent why he had reacted negatively to a seemingly neutral exchange. He continued to be withdrawn when he was being criticized; however, he was more able to observe that his moods sometimes came about from overreacting to his father's comments. He reported being less depressed and anxious at the end of FFT-HR. He continued taking his medications after sessions ended.

In the past 10 years, many papers on bipolar disorder have begun by addressing impairment (e.g., the phrase "bipolar disorder is one of the leading causes of disability" is almost ubiquitous), its association with high rates of suicide, the neurotoxic effects of episodes that predispose patients to future recurrences, and the increased risks of alcohol and substance abuse. Although these are indeed associated features in many patients with BD, they do not tell the whole story: many patients do well over time. In the Course and Outcome of Bipolar Youth Study, about 24% of children or teens who began with active symptoms of bipolar I, II, or not otherwise specified (NOS) disorder showed a "predominantly euthymic" course and 35% a moderately euthymic course over an average of 8 years (Birmaher et al. 2014). Geller et al. (2008) reported that 56% of young adults who had an acute manic or mixed episode in childhood did not have recurrences between 18 and 21 years of age. Thus, the goals of our research should include 1) identifying protective factors that promote remission, well-being, and mood stability over long intervals and 2) developing and testing treatments that augment the effects of protective factors.

An example comes from studies of family environments. It is well known that environments characterized by high levels of parental criticism, hostility, or emotional overinvolvement (high expressed emotion, or EE) are associated with more relapsing outcomes among patients with BD, major depression, schizophrenia, and other disorders (Hooley 2007). However, not all families are high in EE, and some provide protective influences. In a comparison of age-matched teens at risk for BD and teens at risk for psychosis, the former group showed more constructive family communication and lower levels of parent/offspring criticism during laboratory-based family interactions (Salinger et al. 2018). We know comparatively little about why some family environments are low or high in conflict or in constructive communication. Nonetheless, one way to augment the protective effects of the family is to provide interventions that teach skills to reduce familial conflict and promote effective problem solving.

This chapter spells out the rationale for two forms of psychological treatment in the early phases of BD (i.e., childhood or adolescence). In the first section, I focus on family-based treatments that encourage the use of communication or problem-solving skills to blunt the effects of EE or other stressors over time. In the second section, I emphasize individual treatments that attempt to alter the pathway between life events, dysregulated social and circadian rhythms, and mania onset. The primary treatment that has been proposed for mitigating the effects of life events on circadian rhythms is interpersonal and social rhythm therapy (IPSRT), although various forms of cognitive-behavioral therapy also address these targets.

In describing these treatments, I focus on two distinct populations: 1) youth who have already developed BD before the age of 18 (early-onset, syndromal BD I or II) and 2) those with "high risk" (HR) phenotypes that indicate genetic and/or behavioral susceptibility to BD (e.g., subthreshold or "unspecified" BD). HR youth usually have one or more parents with BD. These populations often differ in the degree of medication management that is required in the aftermath of symptomatic phases, ranging from regimens that look similar to those of adults with established BD, to simplified regimens involving mood stabilizer monotherapy, to no pharmacological intervention for youth with minimal symptoms in the pre-onset phase (Schneck et al. 2017).

Family-Focused Therapy

Overview

Family-focused therapy, or FFT, is a direct descendant of behavioral family therapy for schizophrenia. The treatment involves a bipolar patient (or high-risk proband) and his or her parents or primary caregivers, as well as siblings or other relatives in the home. Most commonly, patients receive concurrent pharmacotherapy. Patients usually begin treatment shortly after hospital discharge or after an acute episode has been treated to partial remission on an outpatient basis.

There are three phases to treatment, although the frequency and duration of treatment vary by whether the patients are prodromal and at high risk (i.e., unspecified BD, major depressive disorder with a family history of mania), in which case families are given 12 sessions over 4 months

(FFT-HR); or are adults or adolescents with syndromal BD I or II, in which case they receive 21 sessions over 9 months. Either type of patient can have comorbid conditions such as ADHD or anxiety disorders.

The first phase is *psychoeducation,* during which the patient explores his or her experiences of mania, hypomania, or depression, with a particular focus on the patterning of symptoms, other prodromal features, stressors, and coping strategies that may have preceded the most recent symptom phase. Parents are encouraged to chime in with observations about the child's behavior during this phase. The parents may also share their own experiences with depressive or manic episodes and how they coped with them, even if their episodes occurred years ago. The patient and parents are encouraged to keep a simple mood chart that tracks the patient's ups and downs each week, as well as sleep-wake cycles. Over time, the youth and parents begin to observe patterns in the symptom course, such as the role of sleep or family conflict in precipitating episodes. The major "deliverable" of psychoeducation is a relapse prevention plan in which the family fills out a chart listing the youth's prodromal signs, stressors that often accompany the early stages of an episode, and strategies the child or family could use to intervene with these prodromal symptoms.

In the second phase of treatment, parents and the offspring engage in *communication training* exercises involving using active listening, offering positive or negative feedback, clarifying communication, and making positive requests for changes in one another's behavior. Each skill is taught with in-session role-playing and between-session practice. The aim of skill training is clearly linked to reducing negative or unconstructive family communication, including high EE.

In the third phase, families learn the steps of *problem solving*: defining a specific problem, generating a set of alternative solutions, evaluating the advantages and disadvantages of each proposed solution, discussing hurdles to implementing the solution, and choosing a best solution or series of solutions.

Empirical Studies of Family-Focused Therapy

In studies of adults with BD, FFT plus pharmacotherapy was more effective than brief family education and case management or equally intensive individual psychoeducation plus pharmacotherapy in 1) reducing recurrences of mania or depression over 2 years (number needed to treat: 3.1, 95% confidence interval [CI] 1.9, 8.3), 2) increasing "survival time" prior to recurrences (73.5 weeks for FFT vs. 53.2 weeks for brief family education, hazard ratio=2.6), and 3) enhancing psychosocial functioning (Cohen's

$d=0.80$) (Miklowitz and Chung 2016; Miklowitz et al. 2003; Rea et al. 2003). One study found that adult patients receiving FFT were more consistent in adhering to mood-stabilizing medications than patients receiving brief psychoeducation and case management (Miklowitz et al. 2003).

Randomized trials involving adolescents with bipolar I or II disorder have also yielded positive results, although not as consistently as trials involving adults. In our first trial ($N=58$), adolescents (ages 12–17) in FFT plus pharmacotherapy who began with depressive symptoms had shorter times to remission than adolescents in enhanced care (a three-session family educational treatment) plus pharmacotherapy. Adolescents in FFT also had less time in depressive episodes and more favorable trajectories of depression symptoms over 2 years (Miklowitz et al. 2008). In a replication and extension of this study ($N=145$), conducted across three sites and using more standardized medication regimens, patients in FFT did not differ from those in enhanced care on time to recovery from the initial study episode or recurrence over a 2-year period. Nonetheless, adolescents in FFT showed greater posttreatment stabilization of manic symptoms than those in enhanced care (Miklowitz et al. 2014). Moreover, adolescents in FFT showed greater gains in quality of life related to family functioning and health (O'Donnell et al. 2017).

One open trial (Miklowitz et al. 2011) and one randomized trial (Miklowitz et al. 2013) showed that FFT had benefits when given during the "high-risk" period before the onset of BD (see Table 8–1 later in this chapter). In the randomized controlled trial (RCT), 40 youth between the ages of 9 and 17 were recruited with major depression, cyclothymic disorder, or bipolar disorder not otherwise specified (BD-NOS); all had active mood symptoms and at least one first-degree relative (usually a parent) with bipolar I or II disorder. Youth and parents were randomly assigned to FFT for high-risk youth (FFT-HR), given in 12 sessions, or an educational control (EC) consisting of one to two family sessions of diagnostic clarification, psychoeducation, and clinical referral. About 60% of participants also received pharmacotherapy from study psychiatrists, although in many cases this was a psychostimulant for ADHD.

Over 1 year, youth in FFT-HR showed more rapid attainment of remission of their baseline mood symptoms than youth in EC. They also showed improvements in hypomania scores over the yearlong period. Interestingly, the youth who benefited most from FFT-HR were those with high-EE families (i.e., at least one parent who expressed high criticism toward the patient, hostility, or emotional overinvolvement) at baseline. We found a similar moderating effect of EE in our first study of adolescents with syndromal BD (Miklowitz et al. 2009) and in a study of adults with

BD (Fredman et al. 2015; Kim and Miklowitz 2004). Thus, living in a high-EE household may be an indicator of who will benefit most from FFT. We suspect that the targets of FFT (e.g., conflictual or unclear communication, misunderstanding the illness, and/or attributing negative behaviors of youth to stable personality features) are more salient in high-EE than in low-EE families. The effects of FFT-HR in HR youth are now being investigated more extensively in a three-site randomized trial (see Miklowitz et al. 2017).

Family Interventions for Younger Children With Bipolar Spectrum Disorders

Other investigators have examined family intervention protocols that are more suited to younger bipolar patients. In a wait-list controlled trial, Fristad and colleagues (2009) examined multi-family psychoeducational psychotherapy (MF-PEP) groups versus treatment as usual (TAU) in 165 children (ages 8–12) with bipolar spectrum (70%) or depressive spectrum (30%) disorders. The groups lasted 6 months, with eight 90-minute sessions. MF-PEP was associated with greater improvements in mood severity scores than TAU over the first 12 study months; the TAU participants showed a similar drop in mood severity scores when they received the psychoeducational psychotherapy from 12 to 18 months. Post hoc analyses showed that youth with depressive and transient manic symptoms were four times less likely to transition to bipolar spectrum disorders at 12 months if they received MF-PEP compared with TAU (Nadkarni and Fristad 2010).

An 18-session protocol of individual cognitive-behavioral and family-focused treatment sessions (better known as the "Rainbow" program) was tested in a randomized trial for 69 children with bipolar I/II disorder (38%) or BD-NOS (62%) who were age 12 or younger (West et al. 2014). The program, given weekly for 12 weeks and monthly for 6 months, consisted of alternating child-only, parent-only, and family sessions. A strength of this study is the availability of an attention-matched comparison therapy condition, although it is notable that youth in the Rainbow program attended 11.3 sessions compared with 6.9 sessions in the comparison group. Children in the Rainbow program showed more improvement in parent-reported mania scores, lower parent-reported depression scores, and a steeper response curve for depressive symptoms at the end of treatment and at 6 months.

Several of these investigations have addressed factors that moderate or mediate the effects of family interventions. MF-PEP was associated with improved quality in utilized services accessed by parents for the child, which in turn predicted greater mood improvements in the child (Mendenhall et al. 2009). For the Rainbow program, improvements in parenting skills, family flexibility, and "positive reframing" (i.e., the ability to view illness behaviors or family conflicts in a more positive or workable light) were associated with improved mood and clinician-rated global functioning in children (MacPherson et al. 2016).

Interestingly, children whose parents had higher subthreshold depressive symptoms showed greater improvements in the Rainbow program than in TAU (West et al. 2014). This finding contrasts with those of Garber et al. (2009) who found that among adolescents at risk for major depressive episodes, having a depressed parent was a negative predictor of response to cognitive-behavioral therapy groups.

Individual Modalities: Interpersonal and Social Rhythm Therapy

Separate groups of investigators have examined interpersonal and social rhythm therapy (Frank et al. 2005), an individual therapy for BD based on the interpersonal psychotherapy of depression. IPSRT targets the pathway between life events that disrupt social and circadian rhythms (e.g., transatlantic flights) and manic recurrences (Malkoff-Schwartz et al. 2000). Social rhythm–disrupting events are not always experienced as stressful; they may be subtle changes in the environment that disrupt sleep/wake hours (e.g., a change in job shifts). In IPSRT, patients focus with a clinician on resolving interpersonal problems that may have precipitated the recent mood episode (e.g., ongoing arguments with a parent over autonomy, starting a college semester, problems in the working world). The major goal is to identify stressors that precipitate mood episodes and mood-driven behaviors that precipitate stressors, with the end goal of enhancing interpersonal patterns and habits. A feature of IPSRT for BD is the use of a self-rated social rhythm chart, in which patients keep track of their daily sleep and wake habits—when they eat, exercise, or socialize—and the levels of stimulation provided by each activity. Clinicians assist patients in developing regulated social rhythms, such as going to bed and waking up at standardized times (Frank et al. 2005).

Two large-scale trials in adults with BD found that treatment with IPSRT, given in an acute period after a depressive or manic episode and combined with medication, was associated with greater delays prior to recurrences in up to 2 years of maintenance treatment, compared with an individual "active clinical management" therapy (Frank et al. 2005). Moreover, delays in recurrences were mediated by regulation of daily routines and sleep-wake cycles during acute treatment. In the multisite Systematic Treatment Enhancement Program for Bipolar Disorder, IPSRT was as effective as FFT or cognitive-behavioral therapy in hastening time to recovery among adults with bipolar depression, compared with a minimal psychoeducational intervention (Miklowitz et al. 2007).

IPSRT has been applied to adolescents with BD and adolescents at risk for BD. The model of IPSRT for adolescents was developed by Hlastala et al. (2010), who found symptom benefits in a 20-week open trial. However, a randomized trial of IPSRT in New Zealand, which compared 100 adolescents and young adults with BD (ages 15–36) receiving IPSRT or specialist supportive care over 18 months, found that both treatments were associated with improved depressive symptoms, manic symptoms, and social functioning over 3 years (Inder et al. 2017). There was no differential effect of IPSRT over specialist supportive care, nor was there an independent effect of age. Thus, the effects of IPSRT in adolescent BD are unclear.

Goldstein et al. (2018) examined the effects of an eight-session IPSRT protocol for HR adolescents (ages 12–18) with bipolar parents, given in conjunction with data-informed referral (DIR) and compared with DIR alone. DIR involved referral for services relevant to psychiatric disorders identified in the teen. The trial examined adolescents who were at familial and symptomatic risk for BD but had not developed bipolar spectrum disorders: 42 youth entered the protocol with behavior disorders (50%), anxiety disorders (29%), mood disorders (21%), or no disorders (36%).

Of the eight protocol sessions of IPSRT, adolescents attended a mean of 4.1 sessions. None of the participants developed a new threshold mood episode (mania, hypomania, or depression) over the 6-month study, and there were equal displays of subthreshold symptoms of depression over follow-up. Three adolescents developed subthreshold symptoms of hypomania or mania: two in the DIR-only group, and one in IPSRT plus DIR. Interestingly, IPSRT had a measurable effect on sleep disturbance. When actigraphy data collected during a baseline week were examined, it was found that the IPSRT-plus-DIR group had more time awake after sleep onset compared with DIR only, but had less time awake during a posttreatment week 6 months later. Together with the Frank et al. (2005) results, it appears that changes in sleep/wake functioning and regularity may be important mediators of the clinical effects of IPSRT. Table 8–1 summarizes the findings of studies of early intervention for youth at high risk for BD.

Novel Treatment Methods Under Investigation

There are several models of care for pediatric BD that are in the early testing phases. *Dialectical behavior therapy* (DBT) for adolescents with bipolar I, II, or unspecified type has been used successfully in a pilot RCT ($N=20$) to reduce the severity of depressive symptoms and the frequency and severity of suicidal ideation, compared with a supportive psychosocial treatment (Goldstein et al. 2015). This DBT model, consisting of alternating weekly individual and family skill-training sessions for up to 1 year, is currently being tested in a larger-scale RCT.

Mindfulness-based cognitive therapy (MBCT) is being developed for children and adolescents who are at risk for BD. MBCT, consisting of group sessions that focus on mindfulness meditation and instruction in cognitive-behavioral techniques, has a strong empirical record in the treatment of adult depression and anxiety (Piet and Hougaard 2011). The focus is on regulation of attention and acceptance of one's thoughts, emotions, and experiences, making this approach particularly relevant to the early phases of BD, which often consist of mood instability and anxiety.

In a pilot trial of 12 sessions of MBCT with 10 youth who had a bipolar parent, clinician-rated and youth-rated anxiety both dropped from pre- to posttreatment, whereas parent-rated emotion regulation in the child increased from pre- to posttreatment. The 12-session treatment was well accepted by participants (Cotton et al. 2016). Although based on a small sample, an examination of changes in neural functioning showed that pre- to posttreatment improvements in anxiety correlated with changes in activation in the bilateral insula and anterior cingulate when subjects viewed emotional stimuli (Strawn et al. 2016). These structures are involved in the processing of internal physical cues, a cognitive process that has long been linked to anxiety. Although it is not known whether MBCT will have a long-term impact on childhood anxiety, it is an example of a treatment that may be scalable in the larger at-risk population.

Conclusion and Future Directions

Empirical studies of novel psychosocial interventions for early-onset BD or HR youth are few, with most treatments tested in only one or two trials. Nonetheless, a picture is beginning to emerge of the active ingredients of effective early intervention: psychoeducation, family involvement in therapy and other aspects of care, training in communication and problem-

TABLE 8–1. Psychosocial treatment studies in high-risk offspring of bipolar parents

Study	Sample population and size	Intervention	Design	Outcome
Miklowitz et al. 2011	13 children with a parent with BD I or II and with active mood symptoms	FFT-HR	Open, 12 sessions over 4 months	Improved depression, hypomania, and psychosocial functioning scores over 12 months
Miklowitz et al. 2013	40 youth with BD-NOS, MDD, or cyclothymia with a first-degree relative with BD I or II and active mood symptoms	FFT-HR or EC	RCT of 12 sessions of FFT-HR vs. 1–2 sessions of EC	More rapid recovery from initial mood symptoms, more weeks in remission, and a more favorable trajectory of mania scores over 1 year than youth in EC
Nadkarni and Fristad 2010	165 youth (ages 8–12) with depressive spectrum disorders (with or without transient manic symptoms; $n=50$) or bipolar spectrum disorders ($n=115$)	8 sessions of MF-PEP over 6 months, or wait-list control with 12-month delay	Wait-list controlled: immediate MF-PEP or wait list (MF-PEP delayed by 12 months)	Higher rates of conversion to bipolar spectrum disorders (60%) among youth on the wait list than in MF-PEP (16%)
Goldstein et al. 2014	13 adolescents with a first-degree relative with BD; 50% healthy at baseline, 50% with internalizing/externalizing disorders	IPSRT	Open, 12 sessions over 6 months	High satisfaction but only attended about half of scheduled sessions because of parental BD illness severity; less weekend sleeping in and oversleeping with treatment

TABLE 8–1. Psychosocial treatment studies in high-risk offspring of bipolar parents (*continued*)

Study	Sample population and size	Intervention	Design	Outcome
Goldstein et al. 2018	42 adolescents with a first-degree relative with BD, 64% with internalizing/externalizing disorders at baseline	IPSRT	RCT of IPSRT plus data-informed referral vs. data-informed referral alone	No group differences in symptom severity or new syndromal mood episodes over 6 months, but IPSRT was associated with greater improvements in sleep functioning; patients in IPSRT attended an average of four of eight scheduled sessions
Cotton et al. 2016	10 high-risk offspring with at least one bipolar parent and with anxiety symptoms	Mindfulness-based cognitive therapy for children	Open, pilot 12 weeks	Reduced clinician-rated anxiety and youth-rated trait anxiety; increased parent-rated emotion regulation; increased mindfulness associated with decreased anxiety

Note.   BD=bipolar disorder; BD-NOS=bipolar disorder not otherwise specified; EC=educational control; FFT-HR=family-focused therapy for youth at high risk; IPSRT=interpersonal and social rhythm therapy; MDD=major depressive disorder; MF-PEP=multi-family psychoeducational psychotherapy; RCT=randomized controlled trial.

solving skills (or more broadly, interpersonal skills), and cognitive-behavioral strategies (e.g., mindful acceptance). These treatment elements may all contribute to the outcomes observed over the 6-month to 1-year durations of these studies. Few studies have examined longer-term outcomes, such as whether family psychoeducation or skills training or IPSRT can help delay or prevent the onset of manic episodes.

Successful early interventions should have two key elements. First, they must have clear targets. Knowing that a child has a bipolar parent increases our estimate of risk for bipolar onset; knowing that she also has depression, anxiety, mood instability, or subthreshold manic symptoms increases this estimate considerably (Hafeman et al. 2016). However, these are symptoms of bipolar illness in muted form. Investigators need to have working hypotheses about what features of the child at the neural, biological, or behavioral levels, and what features of the environment, are risk factors for BD onset or recurrence. Our treatments need to be designed to modify these risk factors, or at least reduce their influence. Although not specific to BD, behavioral markers such as sleep/wake disturbance or family conflict and criticism are useful starting points in defining treatment targets.

Second, new treatments must be scalable at the community mental health level. Treatments must be short enough to fit into the formularies of economically strapped clinics or practices, and must not require extensive periods of training and supervision that take clinicians away from their duties. A significant barrier to the uptake of evidence-based psychotherapies—including those described in this chapter—is the skepticism of community clinicians that such practices are relevant to lower-income, under-resourced populations. Convincing community practitioners that preventing BD is a worthwhile goal of treatment may also be difficult. It is the job of treatment researchers to partner with community mental health practitioners and administrators to determine whether evidence-based treatments can be implemented in public health settings, with the patients ordinarily seen there and by the clinicians who work there. These partnerships may lead to modifications of treatment protocols that contribute to scalability and broader population coverage, as well as inform our understanding of factors that affect the onset or course of bipolar illness in multiple contexts.

Clinical Pearls

- Bipolar I and II disorder in children and adolescents can be successfully treated with combinations of pharmacotherapy and family psychosocial interventions.

- There is evidence that youth who are at risk for bipolar disorder can be treated to remission with family-focused treatment and multifamily psychoeducation groups.

- Although less well studied, interpersonal and social rhythm therapy and dialectical behavior therapy have promise as early interventions in bipolar spectrum and high-risk youth.

- Successful psychosocial interventions aim toward improving family communication and problem solving and decreasing conflict in the family, as well as enhancing sleep/wake regularity.

- Reducing parental criticism can be achieved in part through psychoeducation about mood disorders, notably, understanding what behaviors are more versus less controllable by the child.

References

Birmaher B, Gill MK, Axelson DA, et al: Longitudinal trajectories and associated baseline predictors in youths with bipolar spectrum disorders. Am J Psychiatry 171(9):990–999, 2014 24874203

Cotton S, Luberto CM, Sears RW, et al: Mindfulness-based cognitive therapy for youth with anxiety disorders at risk for bipolar disorder: a pilot trial. Early Interv Psychiatry 10(5):426–434, 2016 25582800

Frank E, Kupfer DJ, Thase ME, et al: Two-year outcomes for interpersonal and social rhythm therapy in individuals with bipolar I disorder. Arch Gen Psychiatry 62(9):996–1004, 2005 16143731

Fredman SJ, Baucom DH, Boeding SE, et al: Relatives' emotional involvement moderates the effects of family therapy for bipolar disorder. J Consult Clin Psychol 83(1):81–91, 2015 25198285

Fristad MA, Verducci JS, Walters K, et al: Impact of multifamily psychoeducational psychotherapy in treating children aged 8 to 12 years with mood disorders. Arch Gen Psychiatry 66(9):1013–1021, 2009 19736358

Garber J, Clarke GN, Weersing VR, et al: Prevention of depression in at-risk adolescents: a randomized controlled trial. JAMA 301(21):2215–2224, 2009 19491183

Geller B, Tillman R, Bolhofner K, et al: Child bipolar I disorder: prospective continuity with adult bipolar I disorder; characteristics of second and third episodes; predictors of 8-year outcome. Arch Gen Psychiatry 65(10):1125–1133, 2008 18838629

Goldstein TR, Fersch-Podrat R, Axelson DA, et al: Early intervention for adolescents at high risk for the development of bipolar disorder: pilot study of interpersonal and social rhythm therapy (IPSRT). Psychotherapy 51(1):180–189, 2014 24377402

Goldstein TR, Fersch-Podrat RK, Rivera M, et al: Dialectical behavior therapy for adolescents with bipolar disorder: results from a pilot randomized trial. J Child Adolesc Psychopharmacol 25(2):140–149, 2015 25010702

Goldstein TR, Merranko J, Krantz M, et al: Early intervention for adolescents at-risk for bipolar disorder: A pilot randomized trial of Interpersonal and Social Rhythm Therapy (IPSRT). J Affect Disord 235:348–356, 2018 29665518

Hafeman DM, Merranko J, Axelson D, et al: Toward the definition of a bipolar prodrome: dimensional predictors of bipolar spectrum disorders in at-risk youths. Am J Psychiatry 173(7):695–704, 2016 26892940

Hlastala SA, Kotler JS, McClellan JM, et al: Interpersonal and social rhythm therapy for adolescents with bipolar disorder: treatment development and results from an open trial. Depress Anxiety 27(5):457–464, 2010 20186968

Hooley JM: Expressed emotion and relapse of psychopathology. Annu Rev Clin Psychol 3:329–352, 2007 17716059

Inder ML, Crowe MT, Moor S, et al: Three-year follow-up after psychotherapy for young people with bipolar disorder. Bipolar Disord Dec 22, 2017 [Epub ahead of print] 29271072

Kim EY, Miklowitz DJ: Expressed emotion as a predictor of outcome among bipolar patients undergoing family therapy. J Affect Disord 82(3):343–352, 2004 15555685

MacPherson HA, Weinstein SM, Henry DB, West AE: Mediators in the randomized trial of child- and family-focused cognitive-behavioral therapy for pediatric bipolar disorder. Behav Res Ther 85:60–71, 2016 27567973

Malkoff-Schwartz S, Frank E, Anderson BP, et al: Social rhythm disruption and stressful life events in the onset of bipolar and unipolar episodes. Psychol Med 30(5):1005–1016, 2000 12027038

Mendenhall AN, Fristad MA, Early TJ: Factors influencing service utilization and mood symptom severity in children with mood disorders: effects of multifamily psychoeducation groups (MFPGs). J Consult Clin Psychol 77(3):463–473, 2009 19485588

Miklowitz DJ, Chung B: Family focused therapy for bipolar disorder: reflections on 30 years of research. Fam Process 55(3):483–499, 2016 27471058

Miklowitz DJ, George EL, Richards JA, et al: A randomized study of family focused psychoeducation and pharmacotherapy in the outpatient management of bipolar disorder. Arch Gen Psychiatry 60(9):904–912, 2003 12963672

Miklowitz DJ, Otto MW, Frank E, et al: Psychosocial treatments for bipolar depression: a 1-year randomized trial from the Systematic Treatment Enhancement Program. Arch Gen Psychiatry 64(4):419–426, 2007 17404119

Miklowitz DJ, Axelson DA, Birmaher B, et al: Family focused treatment for adolescents with bipolar disorder: results of a 2-year randomized trial. Arch Gen Psychiatry 65(9):1053–1061, 2008 18762591

Miklowitz DJ, Axelson DA, George EL, et al: Expressed emotion moderates the effects of family focused treatment for bipolar adolescents. J Am Acad Child Adolesc Psychiatry 48(6):643–651, 2009 19454920

Miklowitz DJ, Chang KD, Taylor DO, et al: Early psychosocial intervention for youth at risk for bipolar I or II disorder: a one-year treatment development trial. Bipolar Disord 13(1):67–75, 2011 21320254

Miklowitz DJ, Schneck CD, Singh MK, et al: Early intervention for symptomatic youth at risk for bipolar disorder: a randomized trial of family focused therapy. J Am Acad Child Adolesc Psychiatry 52(2):121–131, 2013 23357439

Miklowitz DJ, Schneck CD, George EL, et al: Pharmacotherapy and family focused treatment for adolescents with bipolar I and II disorders: a 2-year randomized trial. Am J Psychiatry 171(6):658–667, 2014 24626789

Miklowitz DJ, Schneck CD, Walshaw PD, et al: Early intervention for youth at high risk for bipolar disorder: a multisite randomized trial of family focused treatment. Early Interv Psychiatry Aug 4, 2017 [Epub ahead of print] 28776930

Nadkarni RB, Fristad MA: Clinical course of children with a depressive spectrum disorder and transient manic symptoms. Bipolar Disord 12(5):494–503, 2010 20712750

O'Donnell LA, Axelson DA, Kowatch RA, et al: Enhancing quality of life among adolescents with bipolar disorder: a randomized trial of two psychosocial interventions. J Affect Disord 219:201–208, 2017 28570966

Piet J, Hougaard E: The effect of mindfulness-based cognitive therapy for prevention of relapse in recurrent major depressive disorder: a systematic review and meta-analysis. Clin Psychol Rev 31(6):1032–1040, 2011 21802618

Rea MM, Tompson MC, Miklowitz DJ, et al: Family focused treatment versus individual treatment for bipolar disorder: results of a randomized clinical trial. J Consult Clin Psychol 71(3):482–492, 2003 12795572

Salinger JM, O'Brien MP, Miklowitz DJ, et al: Family communication with teens at clinical high-risk for psychosis or bipolar disorder. J Fam Psychol 32(4):507–516, 2018 29389150

Schneck CD, Chang KD, Singh M, et al: A pharmacologic algorithm for youth who are at high risk for bipolar disorder. J Child Adolesc Psychopharmacol 27(9):796–805, 2017 28731778

Strawn JR, Cotton S, Luberto CM, et al: Neural function before and after mindfulness-based cognitive therapy in anxious adolescents at risk for developing bipolar disorder. J Child Adolesc Psychopharmacol 26(4):372–379, 2016 26783833

West AE, Weinstein SM, Peters AT, et al: Child- and family-focused cognitive-behavioral therapy for pediatric bipolar disorder: a randomized clinical trial. J Am Acad Child Adolesc Psychiatry 53(11):1168–1178, 1178.e1, 2014 25440307

9

Pharmacotherapy for Pediatric Depression

Gyung-Mee Kim, M.D., Ph.D.

Raghu Gandhi, M.D.

Kathryn R. Cullen, M.D.

Gabriela is a 14-year-old Hispanic girl who presented to a university outpatient clinic to establish care following a recent hospital admission. The event precipitating the admission was that Gabriela had taken a handful of pills from the medicine cabinet at home with the intent of ending her life. She had been experiencing depressive symptoms for the past 2 years, initially precipitated by the death of her grandmother. Symptoms had worsened in the past 6 months following her father's deportation to Mexico. Symptoms of depression included low mood, irritability, oppositionality (talking back, refusing to do chores), and aggression (picking physical fights with her 11-year-old sibling). She often had difficulty falling asleep, would wake up multiple times during the night, and did not feel rested upon awakening. She complained of poor appetite and had lost 15 pounds. She was struggling academically; she was in a mainstream ninth-grade class but was failing to finish her homework because of a lack of motivation and poor concentration. The school had referred her to a counselor, but she attended only three sessions; neither Gabriela nor her mother had perceived a benefit from therapy. The family doctor had prescribed a low dose of an antidepressant for Gabriela, but she stopped it after 1 week because of perceived inefficacy. When Gabriela was hospitalized, screening laboratory tests, including complete blood count, basic metabolic panel, and thyroid studies, were unremarkable. The inpatient team started fluoxetine and made a referral for step-down to an intensive outpatient program.

At the time of the first clinic visit, Gabriela had been home for 2 weeks. Since the mother primarily spoke Spanish, a Spanish language interpreter was used for the interview. Gabriela was still taking fluoxetine 10 mg daily (it had now been almost 3 weeks); neither Gabriela nor her mother noticed any improvement with the medication. They had decided not to follow through with the intensive outpatient program because they did not feel it would be beneficial. On mental status examination, her speech was soft and slow. She described her mood as "sad," and her affect was blunted and tearful. She denied any suicidal thinking since the attempt before hospitalization. Reasons for not following through on previous recommendations for psychotherapy and intensive outpatient treatment were discussed. Cultural barriers that were identified included stigma about mental illness among family members, Gabriela's fear of being bullied at school if her peers learned about her mental health issues, and lack of clear understanding of the importance and role of psychotherapy in the treatment of depression. These issues were addressed through reassuring Gabriela and her mother about confidentiality and by providing psychoeducation about depression and treatment. The dosage of fluoxetine was increased to 20 mg daily. A referral was made for outpatient cognitive-behavioral therapy (CBT). In addition to history gathering and treatment planning, significant time was devoted to developing rapport and providing psychoeducation about depression and its treatment. A follow-up appointment for medication check was set for 2 weeks.

Although psychoeducation, lifestyle management training, and psychotherapy are the first-line interventions for children and adolescents presenting with depression (Hughes et al. 2007; Lopez et al. 2005), many young patients with severe and/or chronic depression will require pharmacotherapy to achieve response and remission. Selection of the appropriate treatment for a child or adolescent with depression takes into account multiple factors, including the patient's age, the family and social environment, the patient's and family's preferences and expectations, cultural issues, availability of expertise in pharmacotherapy and/or psychotherapy, cognitive development, severity and subtype of depression, chronicity, comorbid conditions, and family psychiatric history. While pharmacotherapy plays an important role in the treatment of many children and adolescents with depression, all treatment phases should include psychoeducation, supportive management, and family and school involvement.

In this chapter, we review available evidence regarding the use of psychotropic medication in the treatment of pediatric depression. (See also Table 4 in Appendix B of this volume for U.S. Food and Drug Administration [FDA] approved, off-label, and emerging pharmacological treatments for pediatric unipolar depression.) In comparison to the large body of evidence on effectiveness of antidepressants for the treatment of depression in adults, knowledge about the use of these medications in children and adolescents has generally lagged behind that in adults. Since the greatest weight of available evidence supports the use of selective serotonin reuptake inhibitors (SSRIs) for the treatment of pediatric depression, we focus on these medications. First, we discuss the general features that are common across SSRI medications (e.g., mechanism of action, pharmacokinetics, side effects, serotonin syndrome, discontinuation syndrome) and then review efficacy data for each medication. When such data are available, we focus on results from double-blind randomized controlled trials (RCTs) in which an antidepressant is tested against placebo and/or a comparison drug. When data from RCTs are not available, we briefly review the highest level of evidence that has been published. Second, following the summary of SSRI medications, we briefly review the available literature on the use of non-SSRI medications in pediatric depression. Third, we discuss the issue of antidepressant suicide risk, the black-box warning, and the lasting impact these issues have had on treating pediatric depression. Fourth, although there has been a paucity of literature on treatment-resistant depression (TRD) in children and adolescents, we review the available information on the pharmacological management of TRD in adolescents. Finally, we discuss pharmacotherapy management once response is achieved: although the vast majority of research studies testing pharmacotherapy options for pediatric depression have focused on the initial phase of treatment, we review the available information (at times relying on expert recommendations rather than prospective data) on the continuation and maintenance phases of treatment. We close with clinical pearls for guidance in treating children and adolescents with depression with psychopharmacology.

Selective Serotonin Reuptake Inhibitors in Pediatric Depression

Overview

Currently marketed SSRIs include fluoxetine, sertraline, paroxetine, fluvoxamine, citalopram, and escitalopram. As of this writing, fluoxetine and escitalopram are the only two FDA-approved antidepressants for the treatment of major depressive disorder (MDD) in youths under 18 years of age. A systematic review and meta-analysis from 13 pediatric MDD trials with a total of 3,004 patients revealed that the greatest improvement with SSRIs versus placebo is observed early in the course of treatment (e.g., within 2 weeks) (Varigonda et al. 2015). There were no significant differences based on maximum SSRI dose or among particular SSRI agents. SSRIs were demonstrated to have a smaller benefit in pediatric compared with adult MDD. The selection of an antidepressant should include consideration of previous antidepressant response, family treatment history, patient/family preference, avoidance of specific side effects, comorbid psychiatric illness, drug-drug interactions, and cost. In general, the doses of SSRIs prescribed for youths are similar to those used for adult patients (Birmaher and Brent 2007). However, in preadolescent youth, these agents are generally started at lower doses and based on weight to ensure tolerability. Clinical response should be assessed at 4- to 6-week intervals, and dosage should be titrated as tolerated and maximized if a complete response has not been obtained.

A summary of SSRIs, including pediatric dose ranges, is presented in Table 9–1.

Mechanism of Action

The SSRIs enhance serotonergic neurotransmission through blockade of the reuptake process on the presynaptic neuron, leading to an acute increase of serotonin in the synapse. In comparison to tricyclic antidepressants (TCAs), which also antagonize muscarinic, histaminergic, and α_1-adrenergic receptors, SSRI medications bind to these receptors much less potently and therefore have fewer anticholinergic, sedative, and cardiovascular side effects.

Pharmacokinetics, Metabolism, and Drug Interactions

Most SSRIs have relatively long half-lives and so are given once daily. An exception is fluvoxamine, which has the shortest half-life (about 14 hours in young people) and so is sometimes prescribed twice daily. Fluoxetine has the longest half-life among SSRIs (1–4 days), and the half-life of its active metabolite is 4–16 days. Food does not appear to affect the systemic bioavailability of fluoxetine, but absorption of sertraline may be slightly enhanced by food. All SSRIs are metabolized in the liver by the cytochrome P450 (CYP) enzymes. Each of the SSRIs has the potential for slowing or

TABLE 9–1. Summary of selective serotonin reuptake inhibitor medications, including dose range

Generic name	Brand name(s)	FDA approval age	Available strengths and dosage forms (generic and brand)	Pediatric dose range
Fluoxetine hydrochloride	Prozac, Sarafem, Selfemra	Acute and maintenance treatment of MDD in adult patients and pediatric patients ages 8–18 years	Fluoxetine: 10 mg, 20 mg, 40 mg, 60 mg tablets and capsules 20 mg/5 mL oral solution 90-mg delayed-release capsule (weekly) Prozac: 10 mg, 20 mg, 40 mg capsules Sarafem: 10 mg, 15 mg, 20 mg tablets Selfemra: 10 mg, 15 mg, 20 mg tablets	5–30 mg/day
Escitalopram oxalate	Lexapro[a]	Approved for treating MDD in patients 12 years and up	Escitalopram: 5 mg, 10 mg, 20 mg tablets 5 mg/5 mL oral solution Lexapro: 5 mg, 10 mg, 20 mg tablets	10–20 mg/day (initial dose)
Citalopram hydrobromide	Celexa	Not approved for pediatric depression	Citalopram: 10 mg, 20 mg, 40 mg tablets 10 mg/5 mL oral solution Celexa: 10, 20, 40 mg tablets	Published studies with pediatric patients have used 20–40 mg/day, with maximum of 40 mg/day in adults
Fluvoxamine maleate	Luvox[a]	Not approved for pediatric depression	Fluvoxamine: 25 mg, 50 mg, 100 mg tablets 100 mg, 150 mg extended-release capsules	50–200 mg/day

TABLE 9–1. Summary of selective serotonin reuptake inhibitor medications, including dose range (*continued*)

Generic name	Brand name(s)	FDA approval age	Available strengths and dosage forms (generic and brand)	Pediatric dose range
Paroxetine hydrochloride	Paxil, Paxil CR	Not approved for pediatric depression	**Paroxetine:** 10 mg, 20 mg, 30 mg, 40 mg tablets 12.5, 25 mg extended-release tablets (24-hour) **Paxil:** 10, 20, 30, 40 mg tablets 10 mg/5 mL oral suspension **Paxil CR:** 12.5 mg, 25 mg, 37.5 mg extended-release tablets (24-hour)	20–50 mg/day in adults Published studies with pediatric patients have used 20–40 mg/day
Paroxetine mesylate	Brisdelle, Pexeva	Not approved for pediatric depression	**Paroxetine:** 7.5 mg capsules **Brisdelle:** 7.5 mg capsules **Pexeva:** 10 mg, 20 mg, 30 mg, 40 mg capsules	
Sertraline hydrochloride	Zoloft	Not approved for pediatric depression	**Sertraline:** 25 mg, 50 mg, 100 mg tablets 20 mg/mL oral concentrate **Zoloft:** 25 mg, 50 mg, and 100 mg tablets 20 mg/mL oral concentrate	25 mg once daily in children (ages 6–12); 50 mg once daily in adolescents (ages 13–17) for OCD

Note. CR=controlled release; FDA=U.S. Food and Drug Administration; MDD=major depressive disorder; OCD=obsessive-compulsive disorder.

[a]Brand discontinued in the United States.

blocking the metabolism of other drugs. For example, fluvoxamine shows clinically significant interactions with theophylline and clozapine through CYP1A2 inhibition, and with clonazepam or alprazolam through CYP3A4 inhibition. Fluoxetine and paroxetine also may interfere with the efficacy of opiate analogs, such as codeine and hydrocodone, through CYP2D6 inhibition. Sertraline, citalopram, and escitalopram have minimal interaction with other drugs.

Side Effects

All SSRIs have similar side-effect profiles, and the SSRIs are better tolerated than TCAs for most patients. The most common side effects of SSRIs are headache and gastrointestinal adverse effects such as nausea, diarrhea, anorexia, vomiting, flatulence, and dyspepsia. Sertraline and fluvoxamine are especially known for inducing gastrointestinal side effects. Headache and initial anorexia are most common with fluoxetine. The SSRIs are associated with an increased risk of gastrointestinal bleeding, because the SSRIs can cause functional impairment of platelet aggregation and bleeding time prolongation (Andrade et al. 2010). In some cases, SSRIs can cause emotional or behavioral adverse effects such as anxiety, emotional blunting, hyperactivity, irritability, hostility, disinhibition, emotional lability, and (as discussed in more detail below) self-harm. Paroxetine, in particular, may cause anticholinergic side effects such as dry mouth, constipation, and sedation.

Serotonin Syndrome

Concurrent administration of monoamine oxidase inhibitors (MAOIs), tryptophan, lithium, or other antidepressants that inhibit reuptake of serotonin can raise plasma serotonin concentration to toxic levels, causing the occurrence of serotonin syndrome. This syndrome is seen with therapeutic medication use, inadvertent interactions between drugs, and intentional self-poisoning. Other agents with serotonergic properties that have been associated with serotonin syndrome include amphetamines, antiemetics, drugs of abuse (e.g., cocaine, 3,4-methylenedioxymethamphetamine [MDMA or ecstasy], lysergic acid diethylamide [LSD]), and over-the-counter drug remedies such as dextromethorphan (Volpi-Abadie et al. 2013). Symptoms of serotonin syndrome include diarrhea, restlessness, agitation, hyperthermia, sweating, tremor, hyperreflexia, myoclonus, seizure, and even lethal conditions such as delirium, coma, status epilepticus, cardiovascular collapse, and death.

SSRI Discontinuation Syndrome

The abrupt discontinuation of SSRIs may result in a withdrawal syndrome, especially with those that have shorter half-lives, including fluvoxamine and paroxetine (half-life 21 hours) (Renoir 2013). Serotonin discontinuation symptoms can include flulike symptoms such as nausea, vomiting, diarrhea, headaches, and sweating, and sleep disturbances such as insomnia, nightmares, and constant sleepiness (Table 9–2). Mood disturbances such as anxiety, rebound depression, and poor concentration are also reported with abrupt SSRI discontinuation. This syndrome can occur within 2–3 days of discontinuing an SSRI and can persist for 2–3 weeks, depending on the half-life of the SSRI. This syndrome is generally mild and self-limited.

Safety in Pregnancy

All SSRIs except paroxetine have been classified as pregnancy category C, which means that animal studies have suggested potential adverse effects to the fetus and that no well-controlled studies have been conducted in humans. In 2005, the FDA changed the classification of paroxetine from pregnancy category C to category D because of concerns about the risk of cardiovascular malformations in neonates exposed to paroxetine during the first trimester. (Notably, in 2015, the FDA changed the labeling from the former pregnancy risk letter categories to the new format described in the Pregnancy and Lactation Labeling (Drugs) Final Rule (U.S. Food and Drug Administration 2014). Subsequent research further investigating cardiac risks associated with paroxetine has led to conflicting results. First, a large, population-based cohort study of 949,504 pregnant women enrolled in the Medicaid program did not find evidence for elevated risk for any cardiac malformation associated with SSRI exposure in the first trimester (relative risk among depressed women was 1.06; 95% confidence interval [95% CI], 0.93–1.22) (Huybrechts et al. 2014). In contrast, a later systematic review reported that paroxetine exposure during the first trimester was associated with an increased risk of major cardiac malformation (pooled odds ratio: 1.28; 95% CI, 1.11–1.47) (Bérard et al. 2016). Similarly, evidence regarding the risk of persistent pulmonary hypertension has been conflicting. According to a review of the literature conducted by the FDA in 2011, although several studies indicated a risk of PPH with SSRI use in pregnancy, three other large studies concluded there was no elevated risk. The FDA concluded: "At present, FDA does not find sufficient evidence to conclude that SSRI use in preg-

TABLE 9–2. FINISH: a mnemonic to remember the SSRI discontinuation syndrome symptoms

F Flulike symptoms, including fatigue, headache/muscle aches, lethargy, general malaise

I Insomnia

N Nausea, vomiting, diarrhea

I Imbalance (dizziness, vertigo, ataxia)

S Sensory disturbances (paresthesia, numbness, tingling, visual disturbance)

H Hyperarousal (anxiety, agitation, irritability, overactivity, aggression, crying spells, low mood)

nancy causes PPHN [persistent pulmonary hypertension in the newborn], and therefore recommends that health care providers treat depression during pregnancy as clinically appropriate" (U.S. Food and Drug Administration 2011).

When the clinician is weighing the options of whether to treat pregnant mothers with depression with SSRIs in the context of these conflicting bodies of evidence, another consideration that must be taken into account is the risks of untreated depression during pregnancy. Risks of untreated depression to the mother may include suicidal ideation and postnatal depression, while risks to the newborn may include low birth weight, preterm delivery, premature death, and admission to the neonatal intensive care unit (Latendresse et al. 2015). Postnatally, untreated depression during pregnancy also may increase the risk to the child of stress-like behaviors during the newborn period, altered functioning in multiple aspects of the central nervous system, internalizing and externalizing problems, and increased salivary cortisol and central adiposity during childhood (Gentile 2017). In some cases, these risks may take greater precedence than the potential harms to the unborn fetus due to the SSRI.

Fluoxetine

Fluoxetine is approved by the FDA for acute and maintenance treatment of MDD in pediatric patients ages 8–18 years. Several RCTs have been published that compared fluoxetine with placebo in the acute treatment of MDD in children and adolescents. In the first reported RCT involving 40 adolescent outpatients with MDD ages 13–18 years, fluoxetine (titrated to 60 mg/day by week 2) was compared with placebo in a 6-week trial. Two-thirds of the patients showed moderate or marked clinical global improvement; although the authors reported that fluoxetine was superior to placebo, the differences were not statistically significant (Simeon et al. 1990). Emslie et al. (1997) were the first to show superiority of fluoxetine over placebo for the treatment of pediatric depression. Ninety-six children and adolescents, ages 7–17 years, with nonpsychotic MDD were randomly assigned to receive 20 mg/day of fluoxetine or placebo. After 5 weeks of treatment, 31% of participants in the fluoxetine group were considered responders compared with 23% in the placebo group. Within the fluoxetine group, four patients dropped out because of side effects (three for manic symptoms, one for a severe rash). In a subsequent study, Emslie et al. (2002) reported on another RCT to confirm efficacy of fluoxetine (fixed dose 20 mg/day) in children and adolescents with MDD. The fluoxetine group showed a significantly greater reduction in depression scores compared with the placebo group, and remission occurred in significantly more patients with fluoxetine (41%) than with placebo (20%) (Emslie et al. 2002). There were no significant differences between treatment groups in discontinuations due to adverse events. Finally, following these placebo-controlled RCTs, a small study compared fluoxetine 40–60 mg/day with fluoxetine 20 mg/day in treating children and adolescents who had not responded to nine-week treatment with fluoxetine 10–20 mg (Heiligenstein et al. 2006). The authors reported that the higher-dose group showed a 71% response rate, while the low-dose group had a 36% response rate, at 10 weeks, and that the groups did not differ in adverse events; however, they also noted that the study was underpowered to detect a significant group difference. In the Treatment for Adolescents with Depression study (TADS), which examined combination treatment (antidepressant + psychotherapy) and whose findings will be discussed in more detail below, the fluoxetine-only treatment arm showed a significantly higher response rate (60.6%) compared with the placebo group (34.8%).

Escitalopram

Escitalopram is approved by the FDA for acute and maintenance treatment of MDD in adolescents ages 12 years and up. Two RCTs have been published that compared escitalopram with placebo in the acute treatment of pediatric MDD. In the first, Wagner et al. (2004) reported on the efficacy and tolerability of flexible-dose (10–20 mg/day) escitalopram versus placebo in children and adolescents, ages 6–17 years, with MDD. Although the main study did not find a significant difference between drug and placebo, a post hoc analysis examining the sample of adolescents separately from the children found that the escitalopram group was superior to placebo in adolescents only, which, in part, explains the FDA indication for escitalopram for depression in youths down to age 12. In the escitalopram group, headache and abdominal pain occurred in >10% of patients. Suicide-related behavior events were observed in three participants (one in the escitalopram group and two in the placebo group); there were no completed suicides. Following this, Emslie et al. (2009) reported results from an 8-week RCT of escitalopram (10–20 mg/day) versus placebo in 312 adolescents (ages 12–17 years) with MDD. The study results indicated that the escitalopram group improved significantly more than the group receiving placebo. Adverse events occurring in at least 10% of escitalopram patients included headache, menstrual cramps, insomnia, and nausea. The incidence of influenza-like symptoms in the escitalopram group was more than twofold that in the placebo group (7.1% vs. 3.2%).

Citalopram

Although citalopram is not approved for pediatric depression by the FDA, there is some evidence supporting its use in pediatric depression, especially for adolescents. Wagner et al. (2004) conducted an RCT testing citalopram (20 mg/day, with the option of increasing the dosage to 40 mg/day at week 4 if clinically indicated) versus placebo in children (ages 7–11) and adolescents (ages 12–17) with MDD. The authors reported significantly greater response rates at week 8 following treatment with citalopram vs. placebo (36% vs. 24%) (Wagner et al. 2004). Citalopram was well tolerated, and the only adverse events to occur with a frequency exceeding 10% were rhinitis, nausea, and abdominal pain, which were not significantly different from rates in the placebo group. There were no serious adverse events and no clinically significant electrocardiographic changes or weight changes in any patient with citalopram in this study. von Knorring et al. (2006) reported on a European, multicenter study in which 244 adolescents with MDD (ages 13–18 years) were randomly assigned to receive treatment with citalopram (n=124) or placebo (n=120) for 12 weeks. The response rate in both groups was about 60%. However, a post hoc analysis that examined the third of all patients who were not also receiving psychotherapy found that in the absence of psychotherapy, the response and remission rates in the citalopram-treated group were significantly higher than those in the placebo group. The most common adverse events in both groups were headache, nausea, and insomnia. Only fatigue was significantly more frequent in the citalopram group than in the placebo group. Hospitalization due to psychiatric disorder was the most common serious adverse event in both groups (14 of 124 and 9 of 120 for citalopram and placebo, respectively). No weight changes, clinically significant changes in laboratory values or vital signs, electrocardiographic changes, or death was shown in either group.

In 2011 and 2012, the FDA issued a black box warning that recommended that citalopram not be used at doses greater than 40 mg/day to avoid the risk of dangerous abnormal heart rhythms such as QT interval prolongation (U.S. Food and Drug Administration 2016). Electrolyte and/or electrocardiographic monitoring is recommended for patients who are taking citalopram, especially if patients experience signs and symptoms of an abnormal heart rate or rhythm such as dizziness, palpitations, or syncope.

Paroxetine

Paroxetine is not approved for pediatric depression by the FDA, possibly for good reason. Two RCTs have been published that compared paroxetine with placebo as an intervention for MDD in children and adolescents. In the first, Keller et al. (2001) tested 8 weeks of paroxetine (20–40 mg) versus placebo, and imipramine (200–300 mg) versus placebo, in 275 adolescents, ages 12–18 years, with MDD. Among the 190 participants who completed 8 weeks of treatment, paroxetine was more effective than both imipramine and placebo. Paroxetine was better tolerated than imipramine and not different from placebo in adverse effects except somnolence (17.2% for paroxetine vs. 3.4% for placebo). Imipramine was not more effective than placebo. Serious adverse events, such as worsening depression, suicidal ideation/gestures, conduct problems or hostility, and euphoria/expansive mood, occurred in 11 of 93 patients in the paroxetine group. However, a later reanalysis of these data concluded that the clinical benefit for either paroxetine or imipramine was not superior to that seen with placebo, and that paroxetine was associated with an increase in suicidal ideation and behavior (Le Noury et al. 2015). A later RCT by Emslie et al. (2006) testing flexible-dose paroxetine versus placebo in children and adolescents, ages 7–17 years, with MDD reported that paroxetine was not more efficacious than placebo.

Sertraline

Although sertraline is not FDA approved for pediatric depression, there is evidence to support its efficacy for treating children and adolescents with MDD. In two multicenter, double-blind, placebo-controlled studies, 376 children and adolescents, ages 6–17 years, with MDD were randomly assigned to receive sertraline (flexible dose, 50–200 mg/day) or placebo

(Wagner et al. 2003). After 10 weeks of treatment, children in the sertraline group showed statistically significantly greater improvement than placebo patients. In this study, sertraline was generally well tolerated, and there was no difference in suicidal ideation between treatment groups. Diarrhea, vomiting, anorexia, and agitation occurred in at least 5% of the sertraline-treated group, and the frequency of these symptoms was at least twice that in the placebo group.

Fluvoxamine

Fluvoxamine is not approved for pediatric depression by the FDA, and no randomized controlled studies have yet investigated its use for treating MDD in children and adolescents.

Non-SSRI Antidepressants

Bupropion

Bupropion weakly inhibits the neuronal uptake of dopamine and norepinephrine but does not inhibit monoamine oxidase or the reuptake of serotonin. No RCTs have been published that have examined bupropion versus placebo in a pediatric sample; the available literature on bupropion for the treatment of pediatric depression is limited to three open-label trials. First, following a 2-week single-blind placebo lead-in, adolescents ages 11–18 years with depression and attention-deficit/hyperactivity disorder (ADHD) treated with open-label, sustained-release bupropion showed significant improvement in depression, ADHD symptoms, and functional impairment (Daviss et al. 2001). Second, an open-label trial of sustained-release bupropion (mean dose 362 mg/day) for adolescents with MDD found significant improvement in depression rating scale scores (Glod et al. 2003). In this study, the most common adverse events were insomnia and weight loss. Finally, another open-label trial of sustained-release bupropion (mean dose 315 mg/day) for the treatment of adolescents with mood disorders, ADHD, and substance use reported that bupropion treatment was associated with significant improvement of symptoms in all of these areas (Solhkhah et al. 2005).

Venlafaxine

Venlafaxine is a serotonin-norepinephrine reuptake inhibitor (SNRI) that selectively inhibits serotonin reuptake at lower doses and acts on both norepinephrine and serotonin reuptake at higher doses (>150 mg/day). Three RCTs have been published that examined the use of venlafaxine versus placebo in children and adolescents with depression. In the first, 33 children and adolescents with MDD were treated with 6 weeks of combination therapy consisting of psychotherapy with either venlafaxine or placebo. In this study, the daily dose for children was 12.5–37.5 mg, and for adolescents 25–75 mg. Both groups showed a significant clinical improvement, and no significant between-group differences in clinical improvement were found (Mandoki et al. 1997). The results of the other two RCTs were published together. These multicenter (50 sites in the United States) studies randomly assigned 334 children and adolescents, ages 7–17 years, with MDD to 8 weeks of venlafaxine extended-release (ER) (flexible-dose, 37.5–225 mg/day) or placebo. Overall results did not show a statistically significant superiority of venlafaxine ER over placebo; however, a post hoc analysis examining adolescents, ages 12–17, separately from children (ages 7–11) found that adolescents randomly assigned to receive venlafaxine ER had a significantly greater clinical improvement than did those receiving placebo, while this finding was absent in children (Emslie et al. 2007). Anorexia and abdominal pain were the most common adverse events, and serious adverse events, including hostility and suicide-related events, were more common in the venlafaxine ER group than in the placebo group. Finally, as discussed below (see section "Treatment-Resistant Depression"), the Treatment of (SSRI) Resistant Depression in Adolescents (TORDIA) study included venlafaxine in two of the study arms (no placebo arm included in this study.)

Duloxetine

Duloxetine is an SNRI that is approved by the FDA for the treatment of depression in adults and for the treatment of generalized anxiety disorder in persons 7 years and older. Two RCTs have been conducted to examine duloxetine in pediatric depression. In a 36-week RCT that included two doses of duloxetine (30 mg and 60 mg), a placebo arm, and a reference fluoxetine control group, Emslie et al. (2014) reported that neither of the duloxetine doses was superior to placebo. Since the reference fluoxetine group also did not separate from placebo, the trial was considered inconclusive with respect to efficacy. Rates of adverse effects were similar to those seen in adult studies. During acute treatment, 6.7% of the patients taking 60 mg of duloxetine and 5.2% of patients taking 30 mg of duloxetine had worsening of suicidal ideation from baseline, but at endpoint, over 80% of those had had improvement in suicidal ideation. The other RCT (10-week acute intervention followed by 26 week open-label extension) reported no significant differences from placebo in clinical improvement after 10 weeks (Atkinson et al. 2014). Similarly, in this study the fluoxetine reference group had also failed to separate from placebo at 10 weeks and so the trial was thought to be inconclusive with respect to efficacy. In this study, more than 80% of the patients with suicidal ideation at baseline had improvement at endpoint during acute treatment, but one in the duloxetine group had treatment-emergent suicidal behavior during the extension period.

Desvenlafaxine

Desvenlafaxine, an SNRI, is a major active metabolite of venlafaxine and has minimal phase I hepatic metabolism by CYP3A4, which provides an advantage over venlafaxine in that desvenlafaxine is less likely to have drug interactions. Desvenlafaxine has been approved by the FDA for the treatment of MDD in adults, but not in children and adolescents. No RCTs examining the efficacy of desvenlafaxine for treating pediatric depression have yet been published. Findling et al. (2014) examined tolerability and safety of desvenlafaxine in children and adolescents, ages 7–17 years, with MDD in an 8-week, multicenter, open-label, fixed-dose study and a 6-month flexible-dose extension study (Findling et al. 2014). In this study, the dosage ranged from 10 to 100 mg/day for children ($n=20$) and from 25 to 200 mg/day for adolescents ($n=20$), and a total of 8 months of desvenlafaxine treatment was generally safe and well tolerated in children and adolescents with MDD. The most common adverse events were upper abdominal pain (15%) and headache (15%) in children, and somnolence (30%) and nausea (20%) in adolescents. Findling et al. also reported the pharmacokinetics of desvenlafaxine: area under the curve (AUC) and maximum serum concentration (C_{max}) increased linearly with dose, and mean oral clearance (CL/F) was generally higher in children than in adolescents (Findling et al. 2016). In this study, 55% of children and 70% of adolescents reported one or more treatment-emergent adverse events, such as headache, upper abdominal pain, vomiting, cough, and oropharyngeal pain with 100 mg of desvenlafaxine in children; and nausea, somnolence, upper abdominal pain, vomiting, and dysmenorrhea with 200 mg of desvenlafaxine in adolescents. There was one reported suicidal ideation after 4 days and after 7 days in an adolescent taking desvenlafaxine 100 mg/day who had had suicidal ideation at baseline. At week 8, depression symptoms were improved. However, two recent RCTs have been conducted that do not support desvenlafaxine's efficacy. One study, using lower-dose (20, 30, or 35 mg/day based on baseline weight) or higher-dose (25, 35, or 50 mg/day based on baseline weight) desvenlafaxine for 8 weeks in 363 children and adolescents, ages 7–17, with MDD, showed that neither of the desvenlafaxine groups had significantly greater clinical improvement compared with placebo (Atkinson et al. 2018). In the second study, 339 children and adolescents (ages 7–17) were randomly assigned to receive 8 weeks of treatment with desvenlafaxine (25–50 mg/day), fluoxetine (20 mg/day), or placebo (Weihs et al. 2018). Since neither the desvenlafaxine group nor the fluoxetine reference group showed significant superiority over placebo, this was considered a failed trial.

Levomilnacipran

Levomilnacipran, an SNRI, is a newer antidepressant that is FDA approved for treating MDD in adults. Although there are not yet any publications from studies examining levomilnacipran in children and adolescents, there are currently two studies investigating the safety and efficacy of this agent in pediatric depression (Allergan 2018; Forest Laboratories 2018).

Tricyclic Antidepressants

TCAs represent the first-generation antidepressants and have historically been used to treat MDD in adults, adolescents, and children. This class of medications includes the agents desipramine, imipramine, nortriptyline, and amitriptyline. One RCT compared desipramine 200 mg daily in divided doses with placebo in 60 adolescents with depression (Kutcher et al. 1994). The desipramine group had a greater number of dropouts, and the response rate (48%) was not significantly superior to that seen with placebo (35%). Imipramine has been used to treat several psychiatric disorders of childhood, including depression, ADHD, obsessive-compulsive disorder (OCD), separation anxiety disorder, and enuresis. In a placebo-controlled RCT conducted by Puig-Antich and colleagues (1987), the study was terminated following a midpoint analysis (38 of 60 prepubertal children with depression had been enrolled) because at that point there was no difference between drug (56%) and placebo (68%) groups, and it was highly improbable that a significant effect versus placebo would have been found had the study continued. As noted earlier, in a study that also examined paroxetine versus placebo, Keller and colleagues (2001) reported that imipramine treatment was not more effective than placebo. In a reanalysis of these data, Le Noury et al. (2015) confirmed that the efficacy of imipramine was not statistically or clinically significantly different from that with placebo for treatment of MDD in children and adolescents and that imipramine treatment was associated with increased cardiovascular problems. As will be discussed below in more detail, in a 10-week RCT of 27 youths with TRD, Birmaher et al. (1998) reported that amitriptyline was no more effective than placebo for reducing depression symptoms. Geller and colleagues (1992) conducted an RCT testing "fixed plasma level" of nortriptyline versus placebo in children with MDD; both groups showed low response rates (31% active vs. 17% placebo) that were not statistically significant. After a systematic review and pooled analysis, Hazell and Mirzaie (2013) concluded that TCAs are not useful in treating depression in children. Given these data suggesting limited evidence for efficacy and considering the higher risk of adverse effects such as change of cardiac conductance and increased risk of seizure, at the current time, TCAs are generally not recommended for treating pediatric depression.

Vortioxetine

Vortioxetine is a multimodal antidepressant that acts as a serotonin (5-HT) 5-HT_3, 5-HT_7, and 5-HT_{1D} receptor antagonist; 5-HT_{1B} receptor partial agonist; 5-HT_{1A} receptor agonist; and inhibitor of the 5-HT transporter in vitro (Bang-Andersen et al. 2011; Mørk et al. 2012; Sanchez et al. 2015). Vortioxetine was approved by the FDA for the treatment of MDD in adults in 2013, but not in children and adolescents. In a recent 14-day, open-label study of pharmacokinetics and safety of vortioxetine in 48 pediatric patients with depressive or anxiety disorder (15 of 48 patients with depressive disorders, 14 of 48 patients with anxiety disorder, and 5 of 48 patients with depressive disorders and anxiety disorders), the C_{max} and AUC_{0-24} of vortioxetine were 30%–40% lower in adolescents than in children, and the median CL/F of vortioxetine was lower in children than in adolescents (Findling et al. 2017). In this study, 79% of children and 75% of adolescents reported treatment-emergent adverse events, and most of these events were mild, except severe headache in one case. The most common adverse events reported were headache (25%), nausea (23%), and sedation (23%). In the 6-month open-label extension study, Findling et al. (2018) concluded that a dosing of 5–20 mg/day for children and adolescents with depressive disorder or anxiety disorder was safe and well tolerated. However, there is no RCT of vortioxetine for treating depressive disorders in children and adolescents.

Vilazodone

Vilazodone, a serotonin modulator/stimulator that has SSRI-like activity and is also a 5-HT_{1A} receptor partial agonist, was approved by the FDA for the treatment of MDD in adults in 2011. It has not yet been approved for treating children and adolescents. Recently, a 10-week, Phase III, double-blind RCT was conducted in 529 adolescents, ages 12–17 years, with a diagnosis with MDD (Durgam et al. 2018). Participants were randomly assigned to receive placebo ($n=174$), vilazodone 15 mg/day ($n=175$), or vilazodone 30 mg/day ($n=180$). In this study, a statistically significant difference between vilazodone and placebo in change from baseline in Children's Depression Rating Scale—Revised score and Clinical Global Impression–Severity score was not observed (Durgam et al. 2018). Although the study results indicated that vilazodone was generally safe and well tolerated, there were no statistically significant group differences in reductions in depression symptoms. Furthermore, there were no significant group differences in suicidal ideation and suicidal behavior in this study. The most common adverse events with vilazodone in this study were nausea (29.1% at 15 mg/day and 27.2% at 30 mg/day) and headache (12.6% at 15 mg/day and 16.1% at 30 mg/day).

Monoamine Oxidase Inhibitors

A case series was conducted in 1988 by Ryan et al. (1988b) that involved 23 adolescents with MDD who had been treated with TCAs; nonresponders were switched to an MAOI, and partial responders had an MAOI added to the TCA. Seventeen of these adolescents showed good or fair antidepressant response to MAOIs. However, there have been no RCTs of MAOIs in depressed children and adolescents, and compliance with dietary restrictions limits suitability for treatment with MAOIs.

Black Box Warning: Risk of Suicidality With Antidepressants in Youth

Pharmacotherapy for pediatric depression has been complicated by concerns about potentially worsening suicidality. In 2004, the FDA issued a public warning about an increased risk of suicidal thoughts or behavior (suicidality) in children and adolescents treated with antidepressant medications (U.S. Food and Drug Administration 2018). The warning was based on the results of a meta-analysis that was conducted by the FDA in collaboration with Columbia University, in which 4,587 pediatric patients in 24 randomized, placebo-controlled antidepressant clinical trials were examined. These studies included children and adolescents with MDD (16 studies), OCD (4 studies), generalized anxiety disorder (2 studies), social anxiety disorder (one study), and ADHD (one study) (Hammad et al. 2006). The rate of suicidal thinking and behavior in this meta-analysis was reported to be 4% in children and adolescents who were assigned to receive active drug compared with 2% in those who were assigned to receive placebo. The FDA reported few suicide attempts and no completions. This meta-analytic study had significant limitations, including failure to include all available RCTs, short-term data, use of relative risk as a metric, inability to generalize the results in populations not included in the RCTs, and multiple comparisons (Hammad et al. 2006). In a case-control study, Olfson et al. (2006) compared the relative risk of suicide attempt and suicide death in severe depression of children and adults who were treated with antidepressants with the risk in those who did not receive antidepressants. The study results suggested that antidepressants were significantly related to suicide attempts or suicide deaths in children but not in adults, so careful clinical monitoring for suicide ideation/suicide attempts in treatment of depressed children and adolescents is recommended. In 2006, the FDA's black box warning was extended to include young adults up to age 25.

Bridge et al. (2007) reanalyzed 27 studies, which included published and unpublished randomized, placebo-controlled, parallel-group trials of second-generation antidepressants such as SSRIs, nefazodone, venlafaxine, and mirtazapine, in children and adolescents with MDD, OCD, or non-OCD anxiety disorders. The risk for suicidal ideation/suicide attempts was 0.7% greater (95% CI, 0.1%–1.3%) for antidepressants versus placebo across all trials; however, risk varied as a function of indication, age, and chronicity. There were no completed suicides. Age-stratified analyses showed that for children younger than 12 years with MDD, only fluoxetine showed benefit over placebo. In MDD trials, efficacy was moderated by age, duration of depression, and number of sites in the treatment trial. The overall number needed to harm (NNH), which is defined as the number of subjects needed to treat in order to observe one adverse event that can be attributed to the active treatment for MDD, was 143. The overall number needed to treat (NNT) for antidepressants in pediatric depression was 10. This number takes into account that some patients respond regardless of medication treatment; an NNT of 10 means that one would need to treat 10 youths with depression in order to have one extra patient respond who would not otherwise have improved (Andrade 2015). Together, this means that nearly 14 times more depressed youths will respond favorably to antidepressants than will spontaneously report suicidality. Results suggested that the benefits of antidepressant medications likely outweigh their risks to children and adolescents with MDD, OCD, and non-OCD anxiety disorders (Bridge et al. 2007).

The black box warning on antidepressants for youths had a major impact on clinical practice (Cheung et al. 2008). The number of SSRI prescriptions for children and adolescents decreased significantly in the United States, Canada, and Europe, and this drop was accompanied by a significant increase in rates of suicide attempts and completed suicides in adolescents (Gibbons et al. 2007; Katz et al. 2008; Lu et al. 2014). Analysis of these data added to findings from multiple prior epidemiological studies that revealed an inverse relationship between number of prescriptions of antidepressants for adolescents and the rate of suicide in the United States (Gibbons et al. 2006; Olfson et al. 2003) and worldwide (Otuyelu et al. 2015).

In a recent review article, Brent (2016) emphasized that youth at high risk for suicidal behaviors have a history of higher levels of suicidal ideation, family conflict, alcohol and substance use, nonsuicidal self-injury, and nonresponse to treatment. Recommendations for minimizing risk for suicidal behaviors during antidepressant treatment included educating youth and their parents about the risk of increased suicidal thoughts or behavior, identifying suicidal risk factors, establishing a safety plan, close clinical monitoring, setting an appropriate dosing schedule, and considering the combination of pharmacotherapy with psychotherapy. Indeed, pivotal studies, including the Treatment for Adolescents with Depression Study (March et al. 2004) and Treatment of Resistant Depression in Adolescents (Brent et al. 2008), have shown that combined treatment with both pharmacotherapy and psychotherapy is more efficacious than monotherapy (March et al. 2006), in terms of, among other outcomes, higher remission rates (Kennard et al. 2006) and rates of symptom reduction (Kratochvil et al. 2006).

Treatment-Resistant Depression

Treatment-resistant depression typically refers to a depression that has been treated with at least one adequate trial of an antidepressant medication, to which the patient had only an insufficient response (Fava 2003). Generally, insufficient response is considered as the failure to achieve at least 50% reduction in depressive symptomatology, though this definition is not always consistent in the field. Adequate antidepressant treatment is defined as at least 8 weeks of treatment, the first 4 weeks at the equivalent dose of 20 mg of fluoxetine and the additional 4 weeks at an increased dose if no response is obtained at the first dosage (Sackeim 2001). About 30%–40% of adolescents with MDD do not show an adequate clinical response to the initial treatment (Maalouf et al. 2011). As always, when faced with treatment resistance, the clinician should reevaluate the clinical picture of diagnosis, comorbidity, and contributing factors, including family dynamics and sociocultural issues.

Poor treatment response in acute adolescent depression treatment is predicted by severity and chronicity of depression, suicidal ideation and nonsuicidal self-injury, and hopelessness (Curry et al. 2006; Wilkinson et al. 2009). The presence of comorbid disorders such as ADHD, dysthymia, anxiety disorders, and substance use disorders has been correlated with poor treatment response. Medical comorbidity, such as anemia, vitamin B$_{12}$ deficiency, hypothyroidism, diabetes mellitus, fibromyalgia, or other chronic medical illness, is also related to functional impairment and may play a role in the aggravation of depressive symptoms in children and adolescents (Lewinsohn et al. 1996). In addition, environmental factors such as history of abuse, family discord, parental depression, bullying at school, and same-sex attraction accompanied by peer victimization or family rejection have been risk factors for depression and predictors of poorer treatment response for depression in adolescents (Brent et al. 2009; Feeny et al. 2009). Two studies have suggested that during treatment of adolescents with depression, cotreatment of insomnia with trazodone may be associated with a poorer antidepressant response (Shamseddeen et al. 2012; Sultan and Courtney 2017). First, in an analysis of data from the TORDIA study, Shamseddeen et al. (2012) reported that adolescents who received trazodone for insomnia showed a lower antidepressant response rate than those who were not taking sleep medication (odds ratio [OR] =0.16, 95% CI, 0.05–0.5, P=0.001) and showed an increased risk of self-harm (OR=3.0, 95% CI=1.1–7.9, P=0.03). Second, Sultan and Courtney (2017) conducted a chart review to investigate the effects of adjunctive trazodone on treatment response rates in adolescents who received either a SSRI or a SNRI. In this study, clinical improvement in adolescents who had been exposed to trazodone was lower than that of adolescents who had not been exposed to trazodone. However, the mechanism underlying the putative lower antidepressant response rate in adolescents receiving cotreatment with trazodone suggested by these preliminary studies is unknown.

Research investigating treatment options for adolescents with TRD is even more scarce than that for first-line interventions. The largest study to date remains the TORDIA study mentioned above. In TORDIA, 334 adolescents (ages 12–18 years) with SSRI-resistant depression were randomly assigned to either a medication switch alone (other SSRI or venlafaxine) or a medication switch plus CBT (Brent et al. 2008). Results indicated that a combination of either an SSRI or venlafaxine plus CBT was significantly more effective than medication alone. At 24 weeks, overall 38.9% of participants had achieved remission, regardless of the initial treatment (Emslie et al. 2010). Similar to the studies examining TCAs as a first-line therapy reviewed earlier in this chapter, an RCT of amitriptyline did not show efficacy versus placebo in a sample of hospitalized adolescents with TRD; both active and placebo groups showed high (70%–80%) rates of response (Birmaher et al. 1998). On the basis of these results, standard clinical practice in child psychiatry in the context of SSRI nonresponse has been to recommend a second SSRI with the addition of CBT.

Consideration should be given to the high placebo rates that have been observed in many pediatric antidepressant trials, which has called into question the efficacy of antidepressants for children and adolescents with depression. Meta-analyses of studies on efficacy of antidepressants for children and adolescents suggest that many of the antidepressants are not more effective than placebo (Cipriani et al. 2016). As recently reviewed by Walkup (2017), one important consideration may have to do with the trial sponsorship; as a general rule, industry-sponsored trials consistently had high placebo response rates (~50%), in contrast to two studies funded by the National Institute of Mental Health (Emslie et al. 1997; March et al. 2004), which had lower placebo response rates (33%–35%). Concerns with industry-sponsored drug trials that could account for high placebo response rates include pressure to recruit a large number of participants in a tight time frame, large numbers of sites with a small number of participants per site, potentially limited experience of the site investigators, inclusion of youths whose symptoms may be more attributable to psychosocial factors than to MDD, and financial incentives to retain participants in the trial (Walkup 2017). Since the gold standard for demonstrating efficacy remains the RCT, these considerations will be important to consider in the future design of treatment studies for pediatric depression.

Unfortunately, in the face of insufficient response following a switch to a second SSRI plus CBT, we reach the end of large, robust studies that have been conducted to provide guidance on where to go next. As noted in the Texas Children's Medication Algorithm Project, at this stage, an augmentation strategy is recommended (Hughes et al. 2007). Most augmentation recommendations are extrapolated from available adult data, which include bupropion and mirtazapine (Trivedi et al. 2006). If there is still treatment resistance, switching to an alternative antidepressant monotherapy may be considered.

Augmentation of antidepressant treatment with lithium is a classic strategy for addressing TRD in adults. Research on lithium augmentation for TRD suggested that this strategy was more effective for patients with a diagnosis of bipolar disorder, for subjects with more than three major depressive episodes, and for those with a family history of MDD or bipolar disorder in a first-degree relative (Sugawara et al. 2010). Several reports have suggested that lithium may be useful as an adjunctive treatment to antidepressants in adolescents with TRD. A case series of lithium augmentation in TCA-refractory depression for 14 adolescents (Ryan et al. 1988a) and a case report of lithium augmentation of venlafaxine in adolescent major depression (Walter et al. 1998) suggested that this strategy may be promising in some adolescents with TRD. In addition, an open trial of lithium augmentation for 24 depressive adolescents who did not respond to 6 weeks of treatment with imipramine (Strober et al. 1992) also yielded favorable results. However, no results from RCTs examining lithium adjunctive treatment in adolescents with TRD have yet been reported.

Augmentation with atypical antipsychotics has been useful for the treatment of adults with depression. A recent systematic review and network meta-analysis study of 16 RCTs of seven different types and dosages of atypical antipsychotics, including quetiapine, aripiprazole, and risperidone, found that augmentation with all standard-dose atypical antipsychotics for adult TRD patients is effective in reducing depressive symptoms (Zhou et al. 2015). In one case series of 10 adolescents with TRD being treated with SSRIs using augmentation with quetiapine, 70% of the patients showed a positive response to treatment with adjunctive quetiapine (mean dose 275 mg/day) (Pathak et al. 2005). However, no RCTs have been published that have examined atypical antipsychotics as an adjunctive treatment for TRD in adolescents.

A classic strategy for addressing TRD in adults is to augment the thyroid system. In the STAR*D (Sequenced Treatment Alternatives to Relieve Depression) study for defining the tolerability and effectiveness of various options of pharmacotherapy in both acute and longer-term treatment in a total of 4,042 adult outpatients with nonpsychotic MDD, the remission rate of T_3 (triiodothyronine, liothyronine) augmentation was 24.7%, which was higher than that of lithium augmentation (13.2%), and fewer participants discontinued T_3 because of adverse effects than discontinued lithium (Rush et al. 2009). However, no publications are available supporting the efficacy of T_3 augmentation for pediatric depression.

Creatine is an organic acid that facilitates recycling of adenosine triphosphate and energy homeostasis primarily in muscle and brain. An open-label study of adjunctive creatine involved five female adolescents who had been treated with fluoxetine for at least 8 weeks and had insufficient response. Following 8 weeks of treatment with creatine 4 g daily, depression scores decreased by 56% (Kondo et al. 2011). A subsequent study by this group enrolled 34 female adolescents with SSRI-resistant depression in a dosing study that included placebo and 2-mg, 4-mg, and 10-mg doses of creatine. Creatine at any of the three doses was not found to separate from placebo in this pilot study (Kondo et al. 2016). The group is currently conducting the next phase of research testing of creatine (10 mg) as a treatment for girls with SSRI-resistant depression (Renshaw 2017).

Lamotrigine, an antiepileptic drug, has known antidepressant effects in both unipolar and bipolar depression in adults and has a lower risk of causing switching to mania in comparison to other antidepressants. A retrospective chart review of 37 adolescents with either unipolar or bipolar depression suggested that lamotrigine was well tolerated and associated with significant clinical improvement at 12 weeks (Shon et al. 2014). However, no RCTs have been conducted testing lamotrigine for TRD in adolescents.

Ketamine, an N-methyl-D-aspartate glutamate receptor antagonist, has been approved by the FDA as an anesthetic for children and adults, and there have been reported RCTs of a rapid-onset antidepressant effect in adults with TRD (McCloud et al. 2015; Murrough et al. 2013; Singh et al. 2016). However, as of the time of this writing, there are no publications yet available about effectiveness of ketamine in adolescents with TRD.

Nonpharmacological somatic options are also a possible consideration for adolescents with TRD. Repetitive transcranial magnetic stimulation (rTMS) of the dorsolateral prefrontal cortex has been approved by the FDA for treatment of TRD in adults, with controlled studies supporting its effectiveness (Avery et al. 2006). While no RCTs have yet been published in children and adolescents, results from an open-label study and several case series are now available about the effectiveness of rTMS for adolescents with TRD. First, in an open-label study using rTMS for treatment of nine adolescents, ages 16–18 years, with TRD, three adolescents met criteria for response after 10 treatments (Bloch et al. 2008). In a 3-year follow-up of this study, eight of these nine patients were reassessed; the improvement of depressive symptoms had been maintained, and there was no observed loss of cognitive function (Mayer et al. 2012). In a case series, two of three adolescents, ages 16–18 years, with TRD who were treated with 10 sessions of rTMS showed reductions in depressive symptoms of 39% and 47% (Walter et al. 2001). The most common adverse effect of TMS is mild headache, but the most significant risk is seizure (approximately 1%). To date, one case of TMS-induced seizure in an adolescent has been reported (Cullen et al. 2016).

Electroconvulsive therapy (ECT) is a gold-standard treatment with unequivocal efficacy for TRD in adults (Pagnin et al. 2004). Although no RCTs have been conducted in children and adolescents, there is some extant literature to support considering ECT in the treatment of TRD in children and adolescents (Bertagnoli and Borchardt 1990; Zhand et al. 2015), especially in patients with bipolar or psychotic depression (Rey and Walter 1997). There have been several observations for effectiveness in the treatment for adolescents with TRD. In an open-label trial, Strober et al. (1998) reported a remission rate of 60% after ECT for 10 adolescents, ages 13–17 years, with treatment-resistant bipolar depression or TRD. Later, in a retrospective study involving a Dutch cohort of adolescents with TRD and/or suicidal behavior, Hegeman et al. (2008) reported that one-third of participants showed an improvement of 60% or more on the Hamilton Rating Scale for Depression or the Montgomery-Åsberg Depression Rating Scale. In a retrospective case report of the efficacy of ECT in six adolescents, ages 14–17 years, with severe TRD, the response rate was 64%, and there were no cognitive deficits after ECT (Ghaziuddin et al. 2011). The Work Group on Quality Issues of the American Academy of Child and Adolescent Psychiatry, in its practice parameter for the use of ECT with adolescents, recommends that ECT be considered after failure of two or more appropriate medication trials, or for adolescents with life-threatening symptoms such as the refusal to eat or drink, severe suicidality, uncontrollable mania, or florid psychosis, with a diagnosis of severe and persistent depression or mania, schizoaffective disorder, or, less often, schizophrenia (Ghaziuddin et al. 2004).

In summary, management of adolescents with TRD requires 1) ongoing and thorough assessment with respect to treatment adherence, adequacy of previous treatments, medical and psychiatric comorbidities, sleep quality, and psychosocial stressors; 2) ongoing psychoeducation to update patient and family expectations regarding disease course and potential risks and benefits of medication treatments; 3) medication optimization; 4) combination of pharmacotherapy with individual and family psychotherapy; and last, but not least, 5) persistence and restoration of hope. *Hope* is defined as positive expectancies for goal attainment. Nearly 50 years ago, Karl Menninger described hope as "a basic but elusive ingredient in our daily work—our teaching, our healing, our diagnosing" (Menninger 1959, p. 481). He asserted that mental illness reflects a lack of hope and that successful treatment involves its restoration (Menninger 1959). In recent decades, psychotherapy researchers have viewed hope as a common factor across successful therapies (Snyder et al. 1991). Such hope taps patients' beliefs that their problems can be resolved and that their futures can and will be better (Snyder et al. 1991). It is of critical importance that the clinician, the patient, and the family remember that although the journey to recovery can be long and arduous, the majority of adolescents with TRD will eventually improve with successive treatments.

Response Achieved—Now What?

In the treatment of pediatric depression, the goals are to achieve response and remission and to prevent future depression episodes (Maalouf and Brent 2012). Since subsyndromal depression is more vulnerable to recurrence, treatment should aim to eliminate or minimize residual symptoms (Brent et al. 2001). Most studies in pediatric depression have evaluated treatments during the acute phase, with fewer studies evaluating continuation-phase treatment (Emslie et al. 2008). In the continuation phase (usually 4–12 months), the goal is to consolidate remission to prevent relapse. In the maintenance phase, which lasts 1 year or longer, the goal is to prevent recurrence, particularly in those with a history of more severe, recurrent, and chronic disorder (Birmaher et al. 2000). There is relatively little information available to guide clinicians on the next steps once a child or adolescent with depression has achieved remission. Best-practice guidelines have recommended that to consolidate the response to the acute treatment and avoid relapses, treatment should always be continued for 6–12 months (Birmaher and Brent 2007). During the continuation phase, antidepressants should be maintained at the same dose, provided there are no significant side effects. Once the patient has been asymptomatic for approximately 6–12 months, the clinician must decide whether maintenance therapy is indicated, and the type and duration of therapy. The discontinuation of medications should be done gradually (generally over a period of 6 weeks) to avoid withdrawal effects.

Maintenance treatment is recommended for patients with a history of at least two major depressive episodes, patients with double depression, patients with severe suicidality, and patients with severe impairment during the episodes (Birmaher and Brent 2007). One severe episode or multiple chronic episodes of depression may require maintenance treatment for longer than 1 year.

Conclusion

Although the knowledge about pharmacological treatment approaches for treating depression in children and adolescents lags behind that in adults, there has been an accumulation of data to guide treatment. At this time, for first-line pharmacotherapy, the evidence is most supportive of SSRIs, and in particular fluoxetine and escitalopram, both of which are approved by the FDA for adolescents. Combined treatment with psychotherapy is generally recommended, especially in cases of patients who have not responded to an adequate trial with an SSRI. More research is needed to guide 1) treatment decisions for adolescents whose depression has failed to respond to multiple interventions and 2) management of the depression once a response is achieved.

Clinical Pearls

- Pharmacotherapy management is optimal only after rapport is established, a full clinical assessment is conducted, and any cultural contributors to the presentation are identified and addressed.

- Factors that may influence help-seeking behavior and treatment receptiveness include cultural beliefs about mental illness, stigma, and culturally sanctioned ways of symptom expression and coping styles.

- Educating the patient and family about what to expect from the different modalities of treatment of depression (both psychotherapy and medication) is critical to ensure engagement and compliance.

- Selective serotonin reuptake inhibitors are the first-line medications for treating depression in youths. While both escitalopram and fluoxetine have U.S. Food and Drug Administration (FDA) approval for adolescents with depression, only fluoxetine is FDA approved for children with depression.

- As a way to avoid side effects and improve adherence, medications are generally started at half the adult starting dose until tolerability is established (≤ 1 week), and then increased gradually to a therapeutic dose with frequent evaluation of tolerability.

- Clinical responses should be assessed at regular intervals to allow adequate time for clinical response at each dosage step. The dose should be adjusted on the basis of clinical response and tolerability.

- In the case of insufficient dose response, dosage should be titrated upward, if necessary to the maximum dose, before a move is made to the next medication.

- Pairing pharmacotherapy with psychotherapy is generally recommended.

- Ongoing psychoeducation, family support, and school involvement are critical parts of a successful pharmacological management plan for pediatric depression.

References

Allergan: Efficacy, safety, and tolerability of levomilnacipran ER in pediatric (7–17 years) with major depressive disorder. NCT03569475. July 25, 2018. Available at: https://clinicaltrials.gov/ct2/show/NCT03569475. Accessed September 18, 2018.

Andrade C: The numbers needed to treat and harm (NNT, NNH) statistics: what they tell us and what they do not. J Clin Psychiatry 76(3):e330–e333, 2015 25830454

Andrade C, Sandarsh S, Chethan KB, et al: Serotonin reuptake inhibitor antidepressants and abnormal bleeding: a review for clinicians and a reconsideration of mechanisms. J Clin Psychiatry 71(12):1565–1575, 2010 21190637

Atkinson SD, Prakash A, Zhang Q, et al: A double-blind efficacy and safety study of duloxetine flexible dosing in children and adolescents with major depressive disorder. J Child Adolesc Psychopharmacol 24(4):180–189, 2014 24813026

Atkinson S, Lubaczewski S, Ramaker S, et al: Desvenlafaxine versus placebo in the treatment of children and adolescents with major depressive disorder. J Child Adolesc Psychopharmacol 28(1):55–65, 2018 29185786

Avery DH, Holtzheimer PE III, Fawaz W, et al: A controlled study of repetitive transcranial magnetic stimulation in medication-resistant major depression. Biol Psychiatry 59(2):187–194, 2006 16139808

Bang-Andersen B, Ruhland T, Jørgensen M, et al: Discovery of 1-[2-(2,4-dimethylphenylsulfanyl)phenyl]piperazine (Lu AA21004): a novel multimodal compound for the treatment of major depressive disorder. J Med Chem 54(9):3206–3221, 2011 21486038

Bérard A, Iessa N, Chaabane S, et al: The risk of major cardiac malformations associated with paroxetine use during the first trimester of pregnancy: a systematic review and meta-analysis. Br J Clin Pharmacol 81(4):589–604, 2016 26613360

Bertagnoli MW, Borchardt CM: A review of ECT for children and adolescents. J Am Acad Child Adolesc Psychiatry 29(2):302–307, 1990 2288556

Birmaher B, Brent D: Practice parameter for the assessment and treatment of children and adolescents with depressive disorders. J Am Acad Child Adolesc Psychiatry 46(11):1503–1526, 2007 18049300

Birmaher B, Waterman GS, Ryan ND, et al: Randomized, controlled trial of amitriptyline versus placebo for adolescents with "treatment-resistant" major depression. J Am Acad Child Adolesc Psychiatry 37(5):527–535, 1998 9585655

Birmaher B, Brent DA, Kolko D, et al: Clinical outcome after short-term psychotherapy for adolescents with major depressive disorder. Arch Gen Psychiatry 57(1):29–36, 2000 10632230

Bloch Y, Grisaru N, Harel EV, et al: Repetitive transcranial magnetic stimulation in the treatment of depression in adolescents: an open-label study. J ECT 24(2):156–159, 2008 18580562

Brent DA: Antidepressants and Suicidality. Psychiatr Clin North Am 39(3):503–512, 2016 27514302

Brent DA, Birmaher B, Kolko D, et al: Subsyndromal depression in adolescents after a brief psychotherapy trial: course and outcome. J Affect Disord 63(1–3):51–58, 2001 11246080

Brent D, Emslie G, Clarke G, et al: Switching to another SSRI or to venlafaxine with or without cognitive behavioral therapy for adolescents with SSRI-resistant depression: the TORDIA randomized controlled trial. JAMA 299(8):901–913, 2008 18314433

Brent DA, Emslie GJ, Clarke GN, et al: Predictors of spontaneous and systematically assessed suicidal adverse events in the Treatment of SSRI-Resistant Depression in Adolescents (TORDIA) study. Am J Psychiatry 166(4):418–426, 2009 19223438

Bridge JA, Iyengar S, Salary CB, et al: Clinical response and risk for reported suicidal ideation and suicide attempts in pediatric antidepressant treatment: a meta-analysis of randomized controlled trials. JAMA 297(15):1683–1696, 2007 17440145

Cheung A, Sacks D, Dewa CS, et al: Pediatric prescribing practices and the FDA black-box warning on antidepressants. J Dev Behav Pediatr 29(3):213–215, 2008 18550990

Cipriani A, Zhou X, Del Giovane C, et al: Comparative efficacy and tolerability of antidepressants for major depressive disorder in children and adolescents: a network meta-analysis. Lancet 388(10047):881–890, 2016 27289172

Cullen KR, Jasberg S, Nelson B, et al: Seizure induced by deep transcranial magnetic stimulation in an adolescent with depression. J Child Adolesc Psychopharmacol 26(7):637–641, 2016 27447245

Curry J, Rohde P, Simons A, et al; TADS Team: Predictors and moderators of acute outcome in the Treatment for Adolescents with Depression Study (TADS). J Am Acad Child Adolesc Psychiatry 45(12):1427–1439, 2006 17135988

Daviss WB, Bentivoglio P, Racusin R, et al: Bupropion sustained release in adolescents with comorbid attention-deficit/hyperactivity disorder and depression. J Am Acad Child Adolesc Psychiatry 40(3):307–314, 2001 11288772

Durgam S, Chen C, Migliore R, et al: A phase 3, double-blind, randomized, placebo-controlled study of vilazodone in adolescents with major depressive disorder. Paediatr Drugs 20(4):353–363, 2018 29633166

Emslie GJ, Rush AJ, Weinberg WA, et al: A double-blind, randomized, placebo-controlled trial of fluoxetine in children and adolescents with depression. Arch Gen Psychiatry 54(11):1031–1037, 1997 9366660

Emslie GJ, Heiligenstein JH, Wagner KD, et al: Fluoxetine for acute treatment of depression in children and adolescents: a placebo-controlled, randomized clinical trial. J Am Acad Child Adolesc Psychiatry 41(10):1205–1215, 2002 12364842

Emslie GJ, Wagner KD, Kutcher S, et al: Paroxetine treatment in children and adolescents with major depressive disorder: a randomized, multicenter, double-blind, placebo-controlled trial. J Am Acad Child Adolesc Psychiatry 45(6):709–719, 2006 16721321

Emslie GJ, Findling RL, Yeung PP, et al: Venlafaxine ER for the treatment of pediatric subjects with depression: results of two placebo-controlled trials. J Am Acad Child Adolesc Psychiatry 46(4):479–488, 2007 17420682

Emslie GJ, Kennard BD, Mayes TL, et al: Fluoxetine versus placebo in preventing relapse of major depression in children and adolescents. Am J Psychiatry 165(4):459–467, 2008 18281410

Emslie GJ, Ventura D, Korotzer A, et al: Escitalopram in the treatment of adolescent depression: a randomized placebo-controlled multisite trial. J Am Acad Child Adolesc Psychiatry 48(7):721–729, 2009 19465881

Emslie GJ, Mayes T, Porta G, et al: Treatment of Resistant Depression in Adolescents (TORDIA): week 24 outcomes. Am J Psychiatry 167(7):782–791, 2010 20478877

Emslie GJ, Prakash A, Zhang Q, et al: A double-blind efficacy and safety study of duloxetine fixed doses in children and adolescents with major depressive disorder. J Child Adolesc Psychopharmacol 24(4):170–179, 2014 24815533

Fava M: Diagnosis and definition of treatment-resistant depression. Biol Psychiatry 53(8):649–659, 2003 12706951

Feeny NC, Silva SG, Reinecke MA, et al: An exploratory analysis of the impact of family functioning on treatment for depression in adolescents. J Clin Child Adolesc Psychol 38(6):814–825, 2009 20183665

Findling RL, Groark J, Chiles D, et al: Safety and tolerability of desvenlafaxine in children and adolescents with major depressive disorder. J Child Adolesc Psychopharmacol 24(4):201–209, 2014 24611442

Findling RL, Groark J, Tourian KA, et al: Pharmacokinetics and tolerability of single-ascending doses of desvenlafaxine administered to children and adolescents with major depressive disorder. J Child Adolesc Psychopharmacol 26(10):909–921, 2016 27428303

Findling RL, Robb AS, DelBello M, et al: Pharmacokinetics and safety of vortioxetine in pediatric patients. J Child Adolesc Psychopharmacol 27(6):526–534, 2017 28333546

Findling RL, Robb AS, DelBello MP, et al: A 6-month open-label extension study of vortioxetine in pediatric patients with depressive or anxiety disorders. J Child Adolesc Psychopharmacol 28(1):47–54, 2018 29035574

Forest Laboratories: Safety and efficacy of levomilnacipran ER in adolescent patients with major depressive disorder. NCT02431806. June 6, 2018. Available at: https://clinicaltrials.gov/ct2/show/NCT02431806. Accessed September 18, 2018.

Geller B, Cooper TB, Graham DL, et al: Pharmacokinetically designed double-blind placebo-controlled study of nortriptyline in 6- to 12-year-olds with major depressive disorder. J Am Acad Child Adolesc Psychiatry 31(1):34–44, 1992 1537779

Gentile S: Untreated depression during pregnancy: short- and long-term effects in offspring—a systematic review. Neuroscience 342:154–166, 2017 26343292

Ghaziuddin N, Kutcher SP, Knapp P, et al; Work Group on Quality Issues; AACAP: Practice parameter for use of electroconvulsive therapy with adolescents. J Am Acad Child Adolesc Psychiatry 43(12):1521–1539, 2004 15564821

Ghaziuddin N, Dumas S, Hodges E: Use of continuation or maintenance electroconvulsive therapy in adolescents with severe treatment-resistant depression. J ECT 27(2):168–174, 2011 21233763

Gibbons RD, Hur K, Bhaumik DK, et al: The relationship between antidepressant prescription rates and rate of early adolescent suicide. Am J Psychiatry 163(11):1898–1904, 2006 17074941

Gibbons RD, Brown CH, Hur K, et al: Early evidence on the effects of regulators' suicidality warnings on SSRI prescriptions and suicide in children and adolescents. Am J Psychiatry 164(9):1356–1363, 2007 17728420

Glod CA, Lynch A, Flynn E, et al: Open trial of bupropion SR in adolescent major depression. J Child Adolesc Psychiatr Nurs 16(3):123–130, 2003 14603988

Hammad TA, Laughren T, Racoosin J: Suicidality in pediatric patients treated with antidepressant drugs. Arch Gen Psychiatry 63(3):332–339, 2006 16520440

Hazell P, Mirzaie M: Tricyclic drugs for depression in children and adolescents. Cochrane Database Syst Rev (6):CD002317, 2013 23780719

Hegeman JM, Doesborgh SJC, van Niel MC, et al: The efficacy of electroconvulsive therapy in adolescents: a retrospective study [in Dutch]. Tijdschr Psychiatr 50(1):23–31, 2008 18188826

Heiligenstein JH, Hoog SL, Wagner KD, et al: Fluoxetine 40–60 mg versus fluoxetine 20 mg in the treatment of children and adolescents with a less-than-complete response to nine-week treatment with fluoxetine 10–20 mg: a pilot study. J Child Adolesc Psychopharmacol 16(1–2):207–217, 2006 16553541

Hughes CW, Emslie GJ, Crismon ML, et al; Texas Consensus Conference Panel on Medication Treatment of Childhood Major Depressive Disorder: Texas Children's Medication Algorithm Project: update from Texas Consensus Conference Panel on Medication Treatment of Childhood Major Depressive Disorder. J Am Acad Child Adolesc Psychiatry 46(6):667–686, 2007 17513980

Huybrechts KF, Palmsten K, Avorn J, et al: Antidepressant use in pregnancy and the risk of cardiac defects. N Engl J Med 370(25):2397–2407, 2014 24941178

Katz LY, Kozyrskyj AL, Prior HJ, et al: Effect of regulatory warnings on antidepressant prescription rates, use of health services and outcomes among children, adolescents and young adults. CMAJ 178(8):1005–1011, 2008 18390943

Keller MB, Ryan ND, Strober M, et al: Efficacy of paroxetine in the treatment of adolescent major depression: a randomized, controlled trial. J Am Acad Child Adolesc Psychiatry 40(7):762–772, 2001 11437014

Kennard B, Silva S, Vitiello B, et al; TADS Team: Remission and residual symptoms after short-term treatment in the Treatment of Adolescents with Depression Study (TADS). J Am Acad Child Adolesc Psychiatry 45(12):1404–1411, 2006 17135985

Kondo DG, Sung YH, Hellem TL, et al: Open-label adjunctive creatine for female adolescents with SSRI-resistant major depressive disorder: a 31-phosphorus magnetic resonance spectroscopy study. J Affect Disord 135(1–3):354–361, 2011 21831448

Kondo DG, Forrest LN, Shi X, et al: Creatine target engagement with brain bioenergetics: a dose-ranging phosphorus-31 magnetic resonance spectroscopy study of adolescent females with SSRI-resistant depression. Amino Acids 48(8):1941–1954, 2016 26907087

Kratochvil C, Emslie G, Silva S, et al; TADS Team: Acute time to response in the Treatment for Adolescents with Depression Study (TADS). J Am Acad Child Adolesc Psychiatry 45(12):1412–1418, 2006 17135986

Kutcher S, Boulos C, Ward B, et al: Response to desipramine treatment in adolescent depression: a fixed-dose, placebo-controlled trial. J Am Acad Child Adolesc Psychiatry 33(5):686–694, 1994 8056732

Latendresse G, Wong B, Dyer J, et al: Duration of maternal stress and depression: predictors of newborn admission to neonatal intensive care unit and postpartum depression. Nurs Res 64(5):331–341, 2015 26325275

Le Noury J, Nardo JM, Healy D, et al: Restoring Study 329: efficacy and harms of paroxetine and imipramine in treatment of major depression in adolescence. BMJ 351:h4320, 2015 26376805

Lewinsohn PM, Seeley JR, Hibbard J, et al: Cross-sectional and prospective relationships between physical morbidity and depression in older adolescents. J Am Acad Child Adolesc Psychiatry 35(9):1120–1129, 1996 8824055

Lopez MA, Toprac MG, Crismon ML, et al: A psychoeducational program for children with ADHD or depression and their families: results from the CMAP feasibility study. Community Ment Health J 41(1):51–66, 2005 15932052

Lu CY, Zhang F, Lakoma MD, et al: Changes in antidepressant use by young people and suicidal behavior after FDA warnings and media coverage: quasi-experimental study. BMJ 348:g3596, 2014 24942789

Maalouf FT, Brent DA: Child and adolescent depression intervention overview: what works, for whom and how well?. Child Adolesc Psychiatr Clin N Am 21(2):299–312, viii, 2012 22537728

Maalouf FT, Atwi M, Brent DA: Treatment-resistant depression in adolescents: review and updates on clinical management. Depress Anxiety 28(11):946–954, 2011 21898710

Mandoki MW, Tapia MR, Tapia MA, et al: Venlafaxine in the treatment of children and adolescents with major depression. Psychopharmacol Bull 33(1):149–154, 1997 9133767

March J, Silva S, Petrycki S, et al; Treatment for Adolescents with Depression Study (TADS) Team: Fluoxetine, cognitive-behavioral therapy, and their combination for adolescents with depression: Treatment for Adolescents With Depression Study (TADS) randomized controlled trial. JAMA 292(7):807–820, 2004 15315995

March J, Silva S, Vitiello B; TADS Team: The Treatment for Adolescents with Depression Study (TADS): methods and message at 12 weeks. J Am Acad Child Adolesc Psychiatry 45(12):1393–1403, 2006 17135984

Mayer G, Faivel N, Aviram S, et al: Repetitive transcranial magnetic stimulation in depressed adolescents: experience, knowledge, and attitudes of recipients and their parents. J ECT 28(2):104–107, 2012 22513510

McCloud TL, Caddy C, Jochim J, et al: Ketamine and other glutamate receptor modulators for depression in bipolar disorder in adults. Cochrane Database Syst Rev (9):CD011611, 2015 26415966

Menninger K: The academic lecture: hope. Am J Psychiatry 116:481–491, 1959

Mørk A, Pehrson A, Brennum LT, et al: Pharmacological effects of Lu AA21004: a novel multimodal compound for the treatment of major depressive disorder. J Pharmacol Exp Ther 340(3):666–675, 2012 22171087

Murrough JW, Iosifescu DV, Chang LC, et al: Antidepressant efficacy of ketamine in treatment-resistant major depression: a two-site randomized controlled trial. Am J Psychiatry 170(10):1134–1142, 2013 23982301

Olfson M, Shaffer D, Marcus SC, et al: Relationship between antidepressant medication treatment and suicide in adolescents. Arch Gen Psychiatry 60(10):978–982, 2003 14557142

Olfson M, Marcus SC, Shaffer D: Antidepressant drug therapy and suicide in severely depressed children and adults: a case-control study. Arch Gen Psychiatry 63(8):865–872, 2006 16894062

Otuyelu E, Foldvari A, Szabo E, et al: Antidepressant drugs and teenage suicide in Hungary: time trend and seasonality analysis. Int J Psychiatry Clin Pract 19(3):221–225, 2015 26058968

Pagnin D, de Queiroz V, Pini S, et al: Efficacy of ECT in depression: a meta-analytic review. J ECT 20(1):13–20, 2004 15087991

Pathak S, Johns ES, Kowatch RA: Adjunctive quetiapine for treatment-resistant adolescent major depressive disorder: a case series. J Child Adolesc Psychopharmacol 15(4):696–702, 2005 16190801

Puig-Antich J, Perel JM, Lupatkin W, et al: Imipramine in prepubertal major depressive disorders. Arch Gen Psychiatry 44(1):81–89, 1987 3541830

Renoir T: Selective serotonin reuptake inhibitor antidepressant treatment discontinuation syndrome: a review of the clinical evidence and the possible mechanisms involved. Front Pharmacol 4:45, 2013 23596418

Renshaw P: Creatine augmentation for adolescent females with treatment-resistant major depressive disorder. NCT02134808. December 7, 2017. Available at: https://clinicaltrials.gov/ct2/show/NCT02134808. Accessed September 18, 2018.

Rey JM, Walter G: Half a century of ECT use in young people. Am J Psychiatry 154(5):595–602, 1997 9137112

Rush AJ, Warden D, Wisniewski SR, et al: STAR*D: revising conventional wisdom. CNS Drugs 23(8):627–647, 2009 19594193

Ryan ND, Meyer V, Dachille S, et al: Lithium antidepressant augmentation in TCA-refractory depression in adolescents. J Am Acad Child Adolesc Psychiatry 27(3):371–376, 1988a 3379022

Ryan ND, Puig-Antich J, Rabinovich H, et al: MAOIs in adolescent major depression unresponsive to tricyclic antidepressants. J Am Acad Child Adolesc Psychiatry 27(6):755–758, 1988b 3198564

Sackeim HA: The definition and meaning of treatment-resistant depression. J Clin Psychiatry 62 (suppl 16):10–17, 2001 11480879

Sanchez C, Asin KE, Artigas F: Vortioxetine, a novel antidepressant with multimodal activity: review of preclinical and clinical data. Pharmacol Ther 145:43–57, 2015 25016186

Shamseddeen W, Clarke G, Keller MB, et al: Adjunctive sleep medications and depression outcome in the treatment of serotonin-selective reuptake inhibitor resistant depression in adolescents study. J Child Adolesc Psychopharmacol 22(1):29–36, 2012 22251024

Shon S-H, Joo Y, Lee J-S, et al: Lamotrigine treatment of adolescents with unipolar and bipolar depression: a retrospective chart review. J Child Adolesc Psychopharmacol 24(5):285–287, 2014 24813210

Simeon JG, Dinicola VF, Ferguson HB, et al: Adolescent depression: a placebo-controlled fluoxetine treatment study and follow-up. Prog Neuropsychopharmacol Biol Psychiatry 14(5):791–795, 1990 2293257

Singh JB, Fedgchin M, Daly EJ, et al: A double-blind, randomized, placebo-controlled, dose-frequency study of intravenous ketamine in patients with treatment-resistant depression. Am J Psychiatry 173(8):816–826, 2016 27056608

Snyder CR, Harris C, Anderson JR, et al: The will and the ways: development and validation of an individual-differences measure of hope. J Pers Soc Psychol 60(4):570–585, 1991 2037968

Solhkhah R, Wilens TE, Daly J, et al: Bupropion SR for the treatment of substance-abusing outpatient adolescents with attention-deficit/hyperactivity disorder and mood disorders. J Child Adolesc Psychopharmacol 15(5):777–786, 2005 16262594

Strober M, Freeman R, Rigali J, et al: The pharmacotherapy of depressive illness in adolescence, II: effects of lithium augmentation in nonresponders to imipramine. J Am Acad Child Adolesc Psychiatry 31(1):16–20, 1992 1537769

Strober M, Rao U, DeAntonio M, et al: Effects of electroconvulsive therapy in adolescents with severe endogenous depression resistant to pharmacotherapy. Biol Psychiatry 43(5):335–338, 1998 9513748

Sugawara H, Sakamoto K, Harada T, et al: Predictors of efficacy in lithium augmentation for treatment-resistant depression. J Affect Disord 125(1–3):165–168, 2010 20089312

Sultan MA, Courtney DB: Adjunctive trazodone and depression outcome in adolescents treated with serotonin re-uptake inhibitors. J Can Acad Child Adolesc Psychiatry 26(3):233–240, 2017 29056986

Trivedi MH, Fava M, Wisniewski SR, et al; STAR*D Study Team: Medication augmentation after the failure of SSRIs for depression. N Engl J Med 354(12):1243–1252, 2006 16554526

U.S. Food and Drug Administration: FDA Drug Safety Communication: Selective serotonin reuptake inhibitor (SSRI) antidepressant use during pregnancy and reports of a rare heart and lung condition in newborn babies. December 14, 2011. Available at: https://www.fda.gov/Drugs/DrugSafety/ucm283375.htm#hcp. Accessed February 25, 2019.

U.S. Food and Drug Administration: Pregnancy and Lactation Labeling (Drugs) Final Rule. December 3, 2014. Available at: https://www.fda.gov/drugs/developmentapprovalprocess/developmentresources/labeling/ucm093307.htm. Accessed February 25, 2019.

U.S. Food and Drug Administration: Clarification of dosing and warning recommendations for Celexa. Center for Drug Evaluation and Research, January 5, 2016. Available at: https://www.fda.gov/Drugs/ResourcesForYou/SpecialFeatures/ucm297764.htm. Accessed September 9, 2018.

U.S. Food and Drug Administration: Suicidality in children and adolescents being treated with antidepressant medications. Center for Drug Evaluation and Research, February 5, 2018. Available at: https://www.fda.gov/drugs/drugsafety/postmarketdrugsafetyinformationforpatientsandproviders/ucm161679.htm. Accessed September 9, 2018.

Varigonda AL, Jakubovski E, Taylor MJ, et al: Systematic review and meta-analysis: early treatment responses of selective serotonin reuptake inhibitors in pediatric major depressive disorder. J Am Acad Child Adolesc Psychiatry 54(7):557–564, 2015 26088660

Volpi-Abadie J, Kaye AM, Kaye AD: Serotonin syndrome. Ochsner J 13(4):533–540, 2013 24358002

von Knorring A-L, Olsson GI, Thomsen PH, et al: A randomized, double-blind, placebo-controlled study of citalopram in adolescents with major depressive disorder. J Clin Psychopharmacol 26(3):311–315, 2006 16702897

Wagner KD, Ambrosini P, Rynn M, et al; Sertraline Pediatric Depression Study Group: Efficacy of sertraline in the treatment of children and adolescents with major depressive disorder: two randomized controlled trials. JAMA 290(8):1033–1041, 2003 12941675

Wagner KD, Robb AS, Findling RL, et al: A randomized, placebo-controlled trial of citalopram for the treatment of major depression in children and adolescents. Am J Psychiatry 161(6):1079–1083, 2004 15169696

Walkup JT: Antidepressant efficacy for depression in children and adolescents: industry- and NIMH-funded studies. Am J Psychiatry 174(5):430–437, 2017 28253735

Walter G, Lyndon B, Kubb R: Lithium augmentation of venlafaxine in adolescent major depression. Aust N Z J Psychiatry 32(3):457–459, 1998 9672738

Walter G, Tormos JM, Israel JA, et al: Transcranial magnetic stimulation in young persons: a review of known cases. J Child Adolesc Psychopharmacol 11(1):69–75, 2001 11322748

Weihs KL, Murphy W, Abbas R, et al: Desvenlafaxine Versus placebo in a fluoxetine-referenced study of children and adolescents with major depressive disorder. J Child Adolesc Psychopharmacol 28(1):36–46, 2018 29189044

Wilkinson P, Dubicka B, Kelvin R, et al: Treated depression in adolescents: predictors of outcome at 28 weeks. Br J Psychiatry 194(4):334–341, 2009 19336785

Zhand N, Courtney DB, Flament MF: Use of electroconvulsive therapy in adolescents with treatment-resistant depressive disorders: a case series. J ECT 31(4):238–245, 2015 25830809

Zhou X, Keitner GI, Qin B, et al: Atypical antipsychotic augmentation for treatment-resistant depression: a systematic review and network meta-analysis. Int J Neuropsychopharmacol 18(11):pyv060, 2015 26012350

10

Pharmacotherapy for Pediatric Bipolar Disorders

Luis R. Patino, M.D., M.Sc.

Melissa P. DelBello, M.D., M.S.

Pediatric bipolar disorder is a chronic, severe, recurrent, and often disabling condition (Chang 2007). The accurate diagnosis of bipolar disorder in children and adolescents is a significant challenge for even the most experienced clinicians, particularly given the frequent psychiatric comorbidities for these patients (Joshi and Wilens 2009). Complicating matters further are the controversies regarding phenomenological presentation and the validity of applying adult-derived criteria to children and adolescents (Axelson et al. 2006). Unlike the distinct episodes of depression and mania often exhibited by adults, bipolar disorder in children and adolescents is often characterized by mixed or dysphoric mood states accompanied by irritability (Geller and Tillman 2005). Children and adolescents may also experience more symptomatic periods and be more susceptible to rapid cycling than their adult counterparts (Geller et al. 2004). Therefore, extrapolating from adult-derived treatment data will likely provide insufficient information regarding effective treatments for pediatric bipolar disorder.

Though diagnosis and treatment can be particularly difficult for this population, these patients require prompt intervention to ameliorate symptoms and reduce the psychosocial morbidity that often accompanies the illness. In fact, early detection and treatment are paramount, because earlier onset and longer duration of illness tend to be associated with poorer rates of recovery (Liu et al. 2011). Currently, there are several pharmacological interventions available for the treatment of pediatric bipolar disorder. Although treatment of acute mania remains the primary treatment target of most clinical trials, there is a need for further clarification of the pharmacotherapy of depression in pediatric bipolar disorder and pharmacotherapy for maintenance treatment.

There are several review articles detailing pharmacological interventions for pediatric bipolar disorder (Chang 2009; Correll et al. 2010; Liu et al. 2011; Peruzzolo et al. 2013). In this chapter, we wish to expand the examination of the efficacy and safety of pharmacological interventions for pediatric bipolar disorder, with particular emphasis on differentiating the mood state treated: depressed, manic, and euthymic/ maintenance. Furthermore, in an attempt to offer a comprehensive collection of the best available evidence, we classify the quality of each study using a two-step evidence-grading scale and determine the strength of the recommendation for each pharmacological agent for the aforementioned mood states.

Methods

PubMed and PsycINFO website searches of literature published through December 2017 were conducted using the individual and two-by-two search terms—"bipolar," "mania," "depression," "maintenance with treatment," "pediatric," "child," "adolescent," "youth," "pharmacologic"—as well as the individual search of specific medication names. We also conducted a search on clinicaltrials.gov for pharmacological trials that included reported results. We reviewed the search results and selected the psychopharmacological intervention trials in children and adolescents that addressed the treatment of acute mania, treatment of acute depression in patients with bipolar disorder, maintenance treatment for bipolar disorder, and treatment of comorbid medical conditions. For maintenance treatment we focused on trials lasting at least 6 months or 26 weeks that evaluated maintenance and/or time to mood event following initial mood stabilization.

TABLE 10–1. Criteria for assigning grade of evidence in relation to type of studies

Grade of evidence[a]	Type of study
A	High-quality RCT[b] or meta-analysis
B	Low-quality RCT[c] or open-label study
C	Case series, retrospective chart review
D	Case reports, expert opinion

Note. RCT=randomized controlled trial.

[a]Once initial grade of individual study is determined: Decrease grade of evidence if study presents: imprecise data (–1); dropout/loss-to-follow-up rate>35% (–1); serious limitations to the study (–2); no intention-to-treat analysis (–1); negative result in double-blind, placebo-controlled trial (–3); inconsistent results (–1). Increase grade if study presents: large effect size response Cohen's $h \geq 0.80$ or remission Cohen's $h \geq 0.60$ (+1); consistent evidence in two or more open-label trials (+1).

[b]Placebo-controlled trial and adequately powered.

[c]Active comparison group or inadequately powered.

We selected the articles that targeted disease-oriented outcomes—specifically, clinical improvement as main outcome—excluding articles in which the treatment of a comorbid condition was the primary outcome or in which changes in measures other than clinical improvement were the main outcome (i.e., neuroimaging, quality of life, adherence, academic performance). Information regarding treatment design and outcomes was extracted from the selected articles. Response and remission rates reported in this review were extracted from the publications following standard definitions (response: $\geq 50\%$ measured symptom reduction from baseline; and remission: Young Mania Rating Scale [YMRS]≤ 12 or Children's Depression Rating Scale [CDRS]≤ 28), or if these standard definitions were unavailable, we used those indicated in the original publications. To obtain comparable effect sizes on these rates, we calculated Cohen's h, a measure of distance between two proportions or probabilities, and estimates of the number needed to treat (NNT) from placebo-controlled trials were included when available.

The selected studies were then classified according to the quality of the evidence based on a ranking system (Table 10–1) adapted from the Grading of Recommendations Assessment, Development and Evaluation (GRADE) (Guyatt et al. 2008). Furthermore, after evaluating all the information, we based conclusions and recommendations using the Strength of Recommendation Taxonomy (SORT) for treatment statements (Ebell et al. 2004) (Table 10–2).

TABLE 10–2.   Level of recommendation, definition, and criteria

	Definition	Evidence required
Level 1	Strong recommendation based on high-quality evidence; further research is unlikely to change the confidence of the evaluated intervention	Based on consistent findings from two or more studies that reach grade A evidence
Level 2	Moderate recommendation; further research is likely to have an important impact on the confidence of recommendation	Based on results of one grade A study or on inconsistent (mixed) findings from two or more grade A studies
Level 3	Weak recommendation; further research is very likely to have an important impact on confidence	Based on studies whose highest level of evidence is B
Level 4	Effect of intervention is uncertain	Based on grade C evidence or lower

Results

A brief overview of the studies selected for this chapter is presented as follows: 1) treatment of mania/hypomania; 2) treatment of bipolar depression; and 3) maintenance treatment. Within these divisions, we organized according to study design: a) randomized controlled trials (RCTs) and meta-analyses; and b) open-label (OL), retrospective, or follow-up studies. Agents presented are in alphabetical order.

Treatments for Bipolar Mania in Youth

Acute mania was found to be the primary treatment focus of most clinical trials.

Randomized Clinical Trials and Meta-analyses

We identified 20 randomized clinical trials, two meta-analyses, and one systematic review exploring the efficacy of pharmacological interventions for acute mania in children and adolescents with bipolar disorder. We removed one study because its primary outcome was based on a comorbid substance use disorder and included a mix of manic, depressed, and euthymic adolescent patients with bipolar disorder. Of the remaining randomized clinical trials, 12 were double-blind, placebo-controlled trials (DBPC trials), 3 were randomized, double-blind, head-to-head comparison trials, 3 were a DBPC trials of a medication added on to an existing treatment, and 1 was a DBPC discontinuation trial that assessed the reemergence of symptoms in treatment responders. A summary of these results can be found in Table 10–3.

Aripiprazole

In a DBPC trial comparing two doses of aripiprazole monotherapy with placebo (Findling et al. 2009), the study authors found significantly greater symptom reduction for both doses compared with placebo (10 mg=−14.2 and 30 mg=−16.5 vs. placebo −8.2; both $P<0.0001$). This study also reported significantly greater response rates (10 mg=44.8% and 30 mg = 63.6% vs. placebo=26.1%; Cohen's h 10 mg=0.39, NNT 10 mg=5.3 and Cohen's h 30 mg=0.77, NNT 30 mg=2.6) and remission rates (10 mg = 25% and 30 mg=47.5% vs. placebo=5.4%; Cohen's h 10 mg=0.57, NNT 10 mg=5.1 and Cohen's h 30 mg=1.0, NNT 30 mg=2.3). Another flexible-dose DBPC trial (Tramontina et al. 2009) in subjects with comorbid ADHD found that aripiprazole monotherapy was superior to placebo in decreasing manic symptoms, with significantly greater response rates (88.9% vs. 52%; Cohen's h=0.85, NNT=2.7), and remission rates (72% vs. 32%; Cohen's h=0.82, NNT=2.5). Common adverse events reported in these studies included sedation, gastrointestinal complaints, headache, and movement symptoms (Findling et al. 2009; Tramontina et al. 2009).

Asenapine

In a large (N=403) 3-week DBPC trial (Findling et al. 2015b) exploring three doses of asenapine as monotherapy (2.5 mg BID, 5 mg BID, and 10 mg BID) for mania, asenapine showed significant decreases in YMRS scores (−12.3 [±9.0], −15.1 [9.5], and −15.9 [9.1] for 2.5, 5, and 10 mg, respectively) as compared with placebo (−9.6 [7.8]; overall mixed model for repeated measures $P<0.001$). Additionally, response rates were significantly higher for active medication (41.5%, 54%, and 52% for 2.5, 5, and 10 mg, respectively; versus 28% placebo; Cohen's h 2.5 mg=0.28, 5 mg=0.53, and 10 mg=0.5; NNT 2.5 mg=7.4, 5 mg=3.8, and 10 mg = 4.2). The side effects most often (>10%) reported by participants in this study included oral hypoesthesia, fatigue (10 mg only), sedation, and somnolence.

Celecoxib

In a small (N=42) 8-week DBPC trial (Mousavi et al. 2017) of inpatient adolescents taking risperidone and lithium, adjunctive celecoxib was supe-

TABLE 10–3. Clinical trials of pharmacological agents for the treatment of pediatric acute mania

	Reference	Design	N	Age, years	Duration	Difference in YMRS score (Cohen's *d*)	Response (NNT)	Remission (NNT)
Aripiprazole	Findling et al. 2009	DBPC 10 mg/day	296	10–17	4 weeks	−6 (0)	45% (5.3)	25% (5.1)
		DBPC 30 mg/day				−8.3 (0)	64% (2.6)	48% (2.3)
	Tramontina et al. 2009	DBPC	43	8–17	6 weeks	N/A	89% (2.7)	72% (2.5)
Asenapine	Findling et al. 2015b	DBPC 2.5 mg BID	403	10–17	3 weeks	−2.7 (0.32)	42% (7.4)	N/A
		DBPC 5 mg BID				−5.5 (0.65)	54% (3.8)	
		DBPC 10 mg BID				−6.3 (0.78)	52% (4.2)	
Celecoxib	Mousavi et al. 2017	DBPC adjunctive lithium and risperidone	42	12–18	8 weeks	−3.9 (0.68)	NS	NS
Divalproex	DelBello et al. 2006b	HtH quetiapine	50	12–18	4 weeks	NS	< Quetiapine	< Quetiapine
	Pavuluri et al. 2010	HtH risperidone	66	8–18	6 weeks	< Risperidone	< Risperidone	< Risperidone
	Wagner et al. 2009	DBPC	150	10–17	4 weeks	NS	NS	NS
Lithium	Findling et al. 2015c	DBPC	81	7–17	8 weeks	−6 (0.53)	32% (9.1)	26% (8.3)

TABLE 10–3. Clinical trials of pharmacological agents for the treatment of pediatric acute mania (*continued*)

	Reference	Design	N	Age, years	Duration	Difference in YMRS score (Cohen's *d*)	Response (NNT)	Remission (NNT)
Olanzapine	Tohen et al. 2007	DBPC	161	13–17	3 weeks	−7.7 (0.84)	45% (3.8)	35% (4.2)
Omega-3	Gracious et al. 2010	DBPC	51	6–17	16 weeks	NS	NS	NS
	Wozniak et al. 2015	HtH+inositol	28	5–12	12 weeks	< combination	< combination	< combination
Oxcarbazepine	Wagner et al. 2006	DBPC	116	7–18	7 weeks	NS	NS	NS
Quetiapine	Pathak et al. 2013	DBPC 400 mg/day	277	10–17	3 weeks	−5.2 (0.53)	55% (3.7)	45% (4.5)
		DBPC 600 mg/day				−6.6 (0.89)	56% (3.6)	52% (3.3)
Risperidone	Haas et al. 2009	DBPC low dose	169	10–17	3 weeks		59% (3.0)	43% (3.7)
		DBPC high dose					63% (2.7)	43% (3.7)
Tamoxifen	Fallah et al. 2016	DBPC adjunctive lithium	44	9–20	4 weeks	N/A	100% (2.2)	N/A
Ziprasidone	Findling et al. 2013a	DBPC	237	10–17	4 weeks	−5.2 (0.5)	53% (3.2)	26% (9.9)

Note. DBPC = randomized, double-blind, placebo-controlled clinical trial; HtH = randomized double-blind, head-to-head controlled clinical trial; N/A=data not available from the study; NNT=number needed to treat; NS=nonsignificant difference; YMRS=Young Mania Rating Scale.

rior to placebo in reducing manic symptoms (YMRS mean difference= –3.85, 95% confidence interval [CI]=0.15–7.54, P=0.04; Cohen's d= 0.68). Celecoxib had a larger response rate (100% vs. 90%) and remission rate (85% vs. 60%), but these differences did not reach statistical significance (P=0.48 and P=0.07, respectively). Frequency of adverse events did not differ between groups, and both creatinine and lithium levels were unaffected by celecoxib.

Divalproex

In a double-blind, head-to-head comparison of quetiapine and divalproex monotherapies, larger response (84% vs. 56%) and remission (60% vs. 28%) rates were seen in the quetiapine group (DelBello et al. 2006b). A second double-blind, head-to-head monotherapy trial (Pavuluri et al. 2010) found greater response to risperidone than to divalproex (78% vs. 46%) and better remission rates (63% vs. 33%). Furthermore, divalproex extended-release monotherapy failed to separate from placebo in a randomized controlled study of the treatment of pediatric mania (Wagner et al. 2009). In this well-powered study, there were no significant group differences in YMRS score reduction (–8.8 divalproex vs. –7.9 placebo), nor were there significant group differences in response (24% vs. 23%) or remission (16% vs. 19%) rates. Common side effects in these studies included gastrointestinal symptoms, sedation, and weight gain. Pancreatitis, hepatotoxicity, alopecia, and thrombocytopenia have also been associated with divalproex, albeit less commonly (Rana et al. 2005). Obtaining complete blood counts and pregnancy tests at baseline and every 6 months thereafter is recommended. Additionally, careful monitoring of menstrual cycles in adolescent females who are prescribed divalproex is strongly warranted, because this medication has been associated with polycystic ovary syndrome (Bilo and Meo 2008).

Lithium

A recent multicenter DBPC trial (Findling et al. 2015c) demonstrated that lithium was significantly superior to placebo in reducing manic symptoms as measured by YMRS scores (P=0.03). In this study, lithium also showed a larger proportion of both treatment response (32% vs. 21%; Cohen's h=0.25, NNT=9.1) and remission (26% vs. 14%; Cohen's h=0.30, NNT=8.3); however, the difference in these rates did not achieve statistical significance. Of note, in this study 30% of the patients in the lithium group dropped out before completing the 8-week trial. In a DBPC discontinuation study (Kafantaris et al. 2004) involving adolescent patients with bipolar disorder who had previously responded to lithium, after discontinuation, lithium failed to significantly separate from placebo with regard to symptom exacerbation postdiscontinuation (62% for placebo vs. 53% for lithium). Common adverse effects associated with lithium include nausea, headache, acne, weight gain, thyroid dysfunction, diabetes insipidus, and tremor. Baseline complete blood counts, thyroid panels, blood urea nitrogen, creatinine, serum calcium, urinalysis, and pregnancy test are recommended prior to initiation of lithium, as well as every 3–6 months thereafter (Findling 2009).

Olanzapine

Olanzapine's efficacy in treating acute mania has been demonstrated in a 3-week DBPC trial (Tohen et al. 2007). In this study, olanzapine was significantly superior to placebo in reducing manic symptoms (-17.6 vs. -9.9, $P<0.001$) and in both response rates (44.8% vs. 18.5%; Cohen's $h=0.56$, NNT=3.8) and remission rates (35.2% vs. 11.1%; Cohen's $h=0.58$, NNT=4.2). Common side effects included sedation, appetite increase, and metabolic changes (McClellan 2007). Weight gain may be of increased significance for this population; in one study, adolescents gained an average of 7.4 kg in 3 weeks, compared with 3.2 kg in adults. Subjects in that study also exhibited pre-/post-trial changes in prolactin, fasting glucose, fasting total cholesterol, uric acid, and hepatic enzymes (Singh et al. 2010).

Omega-3 fatty acids

We identified two RCTs assessing the use of omega-3 fatty acids (Om-3) in bipolar spectrum disorders in subjects displaying acute manic, hypomanic, or mixed symptoms. A 16-week DBPC study using flax oil (which contains the Om-3 alpha-linolenic acid) in 51 children and adolescents found no significant differences in primary clinical outcome measures between Om-3 and placebo (Gracious et al. 2010). In another double-blind study, high-ratio eicosapentaenoic acid (EPA)/docosahexaenoic acid (DHA) Om-3, inositol, and the combination Om-3+inositol were assigned in a randomly double-blind design to 28 subjects with bipolar spectrum disorders; the study authors found response rates of 29% for Om-3 monotherapy and of 60% when Om-3 was combined with inositol ($P<0.05$)(Wozniak et al. 2015).

Oxcarbazepine

Despite initial case reports that hinted toward oxcarbazepine's positive tolerability and its effect in treatment of pediatric mania (Davanzo et al.

2004; Teitelbaum 2001), its efficacy has not been proven in controlled studies. In a DBPC trial (Wagner et al. 2006), no significant difference between oxcarbazepine and placebo was detected in any of the efficacy measures. Remarkably, the study had a very high dropout rate (66% for oxcarbazepine and 60% for placebo). More adverse events in the oxcarbazepine group compared with the placebo group were reported in this study; these included dizziness, nausea, somnolence, diplopia, fatigue, and rash.

Quetiapine

In a DBPC trial, quetiapine was found to be superior to placebo in reducing manic symptoms; furthermore, in terms of improvement of symptoms, quetiapine significantly separated from placebo within the first week of treatment (Pathak et al. 2013). Quetiapine (400 mg/day and 600 mg/day) produced higher response rates and remission rates compared with placebo (400 mg/ day: response rate 55% vs. placebo 28%, Cohen's $h=0.55$, NNT=3.7; remission rate 45% vs. placebo 23%, Cohen's $h=0.47$, NNT=4.5; 600 mg/day: response rate 56%, Cohen's $h=0.58$, NNT=3.6; remission rate 52%, Cohen's $h=0.63$, NNT=3.3). Furthermore, in a head-to-head, randomized, double-blind study comparing quetiapine with divalproex (DelBello et al. 2006b), quetiapine was found to be superior to divalproex with regard to rates of response (84% vs. 56%) and remission (60% vs. 28%). Another RCT study comparing a quetiapine/divalproex combination with divalproex alone (Delbello et al. 2002) found that response rates were significantly higher in the combination group than in the monotherapy group (87% vs. 53%), but that the combination was also associated with greater weight gain (4.2 kg±3.2 vs. 2.5 kg±2.1). Common adverse effects in these studies included sedation, gastrointestinal upset, and weight gain (Fraguas et al. 2011). Quetiapine treatment was associated with an average gain of 1.7 kg in 3 weeks and 3.4 kg in 8 weeks. However, none of these trials reported significant differences in metabolic parameters.

Risperidone

In a three-way DBPC comparison of low-dose risperidone (0.5–2.5 mg/day) and high-dose risperidone (3.0–6.0 mg/day) monotherapy vs. placebo in an adolescent population with acute mania, both active treatment groups experienced significantly decreased manic symptoms (Haas et al. 2009). Response rates for both low (59.2%; Cohen's $h=0.68$, NNT=3.0) and high (63.3%; Cohen's $h=0.76$, NNT=2.7) risperidone dosages were significantly larger than the placebo rate (26.3%). Remission rates were identical for both doses and significantly larger than in the placebo group (43% vs. 16%; Cohen's $h=0.61$, NNT=3.7). Overall, no dose-response differences in efficacy were noted, suggesting that a low dosage may be as effective as higher dosages and, in general, is better tolerated. Additionally, head-to-head comparisons of risperidone to both divalproex (Geller et al. 2012; Pavuluri et al. 2010) and lithium (Geller et al. 2012) have indicated risperidone's superior result. Risperidone use in youth is associated with fatigue, dizziness, extrapyramidal side effects, gastrointestinal symptoms, weight gain, and hyperprolactinemia (Correll and Carlson 2006; dos Santos Júnior et al. 2015; Pappagallo and Silva 2004). Hyperprolactinemia should be monitored closely in pediatric populations, since this may affect bone development, lead to gynecomastia, and bring about undesirable menstrual abnormalities (Pappagallo and Silva 2004).

Tamoxifen

In a small ($N=44$) 4-week DBPC trial of youths hospitalized for acute mania, tamoxifen + lithium treatment was compared with lithium + placebo (Fallah et al. 2016; Findling et al. 2015c). All subjects were started on lithium, with the dose titrated to achieve serum levels between 0.8 and 1.1 mEq/L; those randomly assigned to the active arm ($n=22$) also began receiving tamoxifen at 20 mg/day, with the dose titrated to 40 mg/day. Subjects in the lithium + tamoxifen group displayed a larger reduction in manic symptoms from the first, a difference that was sustained through endpoint. Response rates were also significantly different from the first week (45.5% vs. 9.1%; $P=0.007$; Cohen's $h=0.87$, NNT=2.8), and by the third week all subjects in the lithium + tamoxifen group had achieved clinical response, versus only 54.5% of the control group ($P<0.001$; Cohen's $h>0.9$, NNT=2.2). No information on remission rates was presented in the study. Side effect rates were significantly different between groups, with more subjects reporting at least one side effect in the lithium+placebo group compared with the lithium + tamoxifen group (60% vs. 41%; $P = 0.009$). Side effects associated with tamoxifen use in pediatric populations have not been well established.

A systematic review (Lapid et al. 2013) on the use of tamoxifen for pubertal gynecomastia found that in six studies (total $N=99$), no specific clinical side effects were reported with tamoxifen during the study periods, which ranged from 4 months to 7 years. In a small ($N=28$) OL study on girls with McCune-Albright syndrome, no significant side effects were reported over 12 months of treatment (Eugster et al. 2003). However,

30% of females in a 12-month OL study of tamoxifen therapy for desmoid fibromatosis developed asymptomatic ovarian cysts; of note, the dosage used in this study was much larger (300 mg/day).

Topiramate

We identified a DBPC trial of topiramate for co-occurring pediatric mania and substance abuse in adolescents; however, this study was prematurely terminated by the sponsor because the trials of topiramate in adults with mania showed no efficacy (Delbello et al. 2005). This makes it impossible to draw definite conclusions based on just this study. Common adverse events in pediatric populations include weight decrease, upper respiratory tract infection, paresthesia, decrease appetite, cognitive slowing, and diarrhea (Reith et al. 2003).

Ziprasidone

A DBPC study revealed that subjects treated with ziprasidone monotherapy for 4 weeks (Findling et al. 2013a) displayed a larger decrease in manic symptoms (least squares mean change in YMRS: -13.83 vs. -8.61; $P<0.001$), and that the separation from placebo reached statistical significance as early as week 1. Response rates were also significantly larger in the ziprasidone group compared with the placebo group (53% vs. 22%; Cohen's $h=0.65$, NNT$=3.22$). Interestingly, in this study, subjects who weighed less than 45 kg did not show a significant improvement compared with the placebo control subjects. The most commonly occurring adverse effects included sedation, somnolence, headache, fatigue, and nausea.

Meta-analyses

Two meta-analyses that studied treatment agents for acute mania in children and adolescents were identified. In one meta-analysis reviewing 29 OL studies and 17 RCTs (Liu et al. 2011), the authors found significant mean changes in YMRS scores from baseline to endpoint, with a by-drug-class effect that pointed toward larger effects for second-generation antipsychotics (SGAs). In OL studies, the pooled estimate of the rate of response of all compounds was statistically different from zero (50.6%; $z=14.10$; $P<0.001$). The test of between-study heterogeneity was significant, indicating significant variability in the rate of response to different compounds. When RCTs were considered, the likelihood of response to treatment was two times larger for active medication compared with placebo (odds ratio [OR]$=2.21$; $P<0.001$). This overall significant separation from placebo was mainly accounted for by the highly significant effect of SGAs. A confirmatory analysis demonstrated SGA superiority over other medication compounds.

Another meta-analysis of DBPC trials (Correll et al. 2010) using anti-manic agents in youths showed that YMRS scores improved more significantly with SGAs (effect size [ES]=0.65) than with mood stabilizers (ES=0.24). However, the analysis also indicated there was greater weight gain (ES=0.53 vs. 0.10) and somnolence (number needed to harm=4.7 vs. 9.5) for SGAs than for mood stabilizers. Evaluating the cost-benefit ratio is imperative when determining treatment options for pediatric bipolar mania.

Open-Label Studies

Aripiprazole

We found three OL studies exploring aripiprazole monotherapy in the treatment of acute mania (Biederman et al. 2007a; Findling et al. 2011b; Tramontina et al. 2007). In an 8-week OL trial of 19 bipolar adolescents, response rate was 68% (Biederman et al. 2007a). A 16-week OL conducted in 96 young children with acute mania found that at endpoint symptom response criteria were met in 62.5% of subjects (Findling et al. 2011b). In a 6-week OL of 10 adolescents with acute mania and comorbid ADHD (Tramontina et al. 2007), aripiprazole monotherapy was shown to produce significant improvement in global functioning scores ($F=3.17$; $P=0.01$; ES=0.55), manic symptoms ($F=5.63$; $P<.01$; ES=0.93), and ADHD symptoms ($t=3.42$; $P<0.01$; ES=1.05).

Carbamazepine

In a 6-week monotherapy OL trial in adolescent patients with acute mania (Kowatch et al. 2000), researchers found low response rates for carba-mazepine (38%). Likewise, an OL trial of extended-release carbamaze-pine as monotherapy in younger participants yielded a response rate of 44% (Joshi et al. 2010). To date, no DBPC trials have investigated the use of carbamazepine for the treatment of pediatric bipolar disorder. The most common adverse events associated with carbamazepine include nau-sea and sedation (Joshi et al. 2010). Carbamazepine has also been associ-ated with agranulocytosis and aplastic anemia; thus, blood work should be monitored in these patients (Evans et al. 1987). Furthermore, carbamaz-epine is associated with increased risk for developing Stevens-Johnson syndrome in patients of Asian ancestry (Chong et al. 2014).

Divalproex

Four OL studies using divalproex were identified in our search. At 6-month follow-up, researchers found response rates of 73.5% and remission rates of 52.9% for divalproex (Pavuluri et al. 2005). A 6-week OL random assignment study reported a symptomatic response rate of 53% (Kowatch et al. 2000), while a 2- to 8-week OL trial yielded a 61% response rate (Wagner et al. 2002). In a prospective 6-month OL trial (Pavuluri et al. 2004), 40 subjects were sequentially assigned to receive a combination treatment of either risperidone and lithium or risperidone and divalproex; of the 20 subjects assigned to the risperidone + divalproex group, 80% showed symptomatic response and 60% met remission criteria (results from the risperidone + lithium arm will be discussed below).

Lamotrigine

In an OL 14-week study, 46 children (6–17 years) received lamotrigine, the dosage of which was slowly titrated for 8 weeks (Biederman et al. 2010). In this study, lamotrigine appeared to be effective in maintaining symptom control of manic symptoms in pediatric bipolar disorder, with a response rate of 72% and a remission rate of 56%. Another OL study, which involved 12 weeks of lamotrigine monotherapy in 39 children with bipolar spectrum disorder and acute manic symptoms, found a response rate of 66% and a 36% remission rate (Pavuluri et al. 2009). Common adverse effects of lamotrigine include gastrointestinal symptoms, dizziness, ataxia, tremors, headaches, and skin rashes (Messenheimer et al. 2000). The incidence of serious rashes, including Stevens-Johnson syndrome, was approximately 0.8% in pediatric patients receiving lamotrigine as therapy for epilepsy, 0.08% in adult bipolar patients receiving lamotrigine as monotherapy, and 0.13% as adjunctive therapy in adult bipolar patients, according to the lamotrigine product label (http://www.accessdata.fda.gov/drugsatfda_docs/label/2009/020241s037s038,020764s030s031lbl.pdf).

Lithium

We identified five OL studies that evaluated lithium use in acute pediatric mania. The largest of these studies, which included 100 patients followed up for 4 weeks, reported a response rate of 55% and a remission rate of 26%; in this study, however, 46% of subjects used adjunctive SGAs (Kafantaris et al. 2003). In an 8-week OL dose-escalating trial, of the 61 pediatric subjects in acute mania who received lithium, 62% had a symptomatic response and 28.3% achieved remission (Findling et al. 2011a). In a 6-week random assignment, OL prospective study, of the 14 individuals who received lithium, 38% displayed symptomatic response and 46% were reported as very much improved or much improved according to the Clinical Global Impression—Improvement scale (Kowatch et al. 2000). An additional two OL studies evaluated the effect of lithium in combination with risperidone in a follow up of 6 (Pavuluri et al. 2004) and 12 (Pavuluri et al. 2006) months, showing response rates of 82.4% and 85.7% and remission rates of 64.7% and 57.1% respectively.

Olanzapine

Four OL studies have explored the use of olanzapine in the treatment of pediatric patients with acute mania (Biederman et al. 2005a; DelBello et al. 2006a; Frazier et al. 2001; Wozniak et al. 2009). In an 8-week OL trial of 23 children and adolescents with acute mania, 61% of the youths showed symptom response (Frazier et al. 2001), whereas in a 4-week OL study of 20 adolescents, the response rate was 74% and the remission rate was 54% (DelBello et al. 2006a). An OL comparison of olanzapine and risperidone (Biederman et al. 2005a) for the treatment of acute mania in young children found a response rate of 33% for olanzapine (the results for risperidone are discussed later in this section). Olanzapine was also studied in an 8-week OL trial comparing olanzapine monotherapy with an olanzapine-and-topiramate combination; the study authors found response rates of 47% for monotherapy and 60% in the combination group, but this difference was not statistically significant (Wozniak et al. 2009).

Omega-3 fatty acids

In an 8-week OL study conducted in 20 pediatric patients with bipolar spectrum disorder, Om-3 monotherapy led to 35% response and 10% remission rates (Wozniak et al. 2007). A second OL 6-week study explored the use of Om-3 as an adjunct to standard medication in 18 children and adolescents with bipolar spectrum disorders and mild manic symptoms (Clayton et al. 2009). This study found that Om-3 significantly reduced YMRS symptoms from baseline to endpoint, but none of the patients achieved > 50% reduction of YMRS score.

Paliperidone

In a small ($N=41$) OL study of paliperidone monotherapy, treatment was associated with a 60% response rate and a 40% remission rate (Joshi et al. 2013). However, 40% of patients in the study exhibited clinically significant weight gain (≥7% increase) over just 8 weeks.

Quetiapine

An 8-week OL study in preschool and school-age children with bipolar spectrum disorders and acute mania symptoms found that quetiapine monotherapy led to response rates of 46% in the preschool subjects and 42% in school-age subjects, and a remission rate of 26% in both age groups (Joshi et al. 2012).

Risperidone

We found one OL study of risperidone monotherapy, one OL comparison study, and two OL combination treatment studies in our literature review. In the monotherapy study, 8-week treatment with risperidone in 30 patients led to a 50% response rate (Biederman et al. 2005b). In the OL head-to-head comparison of risperidone and olanzapine, after 8 weeks, 69% of the subjects in the risperidone arm achieved a clinical response according to the study criteria (Biederman et al. 2005a). Risperidone in combination with lithium or divalproex induced response in 85.7% and 80% of patients, respectively, in the OL combination trials (Pavuluri et al. 2004, 2006).

Vitamin D_3

A small ($N=16$) 8-week OL study explored the effect of adjunctive vitamin D_3 on adolescents with bipolar spectrum disorders presenting with manic symptoms (Sikoglu et al. 2015). This study reported that vitamin D_3 supplementation (2,000 IU) decreased baseline manic (YMRS change$=-8.6$; $P=0.002$) and depressive (CDRS change$=-7.9$; $P=0.01$) symptoms.

Ziprasidone

In an 8-week OL study, ziprasidone was evaluated as monotherapy in 21 patients (6–17 years) with a bipolar spectrum diagnosis (17 with acute mania); in this study, ziprasidone produced a response rate of 70% (Biederman et al. 2007b). In an OL trial of an escalating dose of ziprasidone in 63 patients, of which 46 had acute manic episode, ziprasidone monotherapy produced clinically meaningful symptomatic improvements, with a 63% response rate (DelBello et al. 2008).

Treatment of Bipolar Depression in Children and Adolescents

There is a remarkable scarcity of studies on the treatment of bipolar depression in child and adolescent psychiatry. Our search found four randomized clinical trials, five OL studies, and one retrospective chart review.

Randomized Clinical Trials

Lurasidone

A 6-week DBPC trial ($N=374$) in children and adolescents (10–17 years) with acute bipolar depression showed lurasidone to be superior to placebo (DelBello et al. 2017). Subjects treated with a flexible dose of lurasidone (20–80 mg/day) had a larger decrease in depression symptom scores (CDRS mean difference between groups$=-5.7$; Cohen's $d=0.45$) and a higher likelihood of achieving response (59.5% vs. 36.5%; $P<0.0001$; Cohen's $h=0.52$, NNT=5) compared with placebo. Remission rates were also larger in the lurasidone group but did not reach statistical significance (26% vs. 19%; $P=0.08$; Cohen's $h=0.3$, NNT=14); of note, remission was determined using strict criteria (CDRS-Revised score<28, YMRS score<8, and Clinical Global Impression—Severity for Bipolar Disorder depression score<3). More subjects in the lurasidone group than in the placebo group reported having at least one side effect (65% vs. 51%). The most common side effects reported for lurasidone were nausea and somnolence. In March 2018, lurasidone became only the second medication approved by the U.S. Food and Drug Administration (FDA) for the treatment of bipolar depression in children and adolescents.

Olanzapine-fluoxetine combination

An 8-week DBPC trial (Detke et al. 2015) evaluating the olanzapine-fluoxetine combination (OFC) found that patients in active treatment showed a significantly larger decrease in depressive symptomatology (least squares YMRS difference: -28 vs. -23; $P=0.003$). A larger proportion of patients taking OFC compared with placebo achieved remission (59% vs. 43%; Cohen's $h=0.32$, NNT=6.2) or responded (78% vs. 59%; Cohen's $h=0.41$, NNT=5.3). In this study, there was no difference in treatment-emergent suicidal ideation or behavior or worsening of manic symptoms between OFC and placebo. During this study, the most frequent treatment-emergent adverse events in the OFC group were weight gain, increased appetite, and somnolence. Treatment-emergent hyperlipidemia was very common among OFC-treated patients.

Quetiapine

A DBPC trial (DelBello et al. 2009) involving 32 adolescents with bipolar depression found that quetiapine monotherapy failed to separate from placebo in terms of response (quetiapine 71% vs. placebo 67%) and remission (quetiapine 35% vs. placebo 40%) rates. Similar results were found in a large 8-week DBPC clinical trial (Findling et al. 2014) of almost 200 youths, with quetiapine monotherapy failing to differentiate from placebo in reducing depressive symptoms (response: quetiapine 63% vs. placebo 55%; remission: quetiapine 45.7% vs. placebo 34%).

Open-Label Studies

Antidepressants

Two retrospective chart reviews were found in our literature regarding the use of antidepressants in bipolar depressed youth. One retrospective chart review of 59 subjects (Biederman et al. 2000) showed that the use of antidepressants may have led to depressive symptom reduction; nevertheless, bipolar youths treated with antidepressants were up to three times more likely to develop treatment-emergent mania (OR=3.0; 95% CI= 1.2–7.8). Another retrospective chart review of 25 children and adolescents with bipolar depression treated with antidepressants found that 36% of these patients experienced an antidepressant-induced mood switch (Park et al. 2014).

Lamotrigine

OL studies and retrospective evaluation of lamotrigine for pediatric bipolar depression have yielded varying success. Whereas a retrospective chart review (Shon et al. 2014) found only a 43% response rate, other studies have demonstrated a significant reduction in mixed-state depressive symptoms for a large majority (82%) of patients, using lamotrigine plus an SGA (Pavuluri et al. 2009). Another OL study found that lamotrigine as either monotherapy or adjunctive therapy resulted in a response rate of 63% and a remission rate of 58% (Chang et al. 2006).

Lithium

The only published OL study of lithium for bipolar depression in youths (Patel et al. 2006) involved monotherapy treatment in a small sample ($N=27$). The study authors found a large effect (Cohen's $d=1.7$) and high rates of response (48%) and remission (30%).

Uridine

The pyrimidine nucleoside uridine has been studied in adults with bipolar disorder for its role in improving phospholipid metabolism, catecholamine synthesis, and mitochondrial function. A small, 6-week OL prospective study using uridine 500 mg twice daily in seven adolescents with bipolar depression found a mean decrease of –38.4 points in CDRS score and a response rate of 54% (Kondo et al. 2011).

Maintenance Treatment for Bipolar Disorder in Children and Adolescents

Our review of the literature found three RCTs of maintenance treatment and 11 OL studies of long-term treatment/maintenance treatment for children and adolescents with bipolar disorder. Of note, most of the studies represent samples of enriched treatment response (i.e., the patients had previously been stabilized with the medication in question).

Randomized Controlled Trials

Aripiprazole

A 72-week DBPC maintenance study (Findling et al. 2012) found that time to discontinuation due to a mood event was significantly longer for subjects receiving aripiprazole monotherapy than for those receiving placebo (median 6.14 weeks vs. 2.29 weeks); however, there was a substantial rate of withdrawal from treatment in the placebo group (90%), limiting the generalizability of the results. Another DBPC explored the long-term (30-week) efficacy of two doses of aripiprazole monotherapy (Findling et al. 2013b); the study showed aripiprazole to be superior to placebo, yielding a greater reduction in symptoms for those in both the 10-mg group (59%) and the 30-mg group (65%), as compared with the placebo group (30%). Although this DBPC study offered a long-term follow-up, it does not truly represent a maintenance trial because it does not provide measures of recurrence and/or sustained response for those who achieved remission while taking aripiprazole.

Lamotrigine

Following an 18-week OL period, a 36-week DBPC maintenance trial (Findling et al. 2015a) found that lamotrigine added-on to patients' existing medication is effective in increasing time to the occurrence of a mood episode: depressive (155 days [±14.7] vs. 50 days [±3.8]); manic/hypomanic (163 days [±12.2] vs. 120 days [±12.2]); and mixed mood (136 days [±15.4] vs. 107 days [±13.8]). This intervention seemed to be more effective in 13- to 17-year-olds compared with 10- to 12-year-olds.

Lithium or divalproex

One 18-month double-blind RCT comparing lithium and divalproex in patients who had previously been stabilized with the combination of the two drugs found similar relapse rates and time to relapse for both drugs. In this trial, 60% of patients treated with lithium and 66.7% of those treated with divalproex experienced a relapse during the 18-month follow-up and a median time to relapse of 16.3 ± 8.2 weeks and 16 ± 8 weeks, respectively (Findling et al. 2005).

Open-Label Studies

Asenapine

In a 50-week OL extension study that followed a 3-week DBPC trial for pediatric mania (Findling et al. 2016), 241 adolescents who had received asenapine in the DBPC phase continued into the extension phase (As/As), while 81 subjects who had received placebo in the DBPC phase enrolled in the OL extension (PB/As). Those in the As/As group continued to experience a decrease in their YRMS scores (-6.5 [± 10.5]), while those in the PB/As group achieved an average YRMS score decrease of 15.2 [± 5.8] by the end of the yearlong study. The article focused on treatment-emergent side effects; of note, 56.4% of subjects withdrew from the study. Among those who withdrew, 26% did so because of treatment-emergent side effects; 9% because of treatment failure, and 10% because of noncompliance. In terms of side effects, 42% experienced sedation/somnolence, 6% developed extrapyramidal symptoms, and 3% developed akathisia. Furthermore, 35% experienced clinically significant weight gain (increase in z–body mass index equal to 6 percentiles). Among those who achieved response criteria in the acute 3-week DBPC trial and continued in the OL extension ($n=141$), 33% failed to maintain response to manic symptoms after 26 weeks; no reports on rates of treatment-emergent depression were provided.

Divalproex

Two OL studies of long-term use of divalproex in pediatric bipolar disorder were identified. In a 6-month OL prospective trial (Pavuluri et al. 2005), 34 individuals received divalproex and showed a continued decrease in both manic and depressive symptoms. In this small sample, the study authors found that 53% of the patients achieved remission based on a lax definition ($\geq 50\%$ change from baseline on YMRS; ≤ 40 on CDRS-Revised; Clinical Global Impression—Improvement for Bipolar

Disorder score of ≤2; and ≥51 on the Children's Global Assessment Scale). However, the study authors did not report time to relapse or rates of relapse in this small sample. On the other hand, the OL extension study of the DBPC trial of extended-release divalproex monotherapy in acute mania in which the active drug failed to separate from placebo found that subjects did not experience any significant continued decrease in symptoms, with only a minimal (−2.2) change in YMRS score from baseline (Redden et al. 2009).

Lithium

In the 12-month OL study of risperidone augmentation to lithium nonresponders noted in an earlier section (Pavuluri et al. 2006), authors reported that 45% of the lithium monotherapy responders (*n*=38) maintained the effect during follow-up. An 18-month maintenance trial found that of subjects who continued taking lithium monotherapy, only 37.5% experienced a relapse, whereas 92% of those who discontinued lithium experienced a relapse (Strober et al. 1990).

Quetiapine

One small (*N*=21) OL maintenance trial found that 72% of study subjects remained stable for the duration of the 48-week study, suggesting that quetiapine monotherapy may be a viable option for pediatric bipolar maintenance treatment (Duffy et al. 2009).

Ziprasidone

In the 26-week OL extension phase of the ziprasidone monotherapy DBPC trial discussed earlier in this chapter, the study authors found a continued reduction in YMRS scores over time (Findling et al. 2013a). No information on relapses in those who had achieved remission was reported in the article.

Discussion

Although research into the treatment of bipolar disorder in children and adolescents has increased in recent years, many uncertainties remain. Overall, the amount of data on the efficacy of pharmacological interventions is scarce when compared with the adult literature. Moreover, studies for the treatment of manic episodes are by far more abundant than those designed for the treatment of depression or for the maintenance of euthymic mood states. As of this writing, the FDA has approved the following medications for the treatment of pediatric mania: lithium (age 12+ for extended-release formulation and 7+ for immediate-release formulation), aripiprazole (age 10+), asenapine (age 10+), olanzapine (age 13+), quetiapine (age 10+), and risperidone (age 10+).

Youths with bipolar disorder experience full episodes or subsyndromal symptoms of depression nearly 40% of the time. Furthermore, prospective studies have demonstrated that after remission from mania occurs, children and adolescents may be more likely to relapse into a major depressive episode than into a hypomanic, manic, or mixed episode. Unfortunately, there is a paucity of controlled data regarding pharmacotherapy for depression among youths with bipolar disorder. As of this writing, OFC and lurasidone are the only FDA-approved treatments for bipolar depression in children and adolescents. However, examining clinical trial registries revealed that several studies were being conducted to assess different medications for the treatment of bipolar depression (uridine and N-acetylcysteine). Results from these studies will add to the available empirical data and may modify the structure and content of the recommendations for pediatric bipolar depression.

Even though a core aspect of treatment is long-term management of patients with bipolar disorder, only four studies provided information on relapse prevention.

From this review, it is obvious that additional evidence for the pharmacological and nonpharmacological treatments of pediatric bipolar disorder is needed. In addition, because it is highly unlikely that any given medication will be universally effective in youths with bipolar disorder (or in any age group, for that matter), more studies searching for adequate predictors of treatment response are of vital importance to achieve individualized treatment strategies. These predictors can be any clinical or biological factor, ranging from demographic characteristics, symptomatic clusters, family history, pharmacogenetic markers, and cognitive deficits to neuroimaging traits. Moreover, given that no single study will be sufficiently powered to detect predictors of treatment response to all available treatment options, efforts should be taken to have available a pool of data in which to collectively search for those predictors. Systematic data collection, similar data designs, and uniform rater reliability in efficacy measurements should be the initial steps in this endeavor. Vigorous and concerted efforts to address these and other questions will ensure that the momentum of progress in the treatment of pediatric bipolar disorder is sustained over the coming years.

Given the data considered in this chapter and the guidelines in our system for classification of quality of evidence and strength of recommendations, we present the expert opinion of our review.

Expert Opinion

Recommendations for the Treatment of Acute Mania in Children and Adolescents

1. **SGAs should be considered first-line treatment for children and adolescents with acute mania (Level 1).** We have found convergent evidence that, to date, SGAs are more effective than lithium and other mood stabilizers for the treatment of acute mania. In our review of the studies, SGAs show larger effect sizes, display more consistency across studies, and overall are backed by higher quality of evidence. Within the group of currently available SGAs, aripiprazole was the only agent that achieved the highest recommendation grade (Level 1). Second-highest recommendation (Level 2) was achieved by asenapine, quetiapine, and risperidone. Olanzapine is backed by good-quality data and moderate effect size in both response and remission; however, given the important concerns about metabolic side effects, which appear larger than those of other SGAs, recommendation strength was dropped to moderate (Level 3). Similarly, concerns about quality of data downgraded the strength of recommendation of ziprasidone (Level 3), despite its displaying a large effect size; at the time of writing this chapter, another DBPC study of ziprasidone for treatment of acute mania in children and adolescents was being conducted, and the results of this study, when reported, may raise or lower the recommendation. Because of the lack of good-quality data, paliperidone received the lowest recommendation among SGAs (Level 4). Given the well-established weight gain and metabolic adverse effects associated with most SGAs, active surveillance and monitoring are particularly necessary. Much remains unknown regarding the long-term consequences of these side effects in terms of morbidity and mortality when youths who have taken these medications reach adulthood. Currently, a growing number of studies are exploring treatment options for the management of these metabolic side effects, and clinicians should familiarize themselves with such interventions. Unfortunately, a systematic review of the evidence for these interventions goes beyond the scope of this review.

2. **For the treatment of acute mania in children and adolescents, when the use of SGAs is contraindicated or there is failure to achieve the desired response or remission, lithium should be sought as a second-line agent either as monotherapy (Level 3) or in combination with an SGA (Level 2).** Lithium monotherapy displayed a moderate effect size and medium-

quality data but consistency across an RCT and several OL studies. Although there are no DBPC studies for the use of lithium in combination with an SGA, large effect size and consistent findings in OL studies warrant giving this option a moderate recommendation. Furthermore, preliminary data suggest lithium response may run in families (Grof et al. 2002), indicating the potential for genetic determinants in lithium response; also, data in adults point toward a subset of patients who are "super responders"; and lithium has strong and consistent evidence of reducing the risk of suicidal behavior, which was taken into account when we were determining this recommendation. Celecoxib as an adjunct therapy in patients with bipolar disorder appeared to be superior to placebo in a small DBPC trial; however, separation from placebo was achieved only after 8 weeks of treatment.

3. **Divalproex and lamotrigine should be considered third-line agents for the treatment of acute mania in children and adolescents (Level 4).** Negative results from a DBPC study coupled with a demonstrated efficacy that is inferior to that of SGAs (risperidone and quetiapine) led to divalproex being assigned the lowest-grade recommendation (Level 4). Divalproex use for acute mania should be limited to those individuals who have already failed to respond to monotherapy with an SGA or lithium or to the combination of lithium and an SGA. Divalproex use in combination with quetiapine has shown large response and remission rates and may be considered in certain patients. Lamotrigine use for acute mania is limited for practical purposes because of the long period of dose titration required. Lamotrigine also has limited evidence supporting its use in acute mania; therefore, recommendation for its use is low (Level 4).

4. **Further research is required to establish the overall efficacy and safety of a) adjunctive celecoxib to lithium and risperidone combination treatment and b) adjunctive tamoxifen to lithium treatment (Level 3).** Although results from DBPC trials are promising and show robust effect sizes for adjunctive tamoxifen and celecoxib, these samples were small and the overall safety cannot be well established. Given the quality of data and lack of evidence of efficacy, no statement can be made about other pharmacotherapies (i.e., oxcarbazepine, paliperidone, omega-3 fatty acids, vitamin D_3) in the treatment of acute mania.

Recommendations for the Treatment of Bipolar Depression in Children and Adolescents

1. When clinicians determine that the use of a pharmacological intervention for the treatment of bipolar depression in children and adolescents

is warranted, they should consider lurasidone as a first agent (Level 2). Lurasidone recently received FDA approval for use in pediatric bipolar depression (in children 10 years and older). Though effect sizes in terms of response for lurasidone were reported to be in the moderate range, the drug did not separate from placebo in terms of remission rates. Moreover, large placebo responses are particularly common in pediatric bipolar depression, suggesting that psychosocial interventions may be potentially useful as an initial treatment approach in mild to moderate cases.

2. **Olanzapine/fluoxetine combination should be considered a second-line agent for bipolar depression (Level 2).** OFC has been the focus of a large positive DBPC study for the treatment of bipolar depression in children and adolescents. However, the effect size in terms of response and remission was moderate, and there are known concerns about the metabolic and weight gain side effects associated with olanzapine use. For this reason, OFC should be considered a second-line agent in the treatment of youths with bipolar depression, particularly in those who have not responded to psychosocial interventions and lurasidone treatment.

3. **Lithium and lamotrigine should be considered third-line agents for bipolar depression (Level 3).** Lithium has established efficacy in adults with bipolar disorder and in treatment-resistant unipolar depression. Research also suggests that lithium may be particularly effective in preventing suicidal behavior in adults, making it a reasonable treatment option. However, evidence of its efficacy in pediatric bipolar depression is scant at best. Adjunctive lamotrigine, the only antiepileptic medication studied for bipolar depression in youth, yielded positive results in OL studies; however, long titration period and potentially serious side effects limit its use to specific cases.

4. **The use of antidepressants either as add-on or monotherapy should be limited to those patients for whom the potential benefits outweigh the known risks (Level 4).** Antidepressants have been found to be effective and well tolerated for the treatment of unipolar depression in children and adolescents; however, their efficacy in bipolar depression has not been thoroughly examined. The risk of potentially inducing mania must be weighed against the potential therapeutic benefits, as well as the suicide risk that often accompanies severe depression.

Important note: High placebo responses are common in pediatric depression studies, suggesting the need for different study designs in future trials of youths with bipolar depression. Given the paucity of data available, it is prudent for clinicians to be cautious when considering treatment options for depressed children and adolescents with bipolar disorder. Clinicians should also evaluate the efficacy of psychotherapeutic interventions for bipolar depression and weigh them as initial options when clinically appropriate (for a detailed review, see Vallarino et al. 2015).

Recommendations for the Pharmacological Maintenance Treatment of Bipolar Disorder in Children and Adolescents

1. **When selecting an agent for maintenance of euthymic mood state, the clinician should consider aripiprazole monotherapy or lamotrigine as an adjunctive agent as a first-line option (Level 2).** Aripiprazole was found to be superior to placebo in extending time to the emergence of a mood event and showed in an extension study that it can maintain its effect over time. Lamotrigine has evidence of its use as a maintenance agent both as monotherapy and as add-on; stronger evidence supports its use as an add-on agent. Results from these studies show a potential use for this agent, particularly in preventing depressive relapses.
2. **After the patient has achieved stabilization while taking a particular agent, it is reasonable for the patient to continue taking the same agent (Level 3).** Extension studies for aripiprazole, asenapine, quetiapine, and ziprasidone showed that continuing these agents led to maintenance of the response, but as each has only been investigated in one long-term study, their potential is tempered by a lack of replication. Studies evaluating the efficacy of lithium for long-term symptom reduction and relapse prevention for pediatric patients with bipolar disorder have shown moderate success for those who achieved response and remission during the acute phase of treatment.

Important note: Treatments for bipolar maintenance have been evaluated to a limited degree, hampering our ability to provide additional recommendations. Furthermore, given the type of design in these maintenance studies, there are significant concerns over a form of selection bias in which the study samples consist of known responders to the targeted pharmacological agent (as is the case in all of the extension studies). Additional studies to establish the optimal first-line pharmacological strategy for long-term treatment of bipolar disorder in children and adolescents are needed. Current pharmacological agents are still associated with high relapse rates, and residual symptoms are frequent; moreover, as noted, long-term safety and tolerability issues are important to consider. Clinicians must select a treatment for maintenance therapy for each patient on the basis of the available empirical evidence, individual clinical characteristics, and safety concerns.

Limitations of This Review

It is important to note that this review, while extensive, was not a systemic analysis of studies and does not constitute a meta-analytic summary of the data. We attempted to find a balance between simplicity and clarity in our system for grading the quality of evidence and strength of recommendations, based on existing evidence-based medicine systems. We understand quality of evidence falls on a continuum; thus, any discrete categorization involves some degree of arbitrariness. Nevertheless, it is our belief that the advantages of simplicity and transparency outweigh these limitations. However, regardless of how simple or complex a system is, judgments are always required. Although our system provided a framework for a structured reflection of the data, it did not remove the need for judgment when classifying the quality of data and the level of evidence determining our recommendations.

Clinical Pearls

- When the clinician is selecting a pharmacological treatment for a youth with bipolar disorder, it is important to properly identify the patient's current mental status (i.e., what phase of treatment is most appropriate) and determine what, if any, comorbidities are present.

- Independent of mood state or phase of treatment, attentive assessment of treatment response and monitoring for the emergence of side effects should be performed regularly, with special consideration given to treatment adherence.

- Assessment of whether patients are prescribed an adequate dose or whether comorbid conditions or concomitant medication may be complicating the scenario is necessary.

- Psychoeducation and other psychotherapeutic treatments are key components of the treatment of patients and their families.

- At present, treatments for children and adolescents in a manic state have been most extensively studied. A clear pattern has emerged indicating that SGAs are superior to lithium or antiepileptic mood-stabilizing agents. However, continued head-to-head and placebo-controlled trials, most specifically with regard to combination treatments, to determine comparative efficacy are needed.

- Data regarding treatments for depressive states in children and adolescents with bipolar disorder are lacking, and treatments for these illnesses should be an area of focus for research in the near future.

- Large placebo response rates are frequently seen in this population, however, so ascertaining the degree to which a given treatment surpasses placebo is imperative.

- At present, two of the three placebo-controlled trials in this area have failed to find a significant treatment response beyond that seen with placebo. Furthermore, some patients may experience sufficient therapeutic benefit solely from psychosocial interventions. The need for alternative experimental designs is apparent.

- More recently, maintenance of a euthymic mood state in children and adolescents with bipolar disorder has been a focus of treatment studies. Of particular interest are the data from a recently completed investigation of lamotrigine indicating a longer time to a bipolar mood event. Continued research into lamotrigine and other potential maintenance treatments is necessary. Moreover, studies that determine the appropriate treatment duration for a given medication and patient are needed.

- Over the past several years, pediatric bipolarity has been increasingly recognized. Future research endeavors should include studies that allow for personalized treatment strategies, including those based on markers of response and tolerability.

References

Axelson D, Birmaher B, Strober M, et al: Phenomenology of children and adolescents with bipolar spectrum disorders. Arch Gen Psychiatry 63(10):1139–1148, 2006 17015816

Biederman J, Mick E, Spencer TJ, et al: Therapeutic dilemmas in the pharmacotherapy of bipolar depression in the young. J Child Adolesc Psychopharmacol 10(3):185–192, 2000 11052408

Biederman J, Mick E, Hammerness P, et al: Open-label, 8-week trial of olanzapine and risperidone for the treatment of bipolar disorder in preschool-age children. Biol Psychiatry 58(7):589–594, 2005a 16239162

Biederman J, Mick E, Wozniak J, et al: An open-label trial of risperidone in children and adolescents with bipolar disorder. J Child Adolesc Psychopharmacol 15(2):311–317, 2005b 15910215

Biederman J, Mick E, Spencer T, et al: An open-label trial of aripiprazole mono-therapy in children and adolescents with bipolar disorder. CNS Spectr 12(9):683–689, 2007a 17805214

Biederman J, Mick E, Spencer T, et al: A prospective open-label treatment trial of ziprasidone monotherapy in children and adolescents with bipolar disorder. Bipolar Disord 9(8):888–894, 2007b 18076539

Biederman J, Joshi G, Mick E, et al: A prospective open-label trial of lamotrigine monotherapy in children and adolescents with bipolar disorder. CNS Neurosci Ther 16(2):91–102, 2010 20415838

Bilo L, Meo R: Polycystic ovary syndrome in women using valproate: a review. Gynecol Endocrinol 24(10):562–570, 2008 19012099

Chang K: Adult bipolar disorder is continuous with pediatric bipolar disorder. Can J Psychiatry 52(7):418–425, 2007 17688005

Chang K: Challenges in the diagnosis and treatment of pediatric bipolar depression. Dialogues Clin Neurosci 11(1):73–80, 2009 19432389

Chang K, Saxena K, Howe M: An open-label study of lamotrigine adjunct or monotherapy for the treatment of adolescents with bipolar depression. J Am Acad Child Adolesc Psychiatry 45(3):298–304, 2006 16540814

Chong KW, Chan DW, Cheung YB, et al: Association of carbamazepine-induced severe cutaneous drug reactions and HLA-B*1502 allele status, and dose and treatment duration in paediatric neurology patients in Singapore. Arch Dis Child 99(6):581–584, 2014 24225276

Clayton EH, Hanstock TL, Hirneth SJ, et al: Reduced mania and depression in juvenile bipolar disorder associated with long-chain omega-3 polyunsaturated fatty acid supplementation. Eur J Clin Nutr 63(8):1037–1040, 2009 19156158

Correll CU, Carlson HE: Endocrine and metabolic adverse effects of psychotropic medications in children and adolescents. J Am Acad Child Adolesc Psychiatry 45(7):771–791, 2006 16832314

Correll CU, Sheridan EM, DelBello MP: Antipsychotic and mood stabilizer efficacy and tolerability in pediatric and adult patients with bipolar I mania: a comparative analysis of acute, randomized, placebo-controlled trials. Bipolar Disord 12(2):116–141, 2010 20402706

Davanzo P, Nikore V, Yehya N, et al: Oxcarbazepine treatment of juvenile-onset bipolar disorder. J Child Adolesc Psychopharmacol 14(3):344–345, 2004 15650489

Delbello MP, Schwiers ML, Rosenberg HL, et al: A double-blind, randomized, placebo-controlled study of quetiapine as adjunctive treatment for adolescent mania. J Am Acad Child Adolesc Psychiatry 41(10):1216–1223, 2002 12364843

Delbello MP, Findling RL, Kushner S, et al: A pilot controlled trial of topiramate for mania in children and adolescents with bipolar disorder. J Am Acad Child Adolesc Psychiatry 44(6):539–547, 2005 15908836

DelBello MP, Cecil KM, Adler CM, et al: Neurochemical effects of olanzapine in first-hospitalization manic adolescents: a proton magnetic resonance spectroscopy study. Neuropsychopharmacology 31(6):1264–1273, 2006a 16292323

DelBello MP, Kowatch RA, Adler CM, et al: A double-blind randomized pilot study comparing quetiapine and divalproex for adolescent mania. J Am Acad Child Adolesc Psychiatry 45(3):305–313, 2006b 16540815

DelBello MP, Versavel M, Ice K, et al: Tolerability of oral ziprasidone in children and adolescents with bipolar mania, schizophrenia, or schizoaffective disorder. J Child Adolesc Psychopharmacol 18(5):491–499, 2008 18928413

DelBello MP, Chang K, Welge JA, et al: A double-blind, placebo-controlled pilot study of quetiapine for depressed adolescents with bipolar disorder. Bipolar Disord 11(5):483–493, 2009 19624387

DelBello MP, Goldman R, Phillips D, et al: Efficacy and safety of lurasidone in children and adolescents with bipolar I depression: a double-blind, placebo-controlled study. J Am Acad Child Adolesc Psychiatry 56(12):1015–1025, 2017 29173735

Detke HC, DelBello MP, Landry J, et al: Olanzapine/Fluoxetine combination in children and adolescents with bipolar I depression: a randomized, double-blind, placebo-controlled trial. J Am Acad Child Adolesc Psychiatry 54(3):217–224, 2015 25721187

dos Santos Júnior A, Henriques TB, de Mello MP, et al: Hyperprolactinemia in children and adolescents with use of risperidone: clinical and molecular genetics aspects. J Child Adolesc Psychopharmacol 25(10):738–748, 2015 26682995

Duffy A, Milin R, Grof P: Maintenance treatment of adolescent bipolar disorder: open study of the effectiveness and tolerability of quetiapine. BMC Psychiatry 9:4, 2009 19200370

Ebell MH, Siwek J, Weiss BD, et al: Strength of Recommendation Taxonomy (SORT): a patient-centered approach to grading evidence in the medical literature. Am Fam Physician 69(3):548–556, 2004 14971837

Eugster EA, Rubin SD, Reiter EO, et al; McCune-Albright Study Group: Tamoxifen treatment for precocious puberty in McCune-Albright syndrome: a multicenter trial. J Pediatr 143(1):60–66, 2003 12915825

Evans RW, Clay TH, Gualtieri CT: Carbamazepine in pediatric psychiatry. J Am Acad Child Adolesc Psychiatry 26(1):2–8, 1987 3583995

Fallah E, Arman S, Najafi M, et al: Effect of tamoxifen and lithium on treatment of acute mania symptoms in children and adolescents. Iran J Child Neurol 10(2):16–25, 2016 27247580

Findling RL: Safety and tolerability of bipolar disorder treatment in youth. J Clin Psychiatry 70(11):e44, 2009 20031092

Findling RL, McNamara NK, Youngstrom EA, et al: Double-blind 18-month trial of lithium versus divalproex maintenance treatment in pediatric bipolar disorder. J Am Acad Child Adolesc Psychiatry 44(5):409–417, 2005 15843762

Findling RL, Nyilas M, Forbes RA, et al: Acute treatment of pediatric bipolar I disorder, manic or mixed episode, with aripiprazole: a randomized, double-blind, placebo-controlled study. J Clin Psychiatry 70(10):1441–1451, 2009 19906348

Findling RL, Kafantaris V, Pavuluri M, et al: Dosing strategies for lithium monotherapy in children and adolescents with bipolar I disorder. J Child Adolesc Psychopharmacol 21(3):195–205, 2011a 21663422

Findling RL, McNamara NK, Youngstrom EA, et al: An open-label study of aripiprazole in children with a bipolar disorder. J Child Adolesc Psychopharmacol 21(4):345–351, 2011b 21823912

Findling RL, Youngstrom EA, McNamara NK, et al: Double-blind, randomized, placebo-controlled long-term maintenance study of aripiprazole in children with bipolar disorder. J Clin Psychiatry 73(1):57–63, 2012 22152402

Findling RL, Cavus I, Pappadopulos E, et al: Efficacy, long-term safety, and tolerability of ziprasidone in children and adolescents with bipolar disorder. J Child Adolesc Psychopharmacol 23(8):545–557, 2013a 24111980

Findling RL, Correll CU, Nyilas M, et al: Aripiprazole for the treatment of pediatric bipolar I disorder: a 30-week, randomized, placebo-controlled study. Bipolar Disord 15(2):138–149, 2013b 23437959

Findling RL, Pathak S, Earley WR, et al: Efficacy and safety of extended-release quetiapine fumarate in youth with bipolar depression: an 8 week, double-blind, placebo-controlled trial. J Child Adolesc Psychopharmacol 24(6):325–335, 2014 24956042

Findling RL, Chang K, Robb A, et al: Adjunctive maintenance lamotrigine for pediatric bipolar I disorder: a placebo-controlled, randomized withdrawal study. J Am Acad Child Adolesc Psychiatry 54(12):1020.e3–1031.e3, 2015a 26598477

Findling RL, Landbloom RL, Szegedi A, et al: Asenapine for the acute treatment of pediatric manic or mixed episode of bipolar I disorder. J Am Acad Child Adolesc Psychiatry 54(12):1032–1041, 2015b 26598478

Findling RL, Robb A, McNamara NK, et al: Lithium in the acute treatment of bipolar I disorder: a double-blind, placebo-controlled study. Pediatrics 136(5):885–894, 2015c 26459650

Findling RL, Landbloom RL, Mackle M, et al: Long-term safety of asenapine in pediatric patients diagnosed with bipolar I disorder: a 50-week open-label, flexible-dose trial. Paediatr Drugs 18(5):367–378, 2016 27461426

Fraguas D, Correll CU, Merchán-Naranjo J, et al: Efficacy and safety of second-generation antipsychotics in children and adolescents with psychotic and bipolar spectrum disorders: comprehensive review of prospective head-to-head and placebo-controlled comparisons. Eur Neuropsychopharmacol 21(8):621–645, 2011 20702068

Frazier JA, Biederman J, Tohen M, et al: A prospective open-label treatment trial of olanzapine monotherapy in children and adolescents with bipolar disorder. J Child Adolesc Psychopharmacol 11(3):239–250, 2001 11642474

Geller B, Tillman R: Prepubertal and early adolescent bipolar I disorder: review of diagnostic validation by Robins and Guze criteria. J Clin Psychiatry 66 (suppl 7):21–28, 2005 16124838

Geller B, Tillman R, Craney JL, et al: Four-year prospective outcome and natural history of mania in children with a prepubertal and early adolescent bipolar disorder phenotype. Arch Gen Psychiatry 61(5):459–467, 2004 15123490

Geller B, Luby JL, Joshi P, et al: A randomized controlled trial of risperidone, lithium, or divalproex sodium for initial treatment of bipolar I disorder, manic or mixed phase, in children and adolescents. Arch Gen Psychiatry 69(5):515–528, 2012 22213771

Gracious BL, Chirieac MC, Costescu S, et al: Randomized, placebo-controlled trial of flax oil in pediatric bipolar disorder. Bipolar Disord 12(2):142–154, 2010 20402707

Grof P, Duffy A, Cavazzoni P, et al: Is response to prophylactic lithium a familial trait? J Clin Psychiatry 63(10):942–947, 2002 12416605

Guyatt GH, Oxman AD, Vist GE, et al; GRADE Working Group: GRADE: an emerging consensus on rating quality of evidence and strength of recommendations. BMJ 336(7650):924–926, 2008 18436948

Haas M, Delbello MP, Pandina G, et al: Risperidone for the treatment of acute mania in children and adolescents with bipolar disorder: a randomized, double-blind, placebo-controlled study. Bipolar Disord 11(7):687–700, 2009 19839994

Joshi G, Wilens T: Comorbidity in pediatric bipolar disorder. Child Adolesc Psychiatr Clin N Am 18(2):291–319, vii–viii, 2009 19264265

Joshi G, Wozniak J, Mick E, et al: A prospective open-label trial of extended-release carbamazepine monotherapy in children with bipolar disorder. J Child Adolesc Psychopharmacol 20(1):7–14, 2010 20166791

Joshi G, Petty C, Wozniak J, et al: A prospective open-label trial of quetiapine monotherapy in preschool and school age children with bipolar spectrum disorder. J Affect Disord 136(3):1143–1153, 2012 22035648

Joshi G, Petty C, Wozniak J, et al: A prospective open-label trial of paliperidone monotherapy for the treatment of bipolar spectrum disorders in children and adolescents. Psychopharmacology (Berl) 227(3):449–458, 2013 23397049

Kafantaris V, Coletti D, Dicker R, et al: Lithium treatment of acute mania in adolescents: a large open trial. J Am Acad Child Adolesc Psychiatry 42(9):1038–1045, 2003 12960703

Kafantaris V, Coletti DJ, Dicker R, et al: Lithium treatment of acute mania in adolescents: a placebo-controlled discontinuation study. J Am Acad Child Adolesc Psychiatry 43(8):984–993, 2004 15266193

Kondo DG, Sung YH, Hellem TL, et al: Open-label uridine for treatment of depressed adolescents with bipolar disorder. J Child Adolesc Psychopharmacol 21(2):171–175, 2011 21486171

Kowatch RA, Suppes T, Carmody TJ, et al: Effect size of lithium, divalproex sodium, and carbamazepine in children and adolescents with bipolar disorder. J Am Acad Child Adolesc Psychiatry 39(6):713–720, 2000 10846305

Lapid O, van Wingerden JJ, Perlemuter L: Tamoxifen therapy for the management of pubertal gynecomastia: a systematic review. J Pediatr Endocrinol Metab 26(9–10):803–807, 2013 23729603

Liu HY, Potter MP, Woodworth KY, et al: Pharmacologic treatments for pediatric bipolar disorder: a review and meta-analysis. J Am Acad Child Adolesc Psychiatry 50(8):749.e39–762.e39, 2011 21784295

McClellan JM: Olanzapine and pediatric bipolar disorder: evidence for efficacy and safety concerns. Am J Psychiatry 164(10):1462–1464, 2007 17898331

Messenheimer JA, Giorgi L, Risner ME: The tolerability of lamotrigine in children. Drug Saf 22(4):303–312, 2000 10789824

Mousavi SY, Khezri R, Karkhaneh-Yousefi MA, et al: A randomized, double-blind placebo-controlled trial on effectiveness and safety of celecoxib adjunctive therapy in adolescents with acute bipolar mania. J Child Adolesc Psychopharmacol 27(6):494–500, 2017 28409660

Pappagallo M, Silva R: The effect of atypical antipsychotic agents on prolactin levels in children and adolescents. J Child Adolesc Psychopharmacol 14(3):359–371, 2004 15650493

Park KJ, Shon S, Lee HJ, et al: Antidepressant-emergent mood switch in Korean adolescents with mood disorder. Clin Neuropharmacol 37(6):177–185, 2014 25384075

Patel NC, DelBello MP, Bryan HS, et al: Open-label lithium for the treatment of adolescents with bipolar depression. J Am Acad Child Adolesc Psychiatry 45(3):289–297, 2006 16540813

Pathak S, Findling RL, Earley WR, et al: Efficacy and safety of quetiapine in children and adolescents with mania associated with bipolar I disorder: a 3-week, double-blind, placebo-controlled trial. J Clin Psychiatry 74(1):e100–e109, 2013 23419231

Pavuluri MN, Henry DB, Carbray JA, et al: Open-label prospective trial of risperidone in combination with lithium or divalproex sodium in pediatric mania. J Affect Disord 82 (suppl 1):S103–S111, 2004 15571784

Pavuluri MN, Henry DB, Carbray JA, et al: Divalproex sodium for pediatric mixed mania: a 6-month prospective trial. Bipolar Disord 7(3):266–273, 2005 15898964

Pavuluri MN, Henry DB, Carbray JA, et al: A one-year open-label trial of risperidone augmentation in lithium nonresponder youth with preschool-onset bipolar disorder. J Child Adolesc Psychopharmacol 16(3):336–350, 2006 16768641

Pavuluri MN, Henry DB, Moss M, et al: Effectiveness of lamotrigine in maintaining symptom control in pediatric bipolar disorder. J Child Adolesc Psychopharmacol 19(1):75–82, 2009 19232025

Pavuluri MN, Henry DB, Findling RL, et al: Double-blind randomized trial of risperidone versus divalproex in pediatric bipolar disorder. Bipolar Disord 12(6):593–605, 2010 20868458

Peruzzolo TL, Tramontina S, Rohde LA, et al: Pharmacotherapy of bipolar disorder in children and adolescents: an update. Braz J Psychiatry 35(4):393–405, 2013 24402215

Rana M, Khanzode L, Karnik N, et al: Divalproex sodium in the treatment of pediatric psychiatric disorders. Expert Rev Neurother 5(2):165–176, 2005 15853487

Redden L, DelBello M, Wagner KD, et al; Depakote ER Pediatric Mania Group: Long-term safety of divalproex sodium extended-release in children and adolescents with bipolar I disorder. J Child Adolesc Psychopharmacol 19(1):83–89, 2009 19232026

Reith D, Burke C, Appleton DB, et al: Tolerability of topiramate in children and adolescents. J Paediatr Child Health 39(6):416–419, 2003 12919493

Shon SH, Joo Y, Lee JS, et al: Lamotrigine treatment of adolescents with unipolar and bipolar depression: a retrospective chart review. J Child Adolesc Psychopharmacol 24(5):285–287, 2014 24813210

Sikoglu EM, Navarro AA, Starr D, et al: Vitamin D3 supplemental treatment for mania in youth with bipolar spectrum disorders. J Child Adolesc Psychopharmacol 25(5):415–424, 2015 26091195

Singh MK, Ketter TA, Chang KD: Atypical antipsychotics for acute manic and mixed episodes in children and adolescents with bipolar disorder: efficacy and tolerability. Drugs 70(4):433–442, 2010 20205485

Strober M, Morrell W, Lampert C, et al: Relapse following discontinuation of lithium maintenance therapy in adolescents with bipolar I illness: a naturalistic study. Am J Psychiatry 147(4):457–461, 1990 2107763

Teitelbaum M: Oxcarbazepine in bipolar disorder. J Am Acad Child Adolesc Psychiatry 40(9):993–994, 2001 11556642

Tohen M, Kryzhanovskaya L, Carlson G, et al: Olanzapine versus placebo in the treatment of adolescents with bipolar mania. Am J Psychiatry 164(10):1547–1556, 2007 17898346

Tramontina S, Zeni CP, Pheula GF, et al: Aripiprazole in juvenile bipolar disorder comorbid with attention-deficit/hyperactivity disorder: an open clinical trial. CNS Spectr 12(10):758–762, 2007 17934380

Tramontina S, Zeni CP, Ketzer CR, et al: Aripiprazole in children and adolescents with bipolar disorder comorbid with attention-deficit/hyperactivity disorder: a pilot randomized clinical trial. J Clin Psychiatry 70(5):756–764, 2009 19389329

Vallarino M, Henry C, Etain B, et al: An evidence map of psychosocial interventions for the earliest stages of bipolar disorder. Lancet Psychiatry 2(6):548–563, 2015 26360451

Wagner KD, Weller EB, Carlson GA, et al: An open-label trial of divalproex in children and adolescents with bipolar disorder. J Am Acad Child Adolesc Psychiatry 41(10):1224–1230, 2002 12364844

Wagner KD, Kowatch RA, Emslie GJ, et al: A double-blind, randomized, placebo-controlled trial of oxcarbazepine in the treatment of bipolar disorder in children and adolescents. Am J Psychiatry 163(7):1179–1186, 2006 16816222

Wagner KD, Redden L, Kowatch RA, et al: A double-blind, randomized, placebo-controlled trial of divalproex extended-release in the treatment of bipolar disorder in children and adolescents. J Am Acad Child Adolesc Psychiatry 48(5):519–532, 2009 19325497

Wozniak J, Biederman J, Mick E, et al: Omega-3 fatty acid monotherapy for pediatric bipolar disorder: a prospective open-label trial. Eur Neuropsychopharmacol 17(6–7):440–447, 2007 17258897

Wozniak J, Mick E, Waxmonsky J, et al: Comparison of open-label, 8-week trials of olanzapine monotherapy and topiramate augmentation of olanzapine for the treatment of pediatric bipolar disorder. J Child Adolesc Psychopharmacol 19(5):539–545, 2009 19877978

Wozniak J, Faraone SV, Chan J, et al: A randomized clinical trial of high eicosapentaenoic acid omega-3 fatty acids and inositol as monotherapy and in combination in the treatment of pediatric bipolar spectrum disorders: a pilot study. J Clin Psychiatry 76(11):1548–1555, 2015 26646031

11

Longer-Term Management of Mood Disorders in Youth

Rasim Somer Diler, M.D.

Boris Birmaher, M.D.

We start this chapter with a case discussion and then review the risk factors for recurrence and chronicity of unipolar depression, bipolar depression, and mania and the continuation and maintenance treatments to prevent relapses and recurrences of mood episodes. Different studies have defined varying thresholds to report treatment outcomes, but in general, *relapse* indicates a mood episode during the period of remission (no or few mood symptoms and return close to baseline functioning), and *recurrence* indicates the emergence of a mood episode during the period of recovery (absence of significant mood symptoms for more than 2 months) (Birmaher et al. 2007; Diler and Birmaher 2012).

It is important to emphasize that most of the studies reviewed in this chapter involved adolescents because very few studies have been done in children. Also, in this chapter, unless indicated, the word *youth* denotes both children and adolescents.

Case: Recurrent Mood Episodes in Youth With Bipolar Disorder: Long-Term Management Challenges During Follow-Up

John, a 17-year-old male with bipolar I disorder, has been consistently coming to the clinic for the last 6 months for treatment with psychotherapy and the combination of lithium (1,200 mg/day; blood level = 0.8 mEq/L) and risperidone (3 mg/day). He is currently in remission and is not using any recreational drugs. He enjoys bodybuilding and playing guitar with his music band. He wonders how long he needs to take both medications, but his mother is afraid of any changes because she learned that poor adherence to treatment has been associated with mood recurrences.

John was first admitted to a psychiatric hospital 2 years ago with a sudden onset of a manic episode with psychotic features and physical aggression. He responded very well to behavioral interventions combined with risperidone (3 mg/day). However, after he was discharged, he stopped taking the risperidone and engaging in therapy because his father, who also has bipolar disorder, told him that "he needed to act like a man and not use any psychiatric medications." John's father reportedly has a history of good response to lithium, but he refuses to take it.

About 3 months after discontinuing treatment, John had a recurrent episode of mania with psychotic features that required hospitalization. He was started on lithium when he refused risperidone and other second-generation antipsychotics (SGAs) but later agreed to add risperidone when his mood partially improved. However, the symptoms of psychosis persisted. He responded well to the combination of risperidone (3 mg/day) and lithium (1,350 mg/day; blood level=0.9 mEq/L). He continued these medications after discharge with good interepisode recovery and good tolerance, but his adherence to treatment was poor; he failed to take the medications one to three times a week and frequently did not come for therapy. He also started to use marijuana and alcohol a few times a week. Consequently, he had another manic episode with mixed depressive and psychotic symptoms that required hospitalization. He was again quickly stabilized on lithium and risperidone and has been followed up as an outpatient since then. John does not have a history of suicide attempts, self-injurious behaviors, or trauma. Between the second and third hospitalizations, he experienced moderate to severe suicidal ideations, which were accompanied by high levels of anxiety.

Discussion Point: Does John Need One or Two Medications to Prevent Mood Recurrences?

John is a good candidate for long-term lithium treatment because of the following characteristics: no psychiatric history and good premorbid functioning; sudden onset, and the first episode was mania; good interepisode recovery; good response and tolerance to lithium; and family history of positive response to lithium (Berk et al. 2017a; Goldstein et al. 2012). In addition, lithium may help to prevent suicidality, and although evidence is limited, perhaps it can target substance use (Diler and Birmaher 2012; Duffy and Grof 2018; Geller et al. 1998). Thus, lithium can be considered as the primary mood stabilizer for John. Moreover, because he has already had severe manic episodes, he may need long-term maintenance treatment with lithium (as long as he tolerates it and does not develop any medical complications). John and his family were actively included in all decisions regarding his short- and long-term treatment and risk-benefit assessment for medication continuation and changes of dosages or type of medications. If John and his family had demanded to stop medications despite being informed of potential risks, benefits, and alternatives, then the clinician would have needed to work with them to start decreasing the regimen one medication at a time (e.g., risperidone taper before lithium) and one small dose reduction at a time.

Factors suggested that risperidone was indicated for the acute treatment of John's symptomatology. His first manic episode included aggression, and SGAs can show quicker effect than lithium for acute stabilization of a manic episode (Berk et al. 2017a; Diler and Birmaher 2012). In addition, John had psychotic features during his three inpatient admissions, and SGAs are an option to target these symptoms. Considering the limited data about risperidone's effectiveness in preventing future episodes and risk for metabolic side effects, it is advisable to slowly titrate down the risperidone after 6–12 months of mood stability with no psychotic or mixed symptoms and continue with only lithium (Findling et al. 2013b). During this time, John and his family may be educated about "red flags": symptoms that may signal a recurrence. Also, frequent outpatient visits and telephone contacts are recommended.

Clinicians should balance the family's expectations and the youth's autonomy when making long-term treatment decisions and pay attention to the youth's transitional challenges into adulthood. Establishing a therapeutic alliance and providing psychoeducation about early identification of "clinical and subsyndromal" mood symptoms through daily monitoring or charting and about healthy lifestyle approaches (e.g., sleep hygiene, exercise routine, and diet choices) and over-the-counter supplements (e.g., avoiding steroids, considering omega-3) are important for long-term successful maintenance treatment. Medication adherence and comorbid conditions (e.g., substance use and anxiety) also should be the focus of long-term treatment (Diler and Birmaher 2012). Continuation and maintenance treatments for mania (and depression) are detailed in the "Continuation and Maintenance Treatments for Depression and Mania" section later in this chapter.

Risk Factors for Recurrence and Chronicity of Unipolar Depression

Depression is the world's leading cause of morbidity (Lépine and Briley 2011) that usually emerges during adolescence (Thapar et al. 2012). About 20% of adolescents have depression that negatively affects their psychosocial development, school performance, and peer and family relationships (Brent and Birmaher 2006). Furthermore, it significantly increases risks for anxiety, substance use, legal problems, pregnancy, and suicidality, which is the third leading cause of death during adolescence (Brent and Birmaher 2006; Spirito and Esposito-Smythers 2006). Accumulating literature over the past 25 years on identifying etiopathology and improving diagnosis and treatment of depressive disorders in adolescents has suggested that depression is a heterogeneous condition with little evidence about its subtypes and predictors of the outcome (Andersen and Teicher 2008; Emslie et al. 2010; Hamdan et al. 2012; McMakin et al. 2012; Sakolsky and Birmaher 2012; Vitiello et al. 2011). Developmental stage may affect symptom expression and treatment response (e.g., higher placebo response rates and higher suicidality risk with antidepressants in adolescents than in adults) (Sakolsky et al. 2012; Thapar et al. 2012). However, diagnostic criteria for depression in youth are essentially the same as those in adults (i.e., except for irritability in children), and categorical classifications are very limited in informing different etiologies accounting for the different courses and responses to treatment (Aggen et al. 2005; American Psychiatric Association 2000; Thapar et al. 2012). Despite these limitations of categorical approaches, in an attempt to better differentiate chronic depressive presentations, DSM-IV–defined chronic major depressive disorder and dysthymic disorder (lasting for 2 years in adults and 1 year in children) were consolidated into persistent depressive disorder in DSM-5 (American Psychiatric Association 2000, 2013).

Unipolar Depressive Disorders

A significant portion of youth with unipolar depression do not initially respond to pharmacological or psychotherapy interventions, and those who respond still have high risk for relapses and recurrences despite ongoing treatment (Emslie et al. 2010; Maalouf and Brent 2012; Sakolsky and Birmaher 2012; Vitiello et al. 2011). Thus, there has been an increased interest in identifying predictors of recurrence and chronicity of depression that can be used to help clinicians identify these high-risk patients, who might benefit from more intensive treatment (e.g., long-term maintenance treatment).

Twelve-month prevalence of chronic depression was reported as 1.5% for major depression and 0.5% for dysthymia in adults (Blanco et al. 2010), and DSM-5 suggests that there are no clear differences in illness development, course, or family history between DSM-IV dysthymic disorder and chronic major depressive disorder. A recent large community study in adults suggested that 12% of the patients experienced chronic depression over 6 years, and the cumulative recurrence rate for depression in those whose depression remitted was 4.3% at 5 years, 13.4% at 10 years, and 27.1% at 20 years (Ten Have et al. 2018). The same study reported that functioning, clinical characteristics of depression (previous episodes, severity, medication use), psychiatric comorbidity, and mental health use predicted both chronicity and recurrence of depression. In addition, vulnerability characteristics (childhood abuse, negative life events, parental psychopathology) and physical health predicted recurrences. Another large study in adults that used World Mental Health Surveys in 16 countries suggested that early onset, suicidality, severe dysphoria, and anxiety (irritability, panic, nervousness-worry-anxiety) during the index episode of depression predicted both chronicity and recurrences (van Loo et al. 2014).

Studies in youth reported that recovery rates 1 year after treatment onset ranged from 81% to 98%, but recurrence rates ranged from 54% to 60% in 3 years among outpatients and more than 60% in 1 year after inpatient treatment (Emslie et al. 1997; Kovacs 1996). Even effective treatments after remission (e.g., 8 weeks of symptomatic recovery) can be followed by recurrence rates of 30%–40% within 1–2 years, with no treatment yet surpassing others in preventing recurrence, including in the large controlled studies for depression (Birmaher et al. 2000; Curry et al. 2011; Vitiello et al. 2011). The Treatment of (SSRI) Resistant Depression in Adolescents (TORDIA) study suggested that the trajectory of the depressive symptom in the remitters diverged from that in the nonremitters by the first 6 weeks of treatment, suggesting that it may be possible to identify those with chronic course during the early course of the treatment. These studies suggested several predictors of recurrences, including younger age; lower family income; minority ethnicity; severity of depression; longer index episode duration; poorer global functioning; presence of suicidal ideation, hopelessness, melancholic features, and cognitive distortions; comorbid anxiety disorders; comorbid alcohol or substance use; higher number of comorbid disorders; higher parent-child conflict; and lower expectation of improvement (Curry et al. 2011). Interestingly, being overweight or obese was neither a predictor nor a moderator of treatment outcome or of subsequent change in body mass index in the TORDIA study (Mansoor et al. 2013). It is important to consider other studies' contradictory findings that obesity and depression can coexist in youth, which potentially increases treatment resistance (Quek et al. 2017; Schubert et al. 2017), and depression increased risk for the development and persistence of obesity during adolescence (Goodman and Whitaker 2002). These studies suggest the need for careful monitoring of weight (including diet and exercise) in depressed youth.

Subsyndromal Manic Symptoms During Unipolar Depressive Episodes

Identifying subsyndromal manic symptoms in youth with unipolar depression is a challenge but has important clinical significance. Studies have shown that substantial co-occurrence of manic symptoms is found in up to 40% of depressed adults (Angst et al. 2010; Chengappa et al. 2003) and adolescents (Diler et al. 2017b; Scott et al. 2013). Distinguishing manic symptoms that occur within unipolar depression is critical, because this subgroup of nonbipolar depressed individuals with mixed manic symptoms tends to have poorer course and response to available treatments compared with those depressed individuals without manic symptoms (Maalouf et al. 2012; Regeer et al. 2006).

In the DSM-IV classification system, mixed episodes (i.e., equal admixtures of symptoms of mania and depression occurring at the same time) were included as a part of bipolar taxonomy, but the narrow definition was frequently associated with misdiagnosis (Berk et al. 2005) and did not capture the depression spectrum with mixed manic symptoms. Thus, although mania is the hallmark feature of bipolar disorder, recent recommendations in DSM-5 now include an important revision to add "a manic specifier for the depressive disorders" to emphasize the importance of the co-occurrence of subsyndromal manic symptoms in the treatment and course of depressive disorders. However, assessment of manic symptoms in available depression studies has so far not been informative to the field and has been limited to a few screening questions about a manic episode. Consequently, the correlates of a manic presentation in depressed children and adolescents have been largely unexplored.

Furthermore, clinicians need to take into account the developmental progression of subsyndromal manic symptoms: 1) many adolescents experience depression first and before the emergence of mania (Axelson et al. 2011; Chang 2009), 2) the presence of subsyndromal manic symptoms significantly increases the risk for progression to a manic episode (e.g., bipolar) in 1.5 years in 40% of depressed adolescents (Nadkarni and Fristad 2010), and 3) if the mania dimension is ignored or misdiagnosed, then the course of the illness is likely to be recurrent with progressively more severe and refractory episodes of both mania and depression (Geller and Luby 1997). In addition, correct identification of mania is delayed for 7–10 years in the clinics (Bolge et al. 2008; Egeland et al. 2003; Leverich et al. 2007) possibly because of the complexity of ascertainment of mania only with standard clinical instruments (e.g., comorbid conditions and difficulty differentiating normal behavior from aberrant mood in adolescents). This delay may result in many adolescents receiving antidepressant monotherapy during this long hiatus, which may be accompanied by worsening of their mood, impaired psychosocial development, and increased suicidality (Chang 2009). Therefore, improving correct and early identification of manic symptomatology in depressed adolescents is a key goal toward precision medicine (National Research Council of the National Academies 2011) to maximize individual normative developmental capacities (Birmaher and Axelson 2006) and decrease morbidity and mortality risk associated with this co-occurrence.

Risk Factors for Recurrence and Chronicity of Mania and Hypomania

The World Health Organization indicates that bipolar disorder is the sixth leading cause of disability in the world (Gore et al. 2011). Bipolar disorder in youth is increasingly recognized as a significant public health problem that is often associated with impaired family and peer relationships, poor academic performance, high rates of chronic mood symptoms and mixed presentations, psychosis, disruptive behavior disorders, anxiety disorders, substance use disorders, hospitalizations, medical problems (e.g., obesity, thyroid problems, diabetes), and suicide attempts and completions (Diler 2007; Diler and Birmaher 2012). Substantial cumulative research from the United States and abroad is available regarding the phenomenology, differential diagnosis, course, treatment, and neurobiology of mania in children (Diler 2007; Goldstein et al. 2017; Van Meter et al. 2011). Similar to depression, identifying prevalence, associations, and predictors of recurrence and chronicity of mania can help clinicians identify patients who might benefit from more intensive treatment (e.g., more frequent visits to monitor mood symptoms, comorbid conditions, treatment response, and safety); more frequent therapy visits and family involvement to target psychoeducation, coping skills, and adherence; and potentially higher levels of care as necessary (e.g., intensive outpatient treatment, partial hospitalization, or inpatient treatment).

Mania and Hypomania

Studies in adults with bipolar disorder have reported a fluctuating course of illness with about 60% recovery and approximately 48% recurrence during 2-year follow-up (Perlis et al. 2006). In addition, persistent residual depressive or manic symptoms at recovery and proportion of days depressed, manic, or anxious in the preceding year were significantly associated with shorter time to recurrence. Earlier studies in youth suggested high rates of chronicity of manic presentations, such as 14.3% recovery after 6 months (Geller et al. 2000); high rates of rapid cycling (50%) with almost no interepisode recovery (Findling et al. 2001); and only 20% functional recovery in 4 years in those with bipolar disorder and attention-deficit/hyperactivity disorder (ADHD; Biederman et al. 2004). However, it is now agreed that bipolar disorder in youth is characterized by a longitudinal course with recovery and recurrences. These prospective naturalistic studies suggested that 70%–100% of youth with bipolar disorder will recover (e.g., no significant symptoms for 2 months) from their index episode, but up to 80% will experience one or more recurrences in a period of 2–5 years (Birmaher 2007; Birmaher et al. 2009, 2014).

Age at onset has been consistently reported as a significant predictor for persistence of mood symptoms and associated with poor outcome in youth with bipolar disorder. Children with prepubertal-onset bipolar disorder are reported as approximately two times less likely to recover than those with postpubertal-onset bipolar disorder. In addition, patients with prepubertal-onset bipolar disorder had more chronic symptoms, spent more follow-up time with subsyndromal mood symptoms, and had more polarity changes per year than postpubertal-onset bipolar patients (Birmaher et al. 2009; Diler 2007). In addition to early age at onset, index episode of depression instead of mania, mixed or rapid-cycling episodes, long duration of mood symptoms, psychosis, subsyndromal mood symptoms, comorbid disorders, exposure to negative life events, high expressed emotion, low socioeconomic status, and family psychopathology were associated with worse course and outcome, despite the treatment (Birmaher et al. 2009, 2014; DelBello et al. 2007; Diler and Birmaher 2012; Geller et al. 2008; Strober et al. 1995). It is important to take into account that the impairment in psychosocial functioning reported in available studies was not specific to the clinical samples or treatment, because similar findings have been reported in bipolar adolescents never referred for treatment (Lewinsohn et al. 2000).

Focusing on only episodic recovery and recurrences may not give the broader perspective of chronicity of bipolar disorder in youth because of significant subthreshold symptomatology that affects functioning during the course of the illness (Birmaher et al. 2009; DelBello et al. 2007; Geller et al. 2008). Bipolar youth have been reported to have syndromal and subsyndromal bipolar symptoms, particularly depressive and mixed symptoms in about 60% of the follow-up time and within each episode, and youth manifest more fluctuations in mood than do adults with bipolar disorder (Birmaher et al. 2009). In a recent study, Birmaher et al. (2014) used latent class growth analyses to evaluate a more individualized course during a 9-year period and identified four longitudinal mood trajectories: 1) "predominantly euthymic" course (24.0%), 2) "moderately euthymic" course (34.6%), 3) "ill with improving course" (19.1%), and 4) "predominantly ill" course (22.3%). Within each group, youth were euthymic on average 84.4%, 47.3%, 42.8%, and 11.5% of the follow-up time, respectively. Better course was associated with older age at onset of mood symptoms, less lifetime family history of bipolar disorder and substance abuse, and less history at baseline of severe depression, manic symptoms, suicidality, subsyndromal mood episodes, and sexual abuse (Birmaher et al. 2014). Continued syndromal and subsyndromal mood symptoms in all four classes underscore the need to optimize treatment. Treatment optimization is described in the "Improving Treatment Adherence During Long-Term Treatment (Unipolar Depression and Bipolar Mania or Hypomania and Bipolar Depression)" section later in this chapter and includes tailoring the medication and therapy interventions to the youths' and families' long-term expectations, clinical progression, and functioning (e.g., using SGAs for acute intervention and maximizing the first medication to tolerated dose to determine the full efficacy of the medication in the presence of ongoing symptoms before adding a second medication).

Subsyndromal Mania or Hypomania (Bipolar Disorder Not Otherwise Specified) and Developmental Progression

It is important to pay attention to subsyndromal presentation and developmental progression, because they can help guide clinicians about potential "chronicity of these mood symptoms" and other nonspecific clinical presentations. Studies suggest that nonspecific sleep and anxiety problems (Duffy et al. 2010) and a relatively long, predominantly slow-onset mania prodrome, including subthreshold manic and depressive symptoms, appear to be common before the onset of a manic episode (Correll et al. 2014). A large proportion of youth have presentations that do not fulfill the criteria for a manic or hypomanic episode because the duration requirement of 7 days for mania or 4 days for hypomania noted in DSM-IV and DSM-5 is not met (Axelson et al. 2006). These youth with significant manic symptoms that are clustering and episodic usually receive a DSM-IV diagnosis of bipolar disorder not otherwise specified or DSM-5 other specified or unspecified bipolar and related disorder. These subsyndromal youth with bipolar disorder not otherwise specified were phenomenologically in continuum with youth with bipolar I disorder (e.g., similar psychosocial impairment, risk to develop substance abuse and suicidal behaviors, rates of comorbid disorders, and family history for mood disorders); however, they were younger, had a more chronic illness course, were irritable, and had mixed presentations with less euphoric mania as compared with bipolar I disorder (Axelson et al. 2011; Birmaher et al. 2009; Hirneth et al. 2015). Further, about 50% of the youth diagnosed with other specified bipolar and related disorder converted into bipolar I or II disorder when followed up prospectively for approximately 5 years (Axelson et al. 2011). The main predictor of conversion was the presence of a family history of mania in first- or second-degree relatives. In a different study, those offspring of bipolar parents with mood lability, depression or anxiety, subsyndromal manic symptoms, and early-onset parental bipolar disorder were at 50% risk to develop bipolar disorder (Hafeman et al. 2016).

Depression in Youth With and at Risk for Bipolar Disorder

Retrospective studies in adults have reported that as many as 60% experienced the onset of their bipolar disorder before age 20 years, and 10%–20% reported onset before age 10 years (Pavuluri et al. 2005). Depression in youth has a high risk (20%–40%) for switching into bipolar disorder (Pavuluri et al. 2005). Similar to children, studies in adults reported that bipolar depression was less recognized and treated than manic episodes despite the findings that depressive episodes and symptoms dominated the longitudinal course of bipolar disorder and that most suicide-related behaviors occurred during depression (Judd and Akiskal 2003; Thase 2005). Moreover, bipolar depressive episodes in adults have been reported to be more frequent, longer in duration, and less responsive to standard therapies than mania (Thase 2006), and psychosocial impairment has been more strongly predicted by the number of past depressive episodes than by the number of past manias (MacQueen et al. 2000). It has been reported that children with bipolar depression were more likely to have severe depression with suicidality, anhedonia, and hopelessness and had higher rates of comorbid disruptive behavior, anxiety, and substance use disorders compared with children with unipolar depression (Wozniak et al. 2004). Bipolar depressed youth also had lower Global Assessment of Functioning Scale scores and higher rates of hospitalization and psychiatric disorders in first-degree relatives (Wozniak et al. 2004). Adolescents with bipolar depression reported more suicidal behavior (e.g., 60% in bipolar vs. 30% in unipolar major depression) and higher levels of impairment compared with adolescents with other depressive disorders (Karlsson et al. 2007). In addition, depressed youth with bipolar disorder had significantly higher scores in several depressive symptoms and all subsyndromal manic symptoms (with the exception of increased goal-directed activity) compared with youth with unipolar depression as recorded on depression and mania rating scales derived from the Schedule for Affective Disorders and Schizophrenia for Children—Present Version (Axelson et al. 2003; Kaufman et al. 1997) (Diler et al. 2017b). Even the presence of high-risk status for bipolar disorder (without an experience of manic episodes) has indicated differences in mood symptomatology and recurrences: depressed offspring of bipolar parents compared with depressed control patients had a higher number of past depressive episodes; more severe depressive symptoms; a higher percentage of offspring with severe depressive symptoms, especially atypical depressive features; and presence of subsyndromal manic symptoms (Diler et al. 2017a).

Continuation and Maintenance Treatments for Depression and Mania

Clinical Considerations

Available evidence in consensus guidelines varies for long-term management of mood disorders (Parker et al. 2017). Management of mood disorders is strongly informed by the adult literature; however, it is important to note that not all treatments that seem to work or are well tolerated in adults are appropriate for treatment in youth.

During the continuation phase of treatment, which starts soon after the acute treatment of depression, mania, or hypomania to prevent relapse, clinicians usually continue the effective treatment interventions—unless side effects occur—that helped the acute mood episode. After the acute treatment of a mood episode, the clinician should focus on treating the syndromal or subsyndromal mood symptoms, because these symptoms increase the risk for relapse. Treatment also should target other potential comorbid conditions such as ADHD, anxiety disorders, posttraumatic stress disorder, substance use, and sleep disorders to prevent future mood episodes. The clinician should work with the youth and the family to further improve treatment response during the continuation phase (e.g., adding or strengthening therapy approaches and targeting subsyndromal presentations, emphasizing medication adherence, and encouraging healthy lifestyle changes such as good sleep hygiene, exercise, and proper nutrition, and meditation/

yoga) and prepare them for the subsequent maintenance treatment phase that focuses on the prevention of recurrence. Psychotherapy and ongoing psychoeducation sessions should be a part of all long-term interventions for depression and mania.

The optimal duration of psychosocial treatment for pediatric mood disorders has not been established; however, continuing psychosocial interventions for subthreshold symptoms may be helpful beyond acute and continuation phases (Gruber et al. 2011; Miklowitz et al. 2011). It is important to continuously assess the risk of suicide at any phase of treatment, including medication overdose, whether accidental or purposeful. It is reasonable to provide crisis management and booster therapy sessions as appropriate.

Unipolar Depressive Disorders

Overview of Findings

Findings in depression suggested that relapse and recurrences are very common despite ongoing treatment. However, no treatment has shown superiority in preventing recurrence of depression, including in comparisons of two types of psychotherapies (e.g., cognitive-behavioral therapy [CBT], systemic behavioral family therapy, or nondirective supportive therapy), psychotherapy versus medication (fluoxetine, CBT, fluoxetine + CBT, or placebo), and two medications (SSRI vs. serotonin-norepinephrine reuptake inhibitor) (Birmaher et al. 2000; Curry et al. 2011; Vitiello et al. 2011).

Fluoxetine and escitalopram have been shown to be superior to placebo in acute treatment and to be successful in preventing relapses in youth (ages 8–17 years in fluoxetine studies and 12–17 years in escitalopram study) (Emslie et al. 2004, 2008; Findling et al. 2013c). Specifically, in a small 51-week double-blind, multicenter, placebo-controlled fluoxetine study, patients were assigned to continue fluoxetine or switch to placebo for the 32-week relapse-prevention phase (Emslie et al. 2004) (Table 11–1). Relapse occurred in 34% of the fluoxetine group and 60% of the placebo group, and mean time to relapse was significantly longer in the fluoxetine group. In a larger randomized fluoxetine study of 6 months' duration, patients who had an adequate response after 12 weeks with fluoxetine were randomly assigned to receive fluoxetine or placebo, and significantly fewer youth (42%) in the fluoxetine group relapsed compared with those (69%) in the placebo group, and time to relapse was significantly shorter in the placebo group after 6 months (Emslie et al. 2008). One participant in the fluoxetine group was withdrawn after a suicide attempt.

The same authors conducted a follow-up study in depressed youth who responded to fluoxetine for 6 weeks and were later randomly assigned to receive medication management or CBT+medication management for 6 months (Emslie et al. 2015). Although no differences were seen in time to remission between medication and medication+therapy groups (14.3 weeks vs. 18.3 weeks), the medication management group compared with the combination treatment group had a significantly higher risk of relapse throughout the 78-week follow-up period (estimated probability of remission was 96% vs. 92%). In the extension escitalopram study, remission rates were 50.6% for escitalopram and 35.7% for placebo at week 24; although escitalopram responders continued to improve modestly over 24 weeks of treatment, placebo responders did not continue to improve (Findling et al. 2013c). Adverse effects suggestive of self-harm occurred in 5.7% and 7.1% of placebo and escitalopram patients, respectively, and occurrence of suicidal behavior and/or ideation was 10.9% for placebo and 14.5% for escitalopram.

A few large studies have compared different treatment interventions and provided important information about the maintenance treatment of pediatric depression. In the TORDIA study, 334 youth, ages 12–18 years, with major depressive disorder who had failed to respond to an adequate course of SSRI medication were randomly assigned to receive either an alternative SSRI or venlafaxine with or without 12 weeks of adjunctive CBT (Brent et al. 2008; Vitiello et al. 2011). After 12 weeks, the response rate was superior in those who received CBT and either medication (54.8%) compared with those who received a medication alone (40.5%), but there were no differences between the two medication strategies. The cumulative remission rate was 38.9% by 24 weeks, and the strongest predictors of lack of remission were lower rate of response during the first 6 weeks, a diagnosis of dysthymia, high baseline depression, family conflict, and higher drug and alcohol use at the end of acute treatment (Emslie et al. 2010). Among nonresponders, by 12 weeks, subsequent remission was predicted by having received, during the first 12 weeks, either an augmentation of antidepressant treatment with a mood stabilizer or the addition of psychotherapy. By 72 weeks, an estimated 61.1% of the youth had reached remission. Randomly assigned treatment (first 12 weeks) did not influence remission rate or time to remission, but the group assigned to SSRIs had a more rapid decline in self-reported depressive symptoms and suicidal ideation than did those assigned to venlafaxine (Vitiello et al. 2011).

A secondary analysis of TORDIA data with latent class growth analysis used depression scores through 72 weeks from intake to identify three classes: 1) little change in symptomatic status: 24.9% of participants, with

TABLE 11–1. Randomized studies and longitudinal treatment of major depressive disorder and bipolar disorders in youth

Treatment (Study)	Design	Sample	Main outcomes
Fluoxetine (Emslie et al. 2004)	51-week double-blind, multicenter, placebo-controlled fluoxetine study	8- to 17-year-old youth ($N=40$) with major depressive disorder. Patients continued fluoxetine or switched to placebo for the 32-week relapse-prevention phase	Relapse rates: 34% in the fluoxetine vs. 60% in the placebo group. Time to relapse was significantly longer in the fluoxetine group
Fluoxetine (Emslie et al. 2008)	6-month randomized fluoxetine study	8- to 17-year-old youth ($N=102$) with major depressive disorder. Patients who had an adequate response after 12 weeks with fluoxetine were randomly assigned to fluoxetine or placebo	Relapse rates: 42% in the fluoxetine vs. 69% in the placebo group. Time to relapse was significantly longer in the fluoxetine group
Fluoxetine (Emslie et al. 2015)	6-month randomized study involving fluoxetine or CBT+fluoxetine; long-term follow-up assessments at weeks 52 and 78	8- to 17-year-old youth ($N=96$) with major depressive disorder. Patients who had an adequate response after 6 weeks of fluoxetine were randomized.	Relapse rates: 62% for fluoxetine vs. 36% for combination treatment. Most had experienced remission during the 30-week treatment period, and only six additional patients achieved remission during the long-term follow-up. No differences in time to remission between medication and medication+therapy groups

TABLE 11–1. Randomized studies and longitudinal treatment of major depressive disorder and bipolar disorders in youth (*continued*)

Treatment (Study)	Design	Sample	Main outcomes
Escitalopram (Findling et al. 2013c)	16- to 24-week multisite extension trial of randomized escitalopram	12- to 17-year-old youth (*N*=157) with major depressive disorder Patients maintained the same lead-in randomization after 8 weeks of the acute trial (escitalopram or placebo) and dosage	Remission rates: 50.6% for escitalopram vs. 35.7% for placebo
SSRI vs. venlafaxine with or without CBT Treatment of (SSRI) Resistant Depression in Adolescents study (TORDIA; Maalouf et al. 2012; Vitiello et al. 2011)	72-week follow-up study after patients randomly assigned to receive either an alternative SSRI or venlafaxine with or without 12 weeks of adjunctive CBT	12- to 18-year-old youth with major depressive disorder (*N*=334) who had failed to respond to an adequate course of an SSRI	Remission rate: 61.1%, but as-signed treatment (during the first 12 weeks) did not influence re-mission rate or time to remission The group assigned to SSRIs (vs. venlafaxine) had a more rapid decline in self-reported depressive symptoms and suicidal ideation Three trajectories identified: 1) 24.9% with little change in symptomatic status; 2) 47.9% with slow, steady improvement; and 3) 27.2% with rapid symptom response

TABLE 11–1. Randomized studies and longitudinal treatment of major depressive disorder and bipolar disorders in youth (*continued*)

Treatment (Study)	Design	Sample	Main outcomes
Fluoxetine, CBT, or combination Treatment for Adolescents with Depression Study (TADS) (Curry et al. 2011)	5-year longitudinal follow-up in open phase after the acute treatment comparing fluoxetine, CBT, combination treatment (CBT + fluoxetine), and placebo	12- to 17-year-old youth (*N*=196) with major depressive disorder	96.4% recovered from their index depressive episode 46.6% recurrence after remission Acute treatment response and initial combination treatment were not associated with recurrences
Lithium vs. divalproex (Findling et al. 2005)	76-week double-blind study with lithium vs. DVPX monotherapy	5- to 17-year-old youth (*N*=60) with bipolar I or II disorder Patients whose symptoms had previously remitted during combination treatment with lithium and DVPX were randomly assigned to monotherapy with either medication	Lithium and DVPX treatment groups did not differ in survival time until emerging symptoms of relapse or until discontinuation for any reason

TABLE 11–1. Randomized studies and longitudinal treatment of major depressive disorder and bipolar disorders in youth (*continued*)

Treatment (Study)	Design	Sample	Main outcomes
Aripiprazole (Findling et al. 2013a)	26-week double-blind extension study with aripiprazole	10- to 17-year-old youth (*N*=296) with bipolar I disorder (manic or mixed) Patients who completed the 4-week acute phase participated in the extension phase	Response rates: 58.7% in aripiprazole 10-mg group vs. 64.8% in aripiprazole 30-mg group vs. 29.7% in placebo group Greater improvements in global functioning and greater reductions in bipolar severity for aripiprazole groups vs. placebo
Aripiprazole (Findling et al. 2012)	72-week double-blind efficacy study	4- to 9-year-old children (*N*=60) with bipolar spectrum disorders (bipolar I or II disorder and not otherwise specified or cyclothymia) Patients whose symptoms remitted during the 16 weeks of open-label treatment with aripiprazole participated in the long-term study	Relapse: median 6.14 weeks for aripiprazole vs. median 2.29 weeks for placebo groups

TABLE 11–1. Randomized studies and longitudinal treatment of major depressive disorder and bipolar disorders in youth (*continued*)

Treatment (Study)	Design	Sample	Main outcomes
Asenapine (Findling et al. 2016)	50-week longitudinal extension study after 3-week randomized placebo-controlled trial	10- to 17-year-old youth (*N*=321) with bipolar I disorder (manic or mixed) Patients who completed the acute treatment phase (asenapine vs. placebo) were given asenapine during the extension phase	Response rate: 79.2% Relapse rate: 31.1% Mean change in manic symptoms was significantly better at week 50 in the placebo/asenapine group (placebo during the first 3 weeks and asenapine during maintenance) vs. the asenapine/ asenapine group (asenapine during the first 3 weeks and maintenance)
Lithium vs. quetiapine (Berk et al. 2017b)	12-month randomized extension study of lithium vs. quetiapine	15- to 25-year-old individuals with a first manic episode (with bipolar I disorder, *n*=37) and schizoaffective disorder (*n*=2) Patients who were stabilized for 2–3 months after their first manic episode were randomly assigned to lithium or quetiapine monotherapy	Lithium was superior to quetiapine in slowing the progression of white-matter volume reduction after 12 months

TABLE 11–1. Randomized studies and longitudinal treatment of major depressive disorder and bipolar disorders in youth (*continued*)

Treatment (Study)	Design	Sample	Main outcomes
Lurasidone (DelBello et al. 2018)	2-year open-label extension study to continue lurasidone after the placebo-controlled, randomized trial	10- to 17-year-old youth (*N*=347) with acute depressive episode of bipolar I disorder Patients who completed the 6-week acute randomized study of bipolar I depression were continued on lurasidone in a 2-year open-label extension study	Remission rates: 45.7% at week 12, 57.8% at week 28, and 71.6% at week 52

Note. CBT=cognitive-behavioral therapy; DVPX=divalproex.

a 72-week remission rate of 25.3%; 2) slow, steady improvement: 47.9% of participants, with a remission rate of 60.0%; and 3) rapid symptom response: 27.2% of participants, with a remission rate of 85.7%. Higher baseline depression scores and mania scores were the strongest discriminators between slow and rapid responders. In addition, better baseline functioning, lower hopelessness, and lower family conflict and low manic symptoms during follow-up separated rapid responders from the other two groups (Maalouf et al. 2012).

In the Treatment for Adolescents with Depression Study (TADS), the combination treatment (fluoxetine+CBT) was the most efficacious acute treatment compared with fluoxetine, CBT, and a placebo condition (March et al. 2004). Participants were followed up in open phase after the acute treatment. Combination treatment was effective in inducing remission, achieving functional recovery, and reducing suicidal ideation during the acute phase, and early results during follow-up also favored combination treatment for better remission rates (e.g., remission rates of 48% in those who were initially randomly assigned to receive placebo vs. 55%–60% in those who were initially randomly assigned to receive fluoxetine and combination treatments at 9 months) (Kennard et al. 2009b). Although most youth did significantly improve, after 9 months of treatment, 40% of the TADS sample remained symptomatic. In addition, the results from 5-year follow-up indicated 46.6% recurrence after remission (more in females than in males) and failed to confirm that acute treatment response or initial combination treatment predicted recurrences (Curry et al. 2011).

In summary, relapse and recurrences are very common despite ongoing treatment, but SSRIs compared with placebo were helpful in preventing and delaying relapses (Emslie et al. 2004, 2008; Findling et al. 2013c). Combining therapy with medication intervention provided promising results in regard to achieving remission and preventing relapses (Kennard et al. 2009b; Vitiello et al. 2011); however, randomly assigned treatment interventions (medication vs. medication, therapy vs. therapy, therapy vs. medication) did not differ in long-term remission rates.

Considerations for Combination Therapy and Safety During Long-Term Treatment of Unipolar Depression

Treatment should correspond to the level of depression, patient and family preferences, the developmental level of the patient, availability of services, and associated risk factors including safety concerns (e.g., black box warning about antidepressants and suicide risk in youth and young adults) (Clark et al. 2012). Patient and family education about the associated risks and benefits of treatment options, expectations regarding patient monitoring, and follow-up should be provided before acute and maintenance treatment.

In TADS, suicidal ideation decreased in all four treatment groups during the first 12 weeks but less so in the fluoxetine group than in the combination or CBT group (March et al. 2004). After 36 weeks of treatment, no difference was seen in improvement among treatments, but more suicidal events occurred in the medication-only group than in the CBT-only group (Vitiello et al. 2009). Investigators suggested that adding CBT to medication enhanced the safety of fluoxetine; however, others argued against this additional safety effect of CBT during the acute phase of the treatment in TADS (Apter et al. 2005). Most suicidal events in TADS occurred in the context of persistent depression and insufficient improvement, without evidence of medication-induced behavioral activation as a precursor and with no difference in event timing (from 0.4 to 31.1 weeks) for patients receiving medication and those not receiving medication. Severity of self-rated suicidal ideation and depressive symptoms predicted emergence of suicidality during treatment, suggesting the need to carefully monitor suicidality during follow-up (Vitiello et al. 2009).

By contrast, the Adolescent Depression and Psychotherapy study from the United Kingdom reported no differences between community treatment arms in terms of symptom reduction, remission, or incidence of suicidal behavior in patients who received combination (medication+therapy) treatment compared with patients who received medication only (CBT for an additional 16 weeks in addition to their SSRIs vs. those who continued taking SSRIs after 12 weeks of acute treatment) (Goodyer et al. 2007).

In the TORDIA study, the number of therapy sessions and the key components of the therapy were reported as important variables associated with treatment response. Secondary analyses of TORDIA suggested that participants who had more than nine CBT sessions were 2.5 times more likely to have adequate treatment response than were those who had nine or fewer sessions. CBT participants who received problem-solving and social skills treatment components, after the study authors controlled for number of sessions and other confounding variables, were 2.3 and 2.6 times, respectively, more likely to have a positive response (Kennard et al. 2009a). The TORDIA study also suggested overall decline in suicidal ideation throughout the 72-week study, but four subjects attempted suicide during a 48-week period, and those taking venlafaxine compared with SSRIs had higher suicide scores, which all suggests the need for careful long-term monitoring for the risk of suicide in youth with depression (Vitiello et al. 2011).

In summary, although medication-only treatment intervention can be a cost-effective option (Yu et al. 2010), there is no unequivocal support for the superiority of combination treatment. Specifically, in two large controlled trials, TADS and TORDIA, combination treatments had more favorable risk-benefit balance than monotherapy in adolescent depression (Vitiello 2009). It remains to be determined by the treating clinician for which individuals and in which clinical settings these combination treatments are most advantageous.

Bipolar Disorders

Relatively fewer studies have examined continuation and maintenance treatment of bipolar disorder in youth compared with the treatment of unipolar depression, and the data regarding treatment beyond 12 months' duration are especially sparse (Goldstein et al. 2012). Similar to the studies in unipolar depression, available findings in mania suggest that relapse and recurrences (mania or hypomania and depression) are very common despite ongoing treatment (Birmaher et al. 2009; Diler and Birmaher 2012). The Course and Outcome of Bipolar Youth study reported that across all bipolar subtypes during naturalistic follow-up, most syndromal recurrences after the index episode were major depressive episodes (59.5%), followed by hypomanic (20.9%), manic (14.8%), and mixed (4.8%) episodes (Birmaher et al. 2009). However, most treatment studies did not identify differences about relapses and recurrences specific to mania versus depression, and few studies have focused on long-term management of depression in youth with bipolar disorder.

Mania or Hypomania

As for preventing recurrence of mood episodes of bipolar disorder, mood stabilizers such as lithium have been recommended, especially with more pronounced effectiveness after 6 months compared with SGA medications after acute mood stabilization (Berk et al. 2017a; Diler 2007; Duffy and Grof 2018; Parker et al. 2017; Yatham et al. 2016). The relapse rate of mood episodes among patients who discontinued lithium after hospitalization was three times greater than in those who remained adherent with lithium throughout the 18 months (92.3% vs. 37.5%; Strober et al. 1990). Another study randomly assigned 60 youth with bipolar I or II disorder whose symptoms had previously remitted during combination treatment with lithium and divalproex to receive monotherapy with either medication. Treatment proceeded in double-blind fashion for up to 76 weeks. The study authors found a similar survival time to recurrence among those randomly assigned to receive continuation treatment with lithium and those randomly assigned to receive divalproex (114 ± 57 days for lithium and 112 ± 56 days for divalproex) (Findling et al. 2005). In this study, only 10% of the participants remained in each arm at the end of 18 months, and exit reason was mainly lack of efficacy.

In a continuation study, youth with bipolar disorder were maintained on divalproex extended-release following a manic or mixed episode, and mania scores showed a further 12.4-point decrease during the follow-up period (Redden et al. 2009). In a small chart review of youth with bipolar disorder who received divalproex naturalistically for 1.4 ± 1.5 years, 53% were responders, but one-third discontinued the medication because of a side effect such as weight gain (Henry et al. 2003).

Studies in adults suggested that the same effective SGA should be continued after acute treatment, but few long-term studies of SGAs in youth are available (Parker et al. 2017). After a 4-week placebo-controlled acute phase of treatment for mixed or manic episodes with aripiprazole 10 or 30 mg, the study followed up participants for 26 weeks under double-blind conditions (Findling et al. 2013a) (Table 11–1). Greater reductions in manic symptoms were reported for both doses, and time to all-cause discontinuation was longer for both aripiprazole dosages compared with placebo. In addition, aripiprazole 10 mg (58.7%) and 30 mg (64.8%) resulted in significantly greater response rates than for placebo (29.7%) at week 30. Greater improvements in global functioning and greater reductions in clinical global impression bipolar severity also were seen for each of the aripiprazole groups compared with placebo. It is important to note that 32.4% of the participants completed this study.

In another placebo-controlled aripiprazole continuation study, younger children, ages 4–9 years, with bipolar spectrum disorders (bipolar I or II disorder, bipolar disorder not otherwise specified, or cyclothymia) who had responded to open-label treatment with aripiprazole were followed up for 72 weeks (Findling et al. 2012). The study was constrained by high dropout rates within the first 4 weeks (50% and 90% for medication and placebo groups, respectively), but the mean retention duration was 25.9 weeks for aripiprazole and 3 weeks for placebo. Time until discontinuation as a result of a mood event significantly differed between treatment groups (aripiprazole: mean 25.93 ± 5.81 weeks vs. placebo: mean 3.10 ± 0.58 weeks).

A 50-week open-label, flexible-dose asenapine extension study of youth with bipolar I disorder reported improved manic scores at the end of the follow-up (Findling et al. 2016). There were means of 3.2-, 5.3-, and 6.2-point reductions in manic scores for asenapine 2.5-, 5-, and 10-mg twice-daily doses, respectively, at week 3, with response rates of 42%–54%; whereas a mean 9.2-point reduction with 79.2% response rate was found at week 50.

A recent randomized controlled trial reported about maintenance treatment in 15- to 25-year-old patients with bipolar disorder who were stabilized on lithium and quetiapine combination treatment after the first manic episode and then randomly assigned to receive lithium or quetiapine for 12 months (Berk et al. 2017a). Worsening on quetiapine occurred after 6 months, and mood, psychosis, functional outcomes, and quality-of-life measures were better with lithium (0.6–0.8 mEq/L) than with quetiapine (mean dose, 447 mg/day). Furthermore, compared with baseline, lithium was more effective than quetiapine in slowing the progression of white-matter volume reduction after 12 months, suggesting a neuroprotective effect after the first manic episode (Berk et al. 2017b).

Bipolar Depression

Treatment guidelines for bipolar disorder in children and adolescents, much as for BD in adults, discourage antidepressant monotherapy trials in bipolar children and suggest that SSRIs or bupropion may be considered after mood stabilizers (Kowatch et al. 2005) and can be slowly tapered down after the depression remits. In those depressed youth with subsyndromal manic symptoms, treatment response to interventions and potential risk of emergence of mania should be carefully and frequently monitored.

Studies in adults suggested that lamotrigine was successful in preventing depressive episodes in bipolar disorder (Goldstein et al. 2012; Parker et al. 2017). In a 14-weeks open lamotrigine continuation study in youth with mania or hypomania, lamotrigine was slowly titrated to a therapeutic dose over an 8-week period, during which acute symptoms were stabilized with SGAs, followed by a 6-week lamotrigine monotherapy phase (Pavuluri et al. 2009). The remission rate was 56% at 14 weeks, and depressive symptoms were further reduced during the lamotrigine maintenance phase. Among patients who were in remission at 8 weeks, about 23% had relapsed by the end of 14 weeks. Another recent large study of youth with bipolar I disorder randomly assigned participants to lamotrigine or placebo for 36 weeks after acute mood stabilization of at least 6 weeks with combination medication (Findling et al. 2015). The continuation with lamotrigine was superior to placebo in 13- to 17-year–old patients but not in 10- to 12-year-old patients (hazard ratio=0.46 vs. 0.94), but the main analysis did not show significant difference.

Randomized, placebo-controlled studies with olanzapine-fluoxetine combination and lurasidone suggest that these treatments are effective in bipolar I youth with acute depressive episode (DelBello et al. 2017; Detke et al. 2015). However, their long-term use is limited because of potential side effects (e.g., metabolic syndrome) and poor long-term adherence (Brown et al. 2009; Miller et al. 2018), and limited data are available about the long-term effectiveness of SGAs in youth. A recent extension study suggested that lurasidone can be an option in maintenance treatment of bipolar I disorder in youth ages 10–17 years after treatment of an acute depression (DelBello et al. 2018). In this study, 95 of the 155 bipolar I patients who had finished 12 weeks of acute depression treatment with lurasidone were followed up in the extension phase, and mean changes in depression scores at weeks 12, 28, and 52 were −6.2, −10.0, and −10.7, respectively. In addition, remission rates at weeks 12, 28, and 52 were 45.7%, 57.8%, and 71.6%, respectively (DelBello et al. 2018). More studies are needed of monotherapy and adjunct maintenance treatment with lurasidone in youth with bipolar II disorder and other specified bipolar and related disorder.

Finally, an open-label continuation study in youth with bipolar I disorder suggested that medication combinations can help after trying monotherapy first (Kowatch et al. 2003). In this study, 35 young participants (mean age, 11 years), who received 6–8 weeks of acute treatment with a single mood stabilizer (lithium, divalproex, or carbamazepine), received treatment in the extension phase of this open study for 16 weeks. Eighteen responders continued to be responders, whereas 12 of 17 nonresponders later responded to the combination treatment at the end of the trial (Kowatch et al. 2003). Twenty of 35 participants (57%) required treatment with one or two mood stabilizers and either a stimulant, an SGA, or an antidepressant agent. The response rate to combination therapy was very good, with 80% of patients responding to combination therapy with two mood stabilizers after not responding to monotherapy with a mood stabilizer. Two patients required the addition of an antidepressant agent for an episode of major depression. In both cases, an SSRI was added to the single mood stabilizer that the patient was taking (lithium in one patient and divalproex in the other), with a good antidepressant response. The low rate of major depression in this study may have been the result of aggressive treatment with one or two mood stabilizers in all of these patients (Kowatch et al. 2003).

Considerations for Combination Therapy in Bipolar Disorders (Mania or Hypomania and Depression)

Medication-only interventions may be cost-effective, but a combination of psychotherapy and medication may have a more favorable risk-benefit balance than monotherapy, not only for adolescent depression (cognitive-behavioral and interpersonal therapies) but also for youth with and at risk for bipolar disorder (e.g., family-focused therapy [FFT], dialectical behavior therapy [DBT], and interpersonal and social rhythm therapy) (Goldstein et al. 2015, 2018; Miklowitz et al. 2011). During 2-year follow-up, those youth with bipolar disorder who received FFT recovered from their baseline depressive symptoms faster than did control patients, spent fewer weeks in depressive episodes, and had a more favorable trajectory of depression symptoms (Miklowitz et al. 2008). Similarly, adolescents with bipolar disorder receiving DBT had significantly less severe depressive symptoms over 1-year follow-up (Goldstein et al. 2015). Furthermore, in the same study, the DBT group was nearly three times more likely than the control group to show improvement in suicidal ideation. In addition, psychotherapy studies with FFT and interpersonal and social rhythm therapy provide promising results for preventing mood episodes in those at familial risk for developing bipolar disorder (Goldstein et al. 2018; Miklowitz et al. 2017). It remains to be determined by the treating clinician for which individuals and in which clinical settings combination therapy may be most advantageous.

Duration of Bipolar Depression and Mania Treatment

The duration of treatment usually depends on the length and severity of the illness, exposure to stress, the disorders that underlie the severe mood swings, the availability of psychosocial interventions at home and at school, parental psychopathology, social supports, and other family and social conditions (Diler and Birmaher 2012). Although treatment of a depressive episode with antidepressants may continue for 6–12 months after symptomatic recovery, bipolar disorder is generally considered a lifelong illness, and as a consequence, the medications should not be discontinued soon after remission. However, because some bipolar youth have a predominantly euthymic course (Birmaher et al. 2014), clinicians should consider slowly tapering the medications after 12–24 months of the euthymic period, especially if it was a first episode, mild, or short-lived or if the diagnosis of bipolar disorder was questionable. If the child is taking more than one medication, only one medication should be tapered at a time, starting with any medications that could be causing any side effects for the child (e.g., metabolic symptoms with SGAs) or do not seem to be helping.

Limited evidence is available for discontinuation of mood stabilizer treatment in youth. In a discontinuation study with lithium, 40 bipolar adolescents received open treatment with lithium at therapeutic serum levels (0.99 mEq/L) for at least 4 weeks and then responders were randomly assigned to continue or to discontinue lithium during a 2-week double-blind, placebo-controlled phase (Kafantaris et al. 2004). Mean depression scores (58.9% change) and suicide item endorsement declined (95.6% change) significantly at the end of the open lithium treatment. The slightly lower exacerbation rate in the group maintained on lithium (52.6%) compared with the group switched to placebo (61.9%) did not reach statistical significance; however, lithium was discontinued over the course of 3 days, and investigators suggested that a 2-week treatment would not be long enough to demonstrate drug-placebo difference in maintenance treatment (DelBello and Kowatch 2006).

A recent discontinuation study in adults did not find any benefit of continuing risperidone or olanzapine after 6 months of treatment when these SGA medications were combined with lithium or divalproex during maintenance treatment (Yatham et al. 2016). If the symptoms recur, the youth's situation should be reassessed, because the relapse or recurrence may not be a result of the lack of medication but a result of other causes such as medication nonadherence, substance use, adverse life event, or worsening or emergence of comorbid psychiatric (e.g., ADHD or anxiety) or medical conditions (Diler and Birmaher 2012; Goldstein et al. 2012). For cases in which the depressive or manic episode was severe or long and in cases in which the youth had three or more episodes of mania, long-term or even lifelong treatment may be warranted. In this case, as with other chronic illnesses such as epilepsy or diabetes, psychotherapeutic approaches may be beneficial in helping the youth and family gain acceptance of the concept of chronic disease management (Diler and Birmaher 2012; Miklowitz 2016; Miklowitz and Chung 2016).

Improving Treatment Adherence During Long-Term Treatment (Unipolar Depression and Bipolar Mania or Hypomania and Bipolar Depression)

Several factors need to be considered before concluding that a condition is "resistant" to treatment. Some factors include whether the current diagnosis is correct, whether the pharmacological treatment for the diagnosis was the most appropriate, whether the medications were administered for a sufficient length of time, and whether the youth was adherent to the treatment (Diler and Birmaher 2012). Nonadherence in youth with depression and mania is very common, and a recent study in youth with bipolar disorders reported that 41.5% of the doses (58.6% of days) were not taken as prescribed over a mean of 3 months of follow-up, and that the most potent predictor of missed doses was greater overall illness severity (Goldstein et al. 2016). It is important to note that likelihood of achieving long-term remission of adolescent depression and bipolar disorders can be significantly enhanced by treatment adherence (Coletti et al. 2005; Goldstein et al. 2016; Staton 2010). Challenges to adherence are multilevel, some of which are modifiable, such as poor motivation and insight, erroneous beliefs and fears, illness severity, more comorbidity, poor clinician-patient relationship, and low level of family and social support, and others of which are nonmodifiable, such as health insurance and disadvantaged economic circumstances (Staton 2010). Interventions to improve adherence should include establishing effective therapeutic alliances, providing effective patient and family education, providing effective treatment, and attending to relevant factors associated with treatment nonadherence.

Youth are less likely to be compliant if they think that the recommended intervention will be unnecessary or ineffective or interfere with their autonomy or daily routines. The treatment decision process should engage youth and families as active partners and account for their individual and cultural perspectives about health and acceptable treatment options. Ongoing evaluation of treatment adherence (e.g., with motivational interview techniques) and barriers to adherence, including personal/cultural beliefs and experience of side effects (which could considerably reduce adherence, such as acne with lithium, akathisia with aripiprazole, or sexual side effects with SSRIs) and clinically important side effects (e.g., metabolic problems, kidney failure), is warranted (Diler and Birmaher 2012; Staton 2010).

Clinicians must optimize medication treatment to help improve treatment adherence. Because any given medication is unlikely to be effective for all youth with depression or mania, and many youth will still have relapses and recurrences even after good acute treatment response, improved ability to expeditiously identify nonadherence and provide individualized medication optimization is needed. Obtaining a family history of treatment responsiveness is one such strategy but has not been well studied in relation to clinical treatment decisions in youth (Goldstein et al. 2012). For treatment of depression or mania, the minimum clinically effective doses of medications with the fewest side effects should be used to minimize side effects and improve adherence. Unless the medications have significant side effects, the maximum tolerated dose found to be safe in youth should be used to determine the full efficacy of the medication in the presence of ongoing symptoms. This process of dose optimization should be undertaken before adding another medication (Diler and Birmaher 2012).

For youth having no or partial response to initial monotherapy, or for youth having intolerable side effects, monotherapy with another agent is recommended to prevent side effects and to improve adherence. If polypharmacy is indicated, it is important to introduce only one medication at a time to effectively evaluate the response to each medication, except in emergencies. Augmentation strategies, including nutritional interventions (e.g., omega-3, vitamin D or C), light therapy, and healthy lifestyle approaches (especially sleep hygiene and exercise), should be carefully tailored for each individual's clinical picture (Diler and Birmaher 2012; Goldstein et al. 2017).

If necessary, regardless of the youth's age, a responsible adult should oversee the medications, especially in those taking lithium and at higher risk for suicide, such as youth with past suicide attempts, self-injurious behaviors, family history of suicide, recent inpatient admission, mixed mood presentations, and psychotic symptoms. This is also necessary when diversion of medication (e.g., stimulants and benzodiazepines) might be an issue. Providing a limited supply of the medication, changing to another medication, or using pillboxes with monitoring of remaining supplies may be necessary in these cases (Diler and Birmaher 2012). Mood timelines or diaries are very helpful in the assessment and monitoring of mood symptoms as well as suicidal ideations and behaviors. These instruments can help visualize the course of the youth's mood, identify events that may have triggered the mood symptoms and sleep disruptions, and examine the relation between treatment and response. Many of these instruments use colors or ratings from 0 to 10 to chart daily changes in mood along with any corresponding significant stressors, illnesses, and treatments (see, e.g., Diler 2013).

Despite accumulating literature for maintenance treatment of depression and mania in youth, we still need consensus guidelines in adolescents and future studies in children (vs. adolescents) to monitor prospectively long-term (naturalistic and controlled) treatment response and adherence as well as clinical or subclinical and biological correlates of remission and recurrence.

Clinical Pearls

- A significant portion of youth with unipolar depression, bipolar depression, or mania do not initially respond to medication and psychotherapy interventions, and those who respond still have high risk for relapses and recurrences despite ongoing treatment.

- Despite the alarming statistics about relapses and recurrences, most youth with unipolar depression or mania eventually will respond to treatment, but findings suggest the need for individualizing and tailoring maintenance treatment options for the child's and family's needs and expectations, clinical presentation at baseline and progression during follow-up, and available resources.

- It is possible to identify those unipolar depressed youth who will show poorer response during follow-up by baseline severity of clinical characteristics as well as response rates by week 6.

- Baseline characteristics for a poor clinical trajectory in unipolar depression include younger age; lower family income; minority ethnicity; severity of depression; longer index episode duration; poorer global functioning; presence of suicidal ideation, hopelessness, melancholic features, and cognitive distortions; comorbid anxiety disorders; comorbid alcohol or substance use; higher number of comorbid disorders; higher parent-child conflict; lower expectation of improvement; and subsyndromal manic symptoms.

- Baseline characteristics for a poor clinical trajectory in mania include early age at onset, first mood episode of depression instead of mania, mixed or rapid-cycling episodes, long duration of mood symptoms, psychosis, subsyndromal mood symptoms, comorbid disorders, exposure to negative life events, high expressed emotion, low socioeconomic status, and family psychopathology.

- Clinicians must carefully evaluate and monitor developmental progression of bipolar disorder from subsyndromal presentations, especially manic symptoms with or without a depressive episode.

- During the continuation treatment, which starts soon after the acute treatment of a mood episode, clinicians usually continue the effective treatment interventions that were helpful in the acute mood episode.

- It is important to continuously assess the risk of suicide at any phase of the treatment in addition to any potential side effects and emerging or worsening comorbid conditions.

- If medication is needed, a medication combination can offer help, but monotherapy should be tried and optimized first. Unless the medications have significant side effects, the maximum tolerated dose found to be safe in youth should be used to determine the full efficacy of the medication in the presence of ongoing symptoms.

- Psychotherapy interventions may help improve response during acute treatment of unipolar depression, but no medication or combination treatment has yet proven superior to one another (medication, therapy, or combination treatment) in preventing recurrence during long-term follow-up.

- Mood stabilizers such as lithium are recommended for preventing recurrence of depression and mania in bipolar disorder, with more pronounced effectiveness 6 months after acute mood stabilization compared with second-generation antidepressant medications.

- Clinicians should work with the youth and the family to improve long-term treatment response (e.g., adding or strengthening therapy approaches and targeting subsyndromal presentations and comorbid conditions, emphasizing medication adherence, and encouraging healthy lifestyle changes) and adherence (e.g., establishing therapeutic rapport, including youth and families as partners in decision making, monitoring adherence very closely, and focusing on modifiable variables that limit adherence).

References

Aggen SH, Neale MC, Kendler KS: DSM criteria for major depression: evaluating symptom patterns using latent-trait item response models. Psychol Med 35(4):475–487, 2005 15856718

American Psychiatric Association: Diagnostic and Statistical Manual of Mental Disorders, 4th Edition, Text Revision. Washington, DC, American Psychiatric Association, 2000

American Psychiatric Association: Diagnostic and Statistical Manual of Mental Disorders, 5th Edition. Arlington, VA, American Psychiatric Association, 2013

Andersen SL, Teicher MH: Stress, sensitive periods and maturational events in adolescent depression. Trends Neurosci 31(4):183–191, 2008 18329735

Angst J, Cui L, Swendsen J, et al: Major depressive disorder with subthreshold bipolarity in the National Comorbidity Survey Replication. Am J Psychiatry 167(10):1194–1201, 2010 20713498

Apter A, Kronenberg S, Brent D: Turning darkness into light: a new landmark study on the treatment of adolescent depression. Comments on the TADS study (editorial). Eur Child Adolesc Psychiatry 14(3):113–116, 2005 15959656

Axelson D, Birmaher B, Brent D, et al: A preliminary study of the Kiddie Schedule for Affective Disorders and Schizophrenia for School-Age Children mania rating scale for children and adolescents. J Child Adolesc Psychopharmacol 13(4): 463–470, 2003 14977459

Axelson D, Birmaher B, Strober M, et al: Phenomenology of children and adolescents with bipolar spectrum disorders. Arch Gen Psychiatry 63(10):1139–1148, 2006 17015816

Axelson D, Birmaher B, Strober M, et al: Course of subthreshold bipolar disorder in youth: diagnostic progression from bipolar disorder not otherwise specified. J Am Acad Child Adolesc Psychiatry 50(10):1001.e3–1016.e3, 2011 21961775

Berk M, Dodd S, Malhi GS: 'Bipolar missed states': the diagnosis and clinical salience of bipolar mixed states. Aust N Z J Psychiatry 39(4):215–221, 2005
15777356

Berk M, Daglas R, Dandash O, et al: Quetiapine v. lithium in the maintenance
phase following a first episode of mania: randomised controlled trial. Br J
Psychiatry 210(6):413–421, 2017a 28254958

Berk M, Dandash O, Daglas R, et al: Neuroprotection after a first episode of mania: a randomized controlled maintenance trial comparing the effects of lithium and quetiapine on grey and white matter volume. Transl Psychiatry
7(1):e1011, 2017b 28117843

Biederman J, Mick E, Faraone SV, et al: A prospective follow-up study of pediatric bipolar disorder in boys with attention-deficit/hyperactivity disorder.
J Affect Disord 82 (suppl 1):S17–S23, 2004 15571786

Birmaher B: Longitudinal course of pediatric bipolar disorder. Am J Psychiatry
164(4):537–539, 2007 17403961

Birmaher B, Axelson D: Course and outcome of bipolar spectrum disorder in children and adolescents: a review of the existing literature. Dev Psychopathol
18(4):1023–1035, 2006 17064427

Birmaher B, Brent DA, Kolko D, et al: Clinical outcome after short-term psychotherapy for adolescents with major depressive disorder. Arch Gen Psychiatry
57(1):29–36, 2000 10632230

Birmaher B, Brent D, Bernet W, et al; AACAP Work Group on Quality Issues:
Practice parameter for the assessment and treatment of children and adolescents with depressive disorders. J Am Acad Child Adolesc Psychiatry
46(11):1503–1526, 2007 18049300

Birmaher B, Axelson D, Goldstein B, et al: Four-year longitudinal course of children and adolescents with bipolar spectrum disorders: the Course and Outcome of Bipolar Youth (COBY) study. Am J Psychiatry 166(7):795–804,
2009 19448190

Birmaher B, Gill MK, Axelson DA, et al: Longitudinal trajectories and associated
baseline predictors in youths with bipolar spectrum disorders. Am J Psychiatry 171(9):990–999, 2014 24874203

Blanco C, Okuda M, Markowitz JC, et al: The epidemiology of chronic major depressive disorder and dysthymic disorder: results from the National Epidemiologic Survey on Alcohol and Related Conditions. J Clin Psychiatry
71(12):1645–1656, 2010 21190638

Bolge SC, Thompson T, Bourne E, et al: Characteristics and symptomatology of
patients diagnosed with unipolar depression at risk for undiagnosed bipolar
disorder: a bipolar survey. CNS Spectr 13(3):216–224, 2008 18323755

Brent DA, Birmaher B: Treatment-resistant depression in adolescents: recognition
and management. Child Adolesc Psychiatr Clin N Am 15(4):1015–1034, x,
2006 16952773

Brent D, Emslie G, Clarke G, et al: Switching to another SSRI or to venlafaxine with or without cognitive behavioral therapy for adolescents with SSRI-resistant depression: the TORDIA randomized controlled trial. JAMA 299(8):901–913, 2008 18314433

Brown E, Dunner DL, McElroy SL, et al: Olanzapine/fluoxetine combination vs. lamotrigine in the 6-month treatment of bipolar I depression. Int J Neuropsychopharmacol 12(6):773–782, 2009 19079815

Chang K: Challenges in the diagnosis and treatment of pediatric bipolar depression. Dialogues Clin Neurosci 11(1):73–80, 2009 19432389

Chengappa KN, Kupfer DJ, Frank E, et al: Relationship of birth cohort and early age at onset of illness in a bipolar disorder case registry. Am J Psychiatry 160(9):1636–1642, 2003 12944339

Clark MS, Jansen KL, Cloy JA: Treatment of childhood and adolescent depression. Am Fam Physician 86(5):442–448, 2012 22963063

Coletti DJ, Leigh E, Gallelli KA, et al: Patterns of adherence to treatment in adolescents with bipolar disorder. J Child Adolesc Psychopharmacol 15(6):913–917, 2005 16379511

Correll CU, Hauser M, Penzner JB, et al: Type and duration of subsyndromal symptoms in youth with bipolar I disorder prior to their first manic episode. Bipolar Disord 16(5):478–492, 2014 24597782

Curry J, Silva S, Rohde P, et al: Recovery and recurrence following treatment for adolescent major depression. Arch Gen Psychiatry 68(3):263–269, 2011 21041606

DelBello MP, Kowatch RA: Pharmacological interventions for bipolar youth: developmental considerations. Dev Psychopathol 18(4):1231–1246, 2006 17064436

DelBello MP, Hanseman D, Adler CM, et al: Twelve-month outcome of adolescents with bipolar disorder following first hospitalization for a manic or mixed episode. Am J Psychiatry 164(4):582–590, 2007 17403971

DelBello MP, Goldman R, Phillips D, et al: Efficacy and safety of lurasidone in children and adolescents with bipolar I depression: a double-blind, placebo-controlled study. J Am Acad Child Adolesc Psychiatry 56(12):1015–1025, 2017 29173735

DelBello M, Goldman R, Tocco M, et al: Effectiveness of long-term lurasidone in children and adolescents with bipolar depression: interim analysis of year one of a two-year open-label study. Poster presented at the 171st annual meeting of the American Psychiatric Association, New York, NY, May 5–9, 2018

Detke HC, DelBello MP, Landry J, et al: Olanzapine/fluoxetine combination in children and adolescents with bipolar I depression: a randomized, double-blind, placebo-controlled trial. J Am Acad Child Adolesc Psychiatry 54(3):217–224, 2015 25721187

Diler RS: Pediatric Bipolar Disorder: A Global Perspective. New York, Nova Science Publishers, 2007

Diler RS: Mood and energy thermometer. Pittsburgh, PA, Child and Adolescent Bipolar Spectrum Services, Western Psychiatric Institute and Clinic of the University of Pittsburgh, 2013. Available at: https://www.pediatricbipolar.pitt.edu/sites/default/files/Mood%20and%20EnergyThermometer.pdf. Accessed January 17, 2019.

Diler RS, Birmaher B: Bipolar disorder in children and adolescents, in IACAPAP e-Textbook of Child and Adolescent Mental Health. Edited by Ray JN. Geneva, International Child and Adolescent Psychiatry and Allied Professionals, 2012, pp 1–30

Diler RS, Goldstein TR, Hafeman D, et al: Characteristics of depression among offspring at high and low familial risk of bipolar disorder. Bipolar Disord 19(5):344–352, 2017a 28612977

Diler RS, Goldstein TR, Hafeman D, et al: Distinguishing bipolar depression from unipolar depression in youth: preliminary findings. J Child Adolesc Psychopharmacol 27(4):310–319, 2017b 28398819

Duffy A, Grof P: Lithium treatment in children and adolescents. Pharmacopsychiatry 51(5):189–193, 2018 29490377

Duffy A, Alda M, Hajek T, et al: Early stages in the development of bipolar disorder. J Affect Disord 121(1–2):127–135, 2010 19541368

Egeland JA, Shaw JA, Endicott J, et al: Prospective study of prodromal features for bipolarity in well Amish children. J Am Acad Child Adolesc Psychiatry 42(7):786–796, 2003 12819438

Emslie GJ, Rush AJ, Weinberg WA, et al: Recurrence of major depressive disorder in hospitalized children and adolescents. J Am Acad Child Adolesc Psychiatry 36(6):785–792, 1997 9183133

Emslie GJ, Heiligenstein JH, Hoog SL, et al: Fluoxetine treatment for prevention of relapse of depression in children and adolescents: a double-blind, placebo-controlled study. J Am Acad Child Adolesc Psychiatry 43(11):1397–1405, 2004 15502599

Emslie GJ, Kennard BD, Mayes TL, et al: Fluoxetine versus placebo in preventing relapse of major depression in children and adolescents. Am J Psychiatry 165(4):459–467, 2008 18281410

Emslie GJ, Mayes T, Porta G, et al: Treatment of Resistant Depression in Adolescents (TORDIA): week 24 outcomes. Am J Psychiatry 167(7):782–791, 2010 20478877

Emslie GJ, Kennard BD, Mayes TL, et al: Continued effectiveness of relapse prevention cognitive-behavioral therapy following fluoxetine treatment in youth with major depressive disorder. J Am Acad Child Adolesc Psychiatry 54(12):991–998, 2015 26598474

Findling RL, Gracious BL, McNamara NK, et al: Rapid, continuous cycling and psychiatric co-morbidity in pediatric bipolar I disorder. Bipolar Disord 3(4):202–210, 2001 11552959

Findling RL, McNamara NK, Youngstrom EA, et al: Double-blind 18-month trial of lithium versus divalproex maintenance treatment in pediatric bipolar disorder. J Am Acad Child Adolesc Psychiatry 44(5):409–417, 2005 15843762

Findling RL, Youngstrom EA, McNamara NK, et al: Double-blind, randomized, placebo-controlled long-term maintenance study of aripiprazole in children with bipolar disorder. J Clin Psychiatry 73(1):57–63, 2012 22152402

Findling RL, Correll CU, Nyilas M, et al: Aripiprazole for the treatment of pediatric bipolar I disorder: a 30-week, randomized, placebo-controlled study. Bipolar Disord 15(2):138–149, 2013a 23437959

Findling RL, Kafantaris V, Pavuluri M, et al: Post-acute effectiveness of lithium in pediatric bipolar I disorder. J Child Adolesc Psychopharmacol 23(2):80–90, 2013b 23510444

Findling RL, Robb A, Bose A: Escitalopram in the treatment of adolescent depression: a randomized, double-blind, placebo-controlled extension trial. J Child Adolesc Psychopharmacol 23(7):468–480, 2013c 24041408

Findling RL, Chang K, Robb A, et al: Adjunctive maintenance lamotrigine for pediatric bipolar I disorder: a placebo-controlled, randomized withdrawal study. J Am Acad Child Adolesc Psychiatry 54(12):1020.e3–1031.e3, 2015

Findling RL, Landbloom RL, Mackle M, et al: Long-term safety of asenapine in pediatric patients diagnosed with bipolar I disorder: a 50-week open-label, flexible-dose trial. Paediatr Drugs 18(5):367–378, 2016 27461426

Geller B, Luby J: Child and adolescent bipolar disorder: a review of the past 10 years. J Am Acad Child Adolesc Psychiatry 36(9):1168–1176, 1997 9291717

Geller B, Cooper TB, Sun K, et al: Double-blind and placebo-controlled study of lithium for adolescent bipolar disorders with secondary substance dependency. J Am Acad Child Adolesc Psychiatry 37(2):171–178, 1998 9473913

Geller B, Zimerman B, Williams M, et al: Six-month stability and outcome of a prepubertal and early adolescent bipolar disorder phenotype. J Child Adolesc Psychopharmacol 10(3):165–173, 2000 11052406

Geller B, Tillman R, Bolhofner K, et al: Child bipolar I disorder: prospective continuity with adult bipolar I disorder; characteristics of second and third episodes; predictors of 8-year outcome. Arch Gen Psychiatry 65(10):1125–1133, 2008 18838629

Goldstein BI, Sassi R, Diler RS: Pharmacologic treatment of bipolar disorder in children and adolescents. Child Adolesc Psychiatr Clin N Am 21(4):911–939, 2012 23040907

Goldstein BI, Birmaher B, Carlson GA, et al: The International Society for Bipolar Disorders Task Force report on pediatric bipolar disorder: knowledge to date and directions for future research. Bipolar Disord 19(7):524–543, 2017 28944987

Goldstein TR, Fersch-Podrat RK, Rivera M, et al: Dialectical behavior therapy for adolescents with bipolar disorder: results from a pilot randomized trial. J Child Adolesc Psychopharmacol 25(2):140–149, 2015 25010702

Goldstein TR, Krantz M, Merranko J, et al: Medication adherence among adolescents with bipolar disorder. J Child Adolesc Psychopharmacol 26(10):864–872, 2016 27419273

Goldstein TR, Merranko J, Krantz M, et al: Early intervention for adolescents at-risk for bipolar disorder: a pilot randomized trial of interpersonal and social rhythm therapy (IPSRT). J Affect Disord 235:348–356, 2018 29665518

Goodman E, Whitaker RC: A prospective study of the role of depression in the development and persistence of adolescent obesity. Pediatrics 110(3):497–504, 2002 12205250

Goodyer I, Dubicka B, Wilkinson P, et al: Selective serotonin reuptake inhibitors (SSRIs) and routine specialist care with and without cognitive behaviour therapy in adolescents with major depression: randomised controlled trial. BMJ 335(7611):142, 2007 17556431

Gore FM, Bloem PJ, Patton GC, et al: Global burden of disease in young people aged 10–24 years: a systematic analysis. Lancet 377(9783):2093–2102, 2011 21652063

Gruber J, Miklowitz DJ, Harvey AG, et al: Sleep matters: sleep functioning and course of illness in bipolar disorder. J Affect Disord 134(1–3):416–420, 2011 21683450

Hafeman DM, Merranko J, Axelson D, et al: Toward the definition of a bipolar prodrome: dimensional predictors of bipolar spectrum disorders in at-risk youths. Am J Psychiatry 173(7):695–704, 2016 26892940

Hamdan S, Melhem NM, Porta G, et al: The phenomenology and course of depression in parentally bereaved and non-bereaved youth. J Am Acad Child Adolesc Psychiatry 51(5):528–536, 2012 22525959

Henry CA, Zamvil LS, Lam C, et al: Long-term outcome with divalproex in children and adolescents with bipolar disorder. J Child Adolesc Psychopharmacol 13(4):523–529, 2003 14977465

Hirneth SJ, Hazell PL, Hanstock TL, et al: Bipolar disorder subtypes in children and adolescents: demographic and clinical characteristics from an Australian sample. J Affect Disord 175:98–107, 2015 25601309

Judd LL, Akiskal HS: Depressive episodes and symptoms dominate the longitudinal course of bipolar disorder. Curr Psychiatry Rep 5(6):417–418, 2003 14609495

Kafantaris V, Coletti DJ, Dicker R, et al: Lithium treatment of acute mania in adolescents: a placebo-controlled discontinuation study. J Am Acad Child Adolesc Psychiatry 43(8):984–993, 2004 15266193

Karlsson L, Pelkonen M, Heilä H, et al: Differences in the clinical characteristics of adolescent depressive disorders. Depress Anxiety 24(6):421–432, 2007 17051545

Kaufman J, Birmaher B, Brent D, et al: Schedule for Affective Disorders and Schizophrenia for School-Age Children-Present and Lifetime Version (KSADS-PL): initial reliability and validity data [see comments]. J Am Acad Child Adolesc Psychiatry 36(7):980–988, 1997 9204677

Kennard BD, Clarke GN, Weersing VR, et al: Effective components of TORDIA cognitive-behavioral therapy for adolescent depression: preliminary findings. J Consult Clin Psychol 77(6):1033–1041, 2009a 19968380

Kennard BD, Silva SG, Mayes TL, et al; TADS: Assessment of safety and long-term outcomes of initial treatment with placebo in TADS. Am J Psychiatry 166(3):337–344, 2009b 19147693

Kovacs M: Presentation and course of major depressive disorder during childhood and later years of the life span. J Am Acad Child Adolesc Psychiatry 35(6):705–715, 1996 8682751

Kowatch RA, Sethuraman G, Hume JH, et al: Combination pharmacotherapy in children and adolescents with bipolar disorder. Biol Psychiatry 53(11):978–984, 2003 12788243

Kowatch RA, Fristad M, Birmaher B, et al; Child Psychiatric Workgroup on Bipolar Disorder: Treatment guidelines for children and adolescents with bipolar disorder. J Am Acad Child Adolesc Psychiatry 44(3):213–235, 2005 15725966

Lépine JP, Briley M: The increasing burden of depression. Neuropsychiatr Dis Treat 7 (suppl 1):3–7, 2011 21750622

Leverich GS, Post RM, Keck PE Jr, et al: The poor prognosis of childhood-onset bipolar disorder. J Pediatr 150(5):485–490, 2007 17452221

Lewinsohn PM, Klein DN, Seeley JR: Bipolar disorder during adolescence and young adulthood in a community sample. Bipolar Disord 2(3 pt 2):281–293, 2000 11249806

Maalouf FT, Brent DA: Child and adolescent depression intervention overview: what works, for whom and how well? Child Adolesc Psychiatr Clin N Am 21(2):299–312, viii, 2012 22537728

Maalouf FT, Porta G, Vitiello B, et al: Do sub-syndromal manic symptoms influence outcome in treatment resistant depression in adolescents? A latent class analysis from the TORDIA study. J Affect Disord 138(1–2):86–95, 2012 22284022

MacQueen GM, Young LT, Robb JC, et al: Effect of number of episodes on well-being and functioning of patients with bipolar disorder. Acta Psychiatr Scand 101(5):374–381, 2000 10823297

Mansoor B, Rengasamy M, Hilton R, et al: The bidirectional relationship between body mass index and treatment outcome in adolescents with treatment-resistant depression. J Child Adolesc Psychopharmacol 23(7):458–467, 2013 24024532

March J, Silva S, Petrycki S, et al; Treatment for Adolescents with Depression Study (TADS) Team: Fluoxetine, cognitive-behavioral therapy, and their combination for adolescents with depression: Treatment for Adolescents With Depression Study (TADS) randomized controlled trial. JAMA 292(7):807–820, 2004 15315995

McMakin DL, Olino TM, Porta G, et al: Anhedonia predicts poorer recovery among youth with selective serotonin reuptake inhibitor treatment–resistant depression. J Am Acad Child Adolesc Psychiatry 51(4):404–411, 2012 22449646

Miklowitz DJ: Evidence-based family interventions for adolescents and young adults with bipolar disorder. J Clin Psychiatry 77 (suppl E1):e5, 2016 27570931

Miklowitz DJ, Chung B: Family focused therapy for bipolar disorder: reflections on 30 years of research. Fam Process 55(3):483–499, 2016 27471058

Miklowitz DJ, Axelson DA, Birmaher B, et al: Family focused treatment for adolescents with bipolar disorder: results of a 2-year randomized trial. Arch Gen Psychiatry 65(9):1053–1061, 2008 18762591

Miklowitz DJ, Chang KD, Taylor DO, et al: Early psychosocial intervention for youth at risk for bipolar I or II disorder: a one-year treatment development trial. Bipolar Disord 13(1):67–75, 2011 21320254

Miklowitz DJ, Schneck CD, Walshaw PD, et al: Early intervention for youth at high risk for bipolar disorder: a multisite randomized trial of family-focused treatment. Early Interv Psychiatry Aug 4, 2017 [Epub ahead of print] 28776930

Miller S, Do D, Gershon A, et al: Longer-term effectiveness and tolerability of adjunctive open lurasidone in patients with bipolar disorder. J Clin Psychopharmacol 38(3):207–211, 2018 29620693

Nadkarni RB, Fristad MA: Clinical course of children with a depressive spectrum disorder and transient manic symptoms. Bipolar Disord 12(5):494–503, 2010 20712750

National Research Council of the National Academies, Committee on A Framework for Developing a New Taxonomy of Disease: Toward Precision Medicine: Building a Knowledge Network for Biomedical Research and a New Taxonomy of Disease. Washington, DC, National Academies Press, 2011

Parker GB, Graham RK, Tavella G: Is there consensus across international evidence-based guidelines for the management of bipolar disorder? Acta Psychiatr Scand 135(6):515–526, 2017 28260229

Pavuluri MN, Birmaher B, Naylor MW: Pediatric bipolar disorder: a review of the past 10 years. J Am Acad Child Adolesc Psychiatry 44(9):846–871, 2005 16113615

Pavuluri MN, Henry DB, Moss M, et al: Effectiveness of lamotrigine in maintaining symptom control in pediatric bipolar disorder. J Child Adolesc Psychopharmacol 19(1):75–82, 2009 19232025

Perlis RH, Ostacher MJ, Patel JK, et al: Predictors of recurrence in bipolar disorder: primary outcomes from the Systematic Treatment Enhancement Program for Bipolar Disorder (STEP-BD). Am J Psychiatry 163(2):217–224, 2006 16449474

Quek YH, Tam WWS, Zhang MWB, et al: Exploring the association between childhood and adolescent obesity and depression: a meta-analysis. Obes Rev 18(7):742–754, 2017 28401646

Redden L, DelBello M, Wagner KD, et al; Depakote ER Pediatric Mania Group: Long-term safety of divalproex sodium extended-release in children and adolescents with bipolar I disorder. J Child Adolesc Psychopharmacol 19(1):83–89, 2009 19232026

Regeer EJ, Krabbendam L, de Graaf R, et al: A prospective study of the transition rates of subthreshold (hypo)mania and depression in the general population. Psychol Med 36(5):619–627, 2006 16438739

Sakolsky D, Birmaher B: Developmentally informed pharmacotherapy for child and adolescent depressive disorders. Child Adolesc Psychiatr Clin N Am 21(2):313–325, viii, 2012 22537729

Sakolsky DJ, McCracken JT, Nurmi EL: Genetics of pediatric anxiety disorders. Child Adolesc Psychiatr Clin N Am 21(3):479–500, 2012 22800990

Schubert KO, Clark SR, Van LK, et al: Depressive symptom trajectories in late adolescence and early adulthood: a systematic review. Aust N Z J Psychiatry 51(5):477–499, 2017 28415879

Scott EM, Hermens DF, Naismith SL, et al: Distinguishing young people with emerging bipolar disorders from those with unipolar depression. J Affect Disord 144(3):208–215, 2013 22877963

Spirito A, Esposito-Smythers C: Attempted and completed suicide in adolescence. Annu Rev Clin Psychol 2:237–266, 2006 17716070

Staton D: Achieving adolescent adherence to treatment of major depression. Adolesc Health Med Ther 1:73–85, 2010 24600263

Strober M, Morrell W, Lampert C, et al: Relapse following discontinuation of lithium maintenance therapy in adolescents with bipolar I illness: a naturalistic study. Am J Psychiatry 147(4):457–461, 1990 2107763

Strober M, Schmidt-Lackner S, Freeman R, et al: Recovery and relapse in adolescents with bipolar affective illness: a five-year naturalistic, prospective follow-up. J Am Acad Child Adolesc Psychiatry 34(6):724–731, 1995 7608045

Ten Have M, de Graaf R, van Dorsselaer S, et al: Recurrence and chronicity of major depressive disorder and their risk indicators in a population cohort. Acta Psychiatr Scand 137(6):503–515, 2018 29577236

Thapar A, Collishaw S, Pine DS, et al: Depression in adolescence. Lancet 379(9820):1056–1067, 2012 22305766

Thase ME: Bipolar depression: issues in diagnosis and treatment. Harv Rev Psychiatry 13(5):257–271, 2005 16251165

Thase ME: Bipolar depression: diagnostic and treatment considerations. Dev Psychopathol 18(4):1213–1230, 2006 17064435

van Loo HM, Cai T, Gruber MJ, et al: Major depressive disorder subtypes to predict long-term course. Depress Anxiety 31(9):765–777, 2014 24425049

Van Meter AR, Moreira AL, Youngstrom EA: Meta-analysis of epidemiologic studies of pediatric bipolar disorder. J Clin Psychiatry 72(9):1250–1256, 2011 21672501

Vitiello B: Combined cognitive-behavioural therapy and pharmacotherapy for adolescent depression: does it improve outcomes compared with monotherapy? CNS Drugs 23(4):271–280, 2009 19374457

Vitiello B, Silva SG, Rohde P, et al: Suicidal events in the Treatment for Adolescents with Depression Study (TADS). J Clin Psychiatry 70(5):741–747, 2009 19552869

Vitiello B, Emslie G, Clarke G, et al: Long-term outcome of adolescent depression initially resistant to selective serotonin reuptake inhibitor treatment: a follow-up study of the TORDIA sample. J Clin Psychiatry 72(3):388–396, 2011 21208583

Wozniak J, Spencer T, Biederman J, et al: The clinical characteristics of unipolar vs. bipolar major depression in ADHD youth. J Affect Disord 82 (suppl 1):S59–S69, 2004 15571791

Yatham LN, Beaulieu S, Schaffer A, et al: Optimal duration of risperidone or olanzapine adjunctive therapy to mood stabilizer following remission of a manic episode: a CANMAT randomized double-blind trial. Mol Psychiatry 21(8):1050–1056, 2016 26460229

Yu ZJ, Kratochvil CJ, Weller RA, et al: From TADS and SOFTADS to TORDIA and beyond: what's new in the treatment of adolescent depression? Curr Psychiatry Rep 12(2):88–95, 2010 20425292

12

Assessment, Prognosis, and Treatment of Subthreshold Mood Symptoms

Danella Hafeman, M.D., Ph.D.

Meredith Spada, M.D.

A 12-year-old girl presents to your office with periods of depressive symptoms, never lasting more than a few days, during which she is noticeably more irritable, does not enjoy things that she usually does (e.g., dance practice), and has much less energy; she denies other symptoms of depression. These periods occur probably about once every few weeks, but no discernible pattern or clear stressors are evident; they do affect functioning however, because sometimes she will refuse to go to school when she feels this way. When asked about manic symptoms, the patient denies any symptoms. However, her mom reports that she will get extremely silly at times, much more so than her friends or other people around. She will be "bouncing around," "talking my ear off," and much more affectionate than usual. Mom enjoys these times to a point, but after about 30 minutes, they become annoying; they are not always triggered by anything, and the patient seems unable to "tone it down," even in public. The periods never last longer than a few hours. When asked about a family history of mood disorders, her mom notes that her sister (patient's aunt) was diagnosed with bipolar II disorder.

Diagnosis: Other specified depression with subthreshold manic symptoms.

Although diagnostic categories are useful for informing prognosis and treatment, symptoms of depression and mania may be impairing without necessarily meeting full DSM-5 (American Psychiatric Association 2013) criteria for a given disorder. In addition, the presence of these symptoms increases the later chance of developing a full-threshold mood disorder. In this chapter, we describe the epidemiology and prognosis of subthreshold mood symptoms, focusing primarily on the extant literature in pediatric populations. Next, we describe measures and methods for assessing these symptoms; how the concept of a staging model might inform our understanding of subthreshold symptoms; and initial evidence for which treatments might be indicated and efficacious to address these symptoms. We discuss subthreshold depressive and manic symptoms separately but recognize that these symptoms are frequently co-occurring, and the combination likely has the greatest influence on functional impairment.

Subthreshold Depressive Symptoms

Subthreshold depression is defined as the presence of clinically relevant symptoms of major depressive disorder (MDD) that do not meet the full DSM criteria for the disorder (Pincus et al. 1999) (e.g., meeting two to four diagnostic criteria rather than the five required for a diagnosis of MDD) (Meeks et al. 2011). Historically, there has been debate as to whether subthreshold depression represents a distinct entity or a precursor to MDD (Lewinsohn et al. 2000b). Several distinct categories of depressive symptoms not meeting full diagnostic criteria for MDD have previously been described (e.g., minor depression, recurrent brief depression, dysthymia, subthreshold depression). However, overlap of symptomatology among these categories is common (Chen et al. 2000), and contemporary literature lends credence to the concept of depressive symptoms occurring along a continuum, ranging from none to severe (Fergusson et al. 2005; Lewinsohn et al. 2000b), with subthreshold symptoms representing an early stage in the course of depressive illness. As with adults, the concept of depressive symptoms in children and adolescents occurring along a continuum is supported by the literature (Wesselhoeft et al. 2013).

Epidemiology

A growing body of literature has sought to address the prevalence of, risk factors for developing, and subsequent outcomes of subthreshold depression.

Prevalence

Subthreshold depression is at least two to three times more common than major depression in adults (Meeks et al. 2011), and even more striking, a fivefold difference between the prevalence of subthreshold depression (31.1%) and the prevalence of MDD (6.3%) in adults age 65 years and older has previously been reported (Judd and Kunovac 1998). Twelve-month prevalence in children and adolescents has ranged from 3% to 12% in various studies, with lifetime prevalence through late adolescence as high as 26% (Fergusson et al. 2005; Klein et al. 2009; Wittchen et al. 1998). In a large study of 12,395 adolescents from 11 European countries, 29.2% of the participants met criteria for subthreshold depression, whereas 10.5% had symptoms that met full diagnostic criteria for MDD (Balázs et al. 2013).

Risk Factors

Lewinsohn and colleagues (2003) demonstrated that adolescents who have a first-degree relative with MDD are at higher risk for developing subthreshold depression than are those without this family history. Adolescents with subthreshold depression ($n=193$) had more first-degree relatives with MDD than did those adolescents with no mood disorder ($n=221$) (24.3% vs. 20.2%; $P=0.04$); adolescents with MDD ($n=387$) had an even higher rate of MDD in relatives (Lewinsohn et al. 2003). In a sample of 496 female adolescents, Rohde et al. (2009) found that racial and ethnic minority groups were at especially high risk for subthreshold depression, and adolescents with less educated parents had earlier onset. Conflicts with parents and physical abuse in the home are also correlated with subthreshold depression (Jonsson et al. 2011).

Outcomes

Across the life span, multiple studies have indicated that subthreshold depression is associated with poor outcomes (e.g., suicidality and poor psychosocial function) and is predictive of MDD. In a landmark study examining a large community sample ($N=3,003$) of adolescents, adults, and older adults, Lewinsohn and colleagues (2000b) found that subthreshold depressive symptoms were predictive of major depression and psychosocial dysfunction, as well as substance use disorders. Keenan et al. (2008) extended these findings to younger children in a sample of participants from the Pittsburgh Girls Study. In this cohort of 232 girls who had high scores on a depression measure at age 8 years, early depressive symptoms were lasting and conferred risk for depressive disorders and impairment over a 3-year follow-up (Keenan et al. 2008). Similar outcomes have been found even in preschool children. Luby et al. (2014) examined the course of subthreshold depressive symptoms arising in 246 children (3–6 years old) in the Preschool Depression Study. The authors found that preschool-onset depressive symptoms predicted later MDD, even when they controlled for other risk factors, including maternal depression (Luby et al. 2014).

Pine and colleagues (1999) studied longer-term outcomes by following up a sample of 776 young people from New York State from 1983 to 1992 and found that depressive symptoms, even those that were subthreshold, strongly predicted escalation to MDD in adulthood. In a retrospective study of the Baltimore Epidemiologic Catchment Area Community cohort, Wilcox and Anthony (2004) found that 33.3% (50 of 150) of adults with MDD reported at least one depressive symptom before age 19 compared with 7.3% (128 of 1755) of those without MDD. Furthermore, Fergusson et al. (2005) followed up a birth cohort of 1,265 children from New Zealand over 24 years and found that depressive symptoms in adolescence, even those not meeting the full criteria for MDD, increased risk not only for subsequent episodes of MDD and impairment but also for mental health treatment, anxiety disorders, suicidal ideation, and suicide attempts.

Predictors of Progression to Major Depressive Disorder

Increasing numbers of symptoms that cluster predict progression to MDD, and some specific symptoms have particular predictive value. In a prospective study of the Oregon Adolescent Depression Project (OADP) cohort, 1,709 adolescents ages 14 to 18 years participated in initial diagnostic assessments. Of those adolescents, 88% ($n=1,507$) completed follow-up 1 year later. Having seven of nine DSM-III-R (American Psychiatric Association 1987) symptoms of major depression at initial assessment predicted escalation to MDD at follow-up after controlling for depression history and gender. In this study, sad mood added unique variance to the development of major depression (odds ratio=2.01) (Georgiades et al. 2006). On retrospective review of the Baltimore Epidemiologic Catchment Area Community cohort, Wilcox and Anthony (2004) found that the earliest and most common symptoms preceding adult-onset MDD included persistent depressed mood, thoughts of death and suicide, persistent anhedonia, and thoughts of worthlessness. The positive predictive value estimates for persistent anhedonia and feelings of worthlessness were particularly striking: 58% overall for persistent anhedonia (75% in females) and 61% overall for feelings of worthlessness (67% in females).

Comorbidities, family history, and psychosocial stressors also increase the risk for progression to MDD. In the OADP, Klein et al. (2009) examined predictors of conversion to MDD in young adulthood in a sample of 225 adolescents who were followed up from mid-adolescence to age 30. In this sample, the risk for progression to MDD was 67%, with severity of depressive symptoms, medical conditions and symptoms, history of suicidal ideation, history of anxiety disorder, and familial loading for depression all increasing the chances for development of MDD. In adolescents with three or more risk factors, the chance of developing MDD was approximately 90%, versus 47% in participants with fewer than three risk factors, demonstrating that an increasing number of symptoms increases the risk for subsequent development of MDD (Klein et al. 2009). Hill et al. (2014) also examined factors leading to MDD in OADP participants and found that poor friend support was the strongest predictor of progression to MDD. They used decision tree analysis and found that in a subgroup of adolescents with poor friend support, anxiety and substance use were additional predictors of progression to major depression. In a subgroup of adolescents with more friend support, major life events were found to be an important predictor of progression to major depression (Hill et al. 2014). In preschool children, a latent class analysis of data from the Preschool Depression Study found that those with a family history of mood disorder, early childhood social adversity, and preschool-onset externalizing disorders were more likely to be in the class with "high severity depression" over time (Whalen et al. 2016).

Assessment

Here we include a description of instruments that have been used in clinical settings to assess depressive symptoms in youth. This is not a comprehensive list but rather a selection of tools that have been used previously and described in the literature.

- **Children's Depression Inventory (CDI):** This is the child version of the Beck Depression Inventory (BDI, described later in this list) designed for use with children ages 7–18 years. This 27-item self-report scale has three-point answers to evaluate symptoms over the past 2 weeks. Total scores range from 0 to 54 (Kovacs 1985). It is one of the most widely used and studied scales for depression in youth (Stockings et al. 2015).
- **Mood and Feelings Questionnaire (MFQ):** This scale contains 33 questions to measure depressive symptoms over the past 2 weeks in children ages 8–18 years. The items are scored on a three-point scale, with total scores ranging from 0 to 66 (Costello and Angold 1988). The MFQ is recommended by NICE (National Institute for Health and Care Excellence) guidelines for the screening of depression in children and adolescents (Lawton and Moghraby 2016).
- **Reynolds Adolescent Depression Scale (RADS):** This self-report scale is designed to assess depression symptom severity in youth ages 13–18 years. This instrument contains 30 items assessing symptoms (cognitive, somatic, psychomotor, and interpersonal) over the past 2 weeks on a four-point scale, with scores ranging from 30 to 120 (Reynolds 1986; Stockings et al. 2015).
- **Center for Epidemiologic Studies—Depression Scale (CES-D):** This 20-item self-report depression symptom scale intended for the general population assesses six symptom clusters: depressed mood, feelings of guilt/worthlessness, helplessness, psychomotor retardation, loss of appetite, and sleep disturbance. Each of the 20 items is rated on a scale from 0 to 3, with total scores ranging from 0 to 60. Although its use among adults is considered valid and reliable, Radloff established that this scale is suitable for high school students as well but warned that given possible inflation of scores by an excess of transient symptoms, scores of junior high school students must be interpreted with caution (Radloff 1991; Stockings et al. 2015).
- **Beck Depression Inventory (BDI):** This scale was originally developed in 1961 for use in adults but is widely used among both adults and adolescents (Stockings et al. 2015). The BDI comprises 21 items assessing symptoms over the past week: 15 items assess affective or cognitive domains, and 6 items assess vegetative symptoms. The items are scored from 0 to 3, with total scores ranging from 0 to 63 (Beck et al. 1961). Because the scale does not include items pertaining to school, it may not be suitable for use among younger children (Stockings et al. 2015).

Staging Model

A staging approach, which has become standard of care in other areas of medicine (e.g., cancer, heart failure, and chronic kidney disease), involves classifying disease according to phase and severity and using this information to inform prognosis and select treatment approaches that match this classification. Psychiatry has historically lagged behind in developing such a schema for characterizing disorders; however, such a construct has gained footing in recent years.

Given that research findings support the idea of depression as a dimensional construct, the concept of a staging model may be useful. In turn, early identification and treatment can potentially prevent worsening severity and progression to MDD (Cosci and Fava 2013; Hetrick et al. 2008). Fava and Kellner first described a staging model of unipolar depression in 1993, which was subsequently revised in 2007 and again in 2013 (Cosci and Fava 2013; Fava and Kellner 1993; Fava and Tossani 2007). In this staging model, the prodromal stage 1 phase is characterized by anxiety, irritability, anhedonia, and sleep disturbance, with only mild functional change. Subthreshold depression fits into this stage. Stage 2 is characterized by the onset of an episode of major depression, whereas stage 3 marks a residual period that may include no depressive symptoms or dysthymia. Stage 4 signifies a recurrent major or double depression, and stage 5 denotes a chronic major depression lasting at least 2 years without interruption. In this model, the prodromal phase is a potentially critical juncture for intervention. Depressive disorders commonly emerge during adolescence but often remain untreated for several years. Intervening during the early stages may therefore aid in the prevention of escalation to MDD and reduce duration and severity of illness (Fava and Tossani 2007; McGorry et al. 2011). In the subsequent subsection, we review the evidence base for treatment options for youth with subthreshold depression.

Treatment Options

Pharmacotherapy (Not Supported by the Currently Available Literature)

The currently available literature in adults does not support the use of pharmacotherapy as a first-line treatment of subthreshold depression. In a systematic review and meta-analysis of double-blind, randomized controlled trials (RCTs) of patients with subthreshold depression, including 6 studies with 234 patients receiving antidepressants and 234 receiving placebo, Barbui et al. (2011) found no significant difference in terms of failures to respond to treatment (relative risk [RR]=0.94; 95% confidence interval [CI]=0.81–1.08). The authors also extracted data from two studies with a total of 93 patients taking antidepressants and 93 taking placebo that showed no statistically significant difference between antidepressants and placebo in terms of acceptability (RR=1.06; 95% CI=0.65–1.73). No studies have compared benzodiazepines with placebo for the treatment of minor depression (Barbui et al. 2011). To our knowledge, no studies have been published on the use of pharmacological agents in the treatment of subthreshold depression in children and adolescents; however, extrapolating from the adult data, we do not recommend initiation of pharmacological treatment in youth with subthreshold depressive symptoms that do not meet the criteria for MDD. One caveat to this would be in youth with comorbidities for which treatment with an antidepressant is indicated, such as generalized anxiety disorder or panic disorder.

Cognitive-Behavioral Therapy

Although the available literature has not been promising for treatment of subthreshold depression with pharmacological agents, evidence, including a meta-analysis by Cuijpers et al. (2007), has shown that psychological therapies are effective for subthreshold depression in both adult and child populations and may prevent progression to MDD. In an RCT by Clarke and colleagues (1995), the CES-D was administered to 1,652 high school students. Those students with subthreshold depression (i.e., elevated CES-D scores but not meeting full-threshold criteria for a major depressive episode [MDE]; $n=150$) received either a 15-session group cognitive therapy prevention intervention or the usual care control condition. At 12-month follow-up, total incidence rates of affective disorder were 14.5% for active intervention versus 25.7% for control condition, demonstrating a significant improvement in the intervention group (Clarke et al. 1995). Similar effects were found in 94 children ages 13–18 years with subthreshold depressive symptoms with an additional risk factor of a parent receiving treatment for a depressive episode. Compared with usual care, participants randomly assigned to usual care plus a 15-session group cognitive therapy prevention program ($n=45$) showed lower CES-D scores ($P=0.005$) and higher global functioning ($P=0.04$). The cognitive therapy group also showed lower incidence of MDEs (9.3% cumulative major depression incidence in cognitive therapy group vs. 28.8% for usual care group; $P=0.003$) (Clarke et al. 2001).

Along the same lines, in an RCT of 341 adolescents with elevated depressive symptoms randomly assigned to receive one of three interventions (brief group cognitive-behavioral intervention vs. group supportive-expressive intervention vs. bibliotherapy) or assessment-only control condition, those in the brief group cognitive-behavioral intervention showed significantly greater reductions in depressive symptoms, improvements in social adjustment, and reductions in substance use at posttest and 6-month follow-up than did participants in the other three conditions. The brief group cognitive-behavioral intervention (vs. assessment-only control) had a medium effect size ($d = 0.46$) on depressive symptoms (Stice et al. 2008).

Further supporting the efficacy of cognitive-behavioral therapy (CBT) in adolescence, Takagaki and colleagues (2016) conducted a randomized clinical trial in adolescents ages 18–19 with subthreshold depression enrolled as first-year students at Hiroshima University in Japan. Participants were randomly assigned to a treatment group (behavioral activation program conducted once weekly consisting of five 60-minute sessions, $n = 62$) or a control group ($n = 56$). Students in the treatment group showed significant improvements in their depressive symptoms, with a large effect size (Hedges' $g = -0.90$; 95% CI $= -1.28, -0.51$), compared with the control group and also showed significant improvements in self-reported rating of quality of life and in behavioral characteristics (Takagaki et al. 2016). These results support the centrality of behavioral activation to CBT in adolescents with subthreshold symptoms of depression.

Although much of the research on CBT for depression has focused on adults and adolescents, a recent meta-analysis including 10 RCTs with a total of 267 children ages 8–12 years with diagnosed depression or elevated depressive symptoms supported the use of CBT in children with depressive symptoms. The weighted between-group effect size for CBT was $d = 0.66$, whereas the weighted within-group effect size for CBT was $d = 1.02$, indicating a medium and large effect size, respectively (Arnberg and Ost 2014).

CBT in medically complicated youth

CBT targeting individuals with subthreshold depression and concomitant medical illness has shown promise, and because it has been previously reported that medical illness is a risk factor for escalation to MDD in subthreshold depressed youth, interventions for this population are quite clinically relevant (Klein et al. 2009). Szigethy et al. (2007) studied CBT in adolescents ages 11–17 with inflammatory bowel disease (IBD) and mild to moderate subsyndromal depression. Forty-one adolescents were randomly assigned to participate in a CBT protocol (Primary and Secondary Control Enhancement Therapy—Physical Illness, $n=22$), which was modified for youth with IBD, and 19 were randomly assigned to receive treatment as usual plus a depression information sheet. The intervention group showed significantly greater improvement in CDI scores, Children's Global Assessment Scale scores, and Perceived Control Scale for Children scores. Further supporting the benefit of CBT in the treatment of subthreshold depression, in a study of 104 adolescents with newly diagnosed epilepsy, participants deemed to be at increased risk for depression ($n=30$) were randomly assigned to CBT or counseling as usual. Subthreshold depressive disorder significantly improved at 9-month follow-up in the CBT group compared with the treatment as usual group ($P<0.05$) (Martinovic et al. 2006).

CBT: looking to the future

In terms of future directions, the Screening and Training: Enhancing Resilience in Kids study is an RCT targeting children ages 8–17 years, including those with subthreshold depressive symptoms, with parents affected by mood or anxiety disorders. The children were randomly assigned either to participate in 10 weekly individual child CBT sessions and 2 parent sessions or to receive minimal written information. This trial is currently ongoing, and the authors plan to evaluate both the effectiveness and the cost-effectiveness of this intervention (Nauta et al. 2012).

Interpersonal Psychotherapy

Although several studies have reported the utility of CBT in subthreshold depression, evidence also supports the use of interpersonal psychotherapy (IPT) in subthreshold depression. Young et al. (2006) randomly assigned 41 adolescents with elevated depressive symptoms to receive either IPT–Adolescent Skills Training (IPT-AST) or school counseling. IPT-AST showed advantage in terms of significantly fewer depression symptoms, better overall functioning, and fewer depression diagnoses post follow-up at 3 and 6 months (Young et al. 2006). In a more recent exploratory single-blind, randomized controlled crossover trial of Japanese college students ages 20–39 years with subthreshold depressive symptoms, interpersonal counseling ($n=15$) was compared with counseling as usual ($n=16$). Interpersonal counseling resulted in better outcomes, with significantly improved depressive symptoms ($P=0.007$), compared with the control counseling as usual group, as gauged by the Zung Self-Rating Depression Scale total score. In addition, although not statistically significant ($P=0.07$), task-oriented coping (i.e., active problem-solving in stressful situations), as measured by a subscale on the Coping Inventory for Stressful Situations, showed a trend toward a greater increase in the interpersonal counseling group (Yamamoto et al. 2018).

Although the latter study evaluated young adults as opposed to adolescents, these results may be translatable to older adolescents; however, further studies evaluating the effectiveness of IPT in children and adolescents are needed. Moreover, to our knowledge, there have not been any meta-analyses comparing effect sizes between CBT and IPT for subthreshold depressed youth. Such a direct comparison would significantly inform treatment approaches in this population and should be a priority for future research.

Self-Help Strategies

Self-help strategies theoretically decrease the need for interfacing with the mental health care system. These interventions may be an important strategy to consider given the substantial number of people with a continuum of depressive symptoms who need treatment, especially in areas where access to mental health care is limited, and in the current era of medicine in which providing cost-effective care is a matter of importance. Table 12–1 summarizes potential complementary and self-help strategies for the treatment of subthreshold depressive symptoms. Bibliotherapy, computerized interventions, relaxation training, exercise, and light therapy for adolescents with a seasonal component to their depressive symptoms have shown modest benefit in adolescents with depressive symptoms (Morgan and Jorm 2008). In a systematic literature search on the effectiveness of complementary and self-help treatment strategies for depression in children and adolescents, Jorm et al. (2006) found evidence for glutamine, *S*-adenosylmethionine, St. John's wort, vitamin C, omega-3 fatty acids, light therapy, massage, art therapy, bibliotherapy, distraction techniques, exercise, relaxation therapy, and sleep deprivation. However, the studies' quality was noted to be generally poor and the evidence therefore limited. The only intervention found to have "reasonable" support was light therapy for winter depression.

In a large community-based sample of 736 adolescents from the United Kingdom, physical activity did not protect against developing depressive symptoms over the 3-year period studied (Toseeb et al. 2014). However, in a recent systematic review and meta-analysis, Bailey et al. (2018) examined the treatment effect of exercise on depressive symptoms in individuals ages 12–25 years and found a large effect of physical activity on depression symptoms as compared with control subjects (standardized mean difference= -0.82; 95% CI= -1.02, -0.61; $P < 0.05$; $I^2 = 38\%$), but these results should be

TABLE 12–1. Self-help and complementary strategies for the treatment of subthreshold depressive symptoms

Bibliotherapy (e.g., a therapeutic approach that uses literature to bolster mental health)

Computerized interventions

Relaxation training

Light therapy

Art therapy

Massage

Distraction techniques

Exercise

Sleep deprivation

Supplements (e.g., glutamine, S-adenosylmethionine, St. John's wort, vitamin C, omega-3 fatty acids)

---

interpreted with caution, because there was concern about publication bias, and the quality of RCTs included was determined to be low (Bailey et al. 2018). Given the strong biological plausibility that exercise reverses depressive symptoms, there is a clear need to understand the benefits and optimal timing of exercise in developmental populations with depressive symptoms.

Combination Nutraceuticals Plus Psychotherapy

Recent literature indicates that combining nutraceuticals with psychotherapy may prevent escalation to MDD. In a 12-week pilot RCT of 72 youth ages 7–14 with MDD, depression not otherwise specified, or dysthymia, participants were randomly assigned to receive omega-3, psychoeducational psychotherapy (PEP) plus placebo, omega-3 plus PEP, or placebo. The omega-3 versus placebo intervention was double-masked. The individuals who received omega-3 combined with PEP showed greater behavioral improvement and trajectories compared with those taking placebo, with intent-to-treat analyses demonstrating small to medium effects of combined treatment ($d=0.29$) (Fristad et al. 2016).

Combination nutraceuticals plus psychotherapy: looking to the future

Roca et al. (2016) are currently investigating the role of multinutrient supplements (omega-3 fatty acids, calcium, selenium, and vitamins B_{11} and D_3) and food-related behavioral change therapy in the prevention of

MDD in overweight individuals with subthreshold depression in an RCT. The investigators are currently recruiting adults from four European cities, but results from this trial could potentially inform treatment strategies for younger individuals (Roca et al. 2016).

Summary

When clinicians are evaluating youth for depression, the concept of staging can be particularly helpful. The prodromal (subthreshold) phase may be an important time to intervene in order to prevent progression to MDD and decrease severity and length of illness. Pharmacotherapy is not recommended for youth with subthreshold depression, but both CBT and IPT have shown benefit for the treatment of subthreshold depression. Particularly if the child or adolescent has risk factors such as family history or medical illness, the mental health practitioner may want to consider early intervention. Although study quality is generally poor regarding outcomes of self-help strategies in children and adolescents, these strategies may be reasonable first-line interventions in less severe cases of subthreshold depression, particularly if the patient has few risk factors for progression to MDD or if youth live in areas where mental health resources are limited.

Clinical Pearls

- Subthreshold depression is common, and its presence increases the risk for the subsequent development of major depressive disorder (MDD), psychosocial dysfunction, substance use, and many other negative outcomes.

- Risk factors for subthreshold depression include family history of depression, racial/ethnic minority status, conflicts with parents, and physical abuse in the home.

- An increase in the number of symptoms that cluster raises the subthreshold depressed youth's chances of developing MDD.

- One of the following scales should be used to screen for depressive symptoms in youth: the Center for Epidemiologic Studies—Depression Scale, Beck Depression Inventory, Children's Depression Inventory, Reynolds Adolescent Depression Scale, or Mood and Feelings Questionnaire.

- If resources are available, clinicians should intervene early on in the course of depressive illness in youth with subthreshold depression.

- Cognitive-behavioral therapy or interpersonal psychotherapy should be considered for youth with subthreshold depression who are at high risk for subsequent development of MDD.

- Youth with mild subthreshold depressive symptoms should try self-help strategies.

Subthreshold Manic Symptoms

Subthreshold manic symptoms are defined simply as the presence of manic symptoms in the absence of a full-threshold bipolar disorder. They usually are considered to be *episodic* and not explained by other disorders, such as attention-deficit/hyperactivity disorder (ADHD) or anxiety. They also generally must be *clustered* (i.e., temporally co-occurring); thus, increased energy one week and elated mood the next would not qualify in the absence of other symptoms. Beyond these basic criteria, the severity, frequency, and duration of symptoms vary greatly. For example, a child who has periods of excitable mood and hyperactivity lasting just a few hours might be considered, by some standards, to have subthreshold manic symptoms. A child with periods of elation, increased energy, more creativity and productivity, and decreased need for sleep lasting 2 days also would be considered to have subthreshold manic symptoms, because these periods would not meet criteria for hypomania. Clearly, the implications for these two presentations might be very different, and it is thus helpful to think of subthreshold manic symptoms along a continuum.

Here, we distinguish between subthreshold manic *symptoms* and subthreshold manic *episodes*. The latter are defined according to criteria from the Course and Outcome of Bipolar Youth (COBY) study (Birmaher et al. 2006): distinct periods of abnormally elevated or irritable mood plus 1) at least two associated DSM-IV (American Psychiatric Association 1994) manic symptoms (three if the mood is irritable only), 2) a clear change in functioning, and 3) symptom duration of at least 4 hours for a minimum of 4 lifetime days. In contrast, subthreshold manic symptoms are episodic and clustered but do not fit these more stringent criteria. Individuals with subthreshold manic episodes, but not those with just subthreshold manic symptoms, would meet criteria for bipolar disorder not otherwise specified in DSM-IV and other specified bipolar and related disorder in DSM-5.

Epidemiology

Several studies have assessed the rate of subthreshold manic symptoms in the general population. Overall, a surprising finding of these studies is that subthreshold manic symptoms are relatively common in children and adolescents, ranging from 5% to 25.1% (Carlson and Kashani 1988); the rates of subthreshold manic episodes are 1%–2% (Stringaris et al. 2010). Of course, it is fairly difficult to tease out whether these symptoms are episodic, clustered, and not attributable to other disorders in large population-based studies, so this prevalence rate likely includes false-positive results.

Regardless, epidemiological studies generally show that subthreshold manic symptoms are associated with at least some impairment, although the degree of impairment varies greatly by study. Tijssen et al. (2010a) used data from the Early Developmental Stages of Psychopathology study, which included 3,021 adolescents and young adults (14–24 years old), and found that most of the youth who experienced subthreshold manic symptoms, and even full-threshold episodes, never presented for clinical treatment; however, the proportion in treatment did increase with the number of endorsed manic symptoms. In a relatively small study of 150 youth 14–16 years old, Carlson and Kashani (1988) found that the 20 adolescents endorsing manic symptoms also were more likely to have externalizing disorders, anxiety disorders, and psychotic disorders, as well as functional impairment. Similarly, in a community study of 5,326 individuals 8–19 years old, Stringaris and colleagues (2010) found that youth with subthreshold manic episodes were more likely to have externalizing disorders and, even after comorbidity was accounted for, experienced more social impairment than did those who did not have subthreshold manic episodes. Interestingly, there may be different "flavors" of subthreshold manic symptoms that might have very different functional implications. In a factor analysis, Stringaris et al. (2011) found that a certain cluster of manic symptoms ("episodic under control") was associated with impairment in function, whereas another cluster ("exuberance") was not, after adjustment for the first factor; findings were replicated in a population-based study in Brazil (Pan et al. 2014).

Another important question is whether subthreshold manic symptoms, in population-based samples, portend the later development of full-threshold bipolar disorder in adulthood. Epidemiological evidence indicates that most youth with subsyndromal manic symptoms will not develop full-threshold bipolar disorder; however, the presence of such symptoms does seem to increase the probability of this transition. In the Early Developmental Stages of Psychopathology study, Tijssen et al. (2010b) found that even fleeting hypomanic symptoms (experienced by 25% of the sample over two assessments) were associated with a dose-dependent increase in the odds of developing (hypo)manic episodes, and this relationship was even more pronounced with persistent symptoms; however, the absolute risk of hypomania in adulthood was still relatively low (<5%), even in the persistently symptomatic group.

From the Tracking Adolescents' Individual Lives Survey, a prospective community-based survey, authors assessed the relationship between subthreshold manic symptoms at age 11 years (as measured by the Child Behavior Checklist—Mania Scale; CBCL-MS) and bipolar disorder onset by age 19 in 1,429 adolescents. They found that those who were highly symptomatic had a fivefold increased risk of new-onset bipolar disorder compared with the normative group; those with mild symptoms were twice as likely as the normative youth to develop bipolar disorder by age 19 (Papachristou et al. 2017). Even in the 198 highly symptomatic youth, only 15 (7.6%) developed full-threshold bipolar disorder. Lewinsohn et al. (2000a) followed up 1,507 adolescents, 893 into adulthood (24 years old), as part of the OADP; 48 had subthreshold bipolar disorder during adolescence. These authors found that subthreshold bipolar disorder during adolescence was predictive of psychopathology in general, major depression, anxiety, and personality disorders; however, only 2.1% of the adolescents with subsyndromal bipolar disorder developed full-threshold bipolar disorder by early adulthood.

In contrast to the previously described studies, the Longitudinal Investigation of Bipolar Spectrum study found quite high rates of conversion to full-threshold bipolar I and II disorder. This study identified college-age participants whose symptoms met criteria for a subthreshold manic episode ($n=57$), after screening 20,500 college students for elevated manic symptoms, and then conducted diagnostic interviews on a subset of those who screened positive. Over a prospective 4-year follow-up, 52% of these young adults developed full-threshold bipolar I or II disorder within 4.5 years (Alloy et al. 2012). Two possible reasons account for the discrepancy between these conversion rates and those found in other community-recruited samples. First, Alloy and colleagues used a staged approach, screening many students and then performing a full diagnostic interview on participants who screened positive; thus, data quality was likely higher than in pure epidemiological studies that do not involve detailed assessments. Second, this study assessed conversion from subthreshold manic episodes in college students; these episodes in a transitional age range may be more predictive of conversion than in younger samples. This study provides evidence that subthreshold manic episodes in college students, when measured by thorough clinical assessment, are likely to convert to full-threshold bipolar I or II disorder within the next 5 years and thus should be monitored closely.

Family History Studies

One of the most potent risk factors for the development of bipolar disorder in adolescents is familial risk, particularly having a parent with a diagnosis of bipolar disorder. Because of this vulnerability, it is especially important to assess and longitudinally monitor subthreshold manic symptoms in youth with a family history of bipolar disorder. It is also imperative to assess for family history of bipolar disorder in youth, especially when treatment options for other symptoms are being considered. As might be expected, children and adolescents at familial risk for bipolar disorder have higher levels of subthreshold manic symptoms (Shaw et al. 2005).

The effect of these symptoms on the development of bipolar disorder also appears to be more pronounced in youth with a family history of bipolar disorder. In the Pittsburgh Bipolar Offspring Study (BIOS), a prospective study of offspring of bipolar parents and healthy control subjects, subthreshold manic symptoms were found to be an important predictor of progression, particularly during the few years before conversion. Individuals who had new-onset subthreshold manic symptoms, in the context of other risk factors (e.g., mood lability, early age at parental mood onset), had a 50% chance of developing new-onset bipolar spectrum disorder (Hafeman et al. 2016). Also, in the BIOS sample, rates of progression from subthreshold manic episodes to full-threshold bipolar disorder were substantial: of 58 participants with subthreshold manic episodes (i.e., bipolar disorder not otherwise specified), 14 (24.1%) converted to bipolar I or II disorder (Birmaher et al. 2018). In the Dutch Bipolar Offspring Study, participants who developed bipolar I or II disorder ($n = 10$) had higher levels of elated mood and decreased need for sleep (Mesman et al. 2017a).

Clinically Recruited Samples

Although population and family history studies are informative regarding the nosology and epidemiology of disorder, they do not provide accurate information about patients who will present in a clinical setting. A clinical sample is, by definition, selected to have more impairment and often a more pernicious form of the disorder. Just as it is important not to make inferences about the general population based on a clinically recruited sample, the inverse is also true. Indeed, in clinic-based studies, rates of subthreshold manic symptoms are higher, which is unsurprising given that the epidemiological studies show that they cause functional impairment and are associated with a wide range of psychiatric disorders. In the Longitudinal Assessment of Manic Symptoms study, 43% of the youth presenting to outpatient psychiatry clinics had "elevated symptoms of mania" (based on the score of >10 on the Parent General Behavior Inventory–10; PGBI-10, see "Assessment" subsection later in this chapter for details) (Horwitz et al. 2010). Elevated symptoms of mania were associated with greater functional impairment in this clinically recruited sample and higher levels of both internalizing and externalizing symptoms (Findling et al. 2010). Consistent with epidemiological studies that have found high levels of transient manic symptoms in youth, most of the youth with elevated symptoms of mania showed a decrease in these symptoms during the 6–12 months following assessment. However, a sizable minority (15%) did have persistent elevated symptoms of mania, and of these, 18% (18 of 100) converted to bipolar spectrum disorder within the next 48 months (Findling et al. 2013).

Adolescents who present with major depression are also at increased risk for developing bipolar disorder, so subsyndromal manic symptoms are especially important to assess. In one of the first studies to prospectively assess children and adolescents with depression, Strober and Carlson (1982) followed up 60 adolescents, who had been hospitalized for depression, for 3–4 years. They found that 20% of these individuals developed bipolar disorder; psychopharmacologically induced hypomania was an important predictor of conversion, as were rapid onset of symptoms, psychotic features, and family history of mood disorders (especially bipolar disorder) (Strober and Carlson 1982). Similarly, in an RCT testing the effect of multifamily psychoeducational psychotherapy (MF-PEP), Nadkarni and Fristad (2010) assessed youth with major depression for *transient manic symptoms*, defined as at least one manic symptom present for 4 hours or longer (or two episodes lasting 2 hours), associated with functional impairment and not attributable to other psychiatric disorders (e.g., ADHD). The authors found that 48% of 27 youth with major depression and transient manic symptoms converted to bipolar spectrum disorder in 18-month follow-up (Nadkarni and Fristad 2010). Kochman et al. (2005) conducted a 2-year prospective study in 80 children and adolescents with major depression, evaluating dimensional symptoms and cyclothymic-hypersensitive temperament with a questionnaire derived from the Cyclothymic Subscale of the Temperament Evaluation of the Memphis, Pisa, Paris, and San Diego Autoquestionnaire (TEMPS-A); 43% of these youth converted to bipolar disorder during follow-up, and this conversion was more likely in those individuals who had high cyclothymic-hypersensitive temperament scores (64% converted). Studies in adults also indicate that the presence of hypomanic symptoms in individuals with major depression is an important predictor of progression to bipolar disorder (Akiskal et al. 1995; Fiedorowicz et al. 2011; Tohen et al. 2012).

In addition, the rates of progression from subthreshold manic episodes to full-threshold bipolar disorder are quite high in clinically recruited samples. In the COBY study, 45% (63 of 140) of the youth with subthreshold manic episodes at baseline converted to bipolar I or II disorder over a 5-year follow-up period; rates of conversion were even higher (58.5%) in those who had a family history of mania (first- or second-degree relative) (Axelson et al. 2011). In the MF-PEP RCT, as just discussed, 9 of 27 youth (33%) who had subthreshold manic episodes at intake converted to bipolar I or II disorder. Conversion rates were 45%–50% in the subset of youth who had a first-degree relative with bipolar disorder or a "loaded pedigree" for unipolar depression (Martinez and Fristad 2013). These high rates of conversion do call into question whether subsyndromal bipolar disorder is part of the prodrome for bipolar I or II disorder or whether it is in fact a manifestation of the disorder itself. Indeed, youth with sub-threshold manic episodes have a family history of bipolar I or II disorder, risk for suicidality and substance abuse, and psychosocial impairment comparable to those in youth with bipolar I or II disorder (Axelson et al. 2006; Goldstein et al. 2010, 2011; Hafeman et al. 2013).

Summary

Taken together, studies with disparate designs and recruitment strategies point to the following conclusions. First, transient subthreshold manic symptoms are fairly common in childhood and adolescence. These symptoms are associated with functional impairment and both internalizing and externalizing disorders, but they do not necessarily imply a later diagnosis of bipolar I or II disorder, at least in community samples. However, they likely increase risk, particularly if they are persistent. Second, these symptoms are more prevalent in youth with a family history of bipolar disorder and are also more likely to progress to full-threshold bipolar I or II disorder in these youth. Third, subsyndromal manic episodes, particularly those that are severe enough to require clinical treatment, are associated with significant impairment and suicidal ideation and are highly likely to progress to bipolar I or II disorder; rates are even more elevated in those with a family history. One remaining question is whether subthreshold manic episodes in youth who do not require clinical treatment and do not have a family history are likely to progress to full-threshold bipolar I or II disorder. The carefully conducted study in university students discussed earlier, by Alloy and colleagues, showed high rates of conversion, but no comparable study has been done in adolescents younger than 18 years, in whom such episodes may be developmentally limited.

Assessment

The following instruments have been used frequently in clinical settings to assess manic symptoms in youth; note that this list is not comprehensive:

- **Kiddie Schedule for Affective Disorders and Schizophrenia (K-SADS) Mania Rating Scale (KMRS):** This clinician-administered scale derived from the K-SADS Screen and Mania Supplement assesses the presence and severity of individual manic symptoms. This scale has been used in the Pittsburgh BIOS to assess for the presence of manic symptoms longitudinally in at-risk youth, even in the absence of episodes that would meet criteria for bipolar disorder not otherwise specified. KMRS score was found to predict new-onset bipolar disorder in youth at familial risk, especially in the next 2–5 years (Hafeman et al. 2016).

- **Child Behavior Checklist—Mania Scale (parent-report):** The CBCL-MS, developed by Papachristou et al. (2013), is based on 19 items from the Child Behavior Checklist. The scale was found to have high internal consistency and to discriminate between youth with bipolar I disorder and healthy control subjects (area under the curve [AUC] = 0.64). Youth with bipolar I disorder also had higher scores on the CBCL-MS than did youth with anxiety ($P=0.004$) and MDD ($P=0.002$), but not compared with youth with oppositional defiant disorder (ODD) or ADHD. In a longitudinal community study of Dutch adolescents, Papachristou et al. (2017) found that those in mildly and highly symptomatic classes (based on their CBCL-MS scores at age 11) were at a two- and fivefold risk, respectively, to develop new-onset bipolar disorder by age 19 years. After adjustment for confounders, this scale was not predictive of new-onset anxiety or depression, although those youth in the highly symptomatic class were more likely to have diagnoses of ADHD, ODD, and conduct disorder.

- **General Behavioral Inventory, Revised (self-report and parent-report):** This extensive inventory was developed to screen for bipolar disorder and unipolar depression (Depue et al. 1989). It consists of two subscales to assess depression and hypomanic or biphasic symptoms. Several scales have been developed based on the GBI, including shortened scales (Mesman et al. 2017b); a shortened parent-report of the GBI (PGBI-10) (Youngstrom et al. 2008); and a self-report of the GBI in adolescents (Danielson et al. 2003). In the Longitudinal Assessment of

Manic Symptoms study, high or unstable PGBI-10 scores were associated with elevated rates of conversion to bipolar spectrum disorder over a 24-month follow-up ($P < 0.001$) (Findling et al. 2013).

- **Children's Affective Lability Scale (CALS) (self-report and parent-report):** This scale, developed by Gerson et al. (1996), includes both self- and parent-report versions that assess for sudden and intense changes in mood. Based on an analysis from the Pittsburgh BIOS, the CALS has three factors (anxiety/depression, irritability, and mania), all of which were highest in offspring with bipolar disorder, intermediate in nonbipolar offspring of parents with bipolar disorder, and lowest in control offspring; the irritability factor was most important (Birmaher et al. 2013). CALS score also was found to predict new-onset bipolar disorder over follow-up (Hafeman et al. 2016).

- **Cyclothymic-hypersensitive temperament questionnaire (child and adolescent version):** This questionnaire is derived from the TEMPS-A (Kochman et al. 2005) and assesses both cyclothymic and hypersensitivity factors. It has been adapted for adolescents. It assesses primarily mood lability and emotion reactivity. High scores on this scale were found to be predictive of new-onset bipolar disorder in adolescents with major depression.

Assessment of Risk

Although assessing implications for subthreshold manic symptoms on a group level is an important first step, clinically we are most interested in the implications for an individual patient. Given the presence of subthreshold manic symptoms or episodes, what are the chances that disorder will progress? Such information can help when discussing prognosis with a patient and family, as well as making clinical decisions about the frequency of monitoring and possibly the type of treatment indicated (Table 12–2). To this end, risk calculators have been used in other areas of medicine to estimate the probability of a given outcome. In psychiatry, recent work has focused on developing risk calculators for predicting psychosis in clinically defined high-risk populations (Cannon et al. 2016; Carrión et al. 2016) and general outpatient clinics (Fusar-Poli et al. 2017). We recently developed a risk calculator to predict 5-year new-onset bipolar spectrum disorder in 412 youth at familial risk for the disorder (from the BIOS sample) (Figure 12–1). We used predictors identified from a meta-analysis of prodromal symptoms (Van Meter et al. 2011) to build the risk calculator that includes subsyndromal manic symptoms, depressive symptoms, mood lability, anxiety, global psychosocial function, and

TABLE 12–2.   Clinical utility for a risk calculator in practice

If replicated, risk calculators have the potential to inform clinical practice in the following ways:

Inform discussions regarding prognosis—A clinician may or may not provide the actual quantification of risk, so this number can help guide discussion about future expectations.

Inform frequency of follow-up—This might be especially true if starting a patient on an SSRI.

Choose an appropriate therapeutic intervention—If risk is high, the clinician should consider a therapy that is more specific for the prevention of bipolar disorder, such as IPSRT or FFT.

Choose between medication classes —Although this is currently not possible, research using the risk calculator will hopefully inform risks and benefits of SSRIs vs. mood stabilizers in youth who are at low vs. medium vs. high risk for conversion to bipolar disorder.

Note.   FFT=family-focused therapy; IPSRT=interpersonal and social rhythm therapy; SSRI=selective serotonin reuptake inhibitor.

parental age at mood disorder onset. This risk calculator discriminated well between individuals who would develop new-onset bipolar spectrum disorder in the next 5 years and those who would not; the AUC for this model was 0.76, comparable to risk calculators used in other areas of medicine. From the COBY sample, we have built a risk calculator to predict progression from subthreshold manic episodes to bipolar I or II disorder (see Birmaher et al. 2018). Both risk calculators are available for use at www.pediatricbipolar.pitt.edu/resources.

Treatment Options

How does the presence of subthreshold manic symptoms (those not meeting criteria for other specified bipolar and related disorder) affect treatment? This depends in part on family history (when subthreshold manic symptoms are more likely to be a prodrome for bipolar disorder onset) and the accompanying presentation. Data are limited on the treatment of subthreshold manic symptoms in the general population, particularly in youth. However, studies have been done on the treatment of such symptoms in youth with a family history of bipolar disorder. In addition, from the adult literature, there is some evidence for treatment of depression with subthreshold manic symptoms (so-called MDD with mixed features).

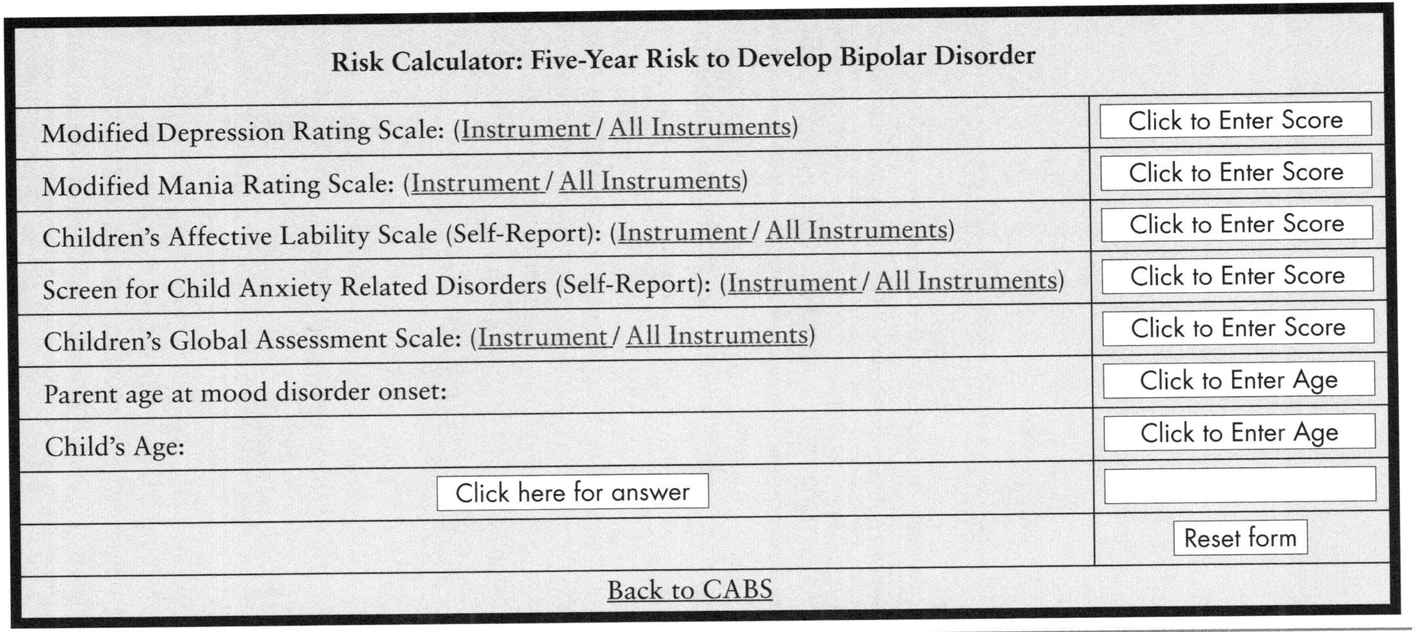

Risk Calculator: Five-Year Risk to Develop Bipolar Disorder

Modified Depression Rating Scale: (Instrument/ All Instruments)	Click to Enter Score
Modified Mania Rating Scale: (Instrument/ All Instruments)	Click to Enter Score
Children's Affective Lability Scale (Self-Report): (Instrument/ All Instruments)	Click to Enter Score
Screen for Child Anxiety Related Disorders (Self-Report): (Instrument/ All Instruments)	Click to Enter Score
Children's Global Assessment Scale: (Instrument/ All Instruments)	Click to Enter Score
Parent age at mood disorder onset:	Click to Enter Age
Child's Age:	Click to Enter Age
Click here for answer	
Back to CABS	Reset form

FIGURE 12–1. Risk calculator to predict 5-year onset of bipolar spectrum disorder in offspring of parents with bipolar disorder. This risk calculator is available at our Web site (www.pediatricbipolar.pitt.edu).

Subthreshold Manic Symptoms With a Major Depressive Episode

In DSM-5, a new specifier for major depression is "with mixed features," which is defined as an MDE with at least three concurrent manic symptoms. Researchers also have regularly included participants with only two concurrent manic features; however, they must be specific and not overlapping with depressive criteria (e.g., Suppes et al. 2016). From the adult literature, evidence indicates that individuals with these mixed features have poorer functioning, are more suicidal, and may have more treatment-resistant symptoms (Dudek et al. 2010; McIntyre et al. 2017). In an inpatient setting, approximately 9% of youth (38 of 407) were found to have symptoms that met criteria for MDD with mixed features, and these youth were found to have more suicidality and anger relative to those with unipolar depression or bipolar disorder (Frazier et al. 2017).

Regarding treatment of major depression in the context of subthreshold manic symptoms, previous work indicates that those with major depression plus subthreshold manic symptoms might have a poorer response to first-line treatments (i.e., selective serotonin reuptake inhibitors [SSRIs]) (Maalouf et al. 2012). Recent evidence indicates that lurasidone may be effective for the treatment of depression with mixed features in adults, associated with a decrease in both depressive and subthreshold manic symptoms (Suppes et al. 2016). No controlled studies have been conducted on the effect of atypical antipsychotics versus antidepressants to treat depression with mixed features in youth. From the current evidence, the standard of care would still be to try an SSRI as first-line treatment, given the evidence for treatment of depression and side-effect profile. An atypical antipsychotic such as lurasidone might be considered in depression with mixed features, particularly following failure of initial treatment with SSRIs, but data to support this approach are limited, especially in children.

Symptoms of Other Psychopathology and Mild Subthreshold Manic Symptoms

Although it would be important to monitor subthreshold manic symptoms closely, treatment in this case would be driven by the presenting problem. For example, the first-line treatment for anxiety with mild subthreshold manic symptoms would be evidence-based therapy (e.g., CBT or IPT), with consideration of an SSRI either in sequence or concomitantly. When considering the risks and benefits of an SSRI, the clinician should highlight the possibility of activation and increase in manic-like symptoms, particularly in someone who is already showing some subthreshold symptoms. A clinician also should consider the presence of family history, which also could increase risk for activation or the development of anti-depressant-related mania-like symptoms. In short, the presence of sub-threshold manic symptoms (even in the context of family history) would not change first-line psychotherapy or psychopharmacology but might influence the decision of whether to start with therapy or medication and the pace of dosing. A similar approach would be used for the treatment of ADHD in the context of subthreshold manic symptoms.

Offspring of Parents With Bipolar Disorder

Given that offspring of parents with bipolar disorder are more likely to have subthreshold manic symptoms and that these symptoms are more likely to progress to bipolar spectrum disorder (Hafeman et al. 2016) and, finally, bipolar I or II disorder (Axelson et al. 2011, 2015), there has been significant interest in testing both psychotherapeutic and pharmacological interventions that might change risk trajectories in those with family loading for bipolar disorder. Although these interventions have been developed specifically for this at-risk sample, they also might ameliorate subthreshold manic symptoms even in the absence of a family history, but this has not been tested.

Psychotherapy Interventions

Interpersonal and social rhythm therapy

Developed initially for adults with bipolar disorder, interpersonal and social rhythm therapy (IPSRT) focuses on regularizing daily routines (social rhythms) and coping with stress that arises from dealing with the illness as well as other sources and is often interpersonal in nature (Frank et al. 2005). In a study of 42 youth, ages 8–17 years, who were offspring of a parent with bipolar disorder, investigators found that IPSRT (vs. evidence-based referral) was associated with a decrease in subthreshold manic symptoms, a finding that was mediated by more regular sleep times (Goldstein et al. 2018).

Family-focused therapy

Initially developed for adolescents with bipolar disorder, family-focused therapy emphasizes psychoeducation, communication, and problem-solving skills in the child and family (Miklowitz et al. 2003). Investigators assessed the efficacy of this 12-week therapy in 9- to 17-year-old offspring of parents with bipolar disorder who had major depression, other specified bipolar and related disorder, or cyclothymia. They found not only that presenting mood symptoms decreased with the intervention (relative to an education control) but also that subthreshold manic (and depressive) symptoms decreased over time (Miklowitz et al. 2013). This was especially true in families with high *expressed emotion*, defined as a high-conflict and high-emotion communication style.

Multifamily psychoeducational psychotherapy

Developed for adolescents with mood disorders, MF-PEP consists of eight 90-minute sessions focused on educating the patient and family about mood disorders, medication, and coping and communication skills (Fristad et al. 2009). An additional post hoc analysis showed that MF-PEP appeared to decrease conversion of major depression plus transient manic symptoms (defined in the "Clinically Recruited Samples" subsection earlier in this chapter) to bipolar spectrum disorders. Of the study completers with this clinical presentation, the illness converted to bipolar spectrum disorders in 60% (9 of 15) of the control group but only 16.7% (2 of 12) of the MF-PEP group (Nadkarni and Fristad 2010).

Pharmacological Interventions

Limited trials have assessed the effect of mood stabilizers in youth with subthreshold manic episodes *and* family history of bipolar disorder, with mixed results. An early open study of quetiapine included 20 youth with affective disorders and a family history of bipolar disorder. Seventy-five percent (15 of 20) responded to quetiapine over the 12-week follow-up period; this response rate was 69.2% (9 of 13) in those with subsyndromal manic episodes (either bipolar disorder not otherwise specified or cyclothymia) (DelBello et al. 2007). However, this has not been replicated in an RCT. In addition, an RCT of divalproex in 56 youth with subsyndromal manic episodes and family history of bipolar I or II disorder yielded negative results; no significant effects were seen on overall discontinuation or discontinuation because of a mood episode ($P > 0.5$) (Findling et al. 2007). More recently, an RCT of aripiprazole (vs. placebo) in youth with subthreshold manic episodes and family history showed a greater decrease in manic symptoms in the active treatment group ($P = 0.005$) (Findling et al. 2017). Thus, even though evidence is limited, there is some indication from both an open trial and an RCT that atypical antipsychotics are effective in these youth; divalproex does not seem to be effective. To our knowledge, lithium has not been evaluated in youth with subthreshold mania but was not effective in prepubertal depressed children with a family history of mood disorder (Geller et al. 1998). In addition, there have not been trials of medication in youth with subsyndromal mania who do not have a positive family history.

Summary

When treatment options are being considered, it is important to consider the presenting problem, the presence and degree of subthreshold manic symptoms and/or episodes, and family history. To determine the proper treatment, it is useful to consider a staging model of subthreshold manic symptoms and episodes. Initial stages might consist of very mild hypomanic symptoms, which perhaps occur for only short periods of time, are not impairing, and do not meet criteria for bipolar spectrum disorder (stage 1a). Later stages would include symptoms that meet criteria for bipolar spectrum disorder, especially in the context of familial risk (stage 1b). On the basis of this model, we consider subthreshold manic symptoms to be an early indicator of possible bipolarity. However, epidemiological and clinical studies indicate that these symptoms also can be nonspecific and transient. Family history provides an important input about whether to simply treat the presenting symptom or perhaps to focus primarily on preventing progression of bipolar disorder. Thus, particularly when pharmacotherapy is being considered, it is important to weigh risks and benefits of each medication class in terms of both bipolar progression and general side-effect burden. In many cases, evidence-based psychotherapy may be tried first and may have a preferable risk-benefit analysis for many patients and families; this is especially true in the context of a family history. We also refer the reader to a previously published treatment algorithm for youth with family history of bipolar I or II disorder (Schneck et al. 2017).

Recommendations regarding psychotherapy

1. For stage 1a plus anxiety or ADHD, consider evidence-based therapies. If family history is positive, consider IPSRT.
2. For stage 1a plus MDE *or* stage 1b, consider MF-PEP. If family history is positive, consider family-focused therapy.

Recommendations regarding pharmacotherapy

1. For stage 1a plus anxiety or ADHD, consider evidence-based treatments (e.g., SSRIs, stimulants). If family history is positive, discuss risks and benefits of these medications with patient and family and alternatives

(e.g., psychotherapy, nonstimulants). Monitor carefully for activation or other side effects of medication.

2. For stage 1a plus MDE, consider SSRIs, which remain the first-line medication in this case, particularly when weighing potential side effects of mood stabilizers. Of note, a recent study in adults showed improvement in "mixed depression" with lurasidone, which has a better side-effect profile than other atypical antipsychotics. Studies have not yet been completed in youth, but this might be considered in the presence of persistent and impairing subthreshold manic symptoms, in the case of a family history, or after initial SSRI treatment failure.

3. For stage 1b, consider mood stabilizers, including atypical antipsychotics, the generally accepted first-line treatment for this stage. In particular, aripiprazole was found to decrease manic symptoms in youth with a family history. In stage 1b, with prominent anxiety or depressive symptoms, an SSRI might be considered; however, this could be associated with treatment-associated activation, and there is at least the theoretical possibility that this could hasten the progression of disorder. Especially for youth who are at stage 1b with a positive family history, the option of a mood stabilizer or an atypical antipsychotic (e.g., lurasidone) might be preferable.

Conclusion

The literature reviewed in this chapter shows that subthreshold mood symptoms are extremely important to assess in child and adolescent patients. These symptoms cause impairment even in the absence of full-threshold disorder, are associated with poor psychosocial function and other sequelae such as substance abuse, and predict further progression of disorder. Identification of subthreshold symptoms, particularly when associated with significant impairment, provides an important opportunity for early intervention. In some cases, the evaluation of these symptoms is critical to choosing the correct psychotropic medication (e.g., for other specified bipolar and related disorder). We have reviewed several measures that can be used to assess these subthreshold mood symptoms, by both self-report and parent report, as well as semi-structured interviews. Future research should focus on improving our ability to identify the youth at greatest risk for progression and use these predictive models to select treatment strategies that are stage-specific and effective.

Clinical Pearls

- Subthreshold mania occurs on a continuum, from transient subthreshold manic symptoms to subthreshold manic episodes, according to duration and symptom count.

- In depressed adolescents, as well as youth with a family history of bipolar disorder (BD), subthreshold manic symptoms may increase the likelihood of future BD onset and so should be assessed and monitored carefully.

- Subthreshold manic episodes cause significant functional impairment and increase the likelihood that a patient will develop BD I/II, particularly in a clinical setting and/or with a family history.

- Several scales are available for the assessment of subthreshold manic symptoms/episodes, including the K-SADS Mania Rating Scale and the General Behavioral Inventory.

- Risk calculators have been developed that can be used to quantify person-level risk for the onset of bipolar spectrum disorder (in youth with a family history) or progression from subthreshold manic episodes to BD I/II. These are freely available at www.pediatricbipolar.pitt.edu.

- Decisions regarding treatment for subthreshold mania should take into account severity of subthreshold mania (e.g., symptoms vs. episodes), other psychopathology, and family history.

References

Akiskal HS, Maser JD, Zeller PJ, et al: Switching from 'unipolar' to bipolar II: an 11-year prospective study of clinical and temperamental predictors in 559 patients. Arch Gen Psychiatry 52(2):114–123, 1995 7848047

Alloy LB, Uroševic S, Abramson LY, et al: Progression along the bipolar spectrum: a longitudinal study of predictors of conversion from bipolar spectrum conditions to bipolar I and II disorders. J Abnorm Psychol 121(1):16–27, 2012 21668080

American Psychiatric Association: Diagnostic and Statistical Manual of Mental Disorders, 3rd Edition, Revised. Washington, DC, American Psychiatric Association, 1987

American Psychiatric Association: Diagnostic and Statistical Manual of Mental Disorders, 4th Edition. Washington, DC, American Psychiatric Association, 1994

American Psychiatric Association: Diagnostic and Statistical Manual of Mental Disorders, 5th Edition. Arlington, VA, American Psychiatric Association, 2013

Arnberg A, Ost LG: CBT for children with depressive symptoms: a meta-analysis. Cogn Behav Ther 43(4):275–288, 2014 25248459

Axelson D, Birmaher B, Strober M, et al: Phenomenology of children and adolescents with bipolar spectrum disorders. Arch Gen Psychiatry 63(10):1139–1148, 2006 17015816

Axelson D, Birmaher B, Strober M, et al: Course of subthreshold bipolar disorder in youth: diagnostic progression from bipolar disorder not otherwise specified. J Am Acad Child Adolesc Psychiatry 50(10):1001.e3–1016.e3, 2011 21961775

Axelson D, Goldstein B, Goldstein T, et al: Diagnostic precursors to bipolar disorder in offspring of parents with bipolar disorder: a longitudinal study. Am J Psychiatry 172(7):638–646, 2015 25734353

Bailey AP, Hetrick SE, Rosenbaum S, et al: Treating depression with physical activity in adolescents and young adults: a systematic review and meta-analysis of randomised controlled trials. Psychol Med 48(7):1068–1083, 2018 28994355

Balázs J, Miklósi M, Keresztény A, et al: Adolescent subthreshold-depression and anxiety: psychopathology, functional impairment and increased suicide risk. J Child Psychol Psychiatry 54(6):670–677, 2013 23330982

Barbui C, Cipriani A, Patel V, et al: Efficacy of antidepressants and benzodiazepines in minor depression: systematic review and meta-analysis. Br J Psychiatry 198(1):11–16, 2011 21200071

Beck AT, Ward CH, Mendelson M, et al: An inventory for measuring depression. Arch Gen Psychiatry 4:561–571, 1961 13688369

Birmaher B, Axelson D, Strober M, et al: Clinical course of children and adolescents with bipolar spectrum disorders. Arch Gen Psychiatry 63(2):175–183, 2006 16461861

Birmaher B, Goldstein BI, Axelson DA, et al: Mood lability among offspring of parents with bipolar disorder and community controls. Bipolar Disord 15(3):253–263, 2013 23551755

Birmaher B, Merranko JA, Goldstein TR, et al: A risk calculator to predict the individual risk of conversion from subthreshold bipolar symptoms to bipolar disorder I or II in youth. J Am Acad Child Adolesc Psychiatry 57(10):755–763.e4, 2018 30274650

Cannon TD, Yu C, Addington J, et al: An individualized risk calculator for research in prodromal psychosis. Am J Psychiatry 173(10):980–988, 2016 27363508

Carlson GA, Kashani JH: Manic symptoms in a non-referred adolescent population. J Affect Disord 15(3):219–226, 1988 2975294

Carrión RE, Cornblatt BA, Burton CZ, et al: Personalized prediction of psychosis: external validation of the NAPLS-2 psychosis risk calculator with the EDIPPP project. Am J Psychiatry 173(10):989–996, 2016 27363511

Chen LS, Eaton WW, Gallo JJ, et al: Empirical examination of current depression categories in a population-based study: symptoms, course, and risk factors. Am J Psychiatry 157(4):573–580, 2000 10739416

Clarke GN, Hawkins W, Murphy M, et al: Targeted prevention of unipolar depressive disorder in an at-risk sample of high school adolescents: a randomized trial of a group cognitive intervention. J Am Acad Child Adolesc Psychiatry 34(3):312–321, 1995 7896672

Clarke GN, Hornbrook M, Lynch F, et al: A randomized trial of a group cognitive intervention for preventing depression in adolescent offspring of depressed parents. Arch Gen Psychiatry 58(12):1127–1134, 2001 11735841

Cosci F, Fava GA: Staging of mental disorders: systematic review. Psychother Psychosom 82(1):20–34, 2013 23147126

Costello EJ, Angold A: Scales to assess child and adolescent depression: checklists, screens, and nets. J Am Acad Child Adolesc Psychiatry 27(6):726–737, 1988 3058677

Cuijpers P, Smit F, van Straten A: Psychological treatments of subthreshold depression: a meta-analytic review. Acta Psychiatr Scand 115(6):434–441, 2007 17498154

Danielson CK, Youngstrom EA, Findling RL, et al: Discriminative validity of the General Behavior Inventory using youth report. J Abnorm Child Psychol 31(1):29–39, 2003 12597697

DelBello MP, Adler CM, Whitsel RM, et al: A 12-week single-blind trial of quetiapine for the treatment of mood symptoms in adolescents at high risk for developing bipolar I disorder. J Clin Psychiatry 68(5):789–795, 2007 17503991

Depue RA, Krauss S, Spoont MR, Arbisi P: General Behavior Inventory identification of unipolar and bipolar affective conditions in a nonclinical university population. J Abnorm Psychol 98(2):117–126, 1989 2708652

Dudek D, Rybakowski JK, Siwek M, et al: Risk factors of treatment resistance in major depression: association with bipolarity. J Affect Disord 126(1–2):268–271, 2010 20381154

Fava GA, Kellner R: Staging: a neglected dimension in psychiatric classification. Acta Psychiatr Scand 87(4):225–230, 1993 8488741

Fava GA, Tossani E: Prodromal stage of major depression. Early Interv Psychiatry 1(1):9–18, 2007 21352104

Fergusson DM, Horwood LJ, Ridder EM, et al: Subthreshold depression in adolescence and mental health outcomes in adulthood. Arch Gen Psychiatry 62(1):66–72, 2005 15630074

Fiedorowicz JG, Endicott J, Leon AC, et al: Subthreshold hypomanic symptoms in progression from unipolar major depression to bipolar disorder. Am J Psychiatry 168(1):40–48, 2011 21078709

Findling RL, Frazier TW, Youngstrom EA, et al: Double-blind, placebo-controlled trial of divalproex monotherapy in the treatment of symptomatic youth at high risk for developing bipolar disorder. J Clin Psychiatry 68(5):781–788, 2007 17503990

Findling RL, Youngstrom EA, Fristad MA, et al: Characteristics of children with elevated symptoms of mania: the Longitudinal Assessment of Manic Symptoms (LAMS) study. J Clin Psychiatry 71(12):1664–1672, 2010 21034685

Findling RL, Jo B, Frazier TW, et al: The 24-month course of manic symptoms in children. Bipolar Disord 15(6):669–679, 2013 23799945

Findling RL, Youngstrom EA, Rowles BM, et al: A double-blind and placebo-controlled trial of aripiprazole in symptomatic youths at genetic high risk for bipolar disorder. J Child Adolesc Psychopharmacol 27(10):864–874, 2017 28759262

Frank E, Kupfer DJ, Thase ME, et al: Two-year outcomes for interpersonal and social rhythm therapy in individuals with bipolar I disorder. Arch Gen Psychiatry 62(9):996–1004, 2005 16143731

Frazier EA, Swenson LP, Mullare T, et al: Depression with mixed features in adolescent psychiatric patients. Child Psychiatry Hum Dev 48(3):393–399, 2017 27349656

Fristad MA, Verducci JS, Walters K, et al: Impact of multifamily psychoeducational psychotherapy in treating children aged 8 to 12 years with mood disorders. Arch Gen Psychiatry 66(9):1013–1021, 2009 19736358

Fristad MA, Vesco AT, Young AS, et al: Pilot randomized controlled trial of omega-3 and individual-family psychoeducational psychotherapy for children and adolescents with depression. J Clin Child Adolesc Psychol 7:1–14, 2016 27819485

Fusar-Poli P, Rutigliano G, Stahl D, et al: Development and validation of a clinically based risk calculator for the transdiagnostic prediction of psychosis. JAMA Psychiatry 74(5):493–500, 2017 28355424

Geller B, Cooper TB, Zimerman B, et al: Lithium for prepubertal depressed children with family history predictors of future bipolarity: a double-blind, placebo-controlled study. J Affect Disord 51(2):165–175, 1998 10743849

Georgiades K, Lewinsohn PM, Monroe SM, et al: Major depressive disorder in adolescence: the role of subthreshold symptoms. J Am Acad Child Adolesc Psychiatry 45(8):936–944, 2006 16865036

Gerson AC, Gerring JP, Freund L, et al: The Children's Affective Lability Scale: a psychometric evaluation of reliability. Psychiatry Res 65(3):189–198, 1996 9029668

Goldstein BI, Shamseddeen W, Axelson DA, et al: Clinical, demographic, and familial correlates of bipolar spectrum disorders among offspring of parents with bipolar disorder. J Am Acad Child Adolesc Psychiatry 49(4):388–396, 2010 20410731

Goldstein TR, Obreja M, Shamseddeen W, et al: Risk for suicidal ideation among the offspring of bipolar parents: results from the Bipolar Offspring Study (BIOS). Arch Suicide Res 15(3):207–222, 2011 21827311

Goldstein TR, Merranko J, Krantz M, et al: Early intervention for adolescents at-risk for bipolar disorder: a pilot randomized trial of interpersonal and social rhythm therapy (IPSRT). J Affect Disord 235:348–356, 2018 29665518

Hafeman D, Axelson D, Demeter C, et al: Phenomenology of bipolar disorder not otherwise specified in youth: a comparison of clinical characteristics across the spectrum of manic symptoms. Bipolar Disord 15(3):240–252, 2013 23521542

Hafeman DM, Merranko J, Axelson D, et al: Toward the definition of a bipolar prodrome: dimensional predictors of bipolar spectrum disorders in at-risk youths. Am J Psychiatry 173(7):695–704, 2016 26892940

Hetrick SE, Parker AG, Hickie IB, et al: Early identification and intervention in depressive disorders: towards a clinical staging model. Psychother Psychosom 77(5):263–270, 2008 18560251

Hill RM, Pettit JW, Lewinsohn PM, et al: Escalation to major depressive disorder among adolescents with subthreshold depressive symptoms: evidence of distinct subgroups at risk. J Affect Disord 158:133–138, 2014 24655777

Horwitz SM, Demeter CA, Pagano ME, et al: Longitudinal Assessment of Manic Symptoms (LAMS) study: background, design, and initial screening results. J Clin Psychiatry 71(11):1511–1517, 2010 21034684

Jonsson U, Bohman H, von Knorring L, et al: Mental health outcome of long-term and episodic adolescent depression: 15-year follow-up of a community sample. J Affect Disord 130(3):395–404, 2011 21112639

Jorm AF, Allen NB, O'Donnell CP, et al: Effectiveness of complementary and self-help treatments for depression in children and adolescents. Med J Aust 185(7):368–372, 2006 17014404

Judd LL, Kunovac JL: Bipolar and unipolar depressive disorders in geriatric patients, in Mental Disorders in the Elderly: New Therapeutic Approaches. Edited by Brunello N, Langer SZ, Racagni G. Basel, S Karger, 1998, pp 1–10

Keenan K, Hipwell A, Feng X, et al: Subthreshold symptoms of depression in preadolescent girls are stable and predictive of depressive disorders. J Am Acad Child Adolesc Psychiatry 47(12):1433–1442, 2008 19034189

Klein DN, Shankman SA, Lewinsohn PM, Seeley JR: Subthreshold depressive disorder in adolescents: predictors of escalation to full-syndrome depressive disorders. J Am Acad Child Adolesc Psychiatry 48(7):703–710, 2009 19465876

Kochman FJ, Hantouche EG, Ferrari P, et al: Cyclothymic temperament as a prospective predictor of bipolarity and suicidality in children and adolescents with major depressive disorder. J Affect Disord 85(1–2):181–189, 2005 15780688

Kovacs M: The Children's Depression Inventory (CDI). Psychopharmacol Bull 21(4):995–998, 1985 4089116

Lawton A, Moghraby OS: Depression in children and young people: identification and management in primary, community and secondary care (NICE guideline CG28). Arch Dis Child Educ Pract Ed 101(4):206–209, 2016 26459492

Lewinsohn PM, Klein DN, Seeley JR: Bipolar disorder during adolescence and young adulthood in a community sample. Bipolar Disord 2(3 pt 2):281–293, 2000a 11249806

Lewinsohn PM, Solomon A, Seeley JR, Zeiss A: Clinical implications of "subthreshold" depressive symptoms. J Abnorm Psychol 109(2):345–351, 2000b 10895574

Lewinsohn PM, Klein DN, Durbin EC, et al: Family study of subthreshold depressive symptoms: risk factor for MDD? J Affect Disord 77(2):149–157, 2003 14607392

Luby JL, Gaffrey MS, Tillman R, et al: Trajectories of preschool disorders to full DSM depression at school age and early adolescence: continuity of preschool depression. Am J Psychiatry 171(7):768–776, 2014 24700355

Maalouf FT, Porta G, Vitiello B, et al: Do sub-syndromal manic symptoms influence outcome in treatment resistant depression in adolescents? A latent class analysis from the TORDIA study. J Affect Disord 138(1–2):86–95, 2012 22284022

Martinez MS, Fristad MA: Conversion from bipolar disorder not otherwise specified (BP-NOS) to bipolar I or II in youth with family history as a predictor of conversion. J Affect Disord 148(2–3):431–434, 2013 22959237

Martinovic Z, Simonovic P, Djokic R: Preventing depression in adolescents with epilepsy. Epilepsy Behav 9(4):619–624, 2006 17049927

McGorry PD, Purcell R, Goldstone S, et al: Age of onset and timing of treatment for mental and substance use disorders: implications for preventive intervention strategies and models of care. Curr Opin Psychiatry 24(4):301–306, 2011 21532481

McIntyre RS, Ng-Mak D, Chuang C-C, et al: Major depressive disorder with subthreshold hypomanic (mixed) features: a real-world assessment of treatment patterns and economic burden. J Affect Disord 210:332–337, 2017 28073041

Meeks TW, Vahia IV, Lavretsky H, et al: A tune in "a minor" can "b major": a review of epidemiology, illness course, and public health implications of subthreshold depression in older adults. J Affect Disord 129(1–3):126–142, 2011 20926139

Mesman E, Nolen WA, Keijsers L, et al: Baseline dimensional psychopathology and future mood disorder onset: findings from the Dutch Bipolar Offspring Study. Acta Psychiatr Scand 136(2):201–209, 2017a 28542780

Mesman E, Youngstrom EA, Juliana NK, et al: Validation of the Seven Up Seven Down Inventory in bipolar offspring: screening and prediction of mood disorders: findings from the Dutch Bipolar Offspring Study. J Affect Disord 207:95–101, 2017b 27718456

Miklowitz DJ, George EL, Richards JA, et al: A randomized study of family focused psychoeducation and pharmacotherapy in the outpatient management of bipolar disorder. Arch Gen Psychiatry 60(9):904–912, 2003 12963672

Miklowitz DJ, Schneck CD, Singh MK, et al: Early intervention for symptomatic youth at risk for bipolar disorder: a randomized trial of family focused therapy. J Am Acad Child Adolesc Psychiatry 52(2):121–131, 2013 23357439

Morgan AJ, Jorm AF: Self-help interventions for depressive disorders and depressive symptoms: a systematic review. Ann Gen Psychiatry 7:13, 2008 18710579

Nadkarni RB, Fristad MA: Clinical course of children with a depressive spectrum disorder and transient manic symptoms. Bipolar Disord 12(5):494–503, 2010 20712750

Nauta MH, Festen H, Reichart CG, et al: Preventing mood and anxiety disorders in youth: a multi-centre RCT in the high risk offspring of depressed and anxious patients. BMC Psychiatry 12:31, 2012 22510426

Pan PM, Salum GA, Gadelha A, et al: Manic symptoms in youth: dimensions, latent classes, and associations with parental psychopathology. J Am Acad Child Adolesc Psychiatry 53(6):625.e2–634.e2, 2014 24839881

Papachristou E, Ormel J, Oldehinkel AJ, et al: Child Behavior Checklist—Mania Scale (CBCL-MS): development and evaluation of a population-based screening scale for bipolar disorder. PLoS One 8(8):e69459, 2013 23967059

Papachristou E, Oldehinkel AJ, Ormel J, et al: The predictive value of childhood subthreshold manic symptoms for adolescent and adult psychiatric outcomes. J Affect Disord 212:86–92, 2017 28157551

Pincus HA, Davis WW, McQueen LE: Subthreshold mental disorders: a review and synthesis of studies on minor depression and other brand names. Br J Psychiatry 174:288–296, 1999 10533546

Pine DS, Cohen E, Cohen P, et al: Adolescent depressive symptoms as predictors of adult depression: moodiness or mood disorder? Am J Psychiatry 156(1):133–135, 1999 9892310

Radloff LS: The use of the Center for Epidemiologic Studies Depression Scale in adolescents and young adults. J Youth Adolesc 20(2):149–166, 1991 24265004

Reynolds W: A model for the screening and identification of depressed children and adolescents in school settings. Professional School Psychology 1(2):117–129, 1986

Roca M, Kohls E, Gili M, et al; MooDFOOD Prevention Trial Investigators: Prevention of depression through nutritional strategies in high-risk persons: rationale and design of the MooDFOOD prevention trial. BMC Psychiatry 16:192, 2016 27277946

Rohde P, Beevers CG, Stice E, et al: Major and minor depression in female adolescents: onset, course, symptom presentation, and demographic associations. J Clin Psychol 65(12):1339–1349, 2009 19827116

Schneck CD, Chang KD, Singh MK, et al: A pharmacologic algorithm for youth who are at high risk for bipolar disorder. J Child Adolesc Psychopharmacol 27(9):796–805, 2017 28731778

Shaw JA, Egeland JA, Endicott J, et al: A 10-year prospective study of prodromal patterns for bipolar disorder among Amish youth. J Am Acad Child Adolesc Psychiatry 44(11):1104–1111, 2005 16239857

Stice E, Rohde P, Seeley JR, et al: Brief cognitive-behavioral depression prevention program for high-risk adolescents outperforms two alternative interventions: a randomized efficacy trial. J Consult Clin Psychol 76(4):595–606, 2008 18665688

Stockings E, Degenhardt L, Lee YY, et al: Symptom screening scales for detecting major depressive disorder in children and adolescents: a systematic review and meta-analysis of reliability, validity and diagnostic utility. J Affect Disord 174:447–463, 2015 25553406

Stringaris A, Santosh P, Leibenluft E, et al: Youth meeting symptom and impairment criteria for mania-like episodes lasting less than four days: an epidemiological enquiry. J Child Psychol Psychiatry 51(1):31–38, 2010 19686330

Stringaris A, Stahl D, Santosh P, et al: Dimensions and latent classes of episodic mania-like symptoms in youth: an empirical enquiry. J Abnorm Child Psychol 39(7):925–937, 2011 21625986

Strober M, Carlson G: Bipolar illness in adolescents with major depression: clinical, genetic, and psychopharmacologic predictors in a three- to four-year prospective follow-up investigation. Arch Gen Psychiatry 39(5):549–555, 1982 7092488

Suppes T, Silva R, Cucchiaro J, et al: Lurasidone for the treatment of major depressive disorder with mixed features: a randomized, double-blind, placebo-controlled study. Am J Psychiatry 173(4):400–407, 2016 26552942

Szigethy E, Kenney E, Carpenter J, et al: Cognitive-behavioral therapy for adolescents with inflammatory bowel disease and subsyndromal depression. J Am Acad Child Adolesc Psychiatry 46(10):1290–1298, 2007 17885570

Takagaki K, Okamoto Y, Jinnin R, et al: Behavioral activation for late adolescents with subthreshold depression: a randomized controlled trial. Eur Child Adolesc Psychiatry 25(11):1171–1182, 2016 27003390

Tijssen MJ, van Os J, Wittchen HU, et al: Evidence that bipolar disorder is the poor outcome fraction of a common developmental phenotype: an 8-year cohort study in young people. Psychol Med 40(2):289–299, 2010a 19515266

Tijssen MJ, van Os J, Wittchen HU, et al: Prediction of transition from common adolescent bipolar experiences to bipolar disorder: 10-year study. Br J Psychiatry 196(2):102–108, 2010b 20118453

Tohen M, Khalsa HK, Salvatore P, et al: Two-year outcomes in first-episode psychotic depression: the McLean-Harvard First-Episode Project. J Affect Disord 136(1–2):1–8, 2012 21943929

Toseeb U, Brage S, Corder K, et al: Exercise and depressive symptoms in adolescents: a longitudinal cohort study. JAMA Pediatr 168(12):1093–1100, 2014 25317674

Van Meter AR, Moreira AL, Youngstrom EA: Meta-analysis of epidemiologic studies of pediatric bipolar disorder. J Clin Psychiatry 72(9):1250–1256, 2011 21672501

Wesselhoeft R, Sørensen MJ, Heiervang ER, Bilenberg N: Subthreshold depression in children and adolescents—a systematic review. J Affect Disord 151(1):7–22, 2013 23856281

Whalen DJ, Luby JL, Tilman R, et al: Latent class profiles of depressive symptoms from early to middle childhood: predictors, outcomes, and gender effects. J Child Psychol Psychiatry 57(7):794–804, 2016 26748606

Wilcox HC, Anthony JC: Child and adolescent clinical features as forerunners of adult-onset major depressive disorder: retrospective evidence from an epidemiological sample. J Affect Disord 82(1):9–20, 2004 15465572

Wittchen HU, Nelson CB, Lachner G: Prevalence of mental disorders and psychosocial impairments in adolescents and young adults. Psychol Med 28(1):109–126, 1998 9483687

Yamamoto A, Tsujimoto E, Taketani R, et al: The effect of interpersonal counseling for subthreshold depression in undergraduates: an exploratory randomized controlled trial. Depress Res Treat 2018:4201897, 2018 29682345

Young JF, Mufson L, Davies M: Efficacy of Interpersonal Psychotherapy–Adolescent Skills Training: an indicated preventive intervention for depression. J Child Psychol Psychiatry 47(12):1254–1262, 2006 17176380

Youngstrom EA, Frazier TW, Demeter C, et al: Developing a 10-item mania scale from the Parent General Behavior Inventory for children and adolescents. J Clin Psychiatry 69(5):831–839, 2008 18452343

13

Management of Suicidal Youth

Stephanie Clarke, Ph.D.

Erica Ragan, Ph.D.

Michele Berk, Ph.D.

Chloe, a 15-year-old girl, was referred for treatment by her school counselor after her teacher saw a series of horizontal scars on Chloe's arm. During the initial intake session, Chloe revealed that she had been cutting herself when she was "really upset about something." She stated that she had never attempted suicide but had thought about trying to overdose on her mother's prescription medication. Chloe's parents reported that Chloe had been skipping class, was not completing homework, and seemed to be up at all hours of the night. Chloe endorsed intense "ups and downs" in her mood and stated that these changes occurred without warning.

Suicide is a leading cause of death among youth in the United States and globally. In this chapter, we begin by reviewing statistics on suicidal behavior in youth in general and in youth with mood disorders. We then review current assessment approaches and best practices, general risk factors, and research examining risk factors in youth with mood disorders. We conclude with treatment recommendations for suicidal youth with mood disorders and clinical considerations in working with suicidal youth.

We use definitions and terminology that are most commonly used in the suicide literature. *Suicide* refers to the act of intentionally ending one's own life. *Suicidal ideation* refers to thoughts about engaging in behavior intended to end one's own life. *Suicide attempt* refers to self-injurious behavior associated with at least some intent to die (Silverman et al. 2007). *Nonsuicidal self-injurious behavior* refers to damage to one's bodily tissue through means such as cutting or burning oneself without intent to die (Nock and Prinstein 2005; Nock et al. 2006). With regard to mood disorders in this chapter, bipolar disorders encompass bipolar I disorder and bipolar II disorder. Depressive disorders include major depressive disorder (MDD) and persistent depressive disorder (dysthymia). Research studies have focused on youth with symptoms that meet diagnostic criteria for specific mood disorders. However, given that mood symptoms, regardless of diagnostic category, are a risk factor, strategies recommended here for youth with specific bipolar and unipolar depressive disorders also should be appropriate for youth with unspecified bipolar and unipolar depressive disorders.

Child and Adolescent Suicide: Overview

Epidemiology

The number of deaths by suicide among children and adolescents in the United States has increased dramatically in recent decades. National Comorbidity Survey Replication Adolescent Supplement (NCS-A; Nock et al. 2013) data show that lifetime prevalence of suicidal ideation is very low (<1%) through age 10 years, with a slow increase through 12 years and a rapid increase between 12 and 17 years. Although suicide attempts are rare before age 12 years, with a rate of 0.17 per 100,000 youth between ages 5 and 11 years (Centers for Disease Control and Prevention 2014), suicide was nevertheless ranked the tenth leading cause of death for elementary-age schoolchildren in 2014.

Death by suicide increases dramatically during adolescence (Glenn et al. 2017; Kõlves and de Leo 2017; Nock et al. 2013) and is the second leading cause of death among 15- to 24-year-old persons and the third leading cause of death for 10- to 14-year-old children in the United States (Centers for Disease Control and Prevention 2017). A 2015 national survey found that 17.7% of high school students had seriously considered making a suicide attempt, and 8.6% had made an attempt (Kann et al. 2016). More than one-third of adolescents who experience suicidal ideation go on to attempt suicide (Nock et al. 2013), and adolescents who experience suicidal ideation are 12 times more likely than adolescents who do not experience suicidal ideation to attempt suicide by age 30 (Reinherz et al. 2006). Furthermore, 86.1% of adolescents make an initial suicide attempt within 12 months of onset of suicidal ideation (Nock et al. 2013), and approximately half of the deaths by suicide in adolescents are the result of an initial attempt (Brent et al. 1988; Marttunen et al. 1991; Shaffer et al. 1996); thus, the need for swift intervention is critical once suicidal ideation has begun.

Mood Disorders

Mood disorders represent a significant risk factor for suicidal thoughts and behavior. A study comparing lethality of suicide attempts found that a mood disorder diagnosis, including unipolar depressive and bipolar disorders, was one of two significant distinguishing factors leading to suicide attempts with greater lethality (Beautrais 2003), the other being male gender, which was directly linked to males' use of lethal methods (e.g., firearms). Given that suicidal behavior is one of the diagnostic criteria for a major depressive episode, the association between mood disorders and suicidal behavior is unsurprising.

The NCS-A (Nock et al. 2013), the first national survey to assess a wide range of psychiatric disorders and suicidal behaviors in youth, found that the most prevalent lifetime disorder among suicidal adolescents was MDD, with 56.8% of youth with suicidal ideation and 75.7% of youth with a history of suicide attempts having symptoms that met diagnostic criteria for MDD or dysthymia. Psychological autopsy studies have shown that up to 60% of adolescents who die by suicide have a depressive disorder at the time of death (Brent et al. 1999; Marttunen et al. 1991; Shaffer et al. 1996). Similarly, other studies have found that a large proportion of adolescents with suicidal ideation or a history of a suicide attempt have symptoms that meet diagnostic criteria for depression (40%–80%; Andrews and Lewinsohn 1992; Beautrais et al. 1998; Goldston et al. 1998; Gould et al. 1998; Lewinsohn et al. 1996; Reinherz et al. 1995; Shaffer et al. 1996). In clinically referred samples, up to 85% of individuals diagnosed with MDD or dysthymia report suicidal ideation, 32% are purported to have made a suicide attempt during adolescence or young adulthood (Kovacs et al. 1993), and 20% will make repeat suicide attempts (Harrington et al. 1994). In summary, although most youth who present with suicidal behavior have symptoms that meet diagnostic criteria for a depressive disorder, two-thirds of adolescents will not go on to attempt suicide. Thus, depressive disorders are a significant risk factor for suicidal behavior; however, more needs to be understood about what leads a subset of adolescents with depressive disorders to go on to engage in suicidal behavior.

The NCS-A data also indicated that the odds of a suicide attempt in youth given a diagnosis of bipolar disorder are highest among all psychiatric disorders, with an odds ratio of 8.8 (Nock et al. 2013). Furthermore, bipolar disorders confer the highest risk for death by suicide among all psychiatric disorders across all age groups (Brent et al. 1993; Stanley et al. 2017). Studies show that up to 50% of youth with bipolar disorders will attempt suicide by age 18 (Bhangoo et al. 2003; Goldstein et al. 2012; Lewinsohn et al. 2003). A 2013 systematic review of more than 14 studies found that 50.4% of youth with bipolar disorder endorsed suicidal ideation, and 25.5% engaged in suicidal behavior; these rates are three times higher than the rates typically found in the general population (Kann et al. 2016). In addition, two longitudinal studies supported significant risk for death by suicide among youth diagnosed with bipolar disorders (Srinath et al. 1998; Welner et al. 1979). For preadolescent children, specifically, with a bipolar disorder diagnosis, studies reported rates of suicidal thoughts and behaviors ranging from 20% to 55% (Algorta et al. 2011; Goldstein et al. 2009; Jolin et al. 2007; Weinstein et al. 2015). A recent meta-analysis of studies comparing risk of suicide attempts in youth with different mood disorder diagnoses found that bipolar disorders represented a significantly higher risk for suicide attempt among adolescents than unipolar depression. Interestingly, bipolar disorders and unipolar depressive disorders were both associated with higher rates of suicide attempts compared with hypomania or mania without major depression (De Crescenzo et al. 2017). This would seem to suggest that dysphoric or depressive mood features are linked to suicidal behavior in mood disorders.

In summary, depressive and bipolar disorders are important risk factors for suicidal behavior in youth. A diagnosis of a bipolar disorder is associated with the highest rate of suicidal behavior and deaths by suicide of any psychiatric disorder across all age groups, whereas MDD is the most common disorder found in individuals who die by suicide. However, the relation between mood disorders and suicidal behavior is complex. For example, even though MDD is commonly found in individuals at risk for suicide, a substantial number of depressed adolescents never go on to experience suicidal behavior. Furthermore, although psychopathology, such as mood disorders, is consistently identified as a significant risk factor for suicide attempts in youth, research shows that suicidal behavior also may occur outside the context of a psychiatric diagnosis. Importantly, the growing consensus is that suicide attempts must be directly targeted in treatment rather than indirectly in the context of treating an underlying psychiatric disorder (Berk and Hughes 2015; Berk et al. 2004; Brent et al. 1997; Emslie et al. 2006; March et al. 2004). That is, simply reducing depressive symptoms may not be sufficient to reduce suicidal thoughts and behaviors.

Adolescent Suicide Assessment

In November 2016, the American Psychological Association released a statement titled "After Decades of Research, Science Is No Better Able to Predict Suicidal Behavior" (Sliwa 2016). Despite significant efforts, a standardized suicide risk assessment that accurately predicts suicidal behavior has not yet been identified. Most risk factors and warning signs have been found to be neither sensitive nor specific enough to accurately predict suicidal behavior (e.g., Lester et al. 2011; Ramchand et al. 2017). Many of the risk factors for suicide are also found in individuals who are not suicidal, resulting in high numbers of false-positive results when attempting to apply a standardized suicide risk assessment (Fowler 2012). The developmental psychopathology principle of *equifinality*—that there are many routes to a particular outcome (Cicchetti and Rogosch 2002)—perhaps best conceptualizes the path to suicidal behavior across the life span. Although actuarial models have been attempted (e.g., Cooper et al. 2006), it has been concluded that assessment and determination of intervention still rely on sound clinical judgment.

Suicide risk assessment should include direct questioning about suicidal ideation and intent, and suicide plans; access to lethal means; history of and current engagement in self-harming and suicidal behavior; and consideration of risk factors. It is important to gather information from the adolescent and caregiver(s), interviewing each independently about these factors, because they may be reluctant to discuss these topics openly and honestly in front of each other. Several structured clinical interviews are available to clinicians to aid with conducting and documenting a comprehensive risk assessment, such as the Columbia–Suicide Severity Rating Scale (Posner et al. 2011), the Linehan Risk Assessment and Management Protocol (Linehan et al. 2012), and the Collaborative Assessment and Management of Suicidal Behavior Framework Suicide Status Form (Jobes 2006). Self-report forms also may be used to gather information, such as the dialectical behavior therapy (DBT) "diary card," the Suicidal Ideation Questionnaire (Pinto et al. 1997), and the Beck Depression Inventory (Steer et al. 1998). Although these instruments may provide additional information to inform risk assessment, no agreed-on heuristic, benchmark, or cutoff scores for suicidal behavior predict which individuals at risk may attempt suicide at any given time.

It is important to document intervention strategies (e.g., written safety plan; see "Written Safety Plan" subsection later in this chapter) used for managing the adolescent's safety during outpatient treatment. It is also helpful to be explicit in documentation regarding decisions about the needed level of care (i.e., outpatient, intensive outpatient, partial hospitalization, inpatient hospitalization, residential treatment). For example, a teenager who agrees to follow a written safety plan and whose parents are willing to monitor her or him closely may be a good candidate for continued care in an outpatient setting, whereas a teenager who feels uncertain about her or his ability to ask for help when needed, who has suicidal ideation with a plan, and whose caregivers are unable to provide close supervision may be better served in a more restrictive level of care, such as an inpatient or a residential facility until the suicidal crisis has been adequately managed. Routine monitoring, assessment, and documentation of suicidal ideation, intent, or plans; nonsuicidal self-injury; and other risk factors for suicide should occur in each clinical contact (Fowler 2012; Rudd et al. 1999). Suicidal behavior should be regularly assessed even after immediate resolution of symptoms, given that suicidal behavior can wax and wane and that previous suicidal behavior is a nonmodifiable risk factor that is the most consistent predictor of future suicidal behavior (Chesin et al. 2017). The initial comprehensive risk assessment therefore serves as an important foundation from which to assess suicidality at each subsequent session throughout treatment.

Risk Factors for Suicidal Behavior in Adolescents

The literature has identified several risk factors for suicidal behavior in adolescents, many of which—but not all—are listed in the following subsections. As previously mentioned, identified risk factors are not sensitive or specific enough to determine risk for suicide attempt in the absence of clinical judgment. Nevertheless, studies generally have found that the probability of a suicide attempt increases as a function of the number of risk factors present (e.g., Lewinsohn et al. 1994). Risk factors have been categorized over the past decade to indicate which are modifiable (i.e., dynamic vs. static; Steele et al. 2018) and when they occur in time prior to suicidal behavior (i.e., distal vs. proximal; Franklin et al. 2017), with clinicians working toward reducing dynamic risk factors (e.g., family conflict;

Holland et al. 2017) for suicidal behavior and identifying proximal risk factors (e.g., sleep disturbance; Goldstein et al. 2008) that may signal an increased risk for imminent suicidal behavior. Researchers are still defining and determining proximal risk factors, and many studies consider a proximal risk factor to be one that occurs within 3–6 months of the suicide attempt (e.g., Czyz and King 2015; Ran et al. 2015; Yen et al. 2013). Several Web sites have lists of warning signs (i.e., behavioral indicators that a suicide attempt is imminent or likely to happen within hours to days; Rudd et al. 2006) for adolescent suicidal behavior, but little research supports these as indicators of an imminent suicidal crisis.

Suicidal Ideation

Longitudinal studies have documented increased risk for suicide attempts among adolescents with more severe (e.g., high intent) and pervasive (high frequency, long duration) suicidal ideation (Lewinsohn et al. 1996; R. Miranda et al. 2014b; Negron et al. 1997; Reinherz et al. 2006).

Previous Suicide Attempt

A previous suicide attempt is among the most consistent predictors of suicidal behavior and death by suicide (Chesin et al. 2017), with increased risk for reattempt persisting for at least 2 years and risk for reattempt highest in the first 3–6 months after the previous attempt (Goldston et al. 1999; Lewinsohn et al. 1996). High medical lethality attempts (e.g., hanging, shooting, or jumping) confer extremely high risk for repeat attempts and death by suicide (Bridge et al. 2006).

Suicidal Intent

The extent to which an individual wishes to die is a significant predictor of repeated suicide attempts and death by suicide (Bridge et al. 2006). For individuals who die by suicide, generally more evidence of planning is found in order to keep suicide plans confidential and reduce risk of detection (Brent et al. 1988).

Nonsuicidal Self-Injury

Nonsuicidal self-injury has been shown to confer a 10-fold risk for death by suicide among adolescents (Brent et al. 2013; Hawton and Harriss 2007). In both community and clinical samples of depressed adolescents, adolescent nonsuicidal self-injury has been shown to be a risk factor for suicide attempt in adolescence and adulthood, even when suicidal intent and previous suicide attempts were controlled for (Asarnow et al. 2011; Chesin et al. 2017; Wilkinson 2011; Wilkinson et al. 2011).

Precipitating Events

Interpersonal conflict and loss are the most common precipitating events for suicide attempts and death by suicide among adolescents (Beautrais 2000). In one study, family conflict was the most common antecedent to death by suicide (Holland et al. 2017), a finding that is consistently found in the psychological literature on adolescent suicide (e.g., Asarnow et al. 1987; Brent 1995; Fergusson and Lynskey 1995; Reinherz et al. 1995; Wilkinson et al. 2011). Several studies have found that loss of a parent through death, divorce, or living away from one or both parents is also a significant risk factor for death by suicide (Agerbo et al. 2002; Brent et al. 1994; Grøholt et al. 1997). When conflict or loss is coupled with substance abuse, risk for suicidal behavior is even greater (e.g., Brent et al. 1999; Gould et al. 1996). Being the victim or perpetrator of bullying also confers risk for suicidal behavior (Kim and Leventhal 2008).

Sexual Orientation and Gender Identity

Nonheterosexual orientation (e.g., gay, lesbian, bisexual) and transgender identity are associated with increased rates of suicide attempts, even when other risk factors, such as depression or alcohol abuse, are controlled for (Russell and Joyner 2001). Studies have found mediating effects of family rejection, victimization, and mood and substance abuse disorders on suicidal behavior among lesbian, gay, bisexual, or transgender–identified youth (Borowsky et al. 2001; Garofalo et al. 1999; Hatzenbuehler 2011; Liu and Mustanski 2012; Mustanski and Liu 2013).

Psychopathology

As discussed earlier, mood disorders confer considerable risk for suicidal behavior among adolescents. Other Axis I psychiatric disorders shown to confer increased risk for suicidal behavior include substance use disorders, attention-deficit/hyperactivity disorder (ADHD), conduct disorder and antisocial behavior, anxiety disorders, posttraumatic stress disorder, psychosis, and eating disorders (e.g., Bridge et al. 2006; Chronis-Tuscano et al. 2010). Psychiatric comorbidity is also a risk factor, with psychological autopsy studies showing that up to 70% of youth who die by suicide have more than one mental health diagnosis (Brent et al. 1999; Shaffer et al. 1996). Furthermore, the combination of mood, disruptive behavior, and substance use disorders is a powerful predictor of suicidal behavior among youth (Brent et al. 1999; Bridge et al. 2006). Similar to findings in adults, personality disorders and personality disorder characteristics are common in adolescents with suicidal behavior. It is estimated that approximately one-third of adolescents who die by suicide have a personality disorder, with antisocial, borderline, histrionic, and narcissistic personality disorders conferring an even greater risk for suicidal behavior (Brent et al. 1994). As previously mentioned, however, a psychiatric diagnosis is not present in all youth who engage in suicidal behavior; in fact, Brent and colleagues (1999) reported that approximately 40% of youth who died by suicide did not have symptoms that met diagnostic criteria for a psychiatric disorder. In these cases, youth were more likely to have engaged in suicidal behavior previously, have legal or disciplinary problems, and have access to a loaded gun (Marttunen et al. 1998).

Psychological and Personality Factors

Studies have shown mixed results regarding personality, cognitive, and other psychological factors in relation to suicidal behavior, with these factors in various contexts and combinations playing more or less of a role in suicidal behavior. Several studies have examined the association between impulsivity and impulsive aggression and suicidal behavior. With regard to impulsivity, a subset of adolescents attempt suicide with relatively little planning (Gunnell et al. 2000; Kashden et al. 1993; Kingsbury et al. 1999). Impulsive aggression, which refers to the tendency to react to provocation or frustration with aggression or hostility, has been shown to predispose individuals to suicidal behavior (Apter et al. 1995). Several studies support the role of impulsive aggression in the familial transmission of suicidal behavior (Brent and Bridge 2003; Brent et al. 1996; Mann 1998; Mann et al. 1999). Other factors under investigation as contributors to suicidal ideation have included constructs such as neuroticism (i.e., temperamental tendency to experience more frequent and prolonged negative affect), low self-esteem (not significant when depression was controlled for in some studies), perceived burdensomeness, poor coping and problem-solving abilities, hopelessness (not significant when depression was controlled for in some studies), perception of expectation of perfectionism, and high levels of anger (Beautrais et al. 1999; Boergers et al. 1998; Enns et al. 2003; Fergusson and Lynskey 1995; Fergusson et al. 2000; Goldston et al. 2001; Lewinsohn et al. 1994; Overholser et al. 1995; Roy 2002; Shaffer et al. 1996; Steele et al. 2018).

Sleep Problems

In both adolescents and adults, multiple studies have demonstrated an association between sleep disturbance and suicidal behavior (Bernert et al. 2015; Drapeau and Nadorff 2017), independent of depressive symptoms. In particular, in both adolescents and adults, insomnia has been shown to be a proximal warning sign of imminent death by suicide (Fawcett et al. 1990; Goldstein et al. 2008). Goldstein and colleagues (2008) used psychological autopsy data from 140 adolescents who had died by suicide and 131 matched control subjects to examine the relation between sleep disturbance and death by suicide. After controlling for severity of depressive symptoms, the study authors found that suicide completers were 10 times more likely than matched control subjects to have overall sleep disturbance within the current episode of mood disorder, 4 times more likely to have sleep problems in the week before death, and 5 times more likely to have insomnia in the week before death (Goldstein et al. 2008). In a large longitudinal study of adults with mood disorders, Fawcett et al. (1990) found that global insomnia was predictive of death by suicide within 1 year. Another study found that suicide attempts among adolescents were predicted by middle insomnia and circadian reversal, and suicidal ideation was associated with terminal insomnia (McGlinchey et al. 2017). Finally, after controlling for factors such as depressed mood and substance use, either short or long sleep duration was associated with suicidal behavior in adolescents, particularly in adolescents with previous suicide attempts (Fitzgerald et al. 2011).

Family History of Suicide

Strong evidence from adoption, twin, and family studies shows that suicidal behavior is transmitted in families, even when taking into account psychopathology and familial transmission of psychopathology (Brent and Mann 2005). In one study, parental history of attempted suicide conferred a nearly fivefold risk for suicide attempt in offspring, even after the investigators controlled for familial transmission of mood disorder (Brent et al. 2015).

Childhood Maltreatment

Physical and sexual abuse are strongly linked to suicide attempts and death by suicide (Borowsky et al. 1999; Brent et al. 1999; Fergusson et al. 1996; Molnar et al. 2001).

Contagion

Studies show that death by suicide among adolescents increases around time (i.e., within a specific time frame) and space (e.g., schools) clusters, supporting the effects of contagion and imitation (Asarnow et al. 2008; Crepeau-Hobson and Leech 2014; Gould et al. 1990). Furthermore, suicidal behavior increases in the presence of a peer who died by suicide, regardless of the quality of the relationship with that peer (Gould 2001).

Risk Factors for Suicidal Behavior Specific to Mood Disorders

Although mood disorders in and of themselves are a well-known risk factor for suicidal behavior, recent literature has examined specific risk factors in the context of mood disorders that are associated with greater risk for suicidal behavior. The presence of a mood disorder (i.e., MDD or bipolar I or II disorder) is associated with greater medical lethality of suicide attempts in youth, particularly in the context of low educational achievement, a recent stressful life event, and a history of psychiatric care (Beautrais 2003). Risk factors for suicidal behavior in youth with mood disorders usually overlap with general suicide risk factors, and most studies of risk factors in depressive or bipolar disorders did not have nondepressed or nonbipolar comparison (e.g., anxiety disorder) or control (i.e., no psychopathology) groups. Therefore, whether identified risk factors in samples of youth with mood disorders are unique to this population remains unclear. However, some important considerations are unique to specific mood disorders.

Depressive Disorders

Suicidal depressed adolescents are not easily distinguishable from nonsuicidal depressed adolescents (e.g., De Wilde et al. 1993). Suicidal behaviors are closely linked to severity of depressive disorder symptoms (Asarnow 1992; Brent et al. 1986, 2009; Esposito and Clum 2002; Wilkinson et al. 2011); however, not all depressed adolescents experience suicidal behavior. With regard to risk factors for suicidal behavior in the context of depression, findings can be difficult to interpret, depending on whether depression was assessed and controlled for. Research in recent years has placed importance on assessing and/or controlling for depression, because many risk factors (e.g., hopelessness) could be accounted for by depression via a third variable effect (e.g., Hetrick et al. 2012). Although further research is needed to determine which risk factors are distinct from depression versus components of depression, these risk factors should be taken into consideration when determining overall risk for a patient.

The major experimental and quasi-experimental treatment trials for depressed youth (i.e., Adolescent Depression Antidepressants and Psychotherapy Trial [Wilkinson et al. 2011]; Treatment of SSRI-Resistant Depression in Adolescents [Asarnow et al. 2011]; Treatment of Adolescent Suicide Attempters [TASA] study [Brent et al. 2009]) have found that severity of depression, as well as risk factors discussed in the previous section, including nonsuicidal self-injury, hopelessness, and previous suicidal behavior, is associated with increased suicidal behavior in samples of depressed youth. Other studies have found associations between suicidal behavior and earlier onset and longer duration of depressive symptoms, comorbid externalizing behaviors, anxiety, substance use, mania, posttraumatic stress disorder symptoms, ADHD, and conduct problems; environmental stress (e.g., breakup of romantic relationship); greater cognitive distortions; less assertiveness; low perceived social support; low family support and cohesiveness; higher levels of anger; experience of being cyberbullied (females only); history of physical and/or sexual abuse; and history of and/or exposure to familial suicide (Asarnow et al. 2011; Bauman et al. 2013; Brent et al. 1990, 2009; Chronis-Tuscano et al. 2010; Fordwood et al. 2007; King et al. 2015; Myers et al. 1991; Reifman and Windle 1995; Thompson et al. 2005; Tuisku et al. 2014).

Bipolar Disorders

With regard to differences in suicidal behavior by type of bipolar diagnosis, studies are mixed (e.g., no difference in suicidal behavior between bipolar I and bipolar II disorder; Goldstein et al. 2012). The most common finding is that mixed states (reflecting a combination of manic and depressive symptoms) are associated with an increase in risk for suicide attempts among adolescents with bipolar disorder (Dilsaver et al. 2005; Goldstein et al. 2005, 2012; Hauser et al. 2013). Other studies have found female sex, early to mid-adolescence (as opposed to preadolescence), earlier illness onset (childhood onset as compared with adolescent onset), higher severity of symptoms, higher frequency of comorbid disorders (e.g., ADHD), substance use, past nonsuicidal self-injury and suicidal behavior, parental depression, quality of life, family history of suicide attempts, and poor family functioning (Algorta et al. 2011; Goldstein et al. 2012; Hauser et al. 2013; Holtzman et al. 2015; Weinstein et al. 2015) all to be associated with increased risk for suicide in youth with bipolar disorders. A recent study of preadolescents with bipolar disorder found that 31% of 7- to 13-year-old children reported active suicidal ideation, which was associated with more depressive symptoms, lower quality of life, hopelessness, low self-esteem, and family rigidity (Weinstein et al. 2015).

Strategies for Managing Suicidal Youth in Outpatient Settings

Regardless of the diagnosis and treatment approach, several strategies can be used to enhance safety and should be routinely applied when working with suicidal adolescents and their families. The ability to implement these strategies effectively plays a critical role in determining the level of care needed (e.g., inpatient vs. outpatient).

Written Safety Plan

Because patients may have difficulty identifying and implementing adaptive coping strategies in the place of self-harm when they are in the midst of a suicidal crisis and overwhelmed by strong negative emotions, it is important to develop a detailed, written safety plan for use in crisis situations (Berk et al. 2004; Stanley et al. 2009; Wenzel et al. 2009). Stanley and Brown (2012) have developed a safety plan template and intervention that has been identified as a "best practice" by the Suicide Prevention Resource Center/American Foundation for Suicide Prevention and can be adapted across settings and populations. This template is available online at http://www.sprc.org/sites/default/files/Brown_StanleySafetyPlanTemplate.pdf. The safety plan template is organized in a stepwise manner and starts with strategies that the youth can implement himself or herself at home and ends with 24-7 emergency contact numbers that can be used when danger is imminent and emergency services are needed.

It is critical to note that the written safety plan is not a "no suicide" contract, which has shown to be ineffective in preventing suicidal behavior and death by suicide (Garvey et al. 2009; Wortzel et al. 2014). A written safety plan is the result of collaboration among the patient, caregiver(s), and clinician. The primary elements of the written safety plan include warning signs of a suicidal crisis, coping skills, and a plan for imminent risk of harming oneself. First, warning signs, or internal thoughts and emotions (e.g., hopelessness, loneliness) and external behaviors (e.g., isolating, destruction of property), that precipitate a suicidal crisis for the patient are documented. It may be helpful to perform a chain analysis of recent suicidal ideation or behaviors to ascertain the internal and external precipitants to suicidal crises. The chain analysis is a detailed, moment-to-moment timeline of emotions, thoughts, behaviors, and situations or contexts that led to past suicidal ideation or a suicidal crisis (Linehan 1993). The chain analysis gives critical information that can be used to attempt to subvert suicidal crises by engaging in coping strategies earlier in the process. Next, specific coping strategies for the adolescent to use when warning signs appear are listed, such as distraction and self-soothing (Linehan 1993). Importantly, the safety plan also includes a list of whom the adolescent can contact in a suicidal crisis, including friends and family members, the therapist, 24-7 crisis hotlines, and 911. It is important to ask the adolescent at each step in the process whether the coping strategy and plans feel feasible and whether he or she can foresee any barriers (e.g., an adolescent may agree to contact the school counselor in a suicidal crisis but on further questioning may state that he or she feels that he or she would be too embarrassed to do this) and to troubleshoot or problem-solve around these barriers (e.g., an adolescent may not feel comfortable raising his or her hand and asking to see the counselor but may feel comfortable giving the teacher a previously agreed-on signal or note indicating that she or he is feeling unsafe and needs to see the counselor). When completed, the safety plan should be reviewed with the adolescent, care-giver(s), and important others (e.g., school counselor), and copies should be given to the adolescent, caregiver(s), and clinician to have on hand.

Means Restriction and Increased Monitoring and Supervision

Means restriction includes removing or limiting access to potentially life-threatening settings or objects, such as firearms, tall buildings, bridges, trains or traffic, sharps, and any medications and toxic substances that could be used to overdose (Miller 2013). Access to firearms is a significant predictor of death by suicide, independent of all other factors (Brent and Bridge 2003). Of note, between 1996 and 2010, firearms were the most common method used in death by suicide in the United States (51%; Fontanella et al. 2015). This is underscored by findings demonstrating that limited access to firearms explains the significantly smaller number of deaths by suicide among on-campus college students, who have a nearly ninefold decrease in access to firearms when compared with age- and gender-matched control subjects (Schwartz 2011). Furthermore, psychological autopsy studies of adolescents who died by suicide in the absence of psychiatric disorders have suggested that access to a loaded firearm is a significant risk factor for death by suicide (Marttunen et al. 1998). In states within the United States and other countries, greater firearm regulations are associated with reductions in suicide deaths by firearms (Lewiecki and Miller 2013).

It has been documented that removing the suicidal individual's access to lethal means is a highly effective suicide prevention strategy with a robust empirical basis (Barber and Miller 2014; Mann et al. 2005). Means restriction assessment and education is a central strategy for suicide prevention for several national organizations' suicide prevention guidelines and best practices (National Registry of Evidence-Based Programs and Practices [Substance Abuse and Mental Health Services Administration 2018]; U.S. Department of Health and Human Services 2012). In clinical practice, this involves recommending that caregivers get rid of firearms and other items entirely and lock up sharps, prescription and nonprescription medications, poisons, and other dangerous items in a safe or lockbox that must be kept in the home.

Several studies have linked low parental supervision and monitoring (i.e., physical supervision of the adolescent as well as awareness of the adolescent's activities and schedule) to increased risk for suicidal behavior among adolescents (King et al. 2001; Kostenuik and Ratnapalan 2010). The American Academy of Child and Adolescent Psychiatry practice parameter for suicidal youth recommends that suicidal children and adolescents be monitored closely by a trustworthy and supportive adult (Shaffer and Pfeffer 2001). In practice, supervision and monitoring can vary in form and intensity, ranging from frequent check-ins, not allowing doors to be locked or closed, and not allowing the adolescent to leave the home unsupervised to constant monitoring, at times including sleeping in the same room as the adolescent. The caregiver's ability to provide close supervision and monitoring may be a deciding factor in whether a suicidal teenager requires a higher level of care (e.g., hospitalization or a more intensive outpatient program, such as an intensive outpatient program or partial hospitalization program) until the suicidal crisis has resolved.

Minimizing Risk Factors

As part of increasing safety, malleable risk factors for suicidal behavior that are systematically identified as stated earlier should be addressed. An important target for increasing immediate safety is the reduction of family conflict in the short term, by asking caregivers to "pick their battles" and put aside any topics typically resulting in conflict to a later time. Reduction of family conflict both reduces the overall amount of negative emotion and increases the likelihood that the youth will go to the parent for help during a suicidal crisis. Treatment manuals for youth with major depression and bipolar disorder also have included reduction of family conflict as a key treatment target and means of reducing symptoms of these disorders (Asarnow et al. 2011; Brent et al. 2009; Miklowitz et al. 2013). It also may be useful to target other major stressors or potential events precipitating suicidal crises, such as academic stress, bullying, and other interpersonal conflict, until the teenager has developed coping strategies and skills to effectively manage these situations. Given the association between sleep disturbance and imminent risk of death by suicide (Goldstein et al. 2008), it is also useful to provide information about sleep hygiene and to connect families with their pediatricians, sleep specialists, and psychiatrists to address sleep difficulties as soon as possible. For individuals with mood disorders, severity of depressive symptoms in depressive disorders and mixed states in bipolar disorder may be indicators of increased risk for suicidal behavior.

Evidence Base for Treatment of Suicidal Behavior in Youth

A 2015 meta-analysis of randomized controlled trials (Ougrin et al. 2015) examining treatments specifically targeting suicidal behavior in adolescents revealed the largest effect sizes for dialectical behavior therapy for adolescents (DBT-A) (Linehan 1993; Miller et al. 1997), an integrated cognitive-behavioral therapy (CBT) intervention for suicidality and substance abuse (I-CBT; Esposito-Smythers et al. 2011), and mentalization-based therapy (Rossouw and Fonagy 2012). Another 2015 review (Berk and Hughes 2015) documented effects of randomized controlled trials for multisystemic therapy (Huey et al. 2004) as well as I-CBT and DBT-A.

At present, DBT-A has the most evidence (Mehlum et al. 2014) for reducing suicidal behavior in adolescents. Standard DBT (Linehan 1993) was developed for adults and is the gold standard treatment approach for adults with suicidal and self-harming behaviors, as well as with a diagnosis of borderline personality disorder. DBT includes weekly individual sessions, weekly skills group, telephone coaching to apply skills outside of treatment sessions, and therapist participation on a consultation team. DBT-A includes weekly individual treatment with the adolescent and weekly multifamily skills group, in which adolescents and caregivers are taught skills in a classroom format. Adolescents have access to their therapist by telephone or pager 24-7 to manage crisis situations and apply skills in context outside of sessions. DBT-A retains a hierarchy of behavioral targets, prioritizing life-interfering behaviors (e.g., suicide attempt, nonsuicidal self-injury), therapy-interfering behavior (e.g., missing treatment sessions), and quality-of-life interfering behavior (e.g., treatment of psychiatric symptoms not prioritized as life-threatening and other behaviors that interfere with one's quality of life). Individuals complete a weekly diary card that includes daily ratings of emotions, suicidal and self-injurious urges and behaviors, skill use, and any other target behaviors that are identified for a particular individual (e.g., substance use). DBT also has been shown to decrease depressive symptoms in adolescents (e.g., Mehlum et al. 2014; Rathus and Miller 2002), although it is not considered a first-line treatment for youth with depression in the absence of suicidal or self-harm behaviors.

Evidence Base for Treatment of Suicidal Behavior in Youth With Mood Disorders

Several studies that found significant treatment effects of CBT for depression in adolescence (Klein et al. 2007) also found a positive effect of CBT on suicidal behavior (Spirito et al. 2011). Brent et al. (1997) compared CBT (involving the adolescent and family, if desired by adolescent and family), systemic behavioral family therapy (i.e., identification of dysfunctional family patterns, teaching problem solving and communication), and nondirective supportive treatment (designed to control for nonspecific aspects of treatment and including focus on patient-therapist alliance and patient-directed efforts to address personal problems). Although CBT outperformed both other conditions in terms of depression level at the conclusion of the study and resulted in more rapid relief of depressive symptoms, suicidal behavior was similarly and significantly reduced in all conditions (Brent et al. 1997). In another study with similar outcomes, depressed adolescents with depressed parents were randomly assigned to participate in a CBT group or to receive treatment as usual, with participants in both conditions showing a similar decline in suicidal behavior posttreatment (Clarke et al. 2002).

The TASA study examined the effect of a suicide-prevention-specific CBT protocol (CBT-SP) on depressed youth with a history of suicide attempt, comparing CBT-SP, CBT-SP plus medication management, and

medication management alone (Stanley et al. 2009). The CBT-SP intervention was administered over approximately 12 sessions and included
chain analysis of index suicide event leading to study eligibility, development of a safety plan, psychoeducation, skill acquisition, family intervention, and relapse prevention. Most participants chose the combined CBT-
SP plus medication management condition, which led to rates of remission
and improvement of depressive symptoms similar to rates in nonsuicidal
depressed adolescents (Vitiello et al. 2009). All conditions led to lowered
suicidal behavior at 6-month follow-up (Brent et al. 2009). Similar studies
comparing CBT, combined CBT plus medication management, and medication management alone have found similar results (selective serotonin
reuptake inhibitors, Melvin et al. 2006; fluoxetine, Goodyer et al. 2007).

A few psychosocial treatments are available for youth with bipolar
disorders (see Fristad and MacPherson 2014 for review), but little work
has examined the effect of these treatments on suicidal behavior. A randomized controlled trial compared child- and family-focused CBT with
treatment as usual in 71 preadolescents ages 7–13 years (Weinstein et al.
2017). Child- and family-focused CBT is a manualized treatment with an
intense family and individual focus. It was developed to be used in conjunction with pharmacotherapy and integrates CBT and positive psychology,
interpersonal, and mindfulness approaches. Child- and family-focused
CBT was not designed to target suicidal behavior directly but targets factors (i.e., emotion regulation, problem solving, hope, self-esteem, family
adaptability, family conflict) found to initiate and maintain suicidal behavior in youth. Results failed to show differences between child- and
family-focused CBT and treatment as usual; however, significant improvement in suicidal ideation among groups suggests that early intervention may serve to protect against the progression from suicidal ideation to
suicidal behavior and death in adolescence, when sharp increases in deaths
by suicide occur.

Goldstein and colleagues (2007) conducted an open DBT trial with 10
adolescents ages 12–18 years with bipolar disorder, 80% of whom had a
history of suicide attempt. Bipolar disorder–specific adjustments—such as
explicitly monitoring and targeting mood, sleep, and medication adherence on the diary card; linking "emotional mind" teaching to depressed,
manic, mixed, and euthymic states; and teaching differential skills application (i.e., coping skills) based on mood states—were made to tailor
treatment to specific issues faced by adolescents with bipolar disorders
and their families. Given the study design, individual family units were
seen for skills training as opposed to attending multifamily skills group.
For the first 6 months of treatment, weekly sessions alternated between

individual and family skills training. For the next 6 months, monthly sessions alternated between individual and family sessions to review skills application and consolidate treatment gains. Results of this study were promising, showing a significant decrease in suicidal behavior, decreases in emotional reactivity, and improvement in depressive symptoms. Additionally, study personnel evaluated treatment as highly feasible to administer, 9 of 10 families completed this yearlong protocol, and satisfaction among adolescents and parents was high.

Medication is commonly considered a central component of treatment for moderate to severe unipolar depression and bipolar disorder. However, at present, no U.S. Food and Drug Administration–approved medication is available for the treatment of suicide-related symptoms or self-harm behaviors in youth (see Chapter 4, "Principles of Treatment of Mood Disorders Across Development"). Moreover, conflicting findings regarding the association of antidepressant use with an increased risk of suicidality mean that psychiatrists must weigh the risk of prescribing antidepressants against the risks of increased suicidality resulting from untreated depressive symptoms (Rihmer and Akiskal 2006). To minimize risk and optimize treatment response, it has been recommended that psychiatrists working with suicidal youth make case-by-case decisions about whether to prescribe medication, as well as 1) provide education to patients and families on the risks and benefits of medications; 2) closely monitor suicidality; 3) take steps to reduce risk of overdose on prescribed psychiatric medications; 4) make timely adjustments to medications if initial strategies were unsuccessful; and 5) guard against polypharmacy, particularly for youth with multiple diagnoses or Axis II traits (see Chapter 4).

Conclusion

Extant research shows that mood disorders play a role in the clinical picture for suicidal youth. The case presented at the start of this chapter represents a fairly common scenario for adolescents who present with suicidality. In Chloe's case, a thorough diagnostic evaluation of underlying psychopathology and treatment course is important, but assessing Chloe's level of suicidality is critical in determining immediate next steps for her. A thorough risk assessment, including direct questioning about suicidal ideation, plans, and intent and previous suicide attempts, must be conducted, interviewing Chloe and her parents separately in case sensitive information is difficult for Chloe to share in front of her parents and vice versa. If Chloe is willing and able to follow a safety plan, the next step will be to create the safety plan, being careful to identify any potential problems with the plan (e.g., What will you do if you cannot reach your parents right away and you need help?). The safety plan can be created with or without Chloe's parents in the room; however, if they are not present, the safety plan should be reviewed with them in detail and copies provided to Chloe and her parents, with extra copies to share with others (e.g., school counselor). If parents become imminently concerned about Chloe's safety, they can take her to their nearest emergency department for evaluation or call 911. Even if Chloe is willing to follow a safety plan, her parents still should restrict her access to lethal means (i.e., sharps, pills, poisons), paying particular attention to means mentioned in any disclosed suicide plans (i.e., pills). Reduction of risk factors associated with suicidality also will be targeted when possible (e.g., discussing decreasing family conflict with family), and treatment planning should include targeted intervention, such as DBT, when appropriate, for Chloe's ongoing nonsuicidal self-injury and suicidality.

Clinical Pearls

- All expressions of suicidality and suicidal behavior among children and adolescents should be taken seriously.

- All youth with mood disorders should be assessed for suicidality given the close linkage between the two.

- Clinicians must ask direct questions about suicidal ideation (e.g., Do you ever have thoughts of wanting to kill yourself or wish you weren't alive?), suicide plans (e.g., Do you have a plan for how you would kill yourself? Do you have access to those items or that place?), and suicidal intent (e.g., How likely are you to carry out this plan in the next week?).

- Suicidal behavior should be targeted directly, because these behaviors may not resolve on their own as mood symptoms improve.

- Suicidal youth should have their access to lethal means restricted, especially firearms, and be closely monitored by parents, the extent of which depends on the level of suicidal ideation, intent, and plans.

- All suicidal youth should have a written safety plan, with copies given to the youth, parents or caregivers, and others in the child's life (e.g., school counselor), if appropriate. Clinicians should ask youth at the end of each session whether they can follow the safety plan until the next session with the provider.

References

Agerbo E, Nordentoft M, Mortensen PB: Familial, psychiatric, and socioeconomic risk factors for suicide in young people: nested case-control study. BMJ 325(7355):74, 2002 12114236

Algorta GP, Youngstrom EA, Frazier TW, et al: Suicidality in pediatric bipolar disorder: predictor or outcome of family processes and mixed mood presentation? Bipolar Disord 13(1):76–86, 2011 21320255

Andrews JA, Lewinsohn PM: Suicidal attempts among older adolescents: prevalence and co-occurrence with psychiatric disorders. J Am Acad Child Adolesc Psychiatry 31(4):655–662, 1992 1644728

Apter A, Gothelf D, Orbach I, et al: Correlation of suicidal and violent behavior in different diagnostic categories in hospitalized adolescent patients. J Am Acad Child Adolesc Psychiatry 34(7):912–918, 1995 7649962

Asarnow JR: Suicidal ideation and attempts during middle childhood: associations with perceived family stress and depression among child psychiatric inpatients. J Clin Child Psychol 21(1):35–40, 1992

Asarnow JR, Carlson GA, Guthrie D: Coping strategies, self-perceptions, hopelessness, and perceived family environments in depressed and suicidal children. J Consult Clin Psychol 55(3):361–366, 1987 3597949

Asarnow JR, Baraff LJ, Berk M, et al: Pediatric emergency department suicidal patients: two-site evaluation of suicide ideators, single attempters, and repeat attempters. J Am Acad Child Adolesc Psychiatry 47(8):958–966, 2008 18596552

Asarnow JR, Porta G, Spirito A, et al: Suicide attempts and nonsuicidal self-injury in the treatment of resistant depression in adolescents: findings from the TORDIA study. J Am Acad Child Adolesc Psychiatry 50(8):772–781, 2011 21784297

Barber CW, Miller MJ: Reducing a suicidal person's access to lethal means of suicide: a research agenda. Am J Prev Med 47(3 suppl 2):S264–S272, 2014 25145749

Bauman S, Toomey RB, Walker JL: Associations among bullying, cyberbullying, and suicide in high school students. J Adolesc 36(2):341–350, 2013 23332116

Beautrais AL: Risk factors for suicide and attempted suicide among young people. Aust N Z J Psychiatry 34(3):420–436, 2000 10881966

Beautrais AL: Suicide and serious suicide attempts in youth: a multiple-group comparison study. Am J Psychiatry 160(6):1093–1099, 2003 12777267

Beautrais AL, Joyce PR, Mulder RT: Psychiatric illness in a New Zealand sample of young people making serious suicide attempts. N Z Med J 111(1060):44–48, 1998 9539914

Beautrais AL, Joyce PR, Mulder RT: Personality traits and cognitive styles as risk factors for serious suicide attempts among young people. Suicide Life Threat Behav 29(1):37–47, 1999 10322619

Berk MS, Hughes J: Cognitive behavioral approaches for treating suicidal behavior in adolescents. Curr Psychiatry Rev 11:1–10, 2015

Berk MS, Henriques GR, Warman DM, et al: A cognitive therapy intervention for suicide attempters: an overview of the treatment case and examples. Cognitive and Behavioral Practice 11(3):265–277, 2004

Bernert RA, Kim JS, Iwata NG, et al: Sleep disturbances as an evidence-based suicide risk factor. Curr Psychiatry Rep 17(3):554, 2015 25698339

Bhangoo RK, Dell ML, Towbin K, et al: Clinical correlates of episodicity in juvenile mania. J Child Adolesc Psychopharmacol 13(4):507–514, 2003 14977463

Boergers J, Spirito A, Donaldson D: Reasons for adolescent suicide attempts: associations with psychological functioning. J Am Acad Child Adolesc Psychiatry 37(12):1287–1293, 1998 9847501

Borowsky IW, Resnick MD, Ireland M, et al: Suicide attempts among American Indian and Alaska Native youth: risk and protective factors. Arch Pediatr Adolesc Med 153(6):573–580, 1999 10357296

Borowsky IW, Ireland M, Resnick MD: Adolescent suicide attempts: risks and protectors. Pediatrics 107(3):485–493, 2001 11230587

Brent DA: Risk factors for adolescent suicide and suicidal behavior: mental and substance abuse disorders, family environmental factors, and life stress. Suicide Life Threat Behav 25(1 suppl):52–63, 1995 8553429

Brent DA, Bridge JA: Firearms availability and suicide: evidence, interventions, and future directions. Am Behav Sci 46:1192–1210, 2003

Brent DA, Mann JJ: Family genetic studies, suicide, and suicidal behavior. Am J Med Genet C Semin Med Genet 133C(1):13–24, 2005 15648081

Brent DA, Kalas R, Edelbrock C, et al: Psychopathology and its relationship to suicidal ideation in childhood and adolescence. J Am Acad Child Psychiatry 25(5):666–673, 1986 3760416

Brent DA, Perper JA, Goldstein CE, et al: Risk factors for adolescent suicide: a comparison of adolescent suicide victims with suicidal inpatients. Arch Gen Psychiatry 45(6):581–588, 1988 3377645

Brent DA, Kolko DJ, Allan MJ, Brown RV: Suicidality in affectively disordered adolescent inpatients. J Am Acad Child Adolesc Psychiatry 29(4):586–593, 1990 2387793

Brent DA, Perper J, Moritz G, et al: Suicide in adolescents with no apparent psychopathology. J Am Acad Child Adolesc Psychiatry 32(3):494–500, 1993 8496111

Brent DA, Perper JA, Moritz G, et al: Familial risk factors for adolescent suicide: a case-control study. Acta Psychiatr Scand 89(1):52–58, 1994 8140907

Brent DA, Bridge J, Johnson BA, Connolly J: Suicidal behavior runs in families: a controlled family study of adolescent suicide victims. Arch Gen Psychiatry 53(12):1145–1152, 1996 8956681

Brent DA, Holder D, Kolko D, et al: A clinical psychotherapy trial for adolescent depression comparing cognitive, family, and supportive therapy. Arch Gen Psychiatry 54(9):877–885, 1997 9294380

Brent DA, Baugher M, Bridge J, et al: Age- and sex-related risk factors for adolescent suicide. J Am Acad Child Adolesc Psychiatry 38(12):1497–1505, 1999 10596249

Brent DA, Bridge J: Firearms availability and suicide: evidence, interventions, and future directions. American Behavioral Scientist 46(9):1192–1210, 2003

Brent DA, Greenhill LL, Compton S, et al: The Treatment of Adolescent Suicide Attempters study (TASA): predictors of suicidal events in an open treatment trial. J Am Acad Child Adolesc Psychiatry 48(10):987–996, 2009 19730274

Brent DA, McMakin DL, Kennard BD, et al: Protecting adolescents from self-harm: a critical review of intervention studies. J Am Acad Child Adolesc Psychiatry 52(12):1260–1271, 2013 24290459

Brent DA, Brunwasser SM, Hollon SD, et al: Effect of a cognitive-behavioral prevention program on depression 6 years after implementation among at-risk adolescents: a randomized clinical trial. JAMA Psychiatry 72(11):1110–1118, 2015 26421861

Bridge JA, Goldstein TR, Brent DA: Adolescent suicide and suicidal behavior. J Child Psychol Psychiatry 47(3–4):372–394, 2006 16492264

Centers for Disease Control and Prevention: Leading causes of death reports, national and regional, 1999–2015. WISQARS. National Center for Injury Prevention and Control, 2014. Available at: http://webappa.cdc.gov/sasweb/ncipc/leadcaus10_us.html. Accessed September 19, 2018.

Centers for Disease Control and Prevention: Fatal injury reports, national, regional, and state, 1981–2016. 2017. Available at: https://www.cdc.gov/injury/wisqars/fatal_injury_reports.html. Accessed September 19, 2018.

Cha CB, Franz PJ, Guzman EM, et al: Annual research review: suicide among youth—epidemiology, (potential) etiology, and treatment. J Child Psychol Psychiatry 59(4):460–482, 2017 29090457

Chesin MS, Galfavy H, Sonmez CC, et al: Nonsuicidal self-injury is predictive of suicide attempts among individuals with mood disorders. Suicide Life Threat Behav 47(5):567–579, 2017 28211201

Chronis-Tuscano A, Molina BS, Pelham WE, et al: Very early predictors of adolescent depression and suicide attempts in children with attention-deficit/hyperactivity disorder. Arch Gen Psychiatry 67(10):1044–1051, 2010 20921120

Cicchetti D, Rogosch FA: A developmental psychopathology perspective on adolescence. J Consult Clin Psychol 70(1):6–20, 2002 10446685

Clarke GN, Hornbrook M, Lynch F, et al: Group cognitive-behavioral treatment for depressed adolescent offspring of depressed parents in a health maintenance organization. J Am Acad Child Adolesc Psychiatry 41(3):305–313, 2002 11886025

Cooper J, Kapur N, Dunning J, et al: A clinical tool for assessing risk after self-harm. Ann Emerg Med 48(4):459–466, 2006 16997684

Crepeau-Hobson MF, Leech NL: The impact of exposure to peer suicidal self-directed violence on youth suicidal behavior: a critical review of the literature. Suicide Life Threat Behav 44(1):58–77, 2014 24033603

Czyz EK, King CA: Longitudinal trajectories of suicidal ideation and subsequent suicide attempts among adolescent inpatients. J Clin Child Adolesc Psychol 44(1):181–193, 2015 24079705

De Crescenzo F, Serra G, Maisto F, et al: Suicide attempts in juvenile bipolar versus major depressive disorders: a systematic review and meta-analysis. J Am Acad Child Adolesc Psychiatry 56(10):825.e3–831.e3, 2017 28942804

De Wilde EJ, Kienhorst IC, Diekstra RF, et al: The specificity of psychological characteristics of adolescent suicide attempters. J Am Acad Child Adolesc Psychiatry 32(1):51–59, 1993 8428884

Dilsaver SC, Benazzi F, Rihmer Z, et al: Gender, suicidality and bipolar mixed states in adolescents. J Affect Disord 87(1):11–16, 2005 15944138

Drapeau CW, Nadorff MR: Suicidality in sleep disorders: prevalence, impact, and management strategies. Nat Sci Sleep 9:213–226, 2017 29075143

Emslie G, Kratochvil C, Vitiello B, et al; Columbia Suicidality Classification Group; TADS Team: Treatment for Adolescents with Depression Study (TADS): safety results. J Am Acad Child Adolesc Psychiatry 45(12):1440–1455, 2006 17135989

Enns MW, Cox BJ, Inayatulla M: Personality predictors of outcome for adolescents hospitalized for suicidal ideation. J Am Acad Child Adolesc Psychiatry 42(6):720–727, 2003 12921480

Esposito CL, Clum GA: Psychiatric symptoms and their relationship to suicidal ideation in a high-risk adolescent community sample. J Am Acad Child Adolesc Psychiatry 41(1):44–51, 2002 11800204

Esposito-Smythers C, Spirito A, Kahler CW, et al: Treatment of co-occurring substance abuse and suicidality among adolescents: a randomized trial. J Consult Clin Psychol 79(6):728–739, 2011 22004303

Fawcett J, Scheftner WA, Fogg L, et al: Time-related predictors of suicide in major affective disorder. Am J Psychiatry 147(9):1189–1194, 1990 2104515

Fergusson DM, Lynskey MT: Childhood circumstances, adolescent adjustment, and suicide attempts in a New Zealand birth cohort. J Am Acad Child Adolesc Psychiatry 34(5):612–622, 1995 7775356

Fergusson DM, Horwood LJ, Lynskey MT: Childhood sexual abuse and psychiatric disorder in young adulthood, II: psychiatric outcomes of childhood sexual abuse. J Am Acad Child Adolesc Psychiatry 35(10):1365–1374, 1996 8885591

Fergusson DM, Woodward LJ, Horwood LJ: Risk factors and life processes associated with the onset of suicidal behaviour during adolescence and early adulthood. Psychol Med 30(1):23–39, 2000 10722173

Fergusson D, Doucette S, Glass KC, et al: Association between suicide attempts and selective serotonin reuptake inhibitors: systematic review of randomised controlled trials. BMJ 330(7488):396, 2005 15718539

Fitzgerald CT, Messias E, Buysse DJ: Teen sleep and suicidality: results from the Youth Risk Behavior Surveys of 2007 and 2009. J Clin Sleep Med 7(4):351–356, 2011 21897771

Fontanella CA, Hiance-Steelesmith DL, Phillips GS, et al: Widening rural-urban disparities in youth suicides, United States, 1996–2010. JAMA Pediatr 169(5):466–473, 2015 25751611

Fordwood SR, Asarnow JR, Huizar DP, Reise SP: Suicide attempts among depressed adolescents in primary care. J Clin Child Adolesc Psychol 36(3):392–404, 2007 17658983

Fowler JC: Suicide risk assessment in clinical practice: pragmatic guidelines for imperfect assessments. Psychotherapy (Chic) 49(1):81–90, 2012 22369082

Franklin JC, Ribeiro JD, Fox KR, et al: Risk factors for suicidal thoughts and behaviors: a meta-analysis of 50 years of research. Psychol Bull 143(2):187–232, 2017 27841450

Fristad MA, MacPherson HA: Evidence-based psychosocial treatments for child and adolescent bipolar spectrum disorders. J Clin Child Adolesc Psychol 43(3):339–355, 2014 23927375

Garofalo R, Wolf RC, Wissow LS, et al: Sexual orientation and risk of suicide attempts among a representative sample of youth. Arch Pediatr Adolesc Med 153(5):487–493, 1999 10323629

Garvey KA, Penn JV, Campbell AL, et al: Contracting for safety with patients: clinical practice and forensic implications. J Am Acad Psychiatry Law 37(3):363–370, 2009 19767501

Glenn CR, Lanzillo EC, Esposito EC, et al: Examining the course of suicidal and nonsuicidal self-injurious thoughts and behaviors in outpatient and inpatient adolescents. J Abnorm Child Psychol 45(5):971–983, 2017 27761783

Goldstein TR, Birmaher B, Axelson D, et al: History of suicide attempts in pediatric bipolar disorder: factors associated with increased risk. Bipolar Disord 7(6):525–535, 2005 16403178

Goldstein TR, Axelson DA, Birmaher B, et al: Dialectical behavior therapy for adolescents with bipolar disorder: a 1-year open trial. J Am Acad Child Adolesc Psychiatry 46(7):820–830, 2007 17581446

Goldstein TR, Bridge JA, Brent DA: Sleep disturbance preceding completed suicide in adolescents. J Consult Clin Psychol 76(1):84–91, 2008 18229986

Goldstein TR, Birmaher B, Axelson D, et al: Family environment and suicidal ideation among bipolar youth. Arch Suicide Res 13(4):378–388, 2009 19813115

Goldstein TR, Ha W, Axelson DA, et al: Predictors of prospectively examined suicide attempts among youth with bipolar disorder. Arch Gen Psychiatry 69(11):1113–1122, 2012 22752079

Goldston DB, Daniel SS, Reboussin BA, et al: Psychiatric diagnoses of previous suicide attempters, first-time attempters, and repeat attempters on an adolescent inpatient psychiatry unit. J Am Acad Child Adolesc Psychiatry 37(9):924–932, 1998 9735612

Goldston DB, Daniel SS, Reboussin DM, et al: Suicide attempts among formerly hospitalized adolescents: a prospective naturalistic study of risk during the first 5 years after discharge. J Am Acad Child Adolesc Psychiatry 38(6):660–671, 1999 10361783

Goldston DB, Daniel SS, Reboussin BA, et al: Cognitive risk factors and suicide attempts among formerly hospitalized adolescents: a prospective naturalistic study. J Am Acad Child Adolesc Psychiatry 40(1):91–99, 2001 11195570

Goodyer I, Dubicka B, Wilkinson P, et al: Selective serotonin reuptake inhibitors (SSRIs) and routine specialist care with and without cognitive behaviour therapy in adolescents with major depression: randomised controlled trial. BMJ 335(7611):142, 2007 17556431

Gould MS: Suicide and the media. Ann N Y Acad Sci 932:200–221, discussion 221–224, 2001 11411187

Gould MS, Wallenstein S, Kleinman MH, et al: Suicide clusters: an examination of age-specific effects. Am J Public Health 80(2):211–212, 1990 2297071

Gould MS, Fisher P, Parides M, et al: Psychosocial risk factors of child and adolescent completed suicide. Arch Gen Psychiatry 53(12):1155–1162, 1996 8956682

Gould MS, King R, Greenwald S, et al: Psychopathology associated with suicidal ideation and attempts among children and adolescents. J Am Acad Child Adolesc Psychiatry 37(9):915–923, 1998 9735611

Grøholt B, Ekeberg O, Wichstrøm L, et al: Youth suicide in Norway, 1990–1992: a comparison between children and adolescents completing suicide and age- and gender-matched controls. Suicide Life Threat Behav 27(3):250–263, 1997 9357080

Gunnell D, Murray V, Hawton K: Use of paracetamol (acetaminophen) for suicide and nonfatal poisoning: worldwide patterns of use and misuse. Suicide Life Threat Behav 30(4):313–326, 2000 11210057

Harrington R, Bredenkamp D, Groothues C, et al: Adult outcomes of childhood and adolescent depression, III: links with suicidal behaviours. J Child Psychol Psychiatry 35(7):1309–1319, 1994 7806612

Hatzenbuehler ML: The social environment and suicide attempts in lesbian, gay, and bisexual youth. Pediatrics 127(5):896–903, 2011 21502225

Hauser M, Galling B, Correll CU: Suicidal ideation and suicide attempts in children and adolescents with bipolar disorder: a systematic review of prevalence and incidence rates, correlates, and targeted interventions. Bipolar Disord 15(5):507–523, 2013 23829436

Hawton K, Harriss L: Deliberate self-harm in young people: characteristics and subsequent mortality in a 20-year cohort of patients presenting to hospital. J Clin Psychiatry 68(10):1574–1583, 2007 17960975

Hetrick SE, Parker AG, Robinson J, et al: Predicting suicidal risk in a cohort of depressed children and adolescents. Crisis 33(1):13–20, 2012 21940241

Holland KM, Vivolo-Kantor AM, Logan JE, et al: Antecedents of suicide among youth aged 11–15: a multistate mixed methods analysis. J Youth Adolesc 46(7):1598–1610, 2017 27844461

Holtzman JN, Miller S, Hooshmand F, et al: Childhood- compared to adolescent-onset bipolar disorder has more statistically significant clinical correlates. J Affect Disord 179:114–120, 2015 25863906

Huey SJ Jr, Henggeler SW, Rowland MD, et al: Multisystemic therapy effects on attempted suicide by youths presenting psychiatric emergencies. J Am Acad Child Adolesc Psychiatry 43(2):183–190, 2004 14726725

Jobes DA: Managing Suicidal Risk. New York, Guilford, 2006

Jolin EM, Weller EB, Weller RA: Suicide risk factors in children and adolescents with bipolar disorder. Curr Psychiatry Rep 9(2):122–128, 2007 17389121

Kann L, McManus T, Harris WA, et al: Youth risk behavior surveillance—United States, 2015. MMWR Surveill Summ 65(6):1–174, 2016 27280474

Kashden J, Fremouw WJ, Callahan TS, et al: Impulsivity in suicidal and nonsuicidal adolescents. J Abnorm Child Psychol 21(3):339–353, 1993 8335767

Kim YS, Leventhal B: Bullying and suicide: a review. Int J Adolesc Med Health 20(2):133–154, 2008 18714552

King CA, Berona J, Czyz E, et al: Identifying adolescents at highly elevated risk for suicidal behavior in the emergency department. J Child Adolesc Psychopharmacol 25(2):100–108, 2015 25746114

King RA, Schwab-Stone M, Flisher AJ, et al: Psychosocial and risk behavior correlates of youth suicide attempts and suicidal ideation. J Am Acad Child Adolesc Psychiatry 40(7):837–846, 2001 11437023

Kingsbury S, Hawton K, Steinhardt K, et al: Do adolescents who take overdoses have specific psychological characteristics? A comparative study with psychiatric and community controls. J Am Acad Child Adolesc Psychiatry 38(9):1125–1131, 1999 10504811

Klein JB, Jacobs RH, Reinecke MA: Cognitive-behavioral therapy for adolescent depression: a meta-analytic investigation of changes in effect-size estimates. J Am Acad Child Adolesc Psychiatry 46(11):1403–1413, 2007 18049290

Kõlves K, de Leo D: Suicide methods in children and adolescents. Eur Child Adolesc Psychiatry 26(2):155–164, 2017 27194156

Kostenuik M, Ratnapalan M: Approach to adolescent suicide prevention. Can Fam Physician 56(8):755–760, 2010 20705879

Kovacs M, Goldston D, Gatsonis C: Suicidal behaviors and childhood-onset depressive disorders: a longitudinal investigation. J Am Acad Child Adolesc Psychiatry 32(1):8–20, 1993 8428888

Lester D, McSwain S, Gunn JF III: A test of the validity of the IS PATH WARM warning signs for suicide. Psychol Rep 108(2):402–404, 2011 21675556

Lewiecki EM, Miller SA: Suicide, guns, and public policy. Am J Public Health 103(1):27–31, 2013 23153127

Lewinsohn PM, Rohde P, Seeley JR: Psychosocial risk factors for future adolescent suicide attempts. J Consult Clin Psychol 62(2):297–305, 1994 8201067

Lewinsohn PM, Rohde P, Seeley JR: Adolescent suicidal ideation and attempts: prevalence, risk factors, and clinical implications. Clinical Psychology: Science and Practice 3:25–36, 1996

Lewinsohn PM, Seeley JR, Klein DN: Bipolar disorder in adolescents: epidemiology and suicidal behavior, in Bipolar Disorder in Childhood and Early Adolescence. Edited by Geller B, DelBello MP. New York, Guilford, 2003, pp 7–24

Linehan MM: Cognitive Behavioral Treatment of Borderline Personality Disorder. New York, Guilford, 1993

Linehan MM, Comtois KA, Ward-Ciesielski EF: Assessing and managing risk with suicidal individuals. Cogn Behav Pract 19(2):218–232, 2012

Liu RT, Mustanski B: Suicidal ideation and self-harm in lesbian, gay, bisexual, and transgender youth. Am J Prev Med 42(3):221–228, 2012 22341158

Mann JJ: The neurobiology of suicide. Nat Med 4(1):25–30, 1998 9427602

Mann JJ, Waternaux C, Haas GL, et al: Toward a clinical model of suicidal behavior in psychiatric patients. Am J Psychiatry 156(2):181–189, 1999 9989552

Mann JJ, Apter A, Bertolote J, et al: Suicide prevention strategies: a systematic review. JAMA 294(16):2064–2074, 2005 16249421

March J, Silva S, Petrycki S, et al; Treatment for Adolescents with Depression Study (TADS) Team: Fluoxetine, cognitive-behavioral therapy, and their combination for adolescents with depression: Treatment for Adolescents with Depression Study (TADS) randomized controlled trial. JAMA 292(7):807–820, 2004 15315995

Marttunen MJ, Aro HM, Henriksson MM, et al: Mental disorders in adolescent suicide: DSM-III-R Axes I and II diagnoses in suicides among 13- to 19-year-olds in Finland. Arch Gen Psychiatry 48(9):834–839, 1991 1929774

Marttunen MJ, Henriksson MM, Isometsä ET, et al: Completed suicide among adolescents with no diagnosable psychiatric disorder. Adolescence 33(131):669–681, 1998 9831884

McGlinchey EL, Courtney-Seidler EA, German M, et al: The role of sleep disturbance in suicidal and nonsuicidal self-injurious behavior among adolescents. Suicide Life Threat Behav 47(1):103–111, 2017 27273654

Mehlum L, Tørmoen AJ, Ramberg M, et al: Dialectical behavior therapy for adolescents with repeated suicidal and self-harming behavior: a randomized trial. J Am Acad Child Adolesc Psychiatry 53(10):1082–1091, 2014 25245352

Melvin GA, Tonge BJ, King NJ, et al: A comparison of cognitive-behavioral therapy, sertraline, and their combination for adolescent depression. J Am Acad Child Adolesc Psychiatry 45(10):1151–1161, 2006 17003660

Miklowitz DJ, Schneck CD, Singh MK, et al: Early intervention for symptomatic youth at risk for bipolar disorder: a randomized trial of family-focused therapy. J Am Acad Child Adolesc Psychiatry 52(5):121–131, 2013 23357439

Miller AL, Rathus JH, Linehan MM, et al: Dialectical behavior therapy adapted for suicidal adolescents. J Psychiatr Pract 3(2):78, 1997

Miller DN: Lessons in suicide prevention from the Golden Gate Bridge: means restriction, public health, and the school psychologist. Contemp School Psychol 17:71–79, 2013

Miranda R, De Jaegere E, Restifo K, et al: Longitudinal follow-up study of adolescents who report a suicide attempt: aspects of suicidal behavior that increase risk of a future attempt. Depress Anxiety 31(1):19–26, 2014a 24105789

Miranda R, Ortin A, Scott M, et al: Characteristics of suicidal ideation that predict the transition to future suicide attempts in adolescents. J Child Psychol Psychiatry 55(11):1288–1296, 2014b 24827817

Molnar BE, Berkman LF, Buka SL: Psychopathology, childhood sexual abuse and other childhood adversities: relative links to subsequent suicidal behaviour in the US. Psychol Med 31(6):965–977, 2001 11513382

Mustanski B, Liu RT: A longitudinal study of predictors of suicide attempts among lesbian, gay, bisexual, and transgender youth. Arch Sex Behav 42(3):437–448, 2013 23054258

Myers K, McCauley E, Calderon R, et al: The 3-year longitudinal course of suicidality and predictive factors for subsequent suicidality in youths with major depressive disorder. J Am Acad Child Adolesc Psychiatry 30(5):804–810, 1991 1938798

Negron R, Piacentini J, Graae F, et al: Microanalysis of adolescent suicide attempters and ideators during the acute suicidal episode. J Am Acad Child Adolesc Psychiatry 36(11):1512–1519, 1997 9394935

Nock MK, Prinstein MJ: Contextual features and behavioral functions self-mutilation among adolescents. J Abnorm Psychol 114:140–146, 2005 15709820

Nock MK, Joiner TE Jr, Gordon KH, et al: Non-suicidal self-injury among adolescents: diagnostic correlates and relation to suicide attempts. Psychiatry Res 144(1):65–72, 2006 16887199

Nock MK, Green JG, Hwang I, et al: Prevalence, correlates, and treatment of lifetime suicidal behavior among adolescents: results from the National Comorbidity Survey Replication Adolescent Supplement. JAMA Psychiatry 70(3):300–310, 2013 23303463

Ougrin D, Tranah T, Stahl D, et al: Therapeutic interventions for suicide attempts and self-harm in adolescents: systematic review and meta-analysis. J Am Acad Child Adolesc Psychiatry 54(2):97–107.e2, 2015 25617250

Overholser JC, Adams DM, Lehnert KL, et al: Self-esteem deficits and suicidal tendencies among adolescents. J Am Acad Child Adolesc Psychiatry 34(7):919–928, 1995 7649963

Pinto A, Whisman A, McCoy MA, et al: Suicidal ideation in adolescents: psychometric properties of the Suicidal Ideation Questionnaire in a clinical sample. Psychol Assess 9(1):63–66, 1997

Posner K, Brown GK, Stanley B, et al: The Columbia–Suicide Severity Rating Scale: initial validity and internal consistency findings from three multisite studies with adolescents and adults. Am J Psychiatry 168(12):1266–1277, 2011 22193671

Ramchand R, Franklin E, Thornton E, et al: Opportunities to intervene? "Warning signs" for suicide in the days before dying. Death Stud 41(6):368–375, 2017 28129088

Ran MS, Zhang Z, Fan M, et al: Risk factors of suicidal ideation among adolescents after Wenchuan earthquake in China. Asian J Psychiatr 13:66–71, 2015 25845324

Rathus JH, Miller AL: Dialectical behavior therapy adapted for suicidal adolescents. Suicide Life Threat Behav 32(2):146–157, 2002 12079031

Reifman A, Windle M: Adolescent suicidal behaviors as a function of depression, hopelessness, alcohol use, and social support: a longitudinal investigation. Am J Community Psychol 23(3):329–354, 1995 7572835

Reinherz HZ, Giaconia RM, Silverman AB, et al: Early psychosocial risks for adolescent suicidal ideation and attempts. J Am Acad Child Adolesc Psychiatry 34(5):599–611, 1995 7775355

Reinherz HZ, Tanner JL, Berger SR, et al: Adolescent suicidal ideation as predictive of psychopathology, suicidal behavior, and compromised functioning at age 30. Am J Psychiatry 163(7):1226–1232, 2006 16816228

Rihmer Z, Akiskal H: Do antidepressants t(h)reat(en) depressives? Toward a clinically judicious formulation of the antidepressant-suicidality FDA advisory in light of declining national suicide statistics from many countries. J Affect Disord 94(1–3):3–13, 2006 16712945

Rossouw TI, Fonagy P: Mentalization-based treatment for self-harm in adolescents: a randomized controlled trial. J Am Acad Child Adolesc Psychiatry 51(12):1304.e3–1313.e3, 2012 23200287

Roy A: Family history of suicide and neuroticism: a preliminary study. Psychiatry Res 110(1):87–90, 2002 12007597

Rudd MD, Joiner TE Jr, Jobes DA, et al: The outpatient treatment of suicidality: an integration of science and recognition of its limitations. Prof Psychol Res Pract 30(5):437–446, 1999

Rudd MD, Berman AL, Joiner TE Jr, et al: Warning signs for suicide: theory, research, and clinical applications. Suicide Life Threat Behav 36(3):255–262, 2006 16805653

Russell ST, Joyner K: Adolescent sexual orientation and suicide risk: evidence from a national study. Am J Public Health 91(8):1276–1281, 2001 11499118

Schwartz AJ: Rate, relative risk, and method of suicide by students at 4-year colleges and universities in the United States, 2004–2005 through 2008–2009. Suicide Life Threat Behav 41(4):353–371, 2011 21535095

Shaffer D, Pfeffer CY; American Academy of Child and Adolescent Psychiatry: Practice parameter for the assessment and treatment of children and adolescents with suicidal behavior. J Am Acad Child Adolesc Psychiatry 40 (7 suppl):24S–51S, 2001 11434483

Shaffer D, Gould MS, Fisher P, et al: Psychiatric diagnosis in child and adolescent suicide. Arch Gen Psychiatry 53(4):339–348, 1996 8634012

Silverman MM, Berman AL, Sanddal ND, et al: Rebuilding the tower of Babel: a revised nomenclature for the study of suicide and suicidal behaviors, Part 2: suicide-related ideations, communications, and behaviors. Suicide Life Threat Behav 37(3):264–277, 2007 17579539

Sliwa J: After decades of research, science is no better able to predict suicidal behavior. November 14, 2016. Available at: http://www.apa.org/press/release/2016/11/suicidal-behaviors.aspx. Accessed September 19, 2018.

Spirito A, Esposito-Smythers C, Wolff J, et al: Cognitive-behavioral therapy for adolescent depression and suicidality. Child Adolesc Psychiatr Clin N Am 20(2):191–204, 2011 21440850

Srinath S, Janardhan Reddy YC, Girimaji SR, et al: A prospective study of bipolar disorder in children and adolescents from India. Acta Psychiatr Scand 98(6):437–442, 1998 9879784

Stanley B, Brown GK: Safety planning intervention: a brief intervention to mitigate suicide risk. Cognitive and Behavioral Practices 19(2):256–264, 2012

Stanley B, Brown G, Brent DA, et al: Cognitive-behavioral therapy for suicide prevention (CBT-SP): treatment model, feasibility, and acceptability. J Am Acad Child Adolesc Psychiatry 48(10):1005–1013, 2009 19730273

Steele IH, Thrower N, Noroian P, et al: Understanding suicide across the lifespan: a United States perspective of suicide risk factors, assessment, and management. J Forensic Sci 63(1):162–171, 2018 28639299

Steer RA, Kumar G, Ranieri WF, et al: Use of the Beck Depression Inventory–II with adolescent psychiatric outpatients. J Psychopathol Behav Assess 20(2):127–139, 1998

Substance Abuse and Mental Health Services Administration: National Registry of Evidence-based Programs and Practices (NREPP). Updated August 7, 2018. Available at: https://www.samhsa.gov/nrepp. Accessed February 6, 2019.

Thompson R, Dubowitz H, English DJ, et al: Suicidal ideation among 8-year-olds who are maltreated and at risk: findings from the LONGSCAN studies. Child Maltreat 10:26–36, 2005 15611324

Tuisku V, Kiviruusu O, Pelkonen M, et al: Depressed adolescents as young adults—predictors of suicide attempt and non-suicidal self-injury during an 8-year follow-up. J Affect Disord 152–154:313–319, 2014 24144580

U.S. Department of Health and Human Services (HHS) Office of the Surgeon General and National Action Alliance for Suicide Prevention: 2012 national strategy for suicide prevention: goals and objectives for action. 2012. Available at: https://www.surgeongeneral.gov/library/reports/national-strategy-suicide-prevention/full-report.pdf. Accessed September 19, 2018.

Vitiello B, Silva SG, Rohde P, et al: Suicidal events in the Treatment for Adolescents With Depression Study (TADS). J Clin Psychiatry 70(5):741–747, 2009 19552869

Weinstein SM, Van Meter A, Katz AC, et al: Cognitive and family correlates of current suicidal ideation in children with bipolar disorder. J Affect Disord 173:15–21, 2015 25462390

Weinstein SM, Cruz RA, Isaia AR, et al: Child- and family focused cognitive behavioral therapy for pediatric bipolar disorder: applications for suicide prevention. Suicide Life Threat Behav Oct 16, 2017 [Epub ahead of print] 29044718

Welner A, Welner Z, Fishman R: Psychiatric adolescent inpatients: eight- to ten-year follow-up. Arch Gen Psychiatry 36(6):698–700, 1979 444023

Wenzel A, Brown GK, Beck AT: Cognitive Therapy for Suicidal Patients: Scientific and Clinical Applications. Washington, DC, American Psychological Association, 2009

Wilkinson PO: Nonsuicidal self-injury: a clear marker for suicide risk. J Am Acad Child Adolesc Psychiatry 50(8):741–743, 2011 21784292

Wilkinson P, Kelvin R, Roberts C, et al: Clinical and psychosocial predictors of suicide attempts and nonsuicidal self-injury in the Adolescent Depression Antidepressants and Psychotherapy Trial (ADAPT). Am J Psychiatry 168(5):495–501, 2011 21285141

Wortzel HS, Homaifar B, Matarazzo B, et al: Therapeutic risk management of the suicidal patient: stratifying risk in terms of severity and temporality. J Psychiatr Pract 20(1):63–67, 2014 24419312

Yen S, Weinstock LM, Andover MS, et al: Prospective predictors of adolescent suicidality: 6-month post-hospitalization follow-up. Psychol Med 43(5):983–993, 2013 22932393

14

Management of Common Co-occurring Conditions in Pediatric Mood Disorders

Daniel Azzopardi-Larios, M.D.
Cathryn A. Galanter, M.D.

In child and adolescent psychiatry, we commonly say that comorbidity is the rule, not the exception. Mood disorders are consistent with this. Comorbidity, or co-occurring conditions, is the simultaneous presence of two or more disorders. As many as 64% of youth with major depressive disorder (MDD) in epidemiological samples (Avenevoli et al. 2015), and in up to 90% of youth with bipolar disorder in clinical samples have co-occurring conditions (Joshi and Wilens 2009).

Evidence on the best approach to treating comorbid conditions is limited because most treatment trials approach one condition. Some of the large, multisite National Institute of Mental Health trials from the turn of the century, such as the Treatment for Adolescents with Depression Study (TADS; March et al. 2004), purposely included co-occurring conditions, allowing us to draw limited conclusions from moderator studies and secondary data analyses. In the case of MDD, we also have guidelines on co-occurring conditions from the Texas Children's Medication Algorithm Project (CMAP; Hughes et al. 2007). For pediatric bipolar disorder, evidence on the treatment of comorbid conditions in children and adolescents is limited, with the notable exception of attention-deficit/hyperactivity disorder (ADHD).

In this chapter, we bring together evidence and clinical practice to provide an evidence-informed approach to treating mood disorders with co-occurring conditions. We recommend using a modified version of the principles of CMAP (Hughes et al. 2007):

1. A comprehensive assessment is the cornerstone of good treatment. It should include a carefully made and accurate diagnosis with evaluation of potential comorbid diagnoses.
2. Standardized measures and rating scales should be used to aid with assessment and to monitor response.
3. A child's social and environmental context is a crucial part of comprehensive assessment and treatment.
4. In many cases, collaboration with a child's school for collateral information as part of assessment and for comprehensive treatment is crucial.
5. Treatment recommendations should be informed by the evidence and include psychopharmacology, psychotherapy, and psychoeducation for both caregivers and youth.
6. Patient and caregiver preferences are important in treatment decisions. Whether to treat symptoms with medication, psychotherapy, or both and how to sequence treatments should be informed by evidence and determined by clinician judgment with discussion, input, consent, and assent from the family and patient.
7. The presence of depression or other psychiatric illness in family members, as well as any family conflict, should be addressed and treated (Birmaher et al. 2000; Brent et al. 1998; Weissman et al. 2006).
8. Complicated or partially and nonresponsive cases, whenever possible, should be referred to a child and adolescent psychiatrist for further assessment and treatment or a second opinion, particularly after adequate trials of the first treatment have been initiated. At this juncture, reassessment of diagnosis and additional assessments of dose, duration, and adherence should be considered.

Depression and Co-occurring Conditions

Addressing the treatment of depression with co-occurring conditions is a common task, given that 40%–90% of children and adolescents with MDD have such conditions (Avenevoli et al. 2015; Birmaher et al. 2007). The first step is always a careful comprehensive assessment to clarify a patient's diagnoses, the target symptoms, and any crucial psychosocial issues. Rating scales are an important part of assessment and future monitoring, because they can help support clinician decision making (Galanter and Jensen 2017). The Texas CMAP update on the medication treatment of childhood disorders (Hughes et al. 2007) offers guidelines and algorithms for treating MDD along with co-occurring conditions.

When choosing a treatment for MDD with co-occurring conditions, we are faced with the option of starting with the treatment for depression, starting with the treatment for the co-occurring condition, or identifying a treatment that might potentially cover both. Given the limited evidence, the "right" choice should be based on the evidence available and adapted to the specific diagnoses as well as the circumstances particular to each child.

Case: Major Depressive Disorder and Attention-Deficit/Hyperactivity Disorder

David, a 14-year-old boy, lived with his parents and attended ninth grade at an academically rigorous high school. He first presented for a psychiatric consultation in December because he "has had a very tumultuous few months and fallen off high school work." His parents were concerned because of his decline in functioning and also because they have a family history of mental illness and want to prevent any adverse outcomes.

David transitioned well to his new school at the beginning of ninth grade. He had always been a high-achieving child who succeeded with very little pressure or intervention from his parents, but transitions were often challenging. About 1 month into school, he had a "meltdown" over a homework assignment. His father became concerned, investigated the online homework log, and found that David had multiple overdue assignments. His parents contacted the school and, with the school's help, instituted a plan of higher supervision for homework and a tutor for math. David appreciated the structure but also was resistant at times; thus, the interventions were only minimally helpful.

David reported that he felt anxious about certain things and could "go into a spiral." He intended to get work done and would spend hours at his desk or the dining room table getting very little done. Although he denied feeling sad, he no longer enjoys activities that used to be fun. Last spring, he quit his travel soccer team to dedicate more time to school and also because he felt that he was no longer one of the best players, and he stopped playing the piano. He denies feeling sad most of the day every day but feels down off and on. In the last few weeks, he has felt "dark and empty" most days. He has always had some difficulty with being fidgety and inattentive, and these problems have worsened drastically this year. He has trouble falling asleep at night but typically sleeps 7 hours. His appetite is good. He has occasionally wished that he were dead when feeling overwhelmed but has not had a wish or an intent to harm himself. He and his parents denied a history of manic symptoms, although at times, he was more energetic and productive.

His psychiatric history is significant for anxiety from a very young age, for which he saw a therapist off and on. He was unable to sleep over at friends' houses or attend sleepaway camp.

Medical history is noncontributory. Developmental milestones were on time. Trauma and substance use were denied. Family history is significant for bipolar disorder, substance use disorder, and anxiety.

David completed a Screen for Child Anxiety Related Emotional Disorders (SCARED; Birmaher et al. 1997) that suggests an anxiety disorder, an Adult ADHD Self-Report Scale (ASRS-v1.1; Adler et al. 2006) that suggests ADHD, and a Patient Health Questionnaire (PHQ-9) Modified for Teens (GLAD-PC Toolkit; available at: http://www.glad-pc.org) that is consistent with moderate depression. David's parents complete a SCARED, which is not consistent with an anxiety disorder, and a Swanson, Nolan and Pelham–IV Questionnaire (SNAP-IV; Bussing et al. 2008), which is consistent with ADHD, inattentive presentation. David is diagnosed with MDD; ADHD; and generalized anxiety disorder, in partial remission.

Treatment Recommendations: Major Depressive Disorder and Attention-Deficit/Hyperactivity Disorder

For children and adolescents with co-occurring ADHD and MDD, the first step is a comprehensive assessment that takes into account the timeline and severity of the symptoms and psychosocial, familial, and academic circumstances of the child. The Texas CMAP (Hughes et al. 2007) offers helpful guidelines for treating co-occurring MDD and ADHD and starts by emphasizing a diagnostic assessment and consulting with the family about a treatment plan. We have included the algorithm in Figure 14–1.

Consistent with the most recent version of the CMAP update on the medication treatment of childhood disorders, we recommend treating the most severe condition first while recognizing that ADHD responds more quickly to psychopharmacological intervention (Hughes et al. 2007). In

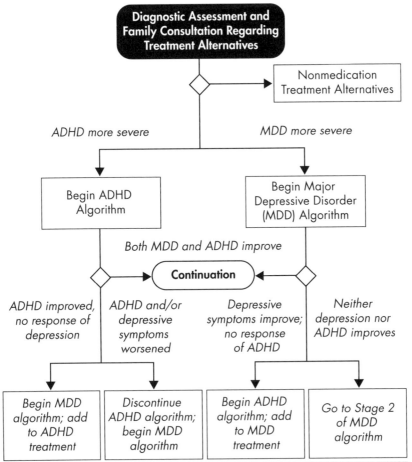

FIGURE 14–1.   Medication algorithm for treating major depressive disorder in children and adolescents whose symptoms also meet criteria for attention-deficit/hyperactivity disorder (ADHD).

Source.   Adapted from the Texas Children's Medication Algorithm Project (CMAP; Hughes et al. 2007).

most cases, we recommend starting only one medication at a time to minimize the chance of overprescribing and adverse effects and to best understand which interventions are effective. Once treatment is initiated, the clinician can reassess symptoms every few weeks.

If starting with a psychopharmacological treatment for depression, we recommend using a selective serotonin reuptake inhibitor (SSRI), and because of the evidence of efficacy for the treatment of depression in both children and adolescents, we typically start with fluoxetine (Emslie et al.

1997). Psychotherapy, such as cognitive-behavioral therapy (CBT) or interpersonal psychotherapy, also may be appropriate first-line treatment for depression, because these therapies have shown efficacy for the treatment of depression (Brent et al. 1998; Dietz et al. 2015; Mufson et al. 1999), although not specifically for MDD with co-occurring ADHD. If starting with treatment for the ADHD, we recommend using first-line ADHD treatments—namely, stimulants (Hughes et al. 2007; Pliszka et al. 2006). Given the evidence for efficacy of SSRIs for treatment of depression (see, e.g., Emslie et al. 1997; March et al. 2004) and lack of evidence for efficacy of noradrenergic antidepressants (e.g., bupropion, desipramine), we prefer an SSRI plus a stimulant, if needed, as opposed to noradrenergic antidepressants.

In some cases, treatment of one disorder leads to improvement of the other. Thus, prescribing additional medication would not be necessary. If symptoms of the first disorder are remitting but other symptoms remain, then the treatment for the second condition should be started in conjunction with the first treatment by following the previously discussed recommendations for a pharmacological approach. If treating the first condition does not lead to improvement of the first condition or worsens the second condition, the clinician should consider discontinuing and switching to the first-line medication for the other condition or trying a different medication for the first condition. CMAP guidelines suggest the first option. For example, adding a stimulant may lead to increased depressive symptoms, and it can be difficult to determine whether the worsening is related to adverse effects of the medication or to the natural course of the underlying condition. Stimulants have been reported to cause depressive symptoms (Lafay-Chebassier et al. 2015). Additionally, SSRIs can cause mild activation and disinhibition, which may look like ADHD (Reinblatt et al. 2009). In these cases, the first step is obtaining a careful history and timeline to determine whether the onset of symptoms coincided with the initiation or dose increase of the medication. If the stimulant may be leading to worsening of depression, given the short half-life, it should be discontinued for at least 1–2 weeks to determine whether the depressive symptoms improve or resolve.

Atomoxetine is a reasonable choice for second-line treatment of ADHD when stimulants are ineffective or lead to adverse effects. We consider atomoxetine after stimulants because of its smaller effect size of 0.62 compared with 0.91 and 0.95 for immediate-release and long-acting stimulants, respectively (Faraone et al. 2006). In a double-blind, randomized treatment trial of atomoxetine to treat ADHD and MDD in adolescents, atomoxetine led to improvement of ADHD but not of depressive symptoms (Bangs et al. 2007). We are unaware of any randomized controlled trials (RCTs) demonstrating efficacy of bupropion for co-occurring MDD and ADHD in children and adolescents. A small open-label trial in children and adolescents with depression (MDD or dysthymia) and ADHD found that bupropion led to improvement in depressive and ADHD symptoms (Daviss et al. 2001). Bupropion has been shown to be only partially effective in treating ADHD in children (Conners et al. 1996) and has smaller effect sizes than those for the stimulants (Stuhec et al. 2015). No RCTs have reported the efficacy of bupropion in treating MDD in youth, but evidence shows that bupropion is effective in treating MDD in adults (Hewett et al. 2010). Thus, further studies are warranted to examine whether bupropion might be an effective treatment of co-occurring ADHD and MDD. It is worth consideration after treatments with more evidence of efficacy have been tried.

Much of the previously described guidance comes from CMAP and clinician consensus. Several secondary data analyses have examined the effect of ADHD on the outcomes of MDD. In TADS, for those patients with MDD and co-occurring ADHD, CBT, fluoxetine alone, and the combined treatments were superior to placebo. In contrast, for participants with MDD without ADHD, only fluoxetine and CBT were more effective than placebo (Curry et al. 2006). At 36 weeks, those adolescents with both MDD and ADHD had improvement trajectories that were similar in all treatment groups (CBT, fluoxetine, combined), in contrast to adolescents with MDD without ADHD, among whom the most rapid improvement occurred with combined treatment (Kratochvil et al. 2009). These analyses examined depressive symptom outcome and not ADHD symptom outcome. They appeared to indicate that CBT may be a viable first-line option for treating depression in patients with co-occurring depression and ADHD. In the Treatment of (SSRI) Resistant Depression in Adolescents (TORDIA) trial, in which participants received either an SSRI or venlafaxine, with or without CBT, improvement of depression correlated with improvement of ADHD diagnoses and symptoms, regardless of the treatment arm, and whether or not adolescents were already taking stimulants for ADHD prior to entering the trial.

> In the case of David, his initial treatment plan included restarting psychotherapy, initiating a low dose (18 mg) of OROS (osmotic-release oral system) methylphenidate, and continuing his tutoring. His stimulant was titrated to 36 mg with good effect. He could more easily concentrate in class, engage with his teachers, and complete his homework. Conflict at home also decreased. He initially complained of no adverse effects other than decreased appetite.

After several months, David's depressive symptoms returned. He began to get overwhelmed in school and stated that he often felt sad for no reason and was often tearful. His psychiatrist prescribed fluoxetine and titrated it up to 20 mg, and his depressive symptoms gradually improved. The following school year, David chose to discontinue his methylphenidate because of the side effects. His attention became mildly impaired but, in his estimation, was "good enough." He continued taking his fluoxetine.

Treatment Recommendations: Major Depressive Disorder and Anxiety Disorders

Depression in children and adolescents is frequently associated with anxiety disorders and anxiety symptoms, with estimates ranging from 15% to 75% (Angold et al. 1999; Yorbik et al. 2004). Despite these high rates of comorbidity, very few RCTs have investigated the treatment of co-occurring MDD and anxiety. Most treatment recommendations are derived from secondary data analyses and clinical consensus. As a result, the choice of initiating medication, psychotherapy, or both may be based on clinical severity, patient preferences, and community resources.

Evidence indicates that both SSRIs and CBT can be used to treat anxiety and MDD and thus should be considered either alone or in combination. This is consistent with recommendations from CMAP (Hughes et al. 2007). Whether therapy, medication, or both should be first line is based on clinical judgment in the absence of evidence. We suggest CBT as first-line treatment for mild to moderate symptoms and a combination for moderate to severe symptoms. This recommendation may be modified according to patient preference and resources available in the community.

We choose fluoxetine as the starting medication because of the data for efficacy in treating both MDD (Cipriani et al. 2016) and anxiety (Birmaher et al. 2007) and the U.S. Food and Drug Administration (FDA) indication for MDD in both children and adolescents 8 years and older. Escitalopram also has been demonstrated to be effective in treating depression in adolescents (Dineen Wagner et al. 2006). There is evidence suggesting efficacy for serotonin-norepinephrine reuptake inhibitors (SNRIs) if first-line SSRIs are not effective. SNRIs have evidence for efficacy for treating anxiety in children and adolescents (March et al. 2007; Rynn et al. 2007; Strawn et al. 2015). In a meta-analysis of double-blind RCTs for the treatment of anxiety disorders, Strawn and colleagues (2018) showed that SSRIs (including fluoxetine) resulted in greater improvement than both placebo and SNRIs. In the TORDIA study, Brent and colleagues (2008) found that when a first SSRI was ineffective, switching to a second medication (a different SSRI or venlafaxine) in combination with CBT was effective. They suggested an SSRI plus

CBT as preferable given that both classes had similar effects but venlafaxine was associated with greater risk of adverse effects (Brent et al. 2008). Thus, given the above evidence, we recommend fluoxetine as the first-line medication for the pharmacological treatment of comorbid depression and anxiety to be taken in combination with psychotherapy, with an alternative SSRI as a second-line, and an SNRI as a third-line, treatment.

No major RCTs have specifically examined the treatment of comorbid MDD and anxiety, but some MDD studies have examined anxiety as a moderator and thus merit mention. In TADS, in which youth ages 12–17 years with MDD were assigned to receive fluoxetine, CBT, both fluoxetine and CBT, or clinical management with pill placebo, comorbid anxiety was a negative predictor and did not moderate treatment outcome (Curry et al. 2006). In studying the efficacy of acute treatment with CBT for depression, investigators found that comorbid anxiety was associated with lessened improvement of depressive symptoms (Clarke et al. 1992). Brent and colleagues (1998) compared three different psychotherapies for adolescents—CBT, systemic behavioral family therapy, and nondirective supportive therapy—and found that those youth receiving CBT were more likely to improve and that comorbid anxiety predicted depression at the end of acute treatment.

In the TORDIA study, in which adolescents were randomly assigned to receive medication alone (SSRI or venlafaxine) or medication combined with CBT, those who received medication and CBT were more likely to be responders (based on Clinical Global Impression [CGI] Scale scores and decreases in depressive symptoms (Brent et al. 2008). Moderator analyses examining the effect of co-occurring conditions found that medication with CBT showed even greater superiority over medication without CBT for those adolescents with comorbid anxiety disorder (Asarnow et al. 2009). Further analysis also showed that an improvement in depression was associated with an improvement in anxiety symptoms and anxiety disorders (Hilton et al. 2013), regardless of the type of treatment received, with no difference between venlafaxine and SSRIs and no added benefit when medication was combined with CBT. Investigators hypothesized that CBT might have shown additive effects on anxiety if it had been included.

Treatment Recommendations: Major Depressive Disorder and Obsessive-Compulsive Disorder

Youth with obsessive-compulsive disorder (OCD) commonly have co-occurring depression at rates of 10%–73% (Farrell et al. 2012). The prevalence of OCD in children with MDD is unknown, but it is lower because OCD is a less common condition.

We are unaware of guidelines for managing MDD with comorbid OCD (Hughes et al. 2007). This may be, in part, because OCD was classified as an anxiety disorder prior to 2013, at which point OCD was separated from anxiety disorders in DSM-5 (American Psychiatric Association 2013).

In the absence of specific research investigating the treatment of co-occurring pediatric depression and OCD, we refer to the algorithm that is used in the treatment of depression and anxiety. As for anxiety, both SSRIs and CBT are effective treatments for both conditions (Curry et al. 2006; Geller and March 2012). With moderate to severe OCD or MDD, we recommend initiating both fluoxetine (based on the evidence of efficacy and an FDA indication for both conditions) and CBT that includes exposure and response prevention (ERP). For mild to moderate OCD and MDD, the decision to start with CBT, an SSRI, or both varies according to patient circumstances, choice, and available resources.

Escitalopram also has evidence for efficacy and FDA approval for the treatment of depression in adolescents (Dineen Wagner et al. 2006). Several double-blind, placebo-controlled studies have demonstrated that SSRIs, including fluoxetine, sertraline, and fluvoxamine, are superior to placebo in treating OCD and have an FDA indication (March et al. 1998; Riddle et al. 1992, 2001).

Several studies have demonstrated the efficacy of CBT and SSRIs in the treatment of OCD and may indicate the added value of combined treatment for youth with co-occurring disorders. The Pediatric OCD Treatment Study II, which excluded patients with co-occurring depression, demonstrated that CBT, sertraline, and combined treatments all led to improvement but that combined treatment was more likely to lead to remission (Franklin et al. 2011). Two studies addressed the effect of depression and depressive symptoms on the response to CBT in the treatment of OCD. Storch and colleagues (2008) treated youth with OCD with family-based CBT that included an exposure component and found that the presence of MDD was associated with lower rates of treatment response and remission. In a different study, Storch and colleagues (2013) compared CBT with and without sertraline in the treatment of OCD. In addition to OCD response, they found a reduction in depressive symptoms across all groups, with a nonsignificant lesser response in the CBT-only group.

Treatment Recommendations: Major Depressive Disorder and Disruptive Behavior Disorders

Disruptive behavior disorders (DBDs), including conduct disorder (CD) and oppositional defiant disorder (ODD), co-occur in 21%–83% of youth with depression (Angold and Costello 1993). Youth with depression and high levels of oppositionality are often particularly difficult to treat (Jacobs et al. 2010). Specific guidelines for the treatment of co-occurring depression and DBD in children and adolescents are not available. We recommend treating the depressive disorder first and then focusing on the ODD or CD.

Pharmacotherapeutic interventions for comorbid depression and DBD have not been well studied. Curry and colleagues (2006) examined whether DBDs (including ODD, CD, and ADHD) moderated the outcome of depressive symptoms in TADS. They found that any co-occurring disorder predicted less improvement in depressive symptoms. However, the specific presence of comorbid DBD did not further moderate which treatment was more or less effective. Jacobs and colleagues (2010) conducted a secondary data analysis from TADS to examine the effect of the different treatment options on co-occurring oppositionality in adolescents with MDD. All treatment arms, especially those that included fluoxetine, led to a reduction in oppositional behavior from clinical to subclinical levels. In patients whose depression was in remission, CBT was better than placebo in improving the symptoms of oppositionality. However, CBT was not better than placebo in patients whose depression was persistent. Results from TORDIA also indicated that remission of treatment-resistant depression had a beneficial effect on disruptive behavior disorder symptoms regardless of the type of treatment (SSRI or venlafaxine alone or medication with CBT) and that there was a nonsignificant trend of SSRIs versus venlafaxine leading to decreased disruptive behavior disorders (Hilton et al. 2013).

Once the depression is treated, we recommend applying the principles from the Treatment Recommendations for the Use of Antipsychotics for Aggressive Youth (TRAAY) and the Treatment of Maladaptive Aggression in Youth (TMAY)—specifically, treating comorbid conditions and using evidence-based psychosocial interventions (Pappadopulos et al. 2003; Scotto Rosato et al. 2012). Evidence-based psychosocial interventions, such as parent management training, have evidence of efficacy (for a review, see Eyberg et al. 2008).

Treatment Recommendations: Major Depressive Disorder and Substance Use Disorders

The comorbidity between depression and substance use disorders is high, with an estimated 20%–30% of depressed adolescents having a substance use disorder (Birmaher et al. 1996). Conversely, MDD may be found in

24%–50% of youth with a substance use disorder (Kaminer et al. 2008). Observational studies suggest that co-occurring depression is associated with worse treatment outcomes for substance use disorders (Zhou et al. 2015).

When treating co-occurring MDD and a substance use disorder in adolescents, we recommend that clinicians perform an initial comprehensive evaluation and periodically reassess for substance use in their patients with depression, because patients may not initially reveal the extent of their use, or may increase use over time. Additionally, youth with treatment-resistant depression may have high rates of substance use (Goldstein et al. 2009).

We are unaware of practice guidelines that specifically address the co-occurring conditions. The volume *Youth Substance Abuse and Co-occurring Disorders* offers one of the most comprehensive reviews (Kaminer 2015). Given limited RCTs targeting the treatment of both disorders, we recommend using evidence-informed treatments provided either by the same clinician with expertise in the treatment of both mood and substance use disorders or by different clinicians, each responsible for one disorder, working in collaboration (Kaminer et al. 2008).

Treatment typically involves a combined pharmacological and psychosocial intervention with psychotherapy that targets both the depression and the substance use disorder. For moderate to severe MDD, we recommend the use of an SSRI. Both fluoxetine and escitalopram have evidence for efficacy in adolescents (Emslie et al. 1997; Dineen Wagner et al. 2006). One meta-analysis examining the efficacy of antidepressants in treating MDD and co-occurring substance use disorders in adolescents and young adults demonstrated that antidepressant medication had a small overall effect in reducing depression, but no significant difference was seen in improving substance abuse symptoms (Zhou et al. 2015). The TORDIA trial excluded youth with substance use disorders by design but found that substance use was common (Goldstein et al. 2009). In their secondary data analysis, investigators found that treatments for MDD (SSRI, venlafaxine, or either medication plus CBT) led to significant improvement in substance-related impairment among adolescents who responded to MDD treatment, and that there were no significant differential effects of specific treatments on substance use.

Several psychotherapeutic interventions for substance use disorders, such as motivational enhancement therapy and CBT, are manualized and have demonstrated efficacy in randomized trials (Dennis et al. 2004). Some evidence indicates that treatment of substance use disorders will result in improvement of depression. In a study of patients with substance use disorders, investigators found that participants in the treatment arm (brief strategic family therapy) and those receiving treatment as usual both had decreases in symptoms of depression and anxiety as well as in rates of probable depressive and anxiety disorders (Horigian et al. 2013).

Cannabinoids have received a great deal of attention over recent years for their possible medicinal uses. At this time, no evidence has supported efficacy of medical marijuana to treat depression. Whiting et al. (2015) conducted a systematic review and meta-analysis of 79 RCTs of cannabinoid use to treat several indications in adults, including depression. Three studies suggested no difference between cannabinoids (dronabinol and nabiximols) and placebo in depression outcomes. A parallel-group trial compared different doses of nabiximols and reported a negative effect at high doses and no difference at low doses when compared with placebo. Evidence shows that cannabis has adverse health effects, and research has indicated an overall medium level of confidence in the association between cannabis use and depression (Levine et al. 2017; Volkow et al. 2014).

Bipolar Disorder and Co-occurring Conditions

The first step to safe and effective treatment of bipolar disorder and co-occurring conditions is a comprehensive assessment. In most cases, the first step of treatment is to assess mania or depression and to stabilize the mood before addressing the co-occurring conditions.

Case: Bipolar Disorder and Attention-Deficit/ Hyperactivity Disorder

Jess, a 15-year-old girl in her sophomore year at parochial school, lives with both of her parents and has an older half-sister in college. Jess is brought in by her mother for a second opinion because of a 1-year history of periods of depressed and elevated mood that coincided with paranoid ideation and visual hallucinations. In the spring of her freshman year, she became disengaged in school, lost interest in previously enjoyable activities, and quit the softball team. Her energy was low, and she withdrew from friends. She felt depressed during most of this period. She had thoughts that she was being videotaped throughout the day by the government. She heard a voice commenting negatively on her appearance and behavior throughout the day, warning her against certain behaviors by saying "bad idea." She saw giant white cats sitting on the hood of a car and denied being intoxicated at the time. She was taking lisdexamfetamine (and had been taking stimulants for several years).

Although mainly depressed for the last 9 months, Jess described a 3-week period during the summer when she experienced elevated mood and energy. She was "laughing, writing, bouncing" throughout this period. She felt "invincible," only needed 4 hours of sleep per night, and felt well rested the next day. She went 2 days without sleep, staying up late and writing poetry that she thought was brilliant, leading her to reach out to an editor at the *New Yorker*. She had pressured speech, and her friends said that she was on "fast forward" and they couldn't press the pause button to slow her down. She reported feeling "horny" and wore more revealing clothes. Her parents did not recall noticing a change in mood or speech at that time. Jess had not been taking a stimulant or any prescribed medication over the summer, because she was on a "medication holiday."

In the fall, Jess felt "down" again. She saw iguanas running all over the drama stage at school. She became angry when she was thrown out of the school play and had several episodes of cutting her thigh without an intent to kill herself. Jess and her mother reported these symptoms to her psychiatrist, who stopped the lisdexamfetamine and referred her for a neurological workup; her magnetic resonance imaging and electroencephalogram were within normal limits. The symptoms continued. She later reported having suicidal ideation and wanting to overdose on her medication, and was admitted to an inpatient psychiatric unit.

Jess was started on aripiprazole, 5 mg/day, with near complete resolution of auditory and visual hallucinations. She continued to have rage symptoms at home, including an episode on New Year's Eve when she was overcome with anger when her parents interfered with her plans to travel to a party. Increase of the aripiprazole to 10 mg led to complete resolution of the hallucinations, rage, and impulsivity.

Jess's history is significant for problems related to attention, distractibility, and difficulty staying on task and organizing activities and assignments. This first became apparent in second grade, and Jess began receiving help at the school learning center. With that support, she was able to function in school until eighth grade. She started taking methylphenidate extended-release tablets in the summer before sixth grade, and the medication was titrated to 54 mg/day with good response. Between eighth and tenth grade, her grades slipped from B's to two C's and three F's. In spring of ninth grade, her psychiatrist stopped the methylphenidate and started the lisdexamfetamine, to which she had little apparent response.

Jess reported having mood instability since third grade, including increased anger and sadness, low energy, frequent crying spells, and onset insomnia. In eighth grade she had depressed mood and visual hallucinations of arrows coming out of stoplights or flickering lights. She also reported periods of anxiety that have waxed and waned.

Jess started smoking marijuana in the fall of her freshman year and has since smoked approximately one to two times per month. At times, the hallucinations occurred while she was using marijuana, but this was not always the case. She denied other substance use other than an occasional drink at parties.

Her father has a chronic medical illness that has at times led to hospitalization, although when healthy, he functions well and works as a graphic designer. Her mother is an advertising executive who has temper problems, ADHD, and bipolar II disorder. Her maternal grandmother and uncle both had mood disorders and died by suicide. No history of diabetes or arrhythmias was found in the family.

Her medical history is unremarkable, and she was on track developmentally with the exception of some early challenges with reading. She had psychological testing done when she was 14 years old that was significant for a Full Scale IQ of 111, with verbal comprehension of 126, perceptual reasoning of 104, working memory of 99, and processing speed of 83.

Jess is well put together, wearing a name-brand warm-up suit and makeup. She appears slightly older than her stated age. She is engaged and cooperative with good eye contact. She can be fidgety, shifting in her seat and tapping her foot. Her speech is of normal rate and volume although slightly monotonous. Her mood is "okay" and her affect, slightly constricted. Her thought process is goal oriented. She denies paranoia, hallucinations, and suicidal and homicidal ideation. Her judgment and insight were fair.

Treatment Recommendations: Bipolar Disorder and Attention-Deficit/Hyperactivity Disorder

Children and adolescents with bipolar disorder often have co-occurring ADHD. A recent meta-analysis found rates as high as 70% (Van Meter et al. 2016). Because ADHD and bipolar disorder have multiple overlapping symptoms, a careful assessment is a key component to effective treatment. This indicates obtaining a timeline of symptoms and discerning whether the patient's symptoms meet full criteria for a manic episode as well as full criteria for ADHD during euthymic periods. The clinician must discern whether this is treatment-emergent mania in a child with ADHD, ADHD with some manic symptoms, or someone who has both ADHD and bipolar disorder. Careful monitoring of baseline symptoms and response using rating scales is important in supporting clinical decision making. Rating scales such as the SNAP-IV (Bussing et al. 2008) and the Child Mania Rating Scale (Pavuluri et al. 2006) are available in the public domain.

When a child with preexisting ADHD develops mania for the first time while taking a stimulant, we recommend discontinuing the stimulant, because stimulants have in rare cases led to manic-like symptoms (Ross 2006). If the manic symptoms resolve, some children may tolerate a carefully monitored rechallenge of the stimulant at a lower dose. Interestingly, data on whether stimulants can cause bipolar disorder are mixed. For example, in a nationwide population-based sample of patients with ADHD in Taiwan, those who took stimulants were less likely to develop bipolar disorder than were those who did not (Wang et al. 2016).

For ADHD with some manic symptoms, stimulants may in fact be helpful. Several studies, including post hoc analyses from the Multimodal

Treatment Study of Children With ADHD, showed that children who had some manic symptoms but whose symptoms did not meet the full criteria for bipolar disorder responded well to treatment with stimulants (Galanter et al. 2003, 2005).

For children and adolescents with both bipolar disorder and ADHD, we recommend first stabilizing the mania. Atypical antipsychotics have the most evidence for efficacy and greatest effect sizes for treating acute mania (Correll et al. 2010; Geller et al. 2012). Lithium also may be a reasonable first-line treatment, especially in patients with nonpsychotic classic mania (Findling et al. 2015). Although atypical antipsychotics have evidence for treating mania, they do not treat ADHD. A randomized pilot study examining the response to aripiprazole compared with placebo in children and adolescents with co-occurring bipolar disorder and ADHD found that those who received aripiprazole had a significantly better improvement in response and remission of manic symptoms but no between-group differences in improvement of ADHD symptoms (Tramontina et al. 2009). Finally, in the Treatment of Early Age Mania (TEAM) study, children and adolescents with bipolar disorder were randomly assigned to receive risperidone, lithium, or divalproex and were most responsive to risperidone (Geller et al. 2012); 93% of the sample had co-occurring ADHD. A moderator analysis showed that those with ADHD in comparison to those without ADHD had a greater probability of improvement of manic symptoms responding to risperidone than to lithium.

Once a patient is euthymic, if ADHD symptoms remain, studies indicate that one can slowly and cautiously initiate a trial with a stimulant. Two small randomized controlled studies showed that after mood stabilization, children and adolescents could undergo safe and effective treatment with mixed amphetamine salts or methylphenidate (Findling et al. 2007; Scheffer et al. 2005), and a third study failed to show efficacy but did not lead to destabilization (Zeni et al. 2009). Scheffer et al. (2005) treated bipolar I disorder and ADHD with divalproex sodium in open treatment, after which euthymic patients participated in a 4-week randomized double-blind, placebo-controlled crossover trial of mixed amphetamine salts versus placebo. The divalproex sodium alone improved ADHD symptoms in a minority of the patients. Mixed amphetamine salts were more effective than placebo without worsening of side effects or manic symptoms. Findling and colleagues (2007) used methylphenidate in a randomized crossover design to treat bipolar spectrum disorders in children and adolescents whose moods had been stabilized with lithium, divalproex sodium, or a combination and found that best-dose methylphenidate was more effective than placebo and was well tolerated. Zeni and colleagues

(2009) stabilized the mood of children and adolescents with bipolar disorder and ADHD with aripiprazole, after which the youth were randomly assigned to methylphenidate or placebo. Methylphenidate was no more effective than placebo in improving manic symptoms, was no more likely to be associated with adverse effects, and significantly improved self-reported depressive symptoms.

Other classes of medications for ADHD have less evidence for safety and efficacy. In open trials, Chang et al. (2009) found that most youth with bipolar disorder and ADHD whose mood had been stabilized responded well to atomoxetine. However, both in their sample and in other reports, atomoxetine was associated with exacerbation of preexisting mania (Chang et al. 2009) and new-onset manic episodes (Peruzzolo et al. 2014). Similarly, we are unaware of any trials showing that α-adrenergic receptor antagonists are more or less likely than stimulants to lead to treatment-emergent mania, although there are case reports of guanfacine leading to mania and hypomania (Horrigan and Barnhill 1999).

Given that stimulants, atomoxetine, and α-antagonists carry with them the risk of precipitating mania, we recommend starting with a stimulant, because it is the first-line treatment for ADHD. Given the risk of destabilization, we recommend starting at a low dose and titrating slowly. In the event that a child has an exacerbation of symptoms such as worsening mood, activation, or agitation, we recommend tapering and possibly discontinuing the stimulant. Once the mood destabilization has resolved, the clinician should consider a retrial with a different stimulant or the same stimulant at a lower dose.

In the case of Jess described earlier in this chapter, several aspects of her treatment are worth noting. Jess had a well-documented history of ADHD and then developed bipolar disorder. Her mood symptoms had been present from a young age but were not detected until adolescence. Her first mood episode was depression, and she then experienced a manic episode. When her psychiatrist became aware of her mood episodes, he wisely discontinued her stimulant to determine whether it was causing or exacerbating her mood symptoms. In her case, removal of the stimulant did not lead to resolution of mood symptoms. She was started on aripiprazole, leading to partial improvement of her mood symptoms. She continued to have irritability and periods of low mood not meeting full criteria for mood episodes. Her psychiatrist at the time recommended evidence-based psychotherapy so that she could develop further skills in managing her mood, but she refused to attend weekly appointments, even though she was willing to come monthly for her medication. Lithium was added, leading to further improvement of her mood. Thereafter, she started taking methylphenidate again, leading to increased attention and ability to complete her schoolwork.

Treatment Recommendations: Bipolar Disorder and Anxiety

Anxiety disorders commonly co-occur in pediatric bipolar disorder, with rates ranging from 23% to 80% (Frías et al. 2015; Van Meter et al. 2016). Anxiety disorders can adversely affect the course of bipolar disorder in youth, as characterized by less follow-up time being asymptomatic and more consistent with syndromal mixed, cycling, and subsyndromal depressive symptomatology (Sala et al. 2014). Anxiety disorders have been shown both to precede the onset of bipolar disorder (Masi et al. 2001) and to develop in youth after bipolar disorder (Sala et al. 2012).

Treating a child with co-occurring bipolar and anxiety disorders poses clinical challenges because of the lack of RCTs. We recommend mood stabilization with pharmacotherapy following treatment guidelines for bipolar disorder as the first goal of treatment, because the symptoms of bipolar disorder produce the most functional impairment.

Once a child's mood symptoms are adequately treated, the focus of treatment can then shift to the anxiety disorder, at which point CBT would be the first-line treatment given the proven efficacy of CBT in the treatment of anxiety (Hofmann et al. 2012) and as an adjunctive treatment for bipolar disorder (Fristad et al. 2011; West et al. 2014), and the risk of the anti-anxiety medication leading to mood destabilization. This sequence of treatment is consistent with the pediatric and adult guidelines (Kowatch et al. 2005; Yatham et al. 2018).

CBT programs developed to treat bipolar and other mood disorders have not been shown to improve anxiety outcomes. Cummings and Fristad (2012) compared multifamily psychoeducational psychotherapy (MF-PEP) with a wait-list control in treating youth with mood disorders. The presence of anxiety symptoms did not impede the response of mood symptoms to MF-PEP. The number of anxiety symptoms decreased in the MF-PEP group and increased in the control group, but this difference did not achieve statistical significance. Similarly, Weinstein and colleagues (2015) examined whether anxiety was a moderator in the response to child- and family-focused CBT and found that the presence of anxiety disorders did not moderate outcome of manic symptom response. In order for anxiety to benefit from CBT, the treatment may need an anxiety focus and elements such as exposure-based CBT, given that exposure has been identified as a key component for the treatment of anxiety (Kendall et al.

2005). Given the evidence for CBT in treating anxiety in the absence of bipolar disorder, we recommend it as the first-line treatment. If the anxiety does not respond to anxiety-targeted CBT, or if CBT is not available, then the clinician may consider other types of psychotherapy.

If psychotherapy, CBT or otherwise, does not lead to improvement of anxiety, we recommend the careful addition of an SSRI. We are unaware of RCTs that investigated whether children or adults with bipolar disorder and anxiety disorders whose moods were first stabilized with a mood stabilizer can be treated safely and effectively with an SSRI. Thus, this recommendation is based on evidence for best practices of treating anxiety. If a clinician decides to treat the comorbid anxiety disorder with an SSRI, the child should be carefully monitored for the potential of manic or hypomanic symptoms. In a naturalistic study, Masi and colleagues (2001) found that for children with bipolar disorder, hypomania after treatment with an antidepressant occurred more frequently in those with comorbid anxiety disorder compared with those without. The authors did not discuss which antidepressants were prescribed and whether they were used to treat anxiety symptoms or depressive symptoms.

SSRIs should be initiated with caution because of the potential risk of destabilization. We do not recommend using an SSRI in the absence of a mood stabilizer to treat anxiety in youth with co-occurring bipolar disorder and anxiety disorders given the risk of precipitating mania. A large study examining the use of antidepressants in children with anxiety and depression drawn from a national medical and prescription claims database demonstrated that manic conversion, defined by a new diagnosis of bipolar disorder, was increased in patients taking SSRIs, tricyclics, or other antidepressants (Martin et al. 2004). Some evidence from adults suggests that giving a mood stabilizer in addition to an antidepressant to treat bipolar depression decreases the risk of a switch to mania and hypomania (Licht et al. 2008; Vázquez et al. 2013), but a meta-analysis concluded that mood stabilizers did not have a significant protective effect (Tondo et al. 2010).

No RCTs have reported on other medications for the treatment of co-occurring bipolar disorder and anxiety. In adults, benzodiazepines are used to treat anxiety. However, evidence of their efficacy in treating anxiety in children is lacking; thus, they should not be considered a first-line treatment (Bernstein and Shaw 1997). Given the lack of evidence for efficacy and potential for abuse and cognitive effects, benzodiazepines should be used only short term (Kowatch et al. 2005). Evidence for the use of other medications is minimal, and thus these agents should only be considered after the treatments discussed above have failed. Adult guidelines have recommended that consideration be given to using a mood-stabilizing agent that also targets the specific comorbid anxiety disorder (Keck et al. 2006). The 2018 Canadian Network for Mood and Anxiety Treatments Task Force recommendations for adults state that quetiapine monotherapy was effective in treating both bipolar depression and symptoms of generalized anxiety disorder and panic disorder (Yatham et al. 2018). Addition of lamotrigine or olanzapine successfully decreased anxiety symptoms in euthymic adults taking lithium. In adults with bipolar depression, olanzapine and fluoxetine, and to a lesser extent olanzapine alone, were effective in decreasing anxiety symptoms. Open-label studies in adults have also found that gabapentin decreases anxiety symptoms when given as adjunctive therapy. However, no available data from studies conducted in children and adolescents at this time support the use of these treatments for co-occurring bipolar disorder and anxiety.

Treatment Recommendations: Bipolar Disorder and Obsessive-Compulsive Disorder

Studies show that in clinical samples of youth with a diagnosis of bipolar disorder, the rate of co-occurring OCD has ranged from 9% to 49% (Amerio et al. 2015; Dineen Wagner et al. 2006). Children with OCD and bipolar disorder compared with those with OCD only have earlier onset of OCD and more impairment (Masi et al. 2004). A comprehensive assessment is an important component of treatment, especially because diagnosis can be challenging. The presentation of one condition may mimic the other: the agitation, racing thoughts, and feelings of distress that may accompany severe OCD could mimic bipolar disorder; conversely, increased goal-directed activity or repetitive, unwanted hypersexual thoughts in bipolar disorder could mimic OCD (Joshi and Wilens 2009).

Best practices for treatment are also challenging given the very limited evidentiary base for specific pharmacological or psychotherapeutic modalities. We recommend first stabilizing bipolar disorder with either atypical antipsychotics or lithium. Joshi and colleagues (2010) conducted a secondary analysis of three open-label trials of olanzapine therapy in youth with bipolar disorder. They concluded that in children and adolescents with bipolar disorder, co-occurring lifetime OCD was associated with poor antimanic response. Response was observed in 25% of youth with comorbid OCD compared with 63% of those without comorbid OCD.

After mood stabilization, we recommend treatment with CBT, including ERP, to target the OCD based on available evidence for efficacy of CBT or ERP to treat OCD and the risk of mood destabilization with SSRIs. If OCD remains problematic after a trial of CBT with ERP, we recommend a trial of an SSRI. The SSRI should be initiated with caution because of the potential risk of destabilization. We do not recommend using an SSRI in the absence of a mood stabilizer to treat anxiety in youth with co-occurring bipolar disorder and anxiety disorders given the risk of precipitating mania. In an observational trial, Masi and colleagues (2004) reported a rate of switching in 30% of the youth with bipolar disorder and OCD comorbidity, compared with 22% of the youth with bipolar disorder alone. Small case series or case reports in adults have suggested the potential benefit of lithium, anticonvulsants, olanzapine, risperidone, quetiapine, or aripiprazole to manage both mood and OCD symptoms (Schaffer et al. 2012).

Treatment Recommendations: Bipolar Disorder and Disruptive Behavior Disorders

Disruptive behavior disorders commonly co-occur with bipolar disorder. A recent meta-analysis of clinical samples showed average rates of ODD in bipolar disorder and bipolar spectrum disorders at 43% and 42% and CD at 20% and 27%, respectively (Van Meter et al. 2016), with other authors reporting even higher rates (Joshi and Wilens 2009).

Most, but not all, studies show that DBDs have a negative effect on the course of bipolar disorder. CD comorbidity has been found to be the most important negative predictor of treatment nonresponse in children and adolescents with bipolar disorder (Masi et al. 2013). Prospective follow-up studies have shown that the presence of DBD in youth with bipolar disorder was associated with a poorer recovery from a manic or mixed episode and more mood episodes at follow-up (DelBello et al. 2007). In contrast, in their treatment trial of bipolar disorder, West and colleagues (2011) found that manic symptoms, as measured by the Young Mania Rating Scale, in youth with DBDs (including ADHD) were more responsive than those in youth with bipolar disorder without DBDs.

Evidence specifically examining treatment of co-occurring bipolar disorder and DBDs is limited. We recommend a sequence of achieving mood stabilization, treating other co-occurring conditions such as ADHD, and approaching the DBDs with behavioral therapy.

Some evidence indicates that atypical antipsychotics, specifically risperidone and quetiapine when used to treat bipolar disorder, improve the symptoms related to ODD or CD. In an RCT of risperidone and valproic acid in youth with bipolar disorder, West and colleagues (2011) examined the effect of DBDs and aggression and found that those with DBDs experienced a greater improvement in their manic symptoms after treatment with risperidone compared with valproic acid, whereas youth who had bipolar disorder without the comorbidity showed similar improvement with either medication. In the TEAM study, risperidone was more effective than lithium and valproic acid in treating bipolar symptoms, and efficacy was not moderated by the presence of ODD or CD (Vitiello et al. 2012). Additionally, ODD symptoms improved in all groups and more for those taking risperidone. In another small RCT comparing risperidone with quetiapine for the treatment of bipolar II disorder and CD in youth, both medications resulted in similar reductions in manic symptoms and aggression, and quetiapine was more effective in improving anxiety and depressive symptoms (Masi et al. 2015). These studies indicate that in youth with bipolar disorder and co-occurring DBDs, treatment with an atypical antipsychotic—risperidone or quetiapine in particular—also may lead to decreased DBD symptoms and aggression. Some evidence of efficacy for valproate also was seen. Barzman and colleagues (2006) conducted an RCT for adolescents with bipolar disorder, DBDs (CD or ODD), and high levels of impulsivity and reactive aggression and found that quetiapine and divalproex were both useful as monotherapy for the treatment of impulsivity and reactive aggression.

After mood stabilization, we recommend using principles from TRAAY and TMAY for treating aggression, including treatment of primary disorders such as ADHD with evidence-based interventions and use of psychosocial interventions, such as evidence-based parent and child skills training (Pappadopulos et al. 2003; Scotto Rosato et al. 2012), Parent Management Training Oregon Model, anger control training, problem-solving skills training, and group assertiveness training, reserved for older youth (Eyberg et al. 2008).

Treatment Recommendations: Bipolar Disorder and Substance Use Disorders

Children and adolescents with bipolar disorder have high rates of comorbid substance use disorder, ranging from 16% to 48% (Frías et al. 2015). The age at onset of bipolar disorder usually precedes the age at onset of the substance use disorder (Geller et al. 1998). Predictors of later substance use disorders in youth with bipolar disorder include alcohol use at intake, CD, ODD, panic disorder, family history of substance use disorders, and absence of antidepressant treatment (Goldstein et al. 2013; Joshi and

Wilens 2009). Substance use disorder can develop before the onset of mood episodes; investigators have found that patients from high-risk samples (with parents affected by bipolar disorder) are at particularly high risk (Duffy et al. 2012).

Treatment should start by ensuring that the patient receives a comprehensive assessment, including determining whether the patient has bipolar disorder or substance/medication-induced bipolar and related disorder. Very limited research is available on the treatment of comorbid bipolar disorder and substance use disorder in youth. Clinicians should address both disorders simultaneously and should involve both medication and psychotherapeutic interventions (Joshi and Wilens 2009).

We are unaware of any recent pharmacological trials examining treatments for substance use disorders in adolescents with co-occurring bipolar disorder. We recommend working with adolescents to discontinue their substance use, because of the risk that it may be exacerbating the mood disorder, and treating bipolar disorder with pharmacotherapy following treatment guidelines for bipolar disorder. Geller and colleagues (1998) compared lithium with placebo in treating bipolar disorder and secondary substance dependency and found that those participants taking lithium had greater improvement as indicated by cleaner drug urine screens and higher scores on Global Assessment of Functioning. Valproic acid also was found to reduce cannabis use significantly in youth with "explosive mood disorder" (Donovan and Nunes 1998). One trial showed efficacy of *N*-acetylcysteine for cannabis use disorders in adolescents without co-occurring psychiatric disorders (Gray et al. 2012).

Psychosocial treatments have been shown to be effective adjuncts in treating bipolar disorder (Fristad 2006) and substance use disorders separately (Dennis et al. 2004). We are unaware of any RCTs for psychotherapy treating adolescents with both conditions. Goldstein and colleagues (2014) examined the treatment of both conditions together in an open trial of family-focused therapy modified to treat bipolar disorder with co-occurring substance use disorders. The treatment included psychoeducation, communication enhancement training, and problem-solving skills training and resulted in significant improvement of mood symptoms and insignificant decreases in cannabis use.

Conclusion

A majority of children and adolescents with mood disorders will also have co-occurring conditions. The treatment of mood disorders and co-occurring conditions can be challenging. Evidence on the best approach to treating comorbid conditions is limited. In the absence of robust clinical guidelines for the management of co-occurring conditions in pediatric mood disorders, we rely on a small number of RCTs, practice guidelines, and expert consensus to assist clinicians in making the informed treatment decisions using the best evidence. Our review highlights clear gaps in the literature that merit attention for future research.

Clinical Pearls

- A comprehensive assessment is a cornerstone of good treatment, especially with co-occurring disorders that can add to complexity. The assessment should include a careful timeline of symptoms, history about social and environmental context, and standardized measures and rating scales to aid in assessment monitoring.

- Treatment recommendations should be informed by the evidence; include consideration of psychotherapy, psychopharmacology, and psychoeducation; and should take into account caregiver and patient preference.

- In treating co-occurring major depressive disorder (MDD) and attention-deficit/hyperactivity disorder (ADHD) we recommend targeting the most severe condition first. Use treatments with efficacy for each condition, such as stimulants, fluoxetine, and empirically based psychotherapies. If prescribing, start one medication at a time so as to minimize the chance of overprescribing and adverse effects.

- For MDD co-occurring with anxiety or obsessive-compulsive disorder (OCD), both selective serotonin reuptake inhibitors (SSRIs) and cognitive-behavioral therapy (CBT) should be considered either alone or in combination. We suggest CBT as first line for mild to moderate symptoms, and in combination with fluoxetine for moderate to severe symptoms.

- When disruptive behavior disorders (DBDs) co-occur with mood disorders, we recommend first treating the mood disorder and then addressing the DBD with behavioral therapy such as parent management training.

- When you suspect mania in child or adolescent with co-occurring conditions, a careful assessment is the first step to determine if the child has true bipolar disorder, manic-like symptoms from the co-occurring condition, or treatment-emergent mania.

- With treatment-emergent mania or manic symptoms with co-occurring ADHD, anxiety disorder, or OCD, strongly consider discontinuing medications that may be activating or precipitating mania such as stimulants or antidepressants.

- For co-occurring bipolar disorder and ADHD, after achieving mood stabilization, studies demonstrate that it is safe to prescribe stimulants for ADHD. Given the risk of destabilization, we recommend starting at a low dose and titrating slowly.

- In co-occurring bipolar disorder and anxiety disorder or OCD, we first recommend mood stabilization with pharmacotherapy and subsequent treatment of anxiety with CBT. SSRIs should only be initiated with caution because of the potential risk of a switch to mania.

References

Adler LA, Spencer T, Faraone SV, et al: Validity of pilot Adult ADHD Self-Report Scale (ASRS) to rate adult ADHD symptoms. Ann Clin Psychiatry 18(3):145–148, 2006 16923651

American Psychiatric Association: Diagnostic and Statistical Manual of Mental Disorders, 5th Edition. Arlington, VA, American Psychiatric Association, 2013

Amerio A, Stubbs B, Odone A, et al: The prevalence and predictors of comorbid bipolar disorder and obsessive-compulsive disorder: a systematic review and meta-analysis. J Affect Disord 186:99–109, 2015 26233320

Angold A, Costello EJ: Depressive comorbidity in children and adolescents: empirical, theoretical, and methodological issues. Am J Psychiatry 150(12):1779–1791, 1993 8238631

Angold A, Costello EJ, Erkanli A: Comorbidity. J Child Psychol Psychiatry 40(1):57–87, 1999 10102726

Asarnow JR, Emslie G, Clarke G, et al: Treatment of selective serotonin reuptake inhibitor–resistant depression in adolescents: predictors and moderators of treatment response. J Am Acad Child Adolesc Psychiatry 48(3):330–339, 2009 19182688

Avenevoli S, Swendsen J, He JP, et al: Major depression in the National Comorbidity Survey–Adolescent Supplement: prevalence, correlates, and treatment. J Am Acad Child Adolesc Psychiatry 54(1):37.e2–44.e2, 2015 25524788

Bangs ME, Emslie GJ, Spencer TJ, et al; Atomoxetine ADHD and Comorbid MDD Study Group: Efficacy and safety of atomoxetine in adolescents with attention-deficit/hyperactivity disorder and major depression. J Child Adolesc Psychopharmacol 17(4):407–420, 2007 17822337

Barzman DH, DelBello MP, Adler CM, et al: The efficacy and tolerability of quetiapine versus divalproex for the treatment of impulsivity and reactive aggression in adolescents with co-occurring bipolar disorder and disruptive behavior disorder(s). J Child Adolesc Psychopharmacol 16(6):665–670, 2006 17201610

Bernstein GA, Shaw K; American Academy of Child and Adolescent Psychiatry: Practice parameters for the assessment and treatment of children and adolescents with anxiety disorders. J Am Acad Child Adolesc Psychiatry 36(10 suppl):69S–84S, 1997 9334566

Birmaher B, Ryan ND, Williamson DE, et al: Childhood and adolescent depression: a review of the past 10 years, part I. J Am Acad Child Adolesc Psychiatry 35(11):1427–1439, 1996 8936909

Birmaher B, Khetarpal S, Brent D, et al: The Screen for Child Anxiety Related Emotional Disorders (SCARED): scale construction and psychometric characteristics. J Am Acad Child Adolesc Psychiatry 36(4):545–553, 1997 9100430

Birmaher B, Brent DA, Kolko D, et al: Clinical outcome after short-term psychotherapy for adolescents with major depressive disorder. Arch Gen Psychiatry 57(1):29–36, 2000 10632230

Birmaher B, Brent D, Bernet W, et al; AACAP Work Group on Quality Issues: Practice parameter for the assessment and treatment of children and adolescents with depressive disorders. J Am Acad Child Adolesc Psychiatry 46(11):1503–1526, 2007 18049300

Brent DA, Kolko DJ, Birmaher B, et al: Predictors of treatment efficacy in a clinical trial of three psychosocial treatments for adolescent depression. J Am Acad Child Adolesc Psychiatry 37(9):906–914, 1998 9735610

Brent D, Emslie G, Clarke G, et al: Switching to another SSRI or to venlafaxine with or without cognitive behavioral therapy for adolescents with SSRI-resistant depression: the TORDIA randomized controlled trial. JAMA 299(8):901–913, 2008 18314433

Bussing R, Fernandez M, Harwood M, et al: Parent and teacher SNAP-IV ratings of attention deficit hyperactivity disorder symptoms: psychometric properties and normative ratings from a school district sample. Assessment 15(3):317–328, 2008 18310593

Chang K, Nayar D, Howe M, et al: Atomoxetine as an adjunct therapy in the treatment of co-morbid attention-deficit/hyperactivity disorder in children and adolescents with bipolar I or II disorder. J Child Adolesc Psychopharmacol 19(5):547–551, 2009 19877979

Cipriani A, Zhou X, Del Giovane C, et al: Comparative efficacy and tolerability of antidepressants for major depressive disorder in children and adolescents: a network meta-analysis. Lancet 388(10047):881–890, 2016 27289172

Clarke G, Hops H, Lewinsohn P, et al: Cognitive-behavioral group treatment of adolescent depression: prediction of outcome. Behav Ther 23:341–354, 1992

Conners CK, Casat CD, Gualtieri CT, et al: Bupropion hydrochloride in attention deficit disorder with hyperactivity. J Am Acad Child Adolesc Psychiatry 35(10):1314–1321, 1996 8885585

Correll CU, Sheridan EM, DelBello MP: Antipsychotic and mood stabilizer efficacy and tolerability in pediatric and adult patients with bipolar I mania: a comparative analysis of acute, randomized, placebo-controlled trials. Bipolar Disord 12(2):116–141, 2010 20402706

Cummings CM, Fristad MA: Anxiety in children with mood disorders: a treatment help or hindrance? J Abnorm Child Psychol 40(3):339–351, 2012 21912843

Curry J, Rohde P, Simons A, et al; TADS Team: Predictors and moderators of acute outcome in the Treatment for Adolescents with Depression Study (TADS). J Am Acad Child Adolesc Psychiatry 45(12):1427–1439, 2006 17135988

Daviss WB, Bentivoglio P, Racusin R, et al: Bupropion sustained release in adolescents with comorbid attention-deficit/hyperactivity disorder and depression. J Am Acad Child Adolesc Psychiatry 40(3):307–314, 2001 11288772

DelBello MP, Hanseman D, Adler CM, et al: Twelve-month outcome of adolescents with bipolar disorder following first hospitalization for a manic or mixed episode. Am J Psychiatry 164(4):582–590, 2007 17403971

Dennis M, Godley SH, Diamond G, et al: The Cannabis Youth Treatment (CYT) Study: main findings from two randomized trials. J Subst Abuse Treat 27(3):197–213, 2004 15501373

Dietz LJ, Weinberg RJ, Brent DA, Mufson L: Family based interpersonal psychotherapy for depressed preadolescents: examining efficacy and potential treatment mechanisms. J Am Acad Child Adolesc Psychiatry 54(3):191–199, 2015 25721184

Dineen Wagner K: Bipolar disorder and comorbid anxiety disorders in children and adolescents. J Clin Psychiatry 67 (suppl 1):16–20, 2006 16426112

Donovan SJ, Nunes EV: Treatment of comorbid affective and substance use disorders: therapeutic potential of anticonvulsants. Am J Addict 7(3):210–220, 1998 9702289

Duffy A, Horrocks J, Milin R, et al: Adolescent substance use disorder during the early stages of bipolar disorder: a prospective high-risk study. J Affect Disord 142(1–3):57–64, 2012 22959686

Emslie GJ, Rush AJ, Weinberg WA, et al: A double-blind, randomized, placebo-controlled trial of fluoxetine in children and adolescents with depression. Arch Gen Psychiatry 54(11):1031–1037, 1997 9366660

Eyberg SM, Nelson MM, Boggs SR: Evidence-based psychosocial treatments for children and adolescents with disruptive behavior. J Clin Child Adolesc Psychol 37(1):215–237, 2008 18444059

Faraone SV, Biederman J, Spencer TJ, et al: Comparing the efficacy of medications for ADHD using meta-analysis. MedGenMed 8(4):4, 2006 17415287

Farrell L, Waters A, Milliner E, et al: Comorbidity and treatment response in pediatric obsessive-compulsive disorder: a pilot study of group cognitive-behavioral treatment. Psychiatry Res 199(2):115–123, 2012 22633155

Findling RL, Short EJ, McNamara NK, et al: Methylphenidate in the treatment of children and adolescents with bipolar disorder and attention-deficit/hyperactivity disorder. J Am Acad Child Adolesc Psychiatry 46(11):1445–1453, 2007 18049294

Findling RL, Robb A, McNamara NK, et al: Lithium in the acute treatment of bipolar I disorder: a double-blind, placebo-controlled study. Pediatrics 136(5):885–894, 2015 26459650

Franklin ME, Sapyta J, Freeman JB, et al: Cognitive behavior therapy augmentation of pharmacotherapy in pediatric obsessive-compulsive disorder: the Pediatric OCD Treatment Study II (POTS II) randomized controlled trial. JAMA 306(11):1224–1232, 2011 21934055

Frías Á, Palma C, Farriols N: Comorbidity in pediatric bipolar disorder: prevalence, clinical impact, etiology and treatment. J Affect Disord 174:378–389, 2015 25545605

Fristad MA: Psychoeducational treatment for school-aged children with bipolar disorder. Dev Psychopathol 18(4):1289–1306, 2006 17064439

Fristad MA, Goldberg Arnold JS, Leffler JM, et al: Psychotherapy for Children With Bipolar and Depressive Disorders. New York, Guilford, 2011

Galanter CA, Jensen PS: Diagnostic Decision Making in the DSM-5 Casebook and Treatment Guide for Child Mental Health. Arlington, VA, American Psychiatric Association Publishing, 2017

Galanter CA, Carlson GA, Jensen PS, et al: Response to methylphenidate in children with attention deficit hyperactivity disorder and manic symptoms in the Multimodal Treatment Study of Children With Attention Deficit Hyperactivity Disorder titration trial. J Child Adolesc Psychopharmacol 13(2):123–136, 2003 12880507

Galanter CA, Pagar DL, Davies M, et al: ADHD and manic symptoms: diagnostic and treatment implications. Clin Neurosci Res 5:283–294, 2005

Geller B, Cooper TB, Sun K, et al: Double-blind and placebo-controlled study of lithium for adolescent bipolar disorders with secondary substance dependency. J Am Acad Child Adolesc Psychiatry 37(2):171–178, 1998 9473913

Geller B, Luby JL, Joshi P, et al: A randomized controlled trial of risperidone, lithium, or divalproex sodium for initial treatment of bipolar I disorder, manic or mixed phase, in children and adolescents. Arch Gen Psychiatry 69(5):515–528, 2012 22213771

Geller DA, March J: Practice parameter for the assessment and treatment of children and adolescents with obsessive-compulsive disorder. J Am Acad Child Adolesc Psychiatry 51(1):98–113, 2012 22176943

Goldstein BI, Shamseddeen W, Spirito A, et al: Substance use and the treatment of resistant depression in adolescents. J Am Acad Child Adolesc Psychiatry 48(12):1182–1192, 2009 19858762

Goldstein BI, Strober M, Axelson D, et al: Predictors of first-onset substance use disorders during the prospective course of bipolar spectrum disorders in adolescents. J Am Acad Child Adolesc Psychiatry 52(10):1026–1037, 2013 24074469

Goldstein BI, Goldstein TR, Collinger KA, et al: Treatment development and feasibility study of family focused treatment for adolescents with bipolar disorder and comorbid substance use disorders. J Psychiatr Pract 20(3):237–248, 2014 24847999

Gray KM, Carpenter MJ, Baker NL, et al: A double-blind randomized controlled trial of N-acetylcysteine in cannabis-dependent adolescents. Am J Psychiatry 169(8):805–812, 2012 22706327

Hewett K, Chrzanowski W, Jokinen R, et al: Double-blind, placebo-controlled evaluation of extended-release bupropion in elderly patients with major depressive disorder. J Psychopharmacol 24(4):521–529, 2010 19164492

Hilton RC, Rengasamy M, Mansoor B, et al: Impact of treatments for depression on comorbid anxiety, attentional, and behavioral symptoms in adolescents with selective serotonin reuptake inhibitor–resistant depression. J Am Acad Child Adolesc Psychiatry 52(5):482–492, 2013 23622849

Hofmann SG, Asnaani A, Vonk IJ, et al: The efficacy of cognitive behavioral therapy: a review of meta-analyses. Cognit Ther Res 36(5):427–440, 2012 23459093

Horigian VE, Weems CF, Robbins MS, et al: Reductions in anxiety and depression symptoms in youth receiving substance use treatment. Am J Addict 22(4):329–337, 2013 23795871

Horrigan JP, Barnhill LJ: Guanfacine and secondary mania in children. J Affect Disord 54(3):309–314, 1999 10467976

Hughes CW, Emslie GJ, Crismon ML, et al; Texas Consensus Conference Panel on Medication Treatment of Childhood Major Depressive Disorder: Texas Children's Medication Algorithm Project: update from Texas Consensus Conference Panel on Medication Treatment of Childhood Major Depressive Disorder. J Am Acad Child Adolesc Psychiatry 46(6):667–686, 2007 17513980

Jacobs RH, Becker-Weidman EG, Reinecke MA, et al: Treating depression and oppositional behavior in adolescents. J Clin Child Adolesc Psychol 39(4):559–567, 2010 20589566

Joshi G, Wilens T: Comorbidity in pediatric bipolar disorder. Child Adolesc Psychiatr Clin N Am 18(2):291–319, vii–viii, 2009 19264265

Joshi G, Mick E, Wozniak J, et al: Impact of obsessive-compulsive disorder on the antimanic response to olanzapine therapy in youth with bipolar disorder. Bipolar Disord 12(2):196–204, 2010 20402712

Kaminer Y: Youth Substance Abuse and Co-occurring Disorders. Washington, DC, American Psychiatric Publishing, 2015

Kaminer Y, Connor DF, Curry JF: Treatment of comorbid adolescent cannabis use and major depressive disorder. Psychiatry (Edgmont) 5(9):34–39, 2008 19727258

Keck PE Jr, Strawn JR, McElroy SL: Pharmacologic treatment considerations in co-occurring bipolar and anxiety disorders. J Clin Psychiatry 67 (suppl 1):8–15, 2006 16426111

Kendall PC, Robin JA, Hedtke KA, et al: Considering CBT with anxious youth? Think exposures. Cognit Behav Pract 12(1):136–150, 2005

Kowatch RA, Fristad M, Birmaher B, et al; Child Psychiatric Workgroup on Bipolar Disorder: Treatment guidelines for children and adolescents with bipolar disorder. J Am Acad Child Adolesc Psychiatry 44(3):213–235, 2005 15725966

Kratochvil CJ, May DE, Silva SG, et al: Treatment response in depressed adolescents with and without co-morbid attention-deficit/hyperactivity disorder in the Treatment for Adolescents with Depression Study. J Child Adolesc Psychopharmacol 19(5):519–527, 2009 19877976

Lafay-Chebassier C, Chavant F, Favrelière S, et al; French Association of Regional Pharmacovigilance Centers: Drug-induced depression: a case/non case study in the French Pharmacovigilance database. Therapie 70(5):425–432, 2015 26056040

Levine A, Clemenza K, Rynn M, et al: Evidence for the risks and consequences of adolescent cannabis exposure. J Am Acad Child Adolesc Psychiatry 56(3):214–225, 2017 28219487

Licht RW, Gijsman H, Nolen WA, et al: Are antidepressants safe in the treatment of bipolar depression? A critical evaluation of their potential risk to induce switch into mania or cycle acceleration. Acta Psychiatr Scand 118(5):337–346, 2008 18754834

March JS, Biederman J, Wolkow R, et al: Sertraline in children and adolescents with obsessive-compulsive disorder: a multicenter randomized controlled trial. JAMA 280(20):1752–1756, 1998 9842950

March J, Silva S, Petrycki S, et al; Treatment for Adolescents with Depression Study (TADS) Team: Fluoxetine, cognitive-behavioral therapy, and their combination for adolescents with depression: Treatment for Adolescents with Depression Study (TADS) randomized controlled trial. JAMA 292(7):807–820, 2004 15315995

March JS, Entusah AR, Rynn M, et al: A randomized controlled trial of venlafaxine ER versus placebo in pediatric social anxiety disorder. Biol Psychiatry 62 (10):1149–1154, 2007 17553467

Martin A, Young C, Leckman JF, et al: Age effects on antidepressant-induced manic conversion. Arch Pediatr Adolesc Med 158(8):773–780, 2004 15289250

Masi G, Toni C, Perugi G, et al: Anxiety disorders in children and adolescents with bipolar disorder: a neglected comorbidity. Can J Psychiatry 46(9):797–802, 2001 11761630

Masi G, Perugi G, Toni C, et al: Obsessive-compulsive bipolar comorbidity: focus on children and adolescents. J Affect Disord 78(3):175–183, 2004 15013241

Masi G, Pisano S, Pfanner C, et al: Quetiapine monotherapy in adolescents with bipolar disorder comorbid with conduct disorder. J Child Adolesc Psychopharmacol 23(8):568–571, 2013 24138010

Masi G, Milone A, Stawinoga A, et al: Efficacy and safety of risperidone and quetiapine in adolescents with bipolar II disorder comorbid with conduct disorder. J Clin Psychopharmacol 35(5):587–590, 2015 26226481

Mufson L, Weissman MM, Moreau D, et al: Efficacy of interpersonal psychotherapy for depressed adolescents. Arch Gen Psychiatry 56(6):573–579, 1999 10359475

Pappadopulos E, Macintyre Ii JC, Crismon ML, et al: Treatment Recommendations for the Use of Antipsychotics for Aggressive Youth (TRAAY): part II. J Am Acad Child Adolesc Psychiatry 42(2):145–161, 2003 12544174

Pavuluri MN, Henry DB, Devineni B, et al: Child Mania Rating Scale: development, reliability, and validity. J Am Acad Child Adolesc Psychiatry 45(5):550–560, 2006 16601399

Peruzzolo TL, Tramontina S, Rodrigues RB, et al: Avoiding stimulants may not prevent manic switch: a case report with atomoxetine. J Neuropsychiatry Clin Neurosci 26(4):E30–E31, 2014 26037880

Pliszka SR, Crismon ML, Hughes CW, et al; Texas Consensus Conference Panel on Pharmacotherapy of Childhood Attention Deficit Hyperactivity Disorder: The Texas Children's Medication Algorithm Project: revision of the algorithm for pharmacotherapy of attention-deficit/hyperactivity disorder. J Am Acad Child Adolesc Psychiatry 45(6):642–657, 2006 16721314

Reinblatt SP, DosReis S, Walkup JT, et al: Activation adverse events induced by the selective serotonin reuptake inhibitor fluvoxamine in children and adolescents. J Child Adolesc Psychopharmacol 19(2):119–126, 2009 19364290

Riddle MA, Scahill L, King RA, et al: Double-blind, crossover trial of fluoxetine and placebo in children and adolescents with obsessive-compulsive disorder. J Am Acad Child Adolesc Psychiatry 31(6):1062–1069, 1992 1429406

Riddle MA, Reeve EA, Yaryura-Tobias JA, et al: Fluvoxamine for children and adolescents with obsessive-compulsive disorder: a randomized, controlled, multicenter trial. J Am Acad Child Adolesc Psychiatry 40(2):222–229, 2001 11211371

Ross RG: Psychotic and manic-like symptoms during stimulant treatment of attention deficit hyperactivity disorder. Am J Psychiatry 163(7):1149–1152, 2006 16816217

Rynn MA, Riddle MA, Yeung PP, Kunz NR: Efficacy and safety of extended-release venlafaxine in the treatment of generalized anxiety disorder in children and adolescents: two placebo-controlled trials. Am J Psychiatry 164:290–300, 2007 17267793

Sala R, Axelson DA, Castro-Fornieles J, et al: Factors associated with the persistence and onset of new anxiety disorders in youth with bipolar spectrum disorders. J Clin Psychiatry 73(1):87–94, 2012 22226375

Sala R, Strober MA, Axelson DA, et al: Effects of comorbid anxiety disorders on the longitudinal course of pediatric bipolar disorders. J Am Acad Child Adolesc Psychiatry 53(1):72–81, 2014 24342387

Schaffer A, McIntosh D, Goldstein BI, et al; Canadian Network for Mood and Anxiety Treatments (CANMAT) Task Force: The CANMAT Task Force recommendations for the management of patients with mood disorders and comorbid anxiety disorders. Ann Clin Psychiatry 24(1):6–22, 2012 22303519

Scheffer RE, Kowatch RA, Carmody T, et al: Randomized, placebo-controlled trial of mixed amphetamine salts for symptoms of comorbid ADHD in pediatric bipolar disorder after mood stabilization with divalproex sodium. Am J Psychiatry 162(1):58–64, 2005 15625202

Scotto Rosato N, Correll CU, Pappadopulos E, et al; Treatment of Maladaptive Aggressive in Youth Steering Committee: Treatment of Maladaptive Aggression in Youth: CERT guidelines II: treatments and ongoing management. Pediatrics 129(6):e1577–e1586, 2012 22641763

Storch EA, Merlo LJ, Larson MJ, et al: Impact of comorbidity on cognitive-behavioral therapy response in pediatric obsessive-compulsive disorder. J Am Acad Child Adolesc Psychiatry 47(5):583–592, 2008 18356759

Storch EA, Bussing R, Small BJ, et al: Randomized, placebo-controlled trial of cognitive-behavioral therapy alone or combined with sertraline in the treatment of pediatric obsessive-compulsive disorder. Behav Res Ther 51(12):823–829, 2013 24184429

Strawn JR, Prakash A, Zhang Q, et al: A randomized, placebo-controlled study of duloxetine for the treatment of children and adolescents with generalized anxiety disorder. J Am Acad Child Adolesc Psychiatry 54(4):283–293, 2015 25791145

Strawn JR, Mills JA, Sauley BA, et al: The impact of antidepressant dose and class on treatment response in pediatric anxiety disorders: a meta-analysis. J Am Acad Child Adolesc Psychiatry 57(4):235–244.e2, 2018 29588049

Stuhec M, Munda B, Svab V, et al: Comparative efficacy and acceptability of atomoxetine, lisdexamfetamine, bupropion and methylphenidate in treatment of attention deficit hyperactivity disorder in children and adolescents: a meta-analysis with focus on bupropion. J Affect Disord 178:149–159, 2015 25813457

Tondo L, Vázquez G, Baldessarini RJ, et al: Mania associated with antidepressant treatment: comprehensive meta-analytic review. Acta Psychiatr Scand 121(6):404–414, 2010 19958306

Tramontina S, Zeni CP, Ketzer CR, et al: Aripiprazole in children and adolescents with bipolar disorder comorbid with attention-deficit/hyperactivity disorder: a pilot randomized clinical trial. J Clin Psychiatry 70(5):756–764, 2009 19389329

Van Meter AR, Burke C, Kowatch RA, et al: Ten-year updated meta-analysis of the clinical characteristics of pediatric mania and hypomania. Bipolar Disord 18(1):19–32, 2016 26748678

Vázquez GH, Tondo L, Undurraga J, et al: Overview of antidepressant treatment of bipolar depression. Int J Neuropsychopharmacol 16(7):1673–1685, 2013 23428003

Vitiello B, Riddle MA, Yenokyan G, et al: Treatment moderators and predictors of outcome in the Treatment of Early Age Mania (TEAM) study. J Am Acad Child Adolesc Psychiatry 51(9):867–878, 2012 22917200

Volkow ND, Baler RD, Compton WM, et al: Adverse health effects of marijuana use. N Engl J Med 370(23):2219–2227, 2014 24897085

Wagner KD, Jonas J, Findling RL, et al: A double-blind, randomized, placebo-controlled trial of escitalopram in the treatment of pediatric depression. J Am Acad Child Adolesc Psychiatry 45(3):280–288, 2006 16540812

Wang LJ, Shyu YC, Yuan SS, et al: Attention-deficit hyperactivity disorder, its pharmacotherapy, and the risk of developing bipolar disorder: a nationwide population-based study in Taiwan. J Psychiatr Res 72:6–14, 2016 26519764

Weinstein SM, Henry DB, Katz AC, et al: Treatment moderators of child- and family focused cognitive-behavioral therapy for pediatric bipolar disorder. J Am Acad Child Adolesc Psychiatry 54(2):116–125, 2015 25617252

Weissman MM, Pilowsky DJ, Wickramaratne PJ, et al: Remissions in maternal depression and child psychopathology: a STAR*D-child report. JAMA 295(12):1389–1398, 2006 16551710

West AE, Weinstein SM, Celio CI, et al: Co-morbid disruptive behavior disorder and aggression predict functional outcomes and differential response to risperidone versus divalproex in pharmacotherapy for pediatric bipolar disorder. J Child Adolesc Psychopharmacol 21(6):545–553, 2011 22136096

West AE, Weinstein SM, Peters AT, et al: Child- and family focused cognitive-behavioral therapy for pediatric bipolar disorder: a randomized clinical trial. J Am Acad Child Adolesc Psychiatry 53(11):1168–1178, 2014 25440307

Whiting PF, Wolff RF, Deshpande S, et al: Cannabinoids for medical use: a systematic review and meta-analysis. JAMA 313(24):2456–2473, 2015 26103030

Yatham LN, Kennedy SH, Parikh SV, et al: Canadian Network for Mood and Anxiety Treatments (CANMAT) and International Society for Bipolar Disorders (ISBD) 2018 guidelines for the management of patients with bipolar disorder. Bipolar Disord 20(2):97–170, 2018 29536616

Yorbik O, Birmaher B, Axelson D, et al: Clinical characteristics of depressive symptoms in children and adolescents with major depressive disorder. J Clin Psychiatry 65(12):1654–1659, quiz 1760–1761, 2004 15641870

Zeni CP, Tramontina S, Ketzer CR, et al: Methylphenidate combined with aripiprazole in children and adolescents with bipolar disorder and attention-deficit/hyperactivity disorder: a randomized crossover trial. J Child Adolesc Psychopharmacol 19(5):553–561, 2009 19877980

Zhou X, Qin B, Del Giovane C, et al: Efficacy and tolerability of antidepressants in the treatment of adolescents and young adults with depression and substance use disorders: a systematic review and meta-analysis. Addiction 110(1):38–48, 2015 25098732

School-Based Interventions for Pediatric-Onset Mood Disorders

Shashank V. Joshi, M.D.

Nadia Jassim, M.F.A.

For clinicians caring for youth with mood disorders, it is crucial to understand educational settings as fully as possible. Teachers and other school staff engage with affected youth on an almost daily basis, and they are key partners to help both clinicians and parents comprehend the social, educational, and cultural context where mood symptoms may manifest. Several interventions have been developed to help affected youth gain better access to the school curriculum, in spite of their mood symptoms. Careful attention should be paid to the *supporting alliance* among parents, teachers, and clinicians (Feinstein et al. 2009) so that members of each of these groups can be resources for one another to best support youth affected by mood conditions (Joshi et al., in press).

Affected students are entitled to several educational interventions through both formal (i.e., legal) and informal mechanisms. Unfortunately, adolescents with mood disorders are at high risk for school problems, including poor attendance, underachievement, and dropping out. In particular, in the midst of an episode, these students can find it especially hard to pay attention, think clearly, solve problems, recall information, engage in group learning activities, and sit still—let alone follow classroom rules (Evans and Andrews 2005; Papolos and Papolos 2002).

Mood disorders can cause at least three types of problems for youth in school settings: 1) those caused by the core symptoms themselves (e.g., difficulty concentrating; Table 15–1), 2) those caused by secondary factors (e.g., peer issues; Table 15–2), and 3) those associated with the treatment itself (e.g., medication side effects; Table 15–3) or life inconveniences associated with treatment (e.g., needing to take medications during the school day or missing school activities to attend therapy appointments) (Fristad and Goldberg Arnold 2004). Youth with mood conditions often struggle with learning issues, and educators would do well to be aware of the additional layers of impaired concentration, reduced motivation, and emotional upheavals that the mood disorder can create (Fristad and Goldberg Arnold 2004).

Online, social media, and book resources are available for both adults and peers who care for these youth, as well as for the affected youth themselves, and these resources are listed at the end of this chapter for further reference.

Case Illustration

James, a 16-year-old second-generation Chinese American teenager, lived in a household with a younger sibling and both parents. He had struggled with sad moods and acculturation stress since middle school but had never talked about these issues with his family or teachers. Several youth from his high school had died by suicide in the previous 3 years and among the victims was James's best friend. School staff members were concerned about James's recent writings and withdrawal from his usual interests, and they asked that the School Mental Health Team consult with him and the family to assess for depression and self-harm potential. After they obtained consent, the team was able to gain the patient's and family's trust quickly by doing the following:

A child and adolescent psychiatry fellow began the consultation by calling the family and outlining the specific steps to School Mental Health

Team consultation, assuring them that although the consult would start at school, steps would be taken to minimize any potential missed time from coursework and to ensure confidentiality.

The child and adolescent psychiatry fellow, Dr. G, gathered as much background information as possible from the school counselor and teacher adviser and then met with James at school that afternoon for an initial meeting with James and his parents together briefly. She then asked to meet the parents alone for about 30 minutes. Dr. G intentionally focused on separate time with the parents, who had immigrated to the United States as adults in their early 20s, to gain their trust and engage them in a culturally focused way: being mindful of the potential for stigma and fears about whether contact with the team might affect James's chances to go to the best college. She approached the family about James's need for treatment by framing his problem in medical terms that were familiar and understandable to them. Dr. G described ways that depression can affect motivation, memory, and general classroom engagement by using a teaching tool that illustrated important pathways for learning, mood, and cognition.[1]

Dr. G highlighted her need to work closely with the school team (especially the guidance counselor) and recommended that family therapy be started to address dysfunctional patterns of family behaviors and communication and to teach new parenting and coping strategies for the mood swings James was experiencing. The school district had a Mandarin-speaking therapist available from a local agency because of the high need for culturally attuned interventions. After appropriate safety planning and after additional history was elicited from James and trusted adults who knew of James's situation, he was given a diagnosis of major depressive disorder and posttraumatic stress symptoms.

After a full discussion of possible therapeutic interventions based on known guidelines (i.e., Texas Children's Medication Algorithm Project; Hughes et al. 2007), Dr. G told James and his family that she would recommend a structured psychotherapy intervention, such as interpersonal therapy (IPT) or cognitive-behavioral therapy (CBT), and that eventually, treatment with a selective serotonin reuptake inhibitor (SSRI) medication (fluoxetine or escitalopram) might be needed. Dr. G was mindful of the potentially good response at lower doses in some Asian patients and also was aware that James's younger sibling had taken medicine for severe anxiety in the past but the family stopped treatment because "he was so sleepy he couldn't do his schoolwork." This was incorporated into the discussion with the family. Dr. G also supported James's and his family's request to continue the omega fatty acid supplement, because they believed that this was important to his overall functioning, and Dr. G believed that it was at least doing no harm and may have carried a "meaning effect." James's best friend who had died had bipolar disorder and was nonadherent with the

---

[1]A useful example of the brain pathway slide that was printed out for the family meeting can be accessed for free at https://slideplayer.com/4292078/14/images/ 40/Dopamine+and+Serotonin.jpg.

TABLE 15–1.　Common problems for youth caused by the core symptoms of a mood disorder

Mood changes	Extremes in mood (sad, excessively giddy, angry) can be especially difficult to manage in school and can severely disrupt the learning process and experience of affected youth.
Loss of interest	Loss of interest may translate to a lack of engagement in school activities and schoolwork. It can create a vicious cycle: not completing work leads to lower grades, which can lead to lower self-worth, loss of motivation, and withdrawal or absenteeism—leading the student to fall behind and feel so overwhelmed that he or she cannot take the first step toward reengagement.
Fatigue	Depression or sleep difficulties during mania can lead to fatigue. School engagement can be quite challenging when a student can barely keep his or her eyes open and has low energy.
Concentration difficulties	Difficulties with concentration can be especially frustrating for youth who would otherwise excel academically but find themselves unable to stay focused and think clearly because of their mood disorder or a medication side effect.
Agitation or retardation	Agitation can cause a constant feeling of having to move (pacing, tapping fingers or feet, restless legs) and can be disruptive to peers. Retardation can make a student feel as if he or she is going "in slow motion." It is normal for people to have specific times of day when they are most efficient ("morning birds" vs. "night owls"). However, students with mood disorders may struggle with dramatic changes in energy level, from hyperactivity to lethargy, and this can make the timely completion of assignments especially hard.
Poor judgment	Mania and hypomania are often associated with questionable decision making, recklessness or impulsivity, and actions or behaviors that will cause later embarrassment (such as making lewd comments, being very daring, or bragging about perceived abilities).
Racing thoughts	Racing thoughts are often associated with mania or hypomania, and they lead to great difficulty with concentration and focus. Thus, listening to and processing school lessons may not be easy.
Loud or pressured speech	Manic or hypomanic states can involve the sensation that words cannot get out fast enough, and result in loud or pressured speech. These patterns often are not noticed by the student but may be noticed or commented on by peers.

Source.　Adapted from Fristad and Goldberg Arnold 2004.

TABLE 15–2. Common problems for youth caused by secondary factors of a mood disorder

Peer problems	Difficulties with peers can be among the most devastating experiences for young people and have long-lasting consequences. Depression is associated with social isolation and withdrawal. As peer networks are ever changing and sometimes fragile, turning down invitations for playdates or hanging out can result in no further invitations from a specific peer. Because youth learn social skills from interacting with one another, lost opportunities to play are also lost opportunities to learn. Age-appropriate social skill development can be delayed and cause affected students to fall further behind socially and to be included less often by peer groups. The quality and quantity of friendships can be affected, because mood-impaired children and teenagers often are drawn to peers with similar problems. Although it is useful to have friends who "get" the student and identify with him or her, having a social network composed exclusively of others with impairing conditions also can be problematic. Helping students make social contacts with those with similar interests and hobbies can help prevent the formation of "moody youth clubs" and "varsity cutting teams."
Other secondary problems	Social isolation resulting from mood disorders causes many other problems. If a student spends the whole morning worrying about whom to play with at recess, he or she will not be focused on the teacher's lessons. Another child might act up just to avoid stressful times of day; being sent to the office or detention may seem easier than facing one's social fears. School staff, parents, and clinicians need to be creative in efforts to understand problems like these to address them properly.

Source. Adapted from Fristad and Goldberg Arnold 2004.

prescribed omega fatty acids and mood stabilizers. James believed that he should "honor the memory" of his friend by trying to take the medicine as prescribed.[2]

---

[2]Meaning effects (Pruett et al. 2010) have been described as phenomena considered to be among "common factors" of effective treatments that may have direct results on adolescent treatment adherence and behavior change because of placebo and positive expectancy effects or a strong therapeutic alliance with the provider (Joshi 2006; Malik et al. 2010; De Nadai et al. 2017).

TABLE 15–3. Common problems for youth caused by treatment of a mood disorder

Medication side effects	Side effects of medications can range from nuisances to significant challenges in getting through the school day. Some side effects are very embarrassing (e.g., lithium treatment leading to bladder accidents), whereas some others may be uncomfortable (e.g., feeling thirsty, having dry mouth, or being dizzy and nauseated). Medication titrations can be associated with headaches or sleepiness that can further interfere with schoolwork.
Other problems associated with treatment	Once-daily dosing is ideal but may not always be possible. If a student takes his or her medication during the school day, there may be challenges around school nurse availability, stigma regarding the need to leave class for medicine, or logistical challenges if a parent needs to obtain an "extra medication bottle" for school. Leaving school activities for therapy or other appointments can cause a student who is already struggling to have even more problems.

Source.   Adapted from Fristad and Goldberg Arnold 2004; Malik et al. 2010.

A student study team was convened by the school, and a 504 plan was developed for James to make in-class accommodations to support his learning and engagement with the curriculum. Examples of accommodations that can be useful for students with mood disorders are listed in Table 15–5. Although James responded to these interventions well, a student with his symptoms might have needed further school-based interventions through an individualized education plan (IEP). Major differences among types of school mental health interventions (IEPs and 504 plans) can be found in Table 15–8.

The supporting alliance (Feinstein et al. 2009) among doctor, parent, family therapist, teachers, and guidance counselor was facilitated by Dr. G, who actively engaged the school to support James and highlighted their role on the team as the "watchful clinical eyes" during the school day. James responded well to a low-dose SSRI and standard-dose omega fatty acids provided by the child and adolescent psychiatry fellow, in conjunction with IPT and family therapy provided by community therapists, and regular mental health checkups with the school counselor. Dr. G continued to see James regularly and had brief telephone meetings with the IPT therapist weekly for the first 6 weeks and monthly thereafter. The parents, although tempted many times to withdraw from this intensity of treatment, kept encouraging James and supporting his continued participation "because Dr. G asked us to make sure he attends all of these meetings (and we participate where needed) and because the treatment may not last forever—it will depend on how he responds. And we trust Dr. G."

Dr. G made it a point to cultivate relationships with school leaders during the course of her work with James. Later in the spring of that school year, Dr. G approached James's team about whether they would be interested in using a brief four-session curriculum to engage all students in teaching about stress, depression, help-seeking, and suicide prevention. The school agreed enthusiastically, because staff wanted to implement universal prevention strategies that would also promote overall wellness. After the director of student services at the central district office reviewed the curriculum, Dr. G received approval to plan the specifics of this with school leadership and helped to implement a best-practices curriculum, *Break Free From Depression* (BFFD; Boston Children's Hospital Neighborhood Partnerships Program 2017).

The goal of BFFD is to raise student cognizance and knowledge about depression and the risk factors working against help-seeking behaviors for the students themselves or others. Delivery of the material consists of an interactive PowerPoint lecture with interactive student components, a documentary film, and group-guided facilitation regarding depression in youth. The BFFD curriculum includes a detailed facilitator's guide and supplementary materials. There is also a group discussion about stigma and other barriers against getting help, how the teenagers in the film negotiated and overcame these barriers, and what finally worked for them. Students are encouraged to seek help for themselves or their peers through a discreet and simple form that is given in each session (Joshi et al. 2015).

Other examples of suicide prevention–focused curricula for high schools include *More Than Sad: Teen Depression* and *More Than Sad: Preventing Teen Suicide* (American Foundation for Suicide Prevention 2014). These programs consist of a 26-minute video and group discussion and another film for staff and parents. The teen video is in docudrama format and features four fictional vignettes of teenagers exhibiting symptoms of depression and anxiety, with voiceover narration regarding symptoms and their medical explanation. Sample depictions feature the help-seeking process in school, confidentiality, and brief glimpses into the counseling and psychotherapy process. The after-video discussion guide emphasizes core themes of depression in youth and highlights the medical aspects of major depression and anxiety and treatments that may be helpful. A mental health clinician might be needed for answering questions not featured in the guide to "frequently asked questions." This program is well received by schools because of the minimal classroom demands and the tailored discussion potential (Joshi et al. 2015).

Another example of a high school curriculum for suicide prevention is *Linking Education and Awareness of Depression and Suicide* (LEADS; Suicide Awareness Voices of Education 2008). The program can be implemented over three 1-hour class periods. The program goal is not only to improve knowledge but also to emphasize the resources available for depression treatment and suicide prevention—and importantly, how to deal with the stigma of mental health difficulties. The materials are currently available on CD (soon to be released online) and include a useful guide for facilitators and handouts for all activities. This prevention curriculum distinguishes itself from others by offering guidelines for school-based management of possible crises. LEADS would be best administered with a mental health professional available, but the detailed instructions that accompany the curriculum could enable most school officials or teachers skilled in classroom discussions to implement it.

These interventions collectively highlight how clinicians can be helpful not only for diagnosing and treating mood disorders in the school setting but also for serving as partners or implementers of best-practices curricula to promote mental health, well-being, and education about the signs and symptoms of mood conditions to mitigate risk from developing serious mood disorders. Previous research (Joshi et al. 2015) led to recommendations against one-and-done presentations, because they may not be effective in changing behavior. Moreover, students (and school staff or parents) should have opportunities for questions, reflection, and follow-up. Thus, all of the curricula described in this section should be delivered over multiple sessions and monitored for effect.

An example of an evidence-supported program to enhance teacher self-efficacy in engaging with high-risk students is Kognito *At-Risk for High School Educators*. This program features interactive role-play simulations that build awareness, knowledge, and skills about mental health and suicide prevention, preparing high school educators to recognize and intervene with students in psychological distress and, if needed, connect them with support services (Kognito 2018).

Examples of school-based depression prevention programs have been summarized nicely in a review by Calear (2012). The author suggests important factors to be considered before implementing a depression prevention program in schools, such as target audience (universal prevention directed to all students, indicated prevention directed to students with elevated symptoms of depression, or selected prevention directed at only students identified as being at high risk for developing depression), program scheduling, support and protocols for referrals, and the assurance of full buy-in from school administrative leaders. Specific programs that are aimed at preventing depression and increasing mental health awareness include the MoodGYM, Penn Resiliency Program, IPT–Adolescent Skills Training (AST), Stress Inoculation Training, Brain Driver's Education, and the Positive Action (Table 15–4).

From Prevention to Classroom Interventions to State Policy and a New Law

In 2016, California became one of the first states to require that all public school districts serving students in grades 7–12 develop a suicide prevention board policy and administrative regulations.

A model suicide prevention policy has been developed by the California Department of Education (2017), and a K-12 Toolkit for Mental Health Promotion and Suicide Prevention (Joshi et al. 2017) lists evidence-based suicide prevention programs and social-emotional learning strategies that can be implemented even earlier than middle school, such as the PAX Good Behavior Game (https://www.goodbehaviorgame.org/pax-science) and Promoting Alternative Thinking Strategies (PATHS; http://www.pathstraining.com/main/curriculum). The Good Behavior Game is a classroom game in which elementary school children are rewarded for displaying appropriate on-task behaviors during instructional times. It has shown long-term benefits in multiple social and emotional domains by strengthening inhibition, extending self-regulation, and improving social-emotional scaffolding, in addition to being associated with significantly decreased suicide risk in later school years by those who participated in this game while in elementary school. PATHS has shown effectiveness in enhancing the educational process and promoting social and emotional competencies in elementary school children, while also reducing aggression and behavior problems.

Engaging With School Settings and Creating Partnerships

Before introducing any intervention in a school setting, clinicians should be aware of previous research that offers guidance on nurturing working relationships and building (and maintaining) trust with school staff and administrators (Bostic and Rauch 1999; Waxman et al. 1999; Weist et al. 2001), especially in the face of tragic events such as a suicide of someone

TABLE 15–4.   Examples of evidence-supported depression prevention and mental health awareness programs developed for schools

MoodGYM (Available for free at https://moodgym.com.au)	Interactive, Internet-based intervention for ages 13–17 years designed to prevent and decrease youth depression. Presented by the classroom teacher for 1 hour weekly over 5 weeks; based on cognitive-behavioral therapy (CBT); contains information, animated demonstrations, quizzes, and homework exercises.
Penn Resiliency Program (Gillham et al. 2007)	12-session group intervention for students ages 10–14 years. Teaches CBT and problem-solving skills. Widely researched and supported by eight randomized controlled trials showing significantly positive results.
Interpersonal Therapy–Adolescent Skills Training (IPT-AST; Young et al. 2006)	IPT-based training in which the goal is to prevent depression by teaching social and communication skills necessary to develop and maintain positive relationships; two individual and eight group sessions for students ages 11–16 years. Significant positive results have been reported at 3- and 6-month follow-ups in the areas of handling interpersonal role disputes, navigating role transitions, and addressing interpersonal deficits.
Stress Inoculation Training (Hains and Ellmann 1994)	CBT-based training that provides individual and group therapy for youth ages 15–18 years; 9–13 sessions are delivered weekly and include a three-phase stress inoculation model: a conceptualization phase, a skill acquisition phase, and a skill application phase. Techniques taught include cognitive restructuring, problem solving, and relaxation. At least two universal school-based trials have found significant results.

TABLE 15–4. Examples of evidence-supported depression prevention and mental health awareness programs developed for schools *(continued)*

Brain Driver's Education (Khan et al. 2014) (https://www.massgeneral.org/psychiatry/assets/pdfs/school-psych/Brain-Drivers-Education-Operators-Guide.pdf)	Program developed by a child and adolescent psychiatrist at the Massachusetts General Hospital School Psychiatry at Harvard Program and an educator in the Boston schools; evidence-informed curriculum on emotional self-regulation. Uses elements of CBT, dialectical behavior therapy, and other widely accepted therapies and approaches for achieving mind-body wellness and healthy interpersonal relationships. Pilot study showed significant positive results regarding emotion regulation and conflict resolution; most students found the curriculum useful for their everyday lives.
Positive Action (Lewis et al. 2013) (https://www.positiveaction.net)	An evidence-based educational program that promotes intrinsic learning while promoting cooperation among peers; embraces the idea that positive actions lead to positive self-perception; adapted for various grade levels; shown to increase academic achievement and reduce problem behaviors; intervention topics address mental health, physical health, behavior, family, academics, and substance use. The program is designed for teachers to run in as little as 15 minutes per school day.

in the school community. The three *R*'s of school consultation (Bostic and Rauch 1999) include the *relationships* that need to be cultivated and fostered, the *recognition* of human motivation during an important or sensitive time, and the *responses* to challenges. For a school mental health consultant, each face-time contact with administration is an opportunity not only to improve the school system and its response to those in greatest need but also to strengthen the system as a whole (Joshi et al. 2015).

First, the consultant strengthens the *relationships* of professionals allied around students, parents, and the greater school community, building bridges among them. This partnership among parents, staff, and therapists for school mental health has been termed the *supporting alliance in school mental health* and has been described previously (Feinstein et al. 2009). Second, the school consultant can foster *recognition* of human motivation and the resistance that may impede healthy changes in the case of introducing organized curricula to educate school communities about mood disorders and suicide prevention. Guiding principles include determining wishes and motives of the student, parent, teacher, and administrator and dismantling any resistance to change. For example, the reluctance to embark on universal suicide prevention strategies often stems from a place of fear (e.g., that such programs may plant the idea of suicide not only in vulnerable youth but also in those who have not considered suicide previously). Third, the school consultant can help the staff create *responses* to challenges. Guiding principles include providing staff new skills to reach and teach distressed students, finding common goals to unite students in the school, reaching parents in the community, and determining the developmental steps toward shared goals (Bostic and Rauch 1999). Finally, the school consultant can leverage the trust he or she has built with school administration and school district leadership to advocate for school climate and other structural changes that have an emerging research base in support of youth mental health. These changes include 1) later school start times to improve total sleep (Adolescent Sleep Working Group 2014); 2) detailed self-study into the sources of major and daily stressful life events for youth (Wagner et al. 1995), such as severe academic stress in communities where youth may see themselves as being evaluated solely in terms of their academic performance, and the pressure to excel is an important measure of their success in school (Ang and Huan 2006); and 3) adoption of formal suicide prevention policies with administrative regulations by local school boards (Joshi et al. 2017). The three empowering principles described above allow the therapeutic skills commonly used in individual and family therapies to be implemented as strategies that can assist education professionals, students, and the larger school community simultaneously (Joshi et al. 2015).

Because teachers are the most present adults controlling the learning environment, it is important to engage with them early and often in order to build a healthy and long-lasting supporting alliance. When children are younger, it may be quite easy for parents or guardians to engage with school staff through volunteering or chaperoning a school field trip, for example. It becomes more difficult to stay engaged as a parent as youth progress through middle and high school.

Table 15–5 lists advice from parents to other parents about simple ways to engage the school team to advocate for a child or teenager who requires school accommodations.

TABLE 15–5.   Engagement strategies for parents with school staff for youth who require school accommodations

Strategy	Explanation
Make extra efforts to get acquainted with each teacher.	Go out of your way to make yourself known and approachable: personally introduce yourself and make eye contact with each teacher, and offer your availability if any problems come up.
After an initial meeting, stay in touch throughout the year.	If a problem develops, give teachers the benefit of the doubt (most are well meaning and want to do right by your child/their student).
Let teachers know when there has been a change in medication or another aspect of treatment.	Like parents, teachers may struggle with dealing with a student's symptoms or with medication side effects. Approach the school staff with a "We're all in this together" demeanor (instead of an accusatory or antagonistic approach), and you're more likely to receive a positive response.
Let teachers know when things are going well.	Occasional thank-you notes or a shout-out to the principal about a specific teacher or staff member will cultivate a sense of teamwork and feed the supporting alliance. Establish yourself as a school asset by volunteering in the office or participating in fund-raising activities. The more you can do to build a positive working relationship with school staff, the more effective you may be when requesting additional services for your student.
In the cases of a difficult relationship with a teacher or school staff member, know what your options are.	Address concerns with a specific staff member gently but directly; if the difficulties continue, engage the principal with your concerns and an attitude of trying to work on the problem together. In the end, it may be necessary to switch classrooms or even find a different school. Your child has enough on his or her plate without having to deal with a teacher who is unwilling or unable to adapt accordingly.

TABLE 15–5. Engagement strategies for parents with school staff for youth who require school accommodations *(continued)*

Strategy	Explanation
Use other strategies.	Explore all possibilities, and ask for all services that are relevant. Be well educated about what has been done for youth with similar conditions in your school district (and elsewhere). Find support from other parents (or join an organization listed at the end of this chapter); be collaborative by making suggestions and also being open to suggestions; know your rights and your child's rights. Keep extensive notes on all interventions and keep them organized in a binder; and be affiliative and show gratitude (e.g., bring baked goods or refreshments to meetings).
Avoid certain behaviors.	Do not be demanding, refuse to listen to alternatives, or make threats.

Source. Evans and Andrews 2005; Fristad and Goldberg Arnold 2004; Parents Helping Parents: http://www.phponline.org); Understood.org 2015.

Table 15–6 features teenagers' comments on when schools have been helpful and what strategies to include and avoid.

As parents engage with schools to advocate for important accommodations for their children with mood conditions, it is important for them to know what their rights and resources are. In the United States, the main laws of relevance are the Individuals With Disabilities Education Act (IDEA), Individuals With Disabilities Education Improvement Act (IDEIA), and Section 504 of the Rehabilitation Act of 1973. IDEA applies to students who have a disability that affects their ability to benefit from general educational services. Section 504 applies to students who are in the general education (mainstream classroom) setting, and its accommodations usually can be implemented in a more timely fashion, because these do not require the same amount of evaluation or intensity of services as compared with IDEA. Table 15–7 lists the major differences between IDEA and Section 504 accommodations. Private schools are not mandated to abide by IDEA or Section 504 to the same degree as public schools but usually will collaborate with families and the local school district to create something

TABLE 15–6. Advice from teenagers to educators

Teenager comments	Application to educators
"It never gets talked about, but it needs to be."	Opportunities for conversations about mental health in the classroom should be created.
"When adults don't listen to youth, youth are also unlikely to listen back."	When adults make obvious efforts to listen, teenagers are more likely to feel respected and valued.
"Schools should listen more closely to students' feedback and should make an effort to incorporate that feedback."	Schools are a major part of a teenager's life; schools can ease stress by taking active steps to ease some of the structural stressors that may make simply going to class difficult (especially for teenagers with mood conditions). This should include having youth leaders involved with small logistical changes and major decisions affecting school life, when possible.
"My school is very competitive, which makes it difficult not to have anxiety or depression at some point."	Stressful school environments can worsen existing mental health conditions and make it hard to maintain overall mental health and wellness; structural changes such as later school start times (Adolescent Sleep Working Group 2014) and offering students free or prep periods can allow them to sleep more and enhance learning.
"Allowing students to leave class for 15 minutes and take a break in our wellness center has been incredible."	Letting students have a safe space to deal with mental health issues and everyday stressors, or even if they just need a break or rest from a bad day, can be very useful and benefit students' mental well-being and readiness to learn.
"In one of my harder classes, my teacher doesn't think I try.... She always calls me out in front of the class and makes me feel even dumber than I am."	Struggling with mental health issues does not mean that students are less intellectual. Teachers misread uncontrollable symptoms of mental illness or severe distress as a sign that students are somehow unable to prosper. It is important for teachers to separate students' mental health from their abilities.

TABLE 15–6.   Advice from teenagers to educators *(continued)*

Teenager comments	Application to educators
"She was calm and had empathy for me."	Having a trusted teacher who can remain calm through difficult times and also listen is crucially important, especially because that teacher may be the *only* person the student is sharing his or her issues with.
"They were open, so I was open back."	Many teenagers agree that teachers make themselves more approachable and seem more trustworthy by being vulnerable and sharing their own stories (this must be done with great care not to overshare and potentially "burden" the student with the teacher's life stressors). Peer consultation can be an essential process if one chooses to share personal stories.
"He took time out of his day to check in with me."	The smallest things can have the largest effect. For students who do not have other resources, knowing that their teacher is thinking about them and has their best interests in mind can be very important and comforting.

Source.   Children's Health Council Teen Wellness Committee 2018.

similar to a formalized IEP to maximize a student's access to the educational curriculum (Evans and Andrews 2005).

For IDEA, students must qualify for at least 1 of 13 categories of disability. The usual categories for getting services for students with major mood disorders are "other health impaired, OHI" and "emotional disturbance, ED." Parents may worry about bias against their students labeled as ED, and teachers at some schools may view these students as "troublemakers." Additionally, these teachers may see disruptive behaviors as willful disobedience (only) and not as symptoms of a biologically based condition. For these reasons, OHI may be a better fit for some students. OHI also includes other conditions, such as attention-deficit/hyperactivity disorder and medical conditions that can affect school performance. This designation not only can reduce stigma attached to mental health conditions but also can encourage the school to consider how the biological aspects of major mood conditions can affect learning, social relationships, and ac-

TABLE 15–7.   Individuals With Disabilities Education Act (IDEA) versus Section 504 of the Rehabilitation Act of 1973

Mechanism	IDEA	Section 504 plan
Eligibility	Must meet at least 1 of 13 qualifying categories	"Substantially limiting" condition (e.g., attention-deficit/hyperactivity disorder, major mood disorder) must be present
Requirements	Written individualized education plan that is based on a multifactored evaluation completed by the school	An agreed-on list of in-class accommodations
Advantages	Federal money goes to the local school district; possibility of extensive modifications and services that are measurable and specific	Expedient and flexible
Disadvantages	Requires more paperwork and time to complete and usually includes psychological testing	No additional money allocated to the school district; easier to design but can be harder to enforce consistently, especially in middle and high schools (multiple classrooms and teachers)

Source.   Fristad and Goldberg Arnold 2004.

cess to the school's offerings overall. It also can help to better inform educational and disciplinary decisions (e.g., highlighting that disruptive behaviors related to the mood disorder may not be under a student's control; Evans and Andrews 2005; Understood.org 2015).

Common Presentations for Mood Disorders in the School Setting

Table 15–8 highlights the educational implications of and classroom strategies for students who struggle with major depressive disorder or pediatric bipolar disorder.

TABLE 15–8. Educational manifestations of mood disorders and classroom strategies

Educational manifestations	Instructional strategies and classroom accommodations
Fluctuations in mood, energy, and motivation that may be seasonal or cyclical (MDD/PBD)	During times of low mood, energy, and motivation, reduce academic workload and demands; adjust accordingly when mood, energy, and motivation increase or are especially high.
Difficulty concentrating or completing assignments (MDD/PBD)	Provide students with audiobooks or recorded instructions when concentration is low.
Difficulty understanding complex instructions; challenges reading long written passages of text (MDD/PBD)	Break assignments into smaller sections and monitor student progress, checking comprehension periodically.
Difficulty with prompt arrival and "readiness to learn" in the early morning because of difficulty sleeping (MDD/PBD)	Accommodate late arrivals by arranging for separate workspace if needed; ensure that IEP or Section 504 plan accounts for this—especially relevant during medication changes.
Easily frustrated and prone to sadness, embarrassment, or rage (MDD/PBD)	Identify a place where student can go for privacy until he or she can regain control.
Difficulty with social skills, boundaries, and peer relationships (MDD/PBD)	Seat student next to peers who the student feels would be helpful to his or her classroom functioning, with changes made as needed.
Fluctuations in cognitive and physical abilities and presence of side effects, especially with medication changes (MDD/PBD)	Adjust the homework and in-class load to prevent the student from becoming overwhelmed; adjust for need for frequent hydration and bathroom breaks.
Impaired planning, organizing, and abstract reasoning (MDD/PBD)	Provide skills training with occupational therapist, school psychologist, or learning specialist to improve these.
Prone to heightened sensitivity to perceived criticism and may react emotionally over seemingly small things (MDD/PBD)	Create a plan for self-calming strategies (journaling, listening to music, drawing, walking out of class or running errands at designated intervals for the teacher).

TABLE 15–8.   Educational manifestations of mood disorders and classroom strategies *(continued)*

Educational manifestations	Instructional strategies and classroom accommodations
Prone to inflated self-esteem and may overestimate their own abilities (PBD)	School staff can ask parents, therapist, or doctor about student's mood cycles and adapt curriculum, class supports, and activities accordingly; problem-solving skills training may be especially helpful. (Adapted from Adolescent Family Focused Therapy for Pediatric Bipolar Disorder, Miklowitz et al. 2013)
May experience high levels of anxiety that interfere with their ability to logically assess a situation; difficulty or shame/self-doubt in communicating educational needs (MDD/PBD)	Have a "lead school staff" whom the students know and trust the most: a guidance counselor, administrator, teacher, or other staff member who could be honest with the student to assist during times of high distress and be the single point of communication.
Marked decreases in interest in schoolwork and activities; especially problematic for group assignments (MDD)	Group student with peers who the student feels would be helpful to his or her classroom functioning, with changes made as needed.
Fluctuations in cognitive and physical abilities and presence of side effects, especially with medication changes (MDD/PBD)	Adjust the homework and in-class load to prevent the student from becoming overwhelmed; adjust for need for frequent hydration and bathroom breaks.
Grades may decline significantly because of lack of interest, loss of motivation, or excessive absences (MDD)	Adjust expectations accordingly, and meet with student, parent, and guidance counselor regularly to review progress; be flexible and realistic about educational goals (school failures and unmet expectations can exacerbate depressive symptoms).
Prone to "all or none" thinking (all bad or all good) (MDD/PBD)	Keep a record of accomplishments to show them at low points.

Note. IEP=individualized education plan; MDD=major depressive disorder; PBD = pediatric bipolar disorder.
Source. California Department of Education 2014; Chokroverty 2010; Papolos and Papolos 2002.

As students transition from elementary to middle to high school, and especially as they transition into young adulthood, mood conditions can become even more difficult to manage in the school setting. Table 15–9 lists some of the unique developmental factors to be considered for all students as they transition at different stages through their school careers.

Self-Care Strategies for Educators

Educators who engage with and teach youth with minor mood conditions and major mood disorders are at risk for compassion fatigue and burnout as a result of a variety of work-related and personal characteristics. Professionalism does not need to be equated with selflessness and deprivation. Student outcomes and parent satisfaction are correlated with teacher well-being and professional satisfaction (Derenne 2018; Feinstein et al. 2009). Several strategies have been described to address these issues. Self-care, resilience, and wellness are interrelated constructs across the educator spectrum, from K-12 to college and professional schools. *Self-care* refers to actions taken to care for oneself. *Wellness* refers to being in a good-enough state of health or well-being and is typically associated with good and consistent self-care strategies. Both self-care and wellness can cultivate *resilience*, which is the ability to manage challenges efficiently without depleting one's inner and external resources (Robinson 2018). Meaningful engagement and connection with colleagues are among the most effective techniques to maintain longevity in high-stress occupations (Adams 2018). Those educators who work in school settings with numerous traumatized students may find themselves at risk for secondary traumatic stress, in which knowing about a traumatic event experienced by a significant other can have emotional consequences. Secondary traumatic stress also can refer to the stress that results from helping (or wanting to help) a traumatized or suffering person (Figley 1995; Hydon et al. 2015).

Table 15–10 reviews strategies to prevent compassion fatigue and burnout among school staff.

TABLE 15–9.   Special challenges in managing mood conditions during the transitions (elementary to middle school, middle to high school, high school to postgraduate years)

Elementary to middle school

Level of responsibility and independence increase.

Relationship changes (family and school) toward greater independence, but student will still need guidance and support.

Stress levels can increase because of transitions in layout of school and need to navigate new physical, personal, and social terrain.

Levels of cognition, reasoning, and planning are higher.

Child is moving away from a strictly self-centered view of the world.

Expectations from parents and teachers shift toward more independence.

Adults need to focus on identifying and documenting learning disabilities and mental health conditions.

Some students start using social media and cell phones.

Puberty/sexuality can accelerate in fourth or fifth grade for some children (body changes/body image concerns).

Bullying and Internet safety need to be attended to.

Parents or guardians should apply for 504 plan or individualized education plan (IEP) if specific accommodations are needed.

Middle school to high school

Transition to independence is even greater, compared with elementary to middle school transition.

Parents need to stay engaged and supportive without being overbearing.

Academic demands increase.

Students are expected to take on more ownership of both academics and behavior.

Learning disabilities can become more evident as academic demands increase.

Potential concerns about social pressures and cultural and social identity arise.

Social media use increases (knowing the pitfalls becomes important for youth; need for Internet safety is crucial).

Puberty/sexuality becomes more relevant (body changes/body image concerns).

Exposure to bullying, drugs, alcohol, and cyberbullying may increase.

Learning disabilities and mental health conditions and 504 plan or IEP must be updated and documented.

TABLE 15–9.   Special challenges in managing mood conditions during the transitions (elementary to middle school, middle to high school, high school to postgraduate years) *(continued)*

High school to post–high school and college

Individuals must take ownership of their future.

Young adults need to learn to recognize mental health issues with greater independence and be open to work with trusted adults to find the best "fit" for college or work setting after graduation.

Parents must keep lines of communication open and plan for emergencies as teenager transitions to "TAY" group (transition-aged youth, 18–25 years old).

Academic demands typically increase.

The emerging young adult must complete the following tasks:

Visiting colleges and asking the right questions to help determine the best fit

Transferring and updating medical records

Preparing for ACT, SAT, college applications, and 4-year plan

Parents and counselors must ensure that students with disabilities have the necessary documentation for standardized tests and college.

Individuals need to know the signs of emotional distress to seek help early.

Young adults should recognize that the risks of depression and anxiety are higher as new life transitions occur (moving away from friends or community).

Students need to update documented learning disabilities and mental health disorders and connect with college resource officers.

Source.   Joshi et al. 2017.

TABLE 15–10. Strategies to prevent compassion fatigue and burnout among school staff

Maintain good boundaries between personal and professional life.

Invest in activities and relationships to increase meaningful engagement and joy.

Practice good and consistent self-care; attend to proper sleep habits, good nutrition, and moderate regular exercise.

Improve self-awareness, interpersonal effectiveness and assertiveness, time management, and organizational skills.

Diversify work to include administrative and leadership roles, in addition to teaching tasks.

Engage in regular supervision and peer support, and cultivate meaningful work relationships.

Take regular vacations at appropriately spaced intervals.

Source.   Adapted from Derenne 2018.

Clinical Pearls

- Children and teenagers spend a significant amount of their waking hours at schools during the week (≥35 hours). Thus, school settings are ideal places for intervening within the context of a child's daily life when he or she has a mood disorder.

- Educators can be the "eyes and ears" and expert consultant for the clinician, in addition to serving roles as trusted adults for affected youth and partners for concerned parents, peers, and others.

- Clinicians can be the expert consultant to help educators reach and teach all students, especially those affected by both minor mood symptoms and major mood conditions.

- With suicide rates rising nationally, it is even more important to promote universal education about stress, distress, and disorders and how educators can participate in "upstream" primary prevention of serious complications from mood disorders, including psychiatric hospitalization and suicide.

- Mood problems usually manifest across home, social, and educational settings, and the range of interventions is often much wider in schools, where staff and school clinicians can help to implement instructional and behavioral strategies to optimize academic and social outcomes and create the best possible "fit" for affected youth.

Useful School Mental Health Web Sites[3]

Center for MH in Schools and Student/Learning Supports at UCLA (http://smhp.psych.ucla.edu): Clearinghouse of important mental health, school, and educational materials.

Collaborative for Academic, Social, and Emotional Learning (CASEL; https://casel.org): "CASEL Select" programs provide outstanding coverage in five essential social-emotional learning skill areas; have at least one well-designed evaluation study demonstrating their effectiveness; and offer professional development supports beyond the initial training.

HEARD Alliance (Health Care Alliance for Response to Adolescent Depression; http:///www.heardalliance.org): A collaborative Web site that features resources for suicide prevention and mental health promotion; features a best-practice K-12 Toolkit for Mental Health Promotion and Suicide Prevention.

LD OnLine (http://www.ldonline.org): Information on classroom changes for students with learning disabilities, including attention-deficit/hyperactivity disorder.11. IDEA Partnership (http://www.ideapartnership.org): Up-to-date information on changes in the Individuals With Disabilities Education Act (IDEA) parameters.

Massachusetts General Hospital School Psychiatry Resource site (https://www.massgeneral.org/psychiatry/services/treatmentprograms.aspx?id=2086): Mental health information for school staff, parents, and clinicians; interventions for psychiatric disorders and symptoms; rating scales to assess disorders and monitor treatments.

National Center for School Mental Health (http://www.schoolmentalhealth.org): A repository of useful resources for school clinicians, educators, families, and students on school mental health.

National Child Traumatic Stress Network (http://www.nctsn.org): Contains very useful resources for educators to reach and teach students with trauma, loss, and anxiety; also has useful tips for speaking with parents, children, and the media about the consequences of human-caused and natural disasters and has resources for preventing burnout in educators.

Promising Practices Network (PPN) on Children, Families and Communities (http://www.promisingpractices.net/programs.asp): The PPN site features summaries of programs and practices that improve outcomes for children.

Suicide Prevention Resource Center: Best Practices Registry for Suicide Prevention (http://www.sprc.org/featured_resources/bpr/index.asp)

What Works Clearinghouse (WWC; http://ies.ed.gov/ncee/wwc): Information on broad categories of findings of "what works" in schools, including academics and mental health.

---

[3]Adapted from Bostic and Hoover 2018.

References

Adams C: 12 smart ways to fight teacher burnout that really work. March 1, 2018. Available at: https://www.weareteachers.com/prevent-teacher-burnout. Accessed September 22, 2018.

Adolescent Sleep Working Group; Committee on Adolescence; Council on School Health: School start times for adolescents. Pediatrics 134(3):642–649, 2014 25156998

American Foundation for Suicide Prevention: More Than Sad Curriculum for Students, Teachers, and Parents. New York, American Foundation for Suicide Prevention, 2014

Ang RP, Huan VSS: Relationship between academic stress and suicidal ideation: testing for depression as a mediator using multiple regression. Child Psychiatry Hum Dev 37(2):133–143, 2006 16858641

Bostic JQ, Hoover SA: School consultation, in Lewis's Child and Adolescent Psychiatry: A Comprehensive Textbook, 5th Edition. Edited by Martin A, Bloch MH, Volkmar F. Philadelphia, PA, Lippincott Williams & Wilkins, 2018, pp 956–974

Bostic JQ, Rauch PK: The 3 R's of school consultation. J Am Acad Child Adolesc Psychiatry 38(3):339–341, 1999 10087697

Boston Children's Hospital Neighborhood Partnerships Program: Break Free From Depression Curriculum, Revised. 2017. Available at: https://www.openpediatrics.org/course/break-free-depression. Accessed September 22, 2018.

Calear AL: Depression in the classroom: considerations and strategies. Child Adolesc Psychiatr Clin N Am 21(1):135–144, x, 2012 22137817

California Department of Education; Placer Co. Office of Education; Minnesota Association for Children's Health: A Guide to Student Mental Health and Wellness in California. St. Paul, Minnesota Association for Children's Health, 2014

California Department of Education: Model Youth Suicide Prevention Policy, 2017. Available at: https://www.cde.ca.gov/ls/cg/mh/suicideprevres.asp. Accessed September 22, 2018.

Children's Health Council Teen Wellness Committee: Just a Thought: Uncensored Narratives on Teen Mental Health. Palo Alto, CA, Children's Health Council, 2018

Chokroverty L: 100 Questions and Answers About Your Child's Depression or Bipolar Disorder. Sudbury, MA, Jones & Bartlett, 2010

De Nadai AS, Karver MS, Murphy TK, et al: Common factors in pediatric psychiatry: a review of essential and adjunctive mechanisms of treatment outcome. J Child Adolesc Psychopharmacol 27(1):10–18, 2017 27128785

Derenne J: Burnout and self-care of clinicians in mental health services, in Student Mental Health: A Guide for Psychiatrists, Psychologists, and Leaders Serving in Higher Education. Edited by Roberts L. Washington, DC, American Psychiatric Association Publishing, 2018, pp 53–65

Evans DW, Andrews LW: If Your Adolescent Has Depression or Bipolar Disorder: An Essential Resource for Parents. New York, Oxford University Press, 2005

Feinstein NR, Fielding K, Udvari-Solner A, et al: The supporting alliance in child and adolescent treatment: enhancing collaboration among therapists, parents, and teachers. Am J Psychother 63(4):319–344, 2009 20131741

Figley CR: Compassion Fatigue: Coping With Secondary Traumatic Stress Disorder in Those Who Treat the Traumatized. London, Psychology Press, 1995

Fristad M, Goldberg Arnold JS: Raising a Moody Child: How to Cope With Depression and Bipolar Disorder. New York, Guilford, 2004

Gillham JE, Reivich KJ, Freres DR, et al: School-based prevention of depressive symptoms: a randomized controlled study of the effectiveness and specificity of the Penn Resiliency Program. J Consult Clin Psychol 75(1):9–19, 2007 17295559

Hains AA, Ellmann SW: Stress inoculation training as a preventative intervention for high school youth. Journal of Cognitive Psychotherapy 8(3):219–228, 230–232, 1994

Hughes CW, Emslie GJ, Crismon ML, et al; Texas Consensus Conference Panel on Medication Treatment of Childhood Major Depressive Disorder: Texas Children's Medication Algorithm Project: update from Texas Consensus Conference Panel on Medication Treatment of Childhood Major Depressive Disorder. J Am Acad Child Adolesc Psychiatry 46(6):667–686, 2007 17513980

Hydon S, Wong M, Langley AK, et al: Preventing secondary traumatic stress in educators. Child Adolesc Psychiatr Clin N Am 24(2):319–333, 2015 25773327

Joshi SV: Teamwork: the therapeutic alliance in pediatric pharmacotherapy. Child Adolesc Psychiatr Clin N Am 15(1):239–262, 2006 16321733

Joshi SV, Hartley SN, Kessler M, Barstead M: School-based suicide prevention: content, process, and the role of trusted adults and peers. Child Adolesc Psychiatr Clin N Am 24(2):353–370, 2015 25773329

Joshi SV, Ojakian M, Lenoir L, Lopez J: K-12 Toolkit for Mental Health Promotion and Suicide Prevention. 2017. Available at: http://www.heardalliance.org/help-toolkit. Accessed September 22, 2018.

Joshi SV, Jassim N, Mani N: Youth depression in school settings: assessment, interventions, and prevention. Child Adolesc Psychiatry Clin N Am (in press)

Khan CK, Peterson AD, Joshi SV: Brain driver education: teaching kids emotion regulation skills through an innovative and integrative curriculum. Presented at the 61st annual meeting of the American Academy of Child and Adolescent Psychiatry, San Diego, CA, October 20–25, 2014

Kognito: At-Risk for High School Educators program. Available at: https://kognito.com/products/at-risk-for-high-school-educators. Accessed September 22, 2018.

Lewis KM, DuBois DL, Bavarian N, et al: Effects of Positive Action on the emotional health of urban youth: a cluster-randomized trial. J Adolesc Health 53:706–711, 2013 23890774

Malik M, Lake J, Lawson WB, Joshi SV: Culturally adapted pharmacotherapy and the integrative formulation. Child Adolesc Psychiatr Clin N Am 19(4):791–814, 2010 21056347

Miklowitz DJ, Schneck CD, Singh MK, et al: Early intervention for symptomatic youth at risk for bipolar disorder: a randomized trial of family focused therapy. J Am Acad Child Adolesc Psychiatry 52(2):121–131, 2013 23357439

Papolos D, Papolos J: The Bipolar Child, Revised Edition. New York, Broadway Books, 2002

Pruett K, Joshi SV, Martin A: Thinking about prescribing: the psychology of psychopharmacology, in Pediatric Psychopharmacology: Principles and Practice, 2nd Edition. Edited by Martin A, Scahill L, Kratochivil C. New York, Oxford University Press, 2010, pp 422–433

Robinson A: Student self-care, wellness, and resilience, in Student Mental Health: A Guide for Psychiatrists, Psychologists, and Leaders Serving in Higher Education. Edited by Roberts LW. Arlington, VA, American Psychiatric Association Publishing, 2018, pp 69–86

Suicide Awareness Voices of Education: The Linking Education and Awareness for Depression and Suicide (LEADS) program for youth, 2008. Available at: https://save.org/what-we-do/education/leads-for-youth-program/. Accessed September 22, 2018.

Understood.org: The difference between IEPs and 504 plans. 2015. Available at: https://www.understood.org/en/school-learning/special-services/504-plan/the-difference-between-ieps-and-504-plans. Accessed September 22, 2018.

Wagner BM, Cole RE, Schwartzman P: Psychosocial correlates of suicide attempts among junior and senior high school youth. Suicide Life Threat Behav 25(3):358–372, 1995 8553416

Waxman RP, Weist MD, Benson DM: Toward collaboration in the growing education–mental health interface. Clin Psychol Rev 19(2):239–253, 1999 10078422

Weist MD, Lowie JA, Flaherty LT, et al: Collaboration among the education, mental health, and public health systems to promote youth mental health. Psychiatr Serv 52(10):1348–1351, 2001 11585951

Young JF, Mufson L, Davies M: Efficacy of Interpersonal Psychotherapy–Adolescent Skills Training: an indicated preventive intervention for depression. J Child Psychol Psychiatry 47(12):1254–1262, 2006 17176380

Preventative and Emerging Pharmacological and Nonpharmacological Treatments

Daniel P. Dickstein, M.D.

Paul E. Croarkin, D.O., M.S.

A 14-year-old female presents with a 3-month history of excessive sleep and fatigue. She also notes irritability with both family and friends. She struggles to complete her schoolwork on a daily basis. She is not suicidal, nor has she ever been. There are no other psychiatric symptoms. The patient has no prior psychiatric history, no history of trauma, and no history of alcohol or substance use. The patient's mother has a history of depression and has been treated effectively with fluoxetine. A paternal uncle has had treatment for bipolar disorder (BD). On interview, the patient's pediatrician does not elicit any history of recent interpersonal stressors, bullying, or cyberbullying. The patient does not have obesity, nor does she have any other medical problems. The patient completes a Patient Health Questionnaire–9 Modified for Teens (PHQ-9 Modified), and her score is a 7. On the basis of the score and clinical interview, the pediatrician explains that the patient has mild symptoms of depression. The pediatrician discusses a number of life-style interventions, such as maintaining a regular sleeping schedule, discontinuing all electronic device use at 7 P.M., and getting daily exercise. The pediatrician emphasizes that exercise does not treat all types of depression and is not universally successful but that it is a reasonable first approach in this circumstance. The patient makes the recommended changes and institutes a program of daily vigorous walking in the morning. At a follow-up appointment 1 month later, the patient's irritable mood and energy are improved. Her PHQ-9 Modified score is 0. The pediatrician discusses the importance of maintaining these healthy lifestyle changes and provides education about the warning signs of depression to monitor for in the future.

Standard psychotherapeutic and pharmacological treatments for child and adolescent mood disorders, including major depressive disorder (MDD) and BD, have advanced considerably over recent decades. Psychotherapy, pharmacological treatments, and the combination offer great benefit for a substantial number of young patients with depressive and bipolar disorders. However, response and remission rates rarely exceed 60% and 30%, respectively, in systematic interventional trials for childhood mood disorders (Birmaher et al. 2007; McClellan et al. 2007). Related side effect burden, unknowns of risk, and the time-intensive nature of psychotherapy are problematic for many patients and families. Contemporary psychiatry increasingly embraces precision medicine and shared-decision-making approaches that place patient and family preferences at the forefront (Gewirtz et al. 2018; Wehry et al. 2018). In this context patients and families often inquire about preventative and alternative approaches. In some circumstances patients and families may prefer such approaches with collective understanding of a limited evidence base.

In this chapter we survey recent understanding of such approaches in child and adolescent mood disorders. Our discussion includes preemptive interventions and novel interventions for treatment-resistant presentations. Often these interventions might best be conceptualized as options either prior to standard treatments recommended in guidelines such as the Texas Children's Medication Algorithm Project or after such recommended treatments have been exhausted.

Exercise and Sleep Hygiene

Patterns of activity, including exercise, sleep hygiene, and interpersonal relationships, are very important to mood disorders, including both MDD and BD. Disturbances in these patterns are often harbingers of worsening mood disorders, including decreased sleep (otherwise known as insomnia) in unipolar depression and decreased need for sleep (meaning getting decreased sleep but not being tired) in mania (Geller et al. 2002). Similarly, changes in activity and energy are core features for both MDD (decreased energy, psychomotor agitation or retardation) and mania (increased energy, psychomotor agitation, and increased goal directed activity). Moreover, actively working to improve these life rhythms is an important treatment target (Swartz et al. 2012).

Exercise

As is true with sleep, changes in physical activity are both sign and symptom of mood disorders, and also a potential treatment target. A recent Cochrane review examined data for the role of physical activity, diet, and other behavioral interventions in improving cognition and school achievement in adolescents with obesity or overweight (Martin et al. 2018). The review authors ultimately included 18 studies covering more than 2,384 children and adolescents. Key take-home points included the fact that physical activity interventions delivered in both school and community settings can improve executive functions and school achievement in children with obesity. The benefits of physical activity on executive functioning have also been shown in children with social, emotional, and behavioral disabilities (Ash et al. 2017). While multiple mechanisms may exist for this benefit, a study by Lubans et al. (2016) summarizing 25 articles reporting data from 22 studies suggested that the strongest evidence was for physical activity improving physical self-perceptions, and thus self-esteem.

With respect to depression, a recent meta-analysis analyzing data from 23 randomized clinical trials (RCTs) involving 977 participants showed that physical exercise had a moderate to large significant effect on depression compared with control conditions ($g=-0.68$) but that the effect became small and not significant at follow-up ($g=-0.22$), potentially because of patients reducing the intensity or frequency of their exercise (Kvam et al. 2016).

Thus, it is important to evaluate typical physical activity in assessing for mood disorders and also in considering treatment options. Such an evaluation will likely include assessing media consumption or screen time that often competes with children's time and interest. It will also include assessing for physical or emotional conditions that would need to be considered in setting up a physical activity plan, or any such conditions that would make the physical activity plan contraindicated, such as prescribing aerobic exercise for someone struggling with an untreated eating disorder. It is likely also a chance to collaborate with the child's or adolescent's primary care providers and caretakers to make exercise a sustainable lifestyle modification, rather than a prescribed intervention that is unlikely to be followed.

Sleep Hygiene

While sleep is very important in the evaluation and treatment of mood disorders, there is still much we do not know about it, particularly in children. For example, we know that children typically need 8–10 hours of sleep each night, and that teenagers need even more (Tarokh et al. 2016). Unfortunately, data show that from childhood to adolescence, youth actually lose sleep—not gain it—because of several factors. These include progressively later natural bedtimes, increased homework load, and earlier school start times as children become adolescents (Wheaton et al. 2016). These trends are not confined to the United States and instead occur worldwide (Yang et al. 2005).

In adults, studies have demonstrated that sleep changes affect cognitive processes, including attention, executive function, reward processing, learning/memory, and overall emotional regulation (Goldstein and Walker 2014; Killgore 2010; Ma et al. 2015; Yang et al. 2005). Studies in adults have shown that sleep can improve these processes, and also that sleep loss can worsen them (Potkin and Bunney 2012). In children and adolescents, the picture is more complicated in that sleep loss may affect some but not all cognitive and emotional processes as uniformly as in adults, potentially because of cognitive and emotional "compensation" from a developing brain (Beebe et al. 2009; Fallone et al. 2001). However, data do seem to support the impairment in mood due to sleep deprivation in children and adolescents, a finding corroborating the experience of clinicians and parents alike (Baum et al. 2014; Talbot et al. 2010).

Therefore, clinicians treating children and adolescents need to pay attention to sleep. Sleep should be monitored in patients with mood disorders. Monitoring includes questions about sleep embedded in many commonly used questionnaires, such as the Child Behavior Checklist (Achenbach and Rescorla 2001), Children's Depression Inventory (Kovacs 1992), or Young Mania Rating Scale (Young et al. 1978), that may be useful during initial evaluation appointments. It also includes use of mood-tracking worksheets or smartphone applications that often track sleep (in terms of duration, onset, and quality) in addition to gathering prospective daily information about mood and other symptoms. Such patterns may be important when clinicians are considering if a child has unipolar MDD or BD.

Beyond monitoring or evaluating, clinicians treating children with mood disorders likely will want to target sleep as part of their care. Clinicians should discuss core principles of sleep hygiene with patients and their families. These include 1) using a bed only for sleep and not for other activity; 2) making regular time to go to sleep and to wake up; 3) reducing exposure to blue light from electronics, especially after dinnertime; 4) turning off social media, texting, and smartphones before bedtime so that sleep is not artificially interrupted; 5) avoiding all-nighters or extreme reductions in sleep; 6) avoiding caffeine and other substances that may alter sleep onset or sleep quality; and 6) making the most of the body's triggers for sleep onset, such as gradually cooling body temperature, by routines involving afternoon exercise and evening showers to warm up the body, and also having a light snack involving a balance of carbohydrates and protein (the so-called Thanksgiving effect) to promote sleep onset at the appropriate time.

Principles of monitoring and improving sleep are embedded in many forms of therapy, but perhaps nowhere as much as in interpersonal and social rhythm therapy (IPSRT). Developed by Ellen Frank, Ph.D., to treat adults with BD, at its core, IPSRT holds that maintaining regular social interaction, exercise, and sleep will result in improved euthymic mood, and that irregularity in those functions is an early warning sign of non–euthymic mood—both worsening depression and mania (Frank 2005). IPSRT in adults is associated with more regular social rhythms and remission from depression (Swartz et al. 2012). Recently, a recent RCT showed that IPSRT was acceptable for adolescents at risk for BD by virtue of having a parent with BD compared with those receiving data-informed referral alone; however, IPSRT was not clearly significantly superior in reducing mood symptoms, with the lack of separation possibly due to small sample size (N=42) (Goldstein et al. 2018).

Nutrition and Nutraceuticals (Omega-3 Fatty Acids)

Nutrition is very important for children and adolescents with mood disorders, providing the substrate for appropriate growth and development of their bodies, brains, and everything in between. Non-euthymic mood states may be associated with changes in eating behavior, including either decreased or increased appetite, eating, and weight in depression, and also changes in eating associated with increased energy or goal-directed activity in mania. Thus, asking about a patient's eating patterns is important in every assessment to get a sense of what is typical for that child, and if it has been recently, episodically altered.

Relatedly, *food insecurity*—defined as being without reliable, regular access to sufficient quantities of affordable, nutritious food—has come into focus as a source of stress for increasing numbers of families. Many researchers hypothesize that the effect of food insecurity is from neural consequences of stress—both acute and chronic—over and above just decreased caloric intake or poor dietary choices. In emerging data, food insecurity has been shown to be associated with negative impact on the home environment. For example, a study of 4,231 mothers of children under age 5 years showed that low and very low food security were significantly associated with higher odds of disciplining children with high frequency (Gill et al. 2018). Interesting new studies are testing the links between the stress of food insecurity and mood disorders, including depression. For example, Dennison et al. (2017) recently showed that among 94 youth ages 6–19 years, maternal food insecurity, but not emotional deprivation or trauma, was associated with impaired reward performance. Moreover, reductions in frontostriatal white-matter integrity mediated the association between food insecurity and depressive symptoms, suggesting distinct behavioral and neurodevelopmental consequences of food insecurity on depression (Dennison et al. 2017). These findings suggest the need to ask detailed questions about how often a particular family is worried about not having enough food for their meals and other questions about periods of financial insecurity when assessing children for mood disorders.

Many families look to natural remedies, including dietary supplements, as potentially preferred treatments for mental health conditions, including mood disorders. There are several reasons for this, including the fact that such natural supplements, also called *nutraceuticals*, are perceived as being natural and thus free of risks and side effects of prescription medications. They also are over the counter and do not require accessing a child psychiatrist, which is often not easy due to stigma, lack of providers, or insurance/financial issues. Thus, families increasingly turn to natural supplements and remedies to address their medical needs (Ekor 2014).

Several nutraceuticals have been studied in the context of mood disorders. These include omega-3 fatty acids, S-adenosylmethionine (SAMe), and St. John's wort.

Omega-3-fatty acids are linked to mood disorders via their role in regulating neurotransmission, including serotonin-, dopamine-, and glutamine-associated signaling, as well as via their role in regulating the hypothalamic-pituitary-adrenal axis (Grosso et al. 2014). For example, a 7-year longitudinal study of young individuals with "ultra-high-risk" phenotypes for psychosis (n=69) showed that a higher polyunsaturated fatty acid (PUFA) ratio of omega-6 to omega-3 at baseline was associated with significantly increased odds for subsequent mood disorder (odds ratio=1.89, P=0.03) despite adjustments for age, gender, smoking, severity of depressive symptoms at baseline, and omega-3 supplementation (Berger et al. 2017). A review of 20 publications published from 1997 through 2016 showed that depletion of omega-3 PUFAs was associated with increased risk of psychiatric disorders compared with controls, though associations with increased risk for suicide itself as an outcome were not necessarily supported (Pompili et al. 2017). Interestingly, a study of 15- to 20-year-olds who had started antidepressant treatment in the prior month (n=88) or had never taken psychiatric medications (n=92) showed that low omega-3 PUFA levels and greater childhood adversity independently correlated with negative emotionality (Coryell et al. 2017).

Several RCTs of omega-3 PUFAs have been conducted in children with mood disorders. A 12-week RCT in 95 youth with mood disorders, including depression, BD not otherwise specified, and cyclothymia, showed that those randomly assigned to receive 1.87 grams of omega-3 daily had significantly greater improvements in the global executive composite, behavior regulation index, and metacognition index of the Behavior Rating Inventory of Executive Functioning (BRIEF) compared with those randomly assigned to receive placebo (Vesco et al. 2018). A similar 12-week RCT in 73 children ages 7–14 years old with MDD, dysthymia, or depression not otherwise specified showed that omega-3 monotherapy, both alone or combined with individual/family psychoeducational psychotherapy, resulted in small to medium effect sizes, but psychotherapy alone had negligible effect size (Fristad et al. 2016). Relatedly, a 16-week RCT in 51 children with symptomatic BD I or II (i.e., mixed, manic, hypomanic, or depressed) comparing 550 mg flax oil with an olive oil placebo found no significant changes in Young Mania Rating Scale, Child Depression Rating Scale, or Clinical Global Impression bipolar ratings (Gracious et al. 2010).

SAMe, another nutraceutical, is primarily produced in the liver, and its metabolic role is as a methyl group donor in metabolic processes, including the synthesis of neurotransmitters and methylation (and regulation) of DNA and RNA and all resultant metabolic cascades. SAMe has been studied in adults with depression with mixed results (Mischoulon and Fava 2002). However, as of this writing, a PubMed search did not reveal any published RCTs evaluating SAMe in the treatment of children with depression or BD.

St. John's wort (*Hypericum perforatum*) is another nutraceutical that has been considered for its potential antidepressant effects. Biochemical studies have shown that St. John's wort inhibits the synaptosomal uptake of serotonin, dopamine, and norepinephrine with equal affinity, and it is also a week inhibitor of monoamine oxidase A and B (Butterweck 2003). In vivo studies have shown that St. John's wort can cause changes in serotonin neurotransmitter concentrations in areas of the rat brain implicated in depression, and that it can protect rats from consequences of stress. However, as of this writing, a PubMed search did not reveal any published RCTs evaluating St. John's wort in children with either unipolar MDD or BD (Jorm et al. 2006).

Taken as a whole, this suggests that although patients may turn to natural remedies for children with mood disorders, there are few compelling data at present to suggest such remedies may be effective. Nevertheless, asking about families' use of these agents in an open, nonjudgmental way is important, as is further research on related agents.

Real-Time Neurofeedback, Transcranial Magnetic Stimulation, and Electroconvulsive Therapy

Real-Time Neurofeedback

Neuroimaging studies continue to suggest that brain networks are organized into centers of neurons with dense intra-connectivity and sparse yet critical interconnectivity. Neurodevelopment most likely involves a substantial reworking of these networks, yet some of this basic organization is continuous through adulthood. Psychiatric disorders such as depression and BD have dysfunctional circuitry correlates among these centers and networks. Safe and noninvasive treatments that might directly impact these underlying pathological correlates are appealing and emerging. The advent of modern positron emission tomography, magnetoencephalography, functional magnetic resonance imaging (fMRI), and quantitative electroencephalography (EEG) techniques have catalyzed this work. Neurofeedback treatments aim to modify brain function through the provision of continuous signals to patients reflective of continuous changes in neurophysiology. Notably, EEG techniques are a relatively inexpensive and accessible modality for this type of work. Waveforms from EEG are generated from brain network synaptic activity and provide a framework for operant conditioning as patients attempt to alter electroencephalographic patterns and ultimately brain function. Recent neurofeedback efforts have also utilized other types of neuroimaging and more recently interleaved EEG-fMRI (Simkin et al. 2014; Thibault et al. 2018).

Early efforts have examined the potential of neurofeedback in childhood neuropsychiatric disorders. General EEG approaches include either 2–4 scalp electrodes with concurrent computer monitoring of brain function or quantitative EEG approaches with low-resolution electromagnetic tomography (LORETA). Contemporary approaches with fMRI neurofeedback are appealing because this modality offers enhanced spatial resolution, greater precision for indexing brain activity through blood oxygen level–dependent (BOLD) signal, and in many cases, improved methodology from early EEG work. Although related literature is rapidly advancing, most work related to mood disorders has focused on adult samples (Simkin et al. 2014; Thibault et al. 2018; Young et al. 2014). One recent study (Alegria et al. 2017) recruited 12- to 17-year-old males ($n=31$) with attention-deficit/hyperactivity disorder (ADHD) for a single-blind RCT examining the efficacy of real-time fMRI neurofeedback of the right inferior prefrontal cortex. The participants receiving fMRI neurofeedback of this region were compared with an active control group receiving fMRI neurofeedback focused on the left parahippocampal gyrus. The feedback intervention used a video of a rocket that participants were asked to move into space. Eleven participants completed a total of 14 neurofeedback sessions, and the overall sample of participants completed an average of 11 neurofeedback sessions. Both groups demonstrated activations in respective brain regions related to repetitive runs, with a concurrent improvement in ADHD symptoms post neurofeedback. Follow-up assessment at 11 months showed that improvement in ADHD symptoms persisted. However, the group with neurofeedback targeting the inferior prefrontal cortex demonstrated improvement in ADHD symptoms, with no concurrent subsequent neurofeedback and increased activation during an inhibitory fMRI paradigm. This exciting work demonstrates feasibility, but many questions remain because the sample size was small, adherence was variable among participants, patients were not all medication naïve, and the study had a single-blind design (Alegria et al. 2017).

Recent work in adults with MDD illustrates how these modalities might be studied and employed in youth. Young and colleagues (2017) enrolled unmedicated adults ages 18–55 ($n=36$) with MDD for a double-blind fMRI neurofeedback intervention focused on the amygdala and autobiographical memory recall. Participants were randomly assigned to two sessions focused on the amygdala ($n=19$) or the parietal cortex ($n=17$) (as a control group because this regions is not involved in emotional processing). The primary outcome measure was the Montgomery-Åsberg Depression Rating Scale

(MADRS). During the neurofeedback intervention, all participants were instructed to recall positive memories while concurrently trying to increase the hemodynamic response (neuronal activation) in their associated brain region. Each run of neurofeedback had a 40-second rest block, positive memories, and then a backward count from 300. There were eight fMRI blocks per run (resting, baseline with no neurofeedback, practice run, three training runs, a transfer run with no neurofeedback, and a final rest run). Participants in the group targeting the amygdala demonstrated increased hemodynamic activity compared with baseline and the control group. This is noteworthy, because depressed patients are thought to have a blunted amygdalar response to positive stimuli. In the group targeting the amygdala, 12 participants had more than a 50% decrease in MADRS scores as compared with two participants in the control group. Six participants in the active group and 1 in the control group had symptoms that met criteria for remission. Active group participants also demonstrated an increase in positive memories retrieved compared with baseline and the control group. These early findings are encouraging and may provide a framework for work with children and adolescents (Young et al. 2017).

In summary, real-time neurofeedback interventions are an appealing and promising area of work. However, this area is primarily investigational at this stage, and there are many unanswered questions and challenges to interpretation of existing work. Replication of behavioral outcomes in existing studies is difficult to demonstrate. Many study designs do not adequately extricate placebo effects. The durability of behavioral or symptomatic gains is also uncertain. With fMRI studies in particular, there are also considerable financial and pragmatic barriers to consider prior to clinical implementation. Rigorously designed, double-blind studies could help answer many of these questions, provide brain-based treatment options for youth with mood disorders, and catalyze further work focused on the cognitive neuroscience of early life mood disorders (Thibault et al. 2018).

Transcranial Magnetic Stimulation

Noninvasive brain stimulation modalities such as repetitive transcranial magnetic stimulation (rTMS) represent another potential brain-based treatment option for adolescents with mood disorders (Croarkin and Rotenberg 2016; Donaldson et al. 2014; Krishnan et al. 2015). High-frequency rTMS has demonstrated efficacy for MDD in adults and is now widely available clinically (George et al. 2010; McClintock et al. 2018; O'Reardon et al. 2007). The treatment of depression with rTMS involves high-frequency trains of magnetic pulses delivered through the scalp that subsequently increase neuronal excitability within the left dorsolateral prefrontal cortex (DLPFC). Treatment typically involves 10-Hz stimulation over the left DLPFC with five daily sessions per week for 6 weeks. Notably, there are a number of alternative dosing regimens with respect to placement and pulsing of the magnetic coil, intensity of stimulation, frequency of treatments, and duration of treatment (Brunoni et al. 2017). This near-infinite parameter space creates challenges and opportunities for further research. Large multisite studies have demonstrated that 35%–40% of adults with MDD reach remission with the standard, U.S. Food and Drug Administration–cleared dosing of rTMS that delivers 10-Hz treatments to the left DLPFC over 4–6 weeks (Brunoni et al. 2017; McClintock et al. 2018). Common side effects include scalp discomfort, headaches, and musculoskeletal discomfort. One very rare but concerning risk is the induction of a seizure. To date, all induced seizures in the literature in adults and adolescents have been self-limited with no ongoing sequelae. The risk for seizures related to rTMS has been estimated at 0.003% per session in adult patients (McClintock et al. 2018). However, this risk may be different in adolescents (Davis 2014; Donaldson et al. 2014; Geddes 2015; McClintock et al. 2018), though similarly low (Allen et al. 2017; Gilbert et al. 2004; Hong et al. 2015; Oberman et al. 2014).

Experience with adults has provided a framework for work with treatment-resistant depression in adolescents. One encouraging finding is that younger age in adults appears to be associated with likelihood for a favorable response to rTMS treatment (Rostami et al. 2017). Several reviews and ethical commentaries have focused on the prospect of rTMS interventions in children and adolescents (Davis 2014; Donaldson et al. 2014; Geddes 2015). Current studies of adolescents with depression treated with rTMS are plagued with methodological concerns. These studies do not include control groups and are often simple adaptations of adult study designs (Croarkin and Rotenberg 2016).

Open-label studies focused on adolescents with depression have often employed 10-Hz stimulation at intensities of 80%–120% of motor threshold and number of sessions ranging from 1 to 30 (Donaldson et al. 2014). Conversely, one open-label study examining rTMS for Tourette syndrome delivered 1-Hz stimulation to the supplementary motor cortex and monitored depressive symptoms as a secondary outcome with the Child Depression Inventory (Donaldson et al. 2014; Le et al. 2013). Participants demonstrated improvement in depressive symptoms, but as with other studies it was unclear if the symptomatic improvement gains were a direct consequence of the rTMS intervention (Croarkin and Rotenberg 2016; Donaldson et al. 2014). This highlights a substantial challenge in the study of rTMS for depression in adolescents. Sessions of rTMS are typically delivered 5 days per week. This treatment regimen provides a substantial amount of structure and nonspecific factors that clinically are quite helpful but represent confounds for research studies. Most rTMS studies of adolescents with depression have employed rTMS as an adjunctive treatment to pharmacotherapy and psychotherapy (Donaldson et al. 2014). However, early landmark adult studies delivered rTMS as monotherapy (George et al. 2010; O'Reardon et al. 2007). Both the positive and the negative aspects of combining rTMS with medications and/or psychotherapy are poorly understood (Croarkin and Rotenberg 2016; Donaldson et al. 2014; McClintock et al. 2018).

Krishnan and colleagues (2015) have provided the largest systematic review of safety of noninvasive brain stimulation techniques in children and adolescents to date. The authors reviewed 48 studies, including more than 500 children and adolescents ranging from ages 2–17 years. This review included studies of both transcranial magnetic stimulation and transcranial current stimulation, with findings that were somewhat encouraging. In general, side effects associated with rTMS were noted to be mild and transient. Common side effects included headaches, scalp discomfort, twitches, mood changes, fatigue, and tinnitus. However, limitations in interpreting the findings of this review include the fact that adverse event data were rarely collected in a systematic fashion and that most studies report only short-term adverse events (Krishnan et al. 2015). One recent case report of a seizure induced by deep transcranial magnetic stimulation in an adolescent with no prior neurological history illustrates the inherent difficulties and pitfalls in adapting adult protocols to adolescents (Cullen 2017).

In summary, although rTMS may represent a future treatment option for child and adolescent mood disorders, existing literature should be interpreted with caution. A multicenter RCT of 10-Hz rTMS applied to the left DLPFC over 6 weeks for adolescents with depression will be completed in late 2018. This study enrolled more than 100 participants and will be the largest database to date for the examination of the efficacy and safety of rTMS in adolescents with depression in a systematic fashion (Neuronetics 2018). Future work will also examine rTMS in the context of neurodevelopmental considerations and tailored treatments with neurophysiological target engagement strategies.

Electroconvulsive Therapy

In contemporary practice, the use of electroconvulsive therapy (ECT) in children and adolescents with mood disorders and other serious psychiatric disorders has decreased over time. In some locations and time periods, ECT has been a relatively controversial and rare treatment approach. There have been concerns about the potential side effects and unknowns related to this treatment in developing children and adolescents. The advent of modern psychopharmacological approaches, negative portrayals of ECT in the media, and active antipsychiatry groups have likely contributed to this decrease in use. As a result, there have been international attempts to prohibit the use of ECT in children and adolescents (Walter et al. 2011). In a number of areas in the United States, ECT is prohibited or restricted by law (Walter et al. 2011).

In the past two decades experts have made strides to define indications for ECT in children and adolescents and have developed guidelines. For example, the American Academy of Child and Adolescent Psychiatry published a practice parameter for the use of ECT in adolescents in 2004 (Ghaziuddin et al. 2004). Unfortunately, published research on the use of ECT in children and adolescents is rare and of low quality. There are no controlled studies, and large, high-quality epidemiological studies are lacking. Often systematic reviews find that there are limited data available for extraction regarding, for example, diagnosis, side effects, and symptomatic improvement. In general, over the past two to three decades the quality of study has improved somewhat (Walter et al. 2011). One study suggested that adolescents are typically referred for ECT for catatonia or suicidal behavior, whereas adults are referred for nonresponse to pharmacotherapy (Bloch et al. 2008).

Recently, Puffer et al. (2016) reviewed the retrospective treatment of 51 adolescents who received ECT. The authors found that ECT was typically recommended for a primary mood, psychotic, or catatonia disorder. Patients in the sample received a mean (SD) of 9.3 (3.5) treatments with initial bitemporal lead placement 71% of the time. On the basis of retrospective evaluation with a Clinical Global Impression—Improvement (CGI-I) scale, 39 patients (77%) were much or very much improved after treatment. Prolonged seizures were somewhat common but appeared to decrease with age.

Another recent retrospective study examined ECT treatments of 36 patients at one center (Maoz et al. 2017). Adolescent patients received a mean number (SD) of 24 (14.2) treatments. The mean CGI-I at the conclusion of an index course of ECT was 2.47 (1.19). After ECT treatment, 26 patients (72.2%) were much or very much improved based on the CGI-I. Five patients had a response after six sessions. Twenty-one patients improved after 12 sessions. On the basis of correlational statistics, early nonresponse did not necessarily appear to predict a failed ECT course. Mitchell and colleagues (2018) recently examined follow-up evaluation of symptoms, attitudes, perception, and functioning of patients who been treated with ECT prior to the age of 18. At the time of follow-up, 59% of the participants had mild or no depression. Notably, the majority of patients (84%) recalled that ECT had improved their overall illness. Many subjects had ongoing impairments in global functioning, but 83% reported adequate academic performance, and 78% reported mild or no suicidality.

Multiple efforts are under way to optimize the delivery of ECT for maximal efficacy and minimal side effect burden. Magnetic seizure therapy (MST) induces seizures in a manner that may ease cognitive side effects. Early work suggested that MST has efficacy in adult patients with treatment-resistant depression, with limited cognitive side effects (Kosel et al. 2003; Lisanby et al. 2003). Larger studies of adults with depression are currently under way (Sun et al. 2016). There is one published case reported describing the delivery of MST to an 18-year-old with treatment-resistant depression in the context of bipolar II disorder. This adolescent had 18 MST treatments and experienced a full remission of clinical symptoms with minimal signs of cognitive impairments. Specifically, his average score on the Montreal Cognitive Assessment was 29 out of 30 during the course of his MST treatments. His Autobiographical Memory Interview—Short Form score decreased from baseline to posttreatment to 6-month follow-up but remained within the normal range. Notably this young man was able to return to studies at a local university after the completion of his MST course (Noda et al. 2014).

In summary, further systematic study of ECT would be helpful, but unfortunately it is very unlikely that controlled trials will be conducted. On the basis of available literature and practice parameters, indications for ECT in adolescents include severe and persistent mood disorders such as MDD and mania with or without psychotic features. The symptom burden should be severe, globally impairing, or life-threatening. In most circumstances, patients should have failed to respond to two adequate trials of indicated psychopharmacological agents of an adequate dose or duration for adolescents being considered for ECT. Pretreatment evaluations should include at least one second opinion from a psychiatrist who is knowledgeable about ECT and mood disorders in adolescents. Initially, unilateral electrode application to the nondominant hemisphere may be the preferred method with brief or ultra-brief pulses at an adequate dose of electricity. Existing guidelines recommend that ECT be administered on an inpatient basis for adolescents (Ghaziuddin et al. 2004; Walter et al. 2011).

Ketamine

There is currently much excitement over the reported antidepressant effects of intravenously administered ketamine (0.5 mg/kg over 40 minutes) for treatment-refractory MDD and bipolar depression (Nemeroff 2018; Sanacora et al. 2017b). Numerous studies have demonstrated marked, albeit transient, effects (Nemeroff 2018). In most cases, clinical effects attenuate within 1 week after the infusion (Vande Voort et al. 2016). A recent RCT with intravenous ketamine versus midazolam also demonstrated ketamine's potential to impact suicidal severity (Grunebaum et al. 2018). An intranasal enantiomer is currently under clinical development for patients with MDD and suicidality (Canuso et al. 2018). Thought leaders in this area have authored expert consensus reports and critical commentaries addressing a number of concerns regarding the apparent rapid clinical implementation of ketamine nationwide (Nemeroff 2018; Sanacora et al. 2017a, 2017b). In this context it is not unexpected that ketamine would also be pondered as a treatment for adolescents with treatment-refractory mood disorders and severe suicidality. It is likely being used on a clinical, off-label basis for adolescents at present throughout the United States. However, publications and rigorous studies focused on the use of ketamine in children and adolescents with mood disorders are limited (Cullen 2017; Dwyer et al. 2017).

Cullen and colleagues recently conducted a pilot open-label study of six subanesthetic ketamine infusions at a dose of 0.5 mg/kg to target treatment-resistant depression in 11 adolescent participants with treatment-refractory depression (Cullen 2017). Treatment response was predefined as a 50% decrease in Children's Depression Rating Scale—Revised (CDRS-R) score from baseline to the day after the final ketamine infusion. Clinical response was reached in 4 of the 11 participants (37%). However, several participants appeared to have subthreshold improvement. The group mean decrease in CDRS-R score was 39%. Notably, in those who had a full response, the clinical effect appeared to be lasting. No severe side effects or serious adverse events were reported in this study (Cullen 2017).

Dwyer and colleagues (2017) reported on the case presentation of a 16-year-old patient with treatment-refractory major depressive disorder and comorbid ADHD and Crohn's disease who was treated with a course of intravenous ketamine infusions. The patient was considered as being at high risk for suicide and had had five inpatient hospitalizations over 13 months. On presentation, he was treated with lithium, aripiprazole, and mixed amphetamine salts. Notably, ECT was strongly considered and discussed with the patient and his family. Given the concerns about cognitive side effects, the patient and family elected to pursue ketamine treatment. The patient received intravenous infusions of ketamine dosed at 0.5 milligrams per kilogram over 40 minutes. He received three infusions during the first week and weekly treatments thereafter, resulting in a total of seven infusions over the course of the hospitalization. He was evaluated with the MADRS and CDRS-R scale. After his first infusion on day 1, he experienced rapid reduction in depressive symptoms, with improvements in both rating scales, and decreased suicidal ideation. He continued to demonstrate improvement over the next two infusions and maintained the improvement throughout his hospitalization. On day 32 he had an exacerbation in depressive symptoms, which was thought to be related to frustration over placement concerns. This increase in symptoms resolved when his placement resolved. He ultimately had an acute recovery with ketamine. After much thought, his follow-up plan included ongoing ketamine infusions every 3–6 weeks as an outpatient with the expectation that the time interval would be gradually increased as tolerated without recurrence of depressive symptoms. He was maintained on his outpatient psychotropic medications. At the time of the publication of the report, the patient had had four subsequent ketamine treatments spaced 6 weeks apart and had not required further hospitalizations; he was living at home and had returned to school full time (Dwyer et al. 2017).

Other authors have examined the idea of intranasal ketamine for the treatment of a pediatric bipolar "fear of harm" (FOH) phenotype. One open-label study examined 12 youth with treatment-refractory BD with a FOH phenotype (10 males and 2 females) ages 6–19 years who received intranasal ketamine at doses ranging from 30 to 120 mg every 3–7 days as indicated based on adjustments every 3–6 days. The authors reported that the intranasal ketamine appeared to be associated with a reduction in measures of mania, aggression, and fear of harm. Other improvements were observed in mood, anxiety, behavior, and attentional symptoms. Executive functioning and insomnia were reported to improve as well. Side effects reported were generally mild and moderate, and none required medical intervention in any patient or at any dose (Papolos et al. 2013). In a follow-up study from the same group of researchers, 45 patients with a diagnosis of juvenile BD with the described FOH phenotype were examined retrospectively. Patients had a mean (SD) age of 15.9 (6.7) years at their first dosing of ketamine. Almost all patients had some improvement, with symptom reductions in multiple categories. There were 14 acute side effects, including a sense of bilateral warmth in over half the patients. Other symptoms included dizziness, disrupted gait, and nasal burning or stinging. Most of the side effects were rated as brief in duration (<20 minutes). Most of the side effects attenuated with continued treatment. Notably two patients did report the persistent of sensory changes. One patient lost temperature sensations throughout his body. The other patient had numbness in the upper extremities. Neurological evaluation determined that these were not progressive deficits in both cases. The patient and family elected to continue with ketamine treatment because they felt the clinical benefits outweighed the risk of persistent side effects (Papolos et al. 2018).

Both of these reports are limited methodologically, because they are retrospective reviews from a single practice without a placebo control or a prospective study design. The authors highlighted that recall bias is likely an important limitation in both efforts (Papolos et al. 2018).

In summary, intravenous ketamine has demonstrated potential for the treatment of adult MDD and suicidality. At this time, there is a multisite trial examining the efficacy and safety of adjunctive intranasal esketamine (the *S*-enantiomer of ketamine) in adolescents ages 12–17 with acute suicidality (Janssen Research and Development 2018). Given ketamine's long track record as an anesthetic in pediatric practice, it is understandable that clinicians will continue to ponder the utility of this intervention for adolescents with treatment-refractory mood disorders as well. Clinical experience suggests that ketamine is already being used in children and adolescents in an off-label fashion nationwide. Conversely, research studies of ketamine for childhood and adolescent mood disorders are limited. Further systematic study of efficacy and safety is critical to optimize practice and better understand numerous safety concerns.

Emerging Cognitive Training and Remediation Strategies

Research during the past two decades has advanced our understanding of the brain and behavioral alterations underlying pediatric mood disorders. While substantial work still needs to be done in this field, including replication and testing of specificity, studies have begun to translate these brain and behavioral alterations into mechanism-targeted treatments.

One important approach in this effort is *cognitive training*, also known as *cognitive remediation*. Cognitive remediation is based on the idea that behavioral treatments can be used to improve cognitive or emotional processes that are impaired in a psychiatric disorder. To do this, one needs to 1) identify the brain or behavioral impairments associated with the illness, 2) devise a training program to build up the skill that has been shown to be impaired in that illness, and 3) evaluate if the training program works—not only in improving the mechanism but also in reducing symptoms or functional impairment.

Cognitive remediation is not a new, twenty-first-century idea. Rather it dates back to the early to mid-twentieth century, when people sought to improve neurocognitive functioning in soldiers who had sustained head injuries in war. Another example from the mid-twentieth century is Wagner's finding that adults with schizophrenia had reduced cognitive function, including attention and abstraction, that improved with positive reinforcement (Frommann et al. 2011). Cognitive remediation typically involves drill-and-practice learning, whereby a patient repeatedly performs each exercise, in the hope that the once-deficient skill will improve, just as one's biceps muscles might get bigger with a regimen of repeated biceps curls with weights.

Cognitive remediation has several potential advantages over traditional medication and psychotherapy treatments. First, it is personalized. Because the cognitive remediation plan was developed to target brain mechanisms specifically impaired in an illness, the hope is that it will be more effective than more general approaches that do not address these biological mechanisms. Second, it is scalable. A cognitive remediation program could potentially overcome the traditional limitations of access to mental health treatment provided by physicians, psychologists, and other therapists, which is typically limited by the 1:1 ratio of treater to patient in individual treatment, or at best 1:10–12 in group therapy. Instead, it is possible that innumerable patients could simultaneously receive the remediation in multiple venues, from a testing center to their smartphone at home, while having their outcomes—including both performance on the remediation and changes in symptoms—monitored by a single professional. Third, it may be more readily accepted than medications by the public, who are sometimes more apprehensive of taking prescribed medications than "more natural" options.

What is known about cognitive remediation in children with mood disorders? As of the writing of this chapter, there are no published RCTs of cognitive remediation for children or adolescents with MDD, BD, or disruptive mood dysregulation disorder (DMDD). As is common in all aspects of research, we know more about cognitive remediation in adults with psychiatric illness than in children.

In depression, one of the most common cognitive remediation approaches being studied is *attention bias modification training* (ABMT). ABMT is based on data implicating frontotemporal circuit alterations underlying perception of negative stimuli, including threatening, negative, and neutral-valenced stimuli such as faces, in depression and anxiety (Beesdo et al. 2009; Hall et al. 2014; Pine et al. 2004; Schaefer et al. 2006). Given this brain/behavior impairment, ABMT seeks to reverse this attention bias by reducing the tendency of depressed people to respond excessively to negatively valenced stimuli. ABMT for depression might have a child play a computer game in which pairs of face stimuli are simultaneously shown on a screen followed by a star on only one side. The child is told to press a button to indicate which side of the screen the star is on. To train away from negatively valenced stimuli, the game would have the star appear mostly on the side with happy, rather than negative or neutral, faces. When the game is played repeatedly, drill-and-practice learning would help the child reduce his or her bias to negative stimuli as evidenced by faster or more accurate response to stars regardless of what side the negative photo is on.

Cognitive remediation studies of young adults with depression have been carried out. Yang et al. (2015) found that ABMT reduced depressive symptoms compared with both the assessment-only and placebo control conditions among college students both after treatment and at 3-month follow-up. Another study, by Baert et al. (2010), showed that ABMT reduced depression among young adults with mild to moderate depression, but increased depression in those with more severe depression, and among those receiving inpatient psychiatric care versus those receiving outpatient care. This suggests that reductions in depression from cognitive remediation might depend on pretreatment depression severity. Ongoing work is evaluating ABMT in younger adolescents and children with MDD, as well as in youth with anxiety disorders. For example, LeMoult et al. (2018) found that six sessions of positive cognitive bias modification training resulted in more positive interpretation of ambiguous scenarios than neutral bias modification training in a sample of adolescents with MDD (total $N=46$) though it did not appear that these effects generalized.

With respect to BD and DMDD, there are several candidate cognitive and emotional processes for cognitive remediation programs based on data using both behavioral tasks and neuroimaging showing impairments in these children, some of which are group specific, and some others of which are shared. These include 1) recognition and response to positively and negatively valenced emotional faces, 2) response inhibition, and 3) cognitive flexibility. Response to positive and negatively valenced emotional stimuli might be an interesting target for cognitive remediation, potentially with use of a variant of ABMT as discussed above, because fMRI studies suggest that the neural circuitry mediating face processing may be different in BD youth with distinct episodes of euphoric or irritable mood compared with those with chronic nonepisodic irritability consistent with DMDD (Brotman et al. 2010; Rich et al. 2008; Thomas et al. 2012).

Response inhibition is the ability to stop actions that might interfere with goal-directed behavior because those actions are incorrect or inappropriate (Brotman et al. 2010; Mostofsky and Simmonds 2008; Rich et al. 2008; Thomas et al. 2012). Response inhibition is linked to impulsivity and ADHD. Studies suggest that BD youth have reduced striatal error signal during failed motor inhibition versus typically developing control (TDC) youth (Leibenluft et al. 2007). Others have found that BD youth have less efficient neural processes underlying response inhibition, as evidenced by greater DLPFC activity to maintain a performance level similar to that of TDC youth (Singh et al. 2010).

Cognitive flexibility is defined as the ability to adapt one's thinking and behavior in response to changing rewards and punishments (Dickstein et al. 2007, 2015). Cognitive flexibility is relevant to BD because clinical features of BD may reflect specific alterations in how reward inaccurately shapes behavior—namely, hyperhedonia in mania (e.g., excessive involvement in pleasurable activities with high potential for painful consequences) and hypohedonia in depression (e.g., anhedonia) (Dickstein et al. 2004, 2007, 2015). Cognitive flexibility can be studied using reversal learning tasks, whereby participants must use trial-and-error learning to first determine which of two simultaneously presented stimuli are initially rewarded. Then, the stimulus/reward relationship reverses without warning, so that the previously rewarded stimulus is now punished, and vice versa. In turn, cognitive flexibility is indexed by how fast the participant can adapt to the new stimulus/reward relationship. Studies suggest that there may be some specificity of both behavioral and fMRI neural alterations underlying reversal learning and cognitive flexibility between BD and DMDD youth that might be useful as a target of cognitive remediation (Adleman et al. 2011; Dickstein et al. 2010; Leibenluft et al. 2007).

In summary, cognitive remediation holds great potential as a brain mechanism targeted treatment for children and adolescents with mood disorders. Moreover, given potential advantages that would improve access to care, it is worthy of continued study (Dickstein et al. 2015).

Conclusion

Treatment options and the evidence base for child and adolescent mood disorders have expanded over recent decades. First-line treatments include psychotherapeutic and pharmacological approaches outlined in previous chapters. For many families, however, additional treatment options are important considerations, because there may be interest in preventative approaches, nontraditional treatments, and options for treatment-resistant mood disorders. Research on exercise, sleep hygiene, nutraceuticals, real-time neurofeedback, transcranial magnetic stimulation, ECT, ketamine, and cognitive remediation is evolving to meet these needs.

Clinical Pearls

- Preventive, nontraditional, emerging, and investigational treatments may be important options for select child and adolescent patients with mood disorders.

- Exercise, sleep hygiene, and stable schedules are important lifestyle interventions for any child or adolescent with a mood disorder both in terms of prevention and coupled with standard psychotherapeutic and pharmacological treatments.

- Although there is much interest in nutraceutical approaches such as omega-3 fatty acids in the treatment of mood disorders, there are few data to support the effectiveness of these approaches. Further research may clarify the role of these agents, and empathic engagement with families about their interest and use of these agents is important for ongoing treatment planning.

- Real-time neurofeedback with electroencephalography and other neuroimaging modalities is an exciting area of research for mood disorders. These modalities have some availability in current clinical practice, but there are many unanswered questions with respect to efficacy and optimal dosing.

- Ketamine and transcranial magnetic stimulation are investigational treatments for treatment-refractory mood disorders. Although both treatments are accessible clinically, systematic data on safety and effectiveness in children and adolescents are lacking.

- Electroconvulsive therapy has been studied retrospectively as an intervention for adolescents with treatment-refractory mood disorders. Based on available data, response and remission rates are likely similar to those in adults. However, large systematic studies and clinical trial data are lacking. Typically, this treatment is initiated during an inpatient hospitalization.

- Cognitive remediation approaches for child and adolescent mood disorders have great promise. Further study is needed to understand and refine these approaches prior to widespread clinical implementation.

References

Achenbach TM, Rescorla LA: Manual for the ASEBA School-Age Forms and Profiles: An Integrated System of Multi-Informant Assessment. Burlington, University of Vermont, Research Center for Children, Youth, and Families, 2001

Adleman NE, Kayser R, Dickstein D, et al: Neural correlates of reversal learning in severe mood dysregulation and pediatric bipolar disorder. J Am Acad Child Adolesc Psychiatry 50(11):1173.e2–1185.e2, 2011 22024005

Alegria AA, Wulff M, Brinson H, et al: Real-time fMRI neurofeedback in adolescents with attention deficit hyperactivity disorder. Hum Brain Mapp 38(6):3190–3209, 2017 28342214

Allen CH, Kluger BM, Buard I: Safety of transcranial magnetic stimulation in children: a systematic review of the literature. Pediatr Neurol 68:3–17, 2017 28216033

Ash T, Bowling A, Davison K, Garcia J: Physical activity interventions for children with social, emotional, and behavioral disabilities—a systematic review. J Dev Behav Pediatr 38(6):431–445, 2017 28671892

Baert S, De Raedt R, Schacht R, et al: Attentional bias training in depression: therapeutic effects depend on depression severity. J Behav Ther Exp Psychiatry 41(3):265–274, 2010 20227062

Baum KT, Desai A, Field J, et al: Sleep restriction worsens mood and emotion regulation in adolescents. J Child Psychol Psychiatry 55(2):180–190, 2014 24889207

Beebe DW, Difrancesco MW, Tlustos SJ, et al: Preliminary fMRI findings in experimentally sleep-restricted adolescents engaged in a working memory task. Behav Brain Funct 5:9, 2009 19228430

Beesdo K, Lau JY, Guyer AE, et al: Common and distinct amygdala-function perturbations in depressed vs anxious adolescents. Arch Gen Psychiatry 66(3):275–285, 2009 19255377

Berger ME, Smesny S, Kim SW, et al: Omega-6 to omega-3 polyunsaturated fatty acid ratio and subsequent mood disorders in young people with at-risk mental states: a 7-year longitudinal study. Transl Psychiatry 7(8):e1220, 2017 28850110

Birmaher B, Brent D, Bernet W, et al; AACAP Work Group on Quality Issues: Practice parameter for the assessment and treatment of children and adolescents with depressive disorders. J Am Acad Child Adolesc Psychiatry 46(11):1503–1526, 2007 18049300

Bloch Y, Sobol D, Levkovitz Y, et al: Reasons for referral for electroconvulsive therapy: a comparison between adolescents and adults. Australas Psychiatry 16(3):191–194, 2008 18568625

Brotman MA, Rich BA, Guyer AE, et al: Amygdala activation during emotion processing of neutral faces in children with severe mood dysregulation versus ADHD or bipolar disorder. Am J Psychiatry 167(1):61–69, 2010 19917597

Brunoni AR, Chaimani A, Moffa AH, et al: Repetitive transcranial magnetic stimulation for the acute treatment of major depressive episodes: a systematic review with network meta-analysis. JAMA Psychiatry 74(2):143–152, 2017 28030740

Butterweck V: Mechanism of action of St John's wort in depression: what is known? CNS Drugs 17(8):539–562, 2003 12775192

Canuso CM, Singh JB, Fedgchin M, et al: Efficacy and safety of intranasal esketamine for the rapid reduction of symptoms of depression and suicidality in patients at imminent risk for suicide: results of a double-blind, randomized, placebo-controlled study. Am J Psychiatry 175(7):620–630, 2018 29656663

Coryell WH, Langbehn DR, Norris AW, et al: Polyunsaturated fatty acid composition and childhood adversity: independent correlates of depressive symptom persistence. Psychiatry Res 256:305–311, 2017 28666200

Croarkin PE, Rotenberg A: Pediatric neuromodulation comes of age. J Child Adolesc Psychopharmacol 26(7):578–581, 2016 27604043

Cullen KR: Ketamine for adolescent treatment-resistant depression. J Am Acad Child Adolesc Psychiatry 56(10S):S345, 2017

Davis NJ: Transcranial stimulation of the developing brain: a plea for extreme caution. Front Hum Neurosci 8:600, 2014 25140146

Dennison MJ, Rosen ML, Sambrook KA, et al: Differential associations of distinct forms of childhood adversity with neurobehavioral measures of reward processing: a developmental pathway to depression. Child Dev Dec 21, 2017 [Epub ahead of print] 29266223

Dickstein DP, Treland JE, Snow J, et al: Neuropsychological performance in pediatric bipolar disorder. Biol Psychiatry 55(1):32–39, 2004 14706422

Dickstein DP, Nelson EE, McClure EB, et al: Cognitive flexibility in phenotypes of pediatric bipolar disorder. J Am Acad Child Adolesc Psychiatry 46(3):341–355, 2007 17314720

Dickstein DP, Finger EC, Skup M, et al: Altered neural function in pediatric bipolar disorder during reversal learning. Bipolar Disord 12(7):707–719, 2010 21040288

Dickstein DP, Cushman GK, Kim KL, et al: Cognitive remediation: potential novel brain-based treatment for bipolar disorder in children and adolescents. CNS Spectr 20(4):382–390, 2015 26135596

Donaldson AE, Gordon MS, Melvin GA, et al: Addressing the needs of adolescents with treatment resistant depressive disorders: a systematic review of rTMS. Brain Stimul 7(1):7–12, 2014 24527502

Dwyer JB, Beyer C, Wilkinson ST, et al: Ketamine as a treatment for adolescent depression: a case report. J Am Acad Child Adolesc Psychiatry 56(4):352–354, 2017 28335880

Ekor M: The growing use of herbal medicines: issues relating to adverse reactions and challenges in monitoring safety. Front Pharmacol 4:177, 2014 24454289

Fallone G, Acebo C, Arndt JT, et al: Effects of acute sleep restriction on behavior, sustained attention, and response inhibition in children. Percept Mot Skills 93(1):213–229, 2001 11693688

Frank E: Treating Bipolar Disorder: A Clinician's Guide to Interpersonal and Social Rhythm Therapy. New York, Guilford, 2005

Fristad MA, Vesco AT, Young AS, et al: Pilot randomized controlled trial of omega-3 and individual-family psychoeducational psychotherapy for children and adolescents with depression. J Clin Child Adolesc Psychol 7:1–14, 2016 27819485

Frommann I, Pukrop R, Brinkmeyer J, et al: Neuropsychological profiles in different at-risk states of psychosis: executive control impairment in the early—and additional memory dysfunction in the late—prodromal state. Schizophr Bull 37(4):861–873, 2011 20053865

Geddes L: Brain stimulation in children spurs hope—and concern. Nature 525(7570):436–437, 2015 26399806

Geller B, Zimerman B, Williams M, et al: DSM-IV mania symptoms in a prepubertal and early adolescent bipolar disorder phenotype compared to attention-deficit hyperactive and normal controls. J Child Adolesc Psychopharmacol 12(1):11–25, 2002 12014591

George MS, Lisanby SH, Avery D, et al: Daily left prefrontal transcranial magnetic stimulation therapy for major depressive disorder: a sham-controlled randomized trial. Arch Gen Psychiatry 67(5):507–516, 2010 20439832

Gewirtz AH, Lee SS, August GJ, He Y: Does giving parents their choice of interventions for child behavior problems improve child outcomes? Prev Sci January 20, 2018 [Epub ahead of print] 29352401

Ghaziuddin N, Kutcher SP, Knapp P, et al; Work Group on Quality Issues; AACAP: Practice parameter for use of electroconvulsive therapy with adolescents. J Am Acad Child Adolesc Psychiatry 43(12):1521–1539, 2004 15564821

Gilbert DL, Garvey MA, Bansal AS, et al: Should transcranial magnetic stimulation research in children be considered minimal risk? Clin Neurophysiol 115(8):1730–1739, 2004 15261851

Gill M, Koleilat M, Whaley SE: The impact of food insecurity on the home emotional environment among low-income mothers of young children. Matern Child Health J 22(8):1146–1153, 2018 29445981

Goldstein AN, Walker MP: The role of sleep in emotional brain function. Annu Rev Clin Psychol 10:679–708, 2014 24499013

Goldstein TR, Merranko J, Krantz M, et al: Early intervention for adolescents at-risk for bipolar disorder: A pilot randomized trial of Interpersonal and Social Rhythm Therapy (IPSRT). J Affect Disord 235:348–356, 2018 29665518

Gracious BL, Chirieac MC, Costescu S, et al: Randomized, placebo-controlled trial of flax oil in pediatric bipolar disorder. Bipolar Disord 12(2):142–154, 2010 20402707

Grosso G, Galvano F, Marventano S, et al: Omega-3 fatty acids and depression: scientific evidence and biological mechanisms. Oxid Med Cell Longev 2014:313570, 2014 24757497

Grunebaum MF, Galfalvy HC, Choo TH, et al: Ketamine for rapid reduction of suicidal thoughts in major depression: a midazolam-controlled randomized clinical trial. Am J Psychiatry 175(4):327–335, 2018 29202655

Hall LM, Klimes-Dougan B, Hunt RH, et al: An fMRI study of emotional face processing in adolescent major depression. J Affect Disord 168:44–50, 2014 25036008

Hong YH, Wu SW, Pedapati EV, et al: Safety and tolerability of theta burst stimulation vs. single and paired pulse transcranial magnetic stimulation: a comparative study of 165 pediatric subjects. Front Hum Neurosci 9:29, 2015 25698958

Janssen Research and Development: Study to evaluate the efficacy and safety of 3 fixed doses of intranasal esketamine in addition to comprehensive standard of care for the rapid reduction of the symptoms of major depressive disorder, including suicidal ideation, in pediatric participants assessed to be at imminent risk for suicide. NCT03185819. August 27, 2018. Available at: https://clinicaltrials.gov/ct2/show/NCT03185819. Accessed September 18, 2018.

Jorm AF, Allen NB, O'Donnell CP, et al: Effectiveness of complementary and self-help treatments for depression in children and adolescents. Med J Aust 185(7):368–372, 2006 17014404

Killgore WD: Effects of sleep deprivation on cognition. Prog Brain Res 185:105–129, 2010 21075236

Kosel M, Frick C, Lisanby SH, et al: Magnetic seizure therapy improves mood in refractory major depression. Neuropsychopharmacology 28(11):2045–2048, 2003 12942146

Kovacs M: The Children's Depression Inventory Manual. Toronto, ON, Canada, Multi-Health Systems, 1992

Krishnan C, Santos L, Peterson MD, et al: Safety of noninvasive brain stimulation in children and adolescents. Brain Stimul 8(1):76–87, 2015 25499471

Kvam S, Kleppe CL, Nordhus IH, et al: Exercise as a treatment for depression: a meta-analysis. J Affect Disord 202:67–86, 2016 27253219

Le K, Liu L, Sun M, et al: Transcranial magnetic stimulation at 1 Hertz improves clinical symptoms in children with Tourette syndrome for at least 6 months. J Clin Neurosci 20(2):257–262, 2013 23238046

Leibenluft E, Rich BA, Vinton DT, et al: Neural circuitry engaged during unsuccessful motor inhibition in pediatric bipolar disorder. Am J Psychiatry 164(1):52–60, 2007 17202544

LeMoult J, Colich N, Joormann J, et al: Interpretation bias training in depressed adolescents: near- and far-transfer effects. J Abnorm Child Psychol 46(1):159–167, 2018 28299526

Lisanby SH, Luber B, Schlaepfer TE, et al: Safety and feasibility of magnetic seizure therapy (MST) in major depression: randomized within-subject comparison with electroconvulsive therapy. Neuropsychopharmacology 28(10):1852–1865, 2003 12865903

Lubans D, Richards J, Hillman C, et al: Physical activity for cognitive and mental health in youth: a systematic review of mechanisms. Pediatrics 138(3):e20161642, 2016 27542849

Ma N, Dinges DF, Basner M, et al: How acute total sleep loss affects the attending brain: a meta-analysis of neuroimaging studies. Sleep 38(2):233–240, 2015 25409102

Maoz H, Nitzan U, Goldwyn Y, et al: When can we predict the outcome of an electroconvulsive therapy course in adolescents? A retrospective study. J ECT 34(2):104–107, 2017 29219862

Martin A, Booth JN, Laird Y, et al: Physical activity, diet and other behavioural interventions for improving cognition and school achievement in children and adolescents with obesity or overweight. Cochrane Database Syst Rev 3:CD009728, 2018 29499084

McClellan J, Kowatch R, Findling RL; Work Group on Quality Issues: Practice parameter for the assessment and treatment of children and adolescents with bipolar disorder. J Am Acad Child Adolesc Psychiatry 46(1):107–125, 2007 17195735

McClintock SM, Reti IM, Carpenter LL, et al; National Network of Depression Centers rTMS Task Group; American Psychiatric Association Council on Research Task Force on Novel Biomarkers and Treatments: Consensus recommendations for the clinical application of repetitive transcranial magnetic stimulation (rTMS) in the treatment of depression. J Clin Psychiatry 79(1):16cs10905, 2018 28541649

Mischoulon D, Fava M: Role of S-adenosyl-L-methionine in the treatment of depression: a review of the evidence. Am J Clin Nutr 76(5):1158S–1161S, 2002 12420702

Mitchell S, Hassan E, Ghaziuddin N: A follow-up study of electroconvulsive therapy in children and adolescents. J ECT 34(1):40–44, 2018 28937548

Mostofsky SH, Simmonds DJ: Response inhibition and response selection: two sides of the same coin. J Cogn Neurosci 20(5):751–761, 2008 18201122

Nemeroff CB: Ketamine: quo vadis? Am J Psychiatry 175(4):297–299, 2018 29606064

Neuronetics: Safety and effectiveness of NeuroStar transcranial magnetic stimulation (TMS) therapy in depressed adolescents. NCT02586688. February 2, 2018. Available at: https://clinicaltrials.gov/ct2/show/NCT02586688. Accessed September 18, 2018.

Noda Y, Daskalakis ZJ, Downar J, et al: Magnetic seizure therapy in an adolescent with refractory bipolar depression: a case report. Neuropsychiatr Dis Treat 10:2049–2055, 2014 25382978

Oberman LM, Pascual-Leone A, Rotenberg A: Modulation of corticospinal excitability by transcranial magnetic stimulation in children and adolescents with autism spectrum disorder. Front Hum Neurosci 8:627, 2014 25165441

O'Reardon JP, Solvason HB, Janicak PG, et al: Efficacy and safety of transcranial magnetic stimulation in the acute treatment of major depression: a multisite randomized controlled trial. Biol Psychiatry 62(11):1208–1216, 2007 17573044

Papolos DF, Teicher MH, Faedda GL, et al: Clinical experience using intranasal ketamine in the treatment of pediatric bipolar disorder/fear of harm phenotype. J Affect Disord 147(1–3):431–436, 2013 23200737

Papolos D, Frei M, Rossignol D, et al: Clinical experience using intranasal ketamine in the longitudinal treatment of juvenile bipolar disorder with fear of harm phenotype. J Affect Disord 225:545–551, 2018 28866299

Pine DS, Lissek S, Klein RG, et al: Face-memory and emotion: associations with major depression in children and adolescents. J Child Psychol Psychiatry 45(7):1199–1208, 2004 15335340

Pompili M, Longo L, Dominici G, et al: Polyunsaturated fatty acids and suicide risk in mood disorders: a systematic review. Prog Neuropsychopharmacol Biol Psychiatry 74:43–56, 2017 27940200

Potkin KT, Bunney WE Jr: Sleep improves memory: the effect of sleep on long term memory in early adolescence. PLoS One 7(8):e42191, 2012 22879917

Puffer CC, Wall CA, Huxsahl JE, et al: A 20-year practice review of electroconvulsive therapy for adolescents. J Child Adolesc Psychopharmacol 26(7):632–636, 2016 26784386

Rich BA, Grimley ME, Schmajuk M, et al: Face emotion labeling deficits in children with bipolar disorder and severe mood dysregulation. Dev Psychopathol 20(2):529–546, 2008 18423093

Rostami R, Kazemi R, Nitsche MA, et al: Clinical and demographic predictors of response to rTMS treatment in unipolar and bipolar depressive disorders. Clin Neurophysiol 128(10):1961–1970, 2017 28829979

Sanacora G, Frye MA, McDonald W, et al; American Psychiatric Association (APA) Council of Research Task Force on Novel Biomarkers and Treatments: a consensus statement on the use of ketamine in the treatment of mood disorders. JAMA Psychiatry 74(4):399–405, 2017a 28249076

Sanacora G, Heimer H, Hartman D, et al: Balancing the promise and risks of ketamine treatment for mood disorders. Neuropsychopharmacology 42(6):1179–1181, 2017b 27640324

Schaefer HS, Putnam KM, Benca RM, et al: Event-related functional magnetic resonance imaging measures of neural activity to positive social stimuli in pre- and post-treatment depression. Biol Psychiatry 60(9):974–986, 2006 16780808

Simkin DR, Thatcher RW, Lubar J: Quantitative EEG and neurofeedback in children and adolescents: anxiety disorders, depressive disorders, comorbid addiction and attention-deficit/hyperactivity disorder, and brain injury. Child Adolesc Psychiatr Clin N Am 23(3):427–464, 2014 24975621

Singh MK, Chang KD, Mazaika P, et al: Neural correlates of response inhibition in pediatric bipolar disorder. J Child Adolesc Psychopharmacol 20(1):15–24, 2010 20166792

Sun Y, Farzan F, Mulsant BH, et al: Indicators for remission of suicidal ideation following magnetic seizure therapy in patients with treatment-resistant depression. JAMA Psychiatry 73(4):337–345, 2016 26981889

Swartz HA, Levenson JC, Frank E: Psychotherapy for bipolar II disorder: the role of interpersonal and social rhythm therapy. Prof Psychol Res Pr 43(2):145–153, 2012 26612968

Talbot LS, McGlinchey EL, Kaplan KA, et al: Sleep deprivation in adolescents and adults: changes in affect. Emotion 10(6):831–841, 2010 21058849

Tarokh L, Saletin JM, Carskadon MA: Sleep in adolescence: physiology, cognition and mental health. Neurosci Biobehav Rev 70:182–188, 2016 27531236

Thibault RT, MacPherson A, Lifshitz M, et al: Neurofeedback with fMRI: a critical systematic review. Neuroimage 172:786–807, 2018 29288868

Thomas LA, Brotman MA, Muhrer EJ, et al: Parametric modulation of neural activity by emotion in youth with bipolar disorder, youth with severe mood dysregulation, and healthy volunteers. Arch Gen Psychiatry 69(12):1257–1266, 2012 23026912

Vande Voort JL, Morgan RJ, Kung S, et al: Continuation phase intravenous ketamine in adults with treatment-resistant depression. J Affect Disord 206:300–304, 2016 27656788

Vesco AT, Young AS, Arnold LE, et al: Omega-3 supplementation associated with improved parent-rated executive function in youth with mood disorders: secondary analyses of the omega 3 and therapy (OATS) trials. J Child Psychol Psychiatry 59(6):628–636, 2018 29063592

Walter G, Rey JM, Ghaziuddin N, Loo C: Electroconvulsive therapy, transcranial magnetic stimulation, and vagus nerve stimulation, in Pediatric Psychopharmacology, 2nd Edition. Edited by Martin A, Scahill L, Kratochvil CJ. New York, Oxford, 2011, pp 363–373

Wehry AM, Ramsey L, Dulemba SE, et al: Pharmacogenomic testing in child and adolescent psychiatry: an evidence-based review. Curr Probl Pediatr Adolesc Health Care 48(2):40–49, 2018 29325731

Wheaton AG, Olsen EO, Miller GF, et al: Sleep Duration and Injury-Related Risk Behaviors Among High School Students—United States, 2007–2013. MMWR Morb Mortal Wkly Rep 65(13):337–341, 2016 27054407

Yang CK, Kim JK, Patel SR, et al: Age-related changes in sleep/wake patterns among Korean teenagers. Pediatrics 115(1, suppl):250–256, 2005 15866859

Yang W, Ding Z, Dai T, et al: Attention bias modification training in individuals with depressive symptoms: a randomized controlled trial. J Behav Ther Exp Psychiatry 49 (Pt A):101–111, 2015 25245928

Young KD, Zotev V, Phillips R, et al: Real-time FMRI neurofeedback training of amygdala activity in patients with major depressive disorder. PLoS One 9(2):e88785, 2014 24523939

Young KD, Siegle GJ, Zotev V, et al: Randomized clinical trial of real-time fMRI amygdala neurofeedback for major depressive disorder: effects on symptoms and autobiographical memory recall. Am J Psychiatry 174(8):748–755, 2017 28407727

Young RC, Biggs JT, Ziegler VE, et al: A rating scale for mania: reliability, validity and sensitivity. Br J Psychiatry 133:429–435, 1978 728692

Part 3
Appendixes
RESOURCES AND READINGS AND QUICK REFERENCE FACTS

Appendix A

Resources and Readings

Manpreet Kaur Singh, M.D., M.S.

This appendix provides a quick reference for useful resources and relevant readings for information about pediatric-onset mood disorders, to support the clinician's task of providing psychoeducation and bibliotherapy resources to patients and families.

Nationwide and Online Resources

- American Academy of Child and Adolescent Psychiatry: https://www.aacap.org
- Parents Helping Parents: http://www.phponline.org
- American Foundation for Suicide Prevention: https://afsp.org
- Child and Adolescent Bipolar Foundation: (847) 492-8519
- NAMI: National Alliance on Mental Illness: (800) 950-6264; https://www.nami.org
- Depression and Bipolar Support Alliance: (800) 826-3632
- Mental Health America: (703) 684-7722; http://www.mentalhealthamerica.net
- The Balanced Mind Foundation: (847) 492-8510
- Juvenile Bipolar Research Foundation: https://www.jbrf.org

- Wrightslaw: http://www.wrightslaw.com (for information regarding special education)
- National Dissemination Center for Children with Disabilities: https://www.parentcenterhub.org/nichcy-gone/
- American Psychiatric Association's Healthy Minds (website for teens about mental health)
- The Ryan Licht Sang Bipolar Foundation: http://www.ryanlichtsangbipolarfoundation.org (Dedicated to fostering awareness, understanding and research for child and adolescent bipolar disorder. The Foundation is on a "Quest For The Test™" to find an empirical test for bipolar disorder so that early detection and intervention become a reality.)

Book and Journal Resources

Readings for Clinicians

Cheung AH, Zuckerbrot RA, Jensen PS, et al; GLAD-PC Steering Group: Guidelines for Adolescent Depression in Primary Care (GLAD-PC), Part II: treatment and ongoing management. Pediatrics 141(3), pii: e20174082, 2018. Available at: http://pediatrics.aappublications.org/content/141/3/e20174082.

Findling RL, Kowatch RA, Post RM: Pediatric Bipolar Disorder: A Handbook for Clinicians. London, Martin Dunitz, 2003

Fristad MA, Goldberg Arnold JS, Leffler J: Psychotherapy for Children With Bipolar and Depressive Disorders. New York, Guilford, 2011

Geller B, Delbello MP (eds): Bipolar Disorder in Childhood and Early Adolescence. New York, Guilford, 2003

McClellan J, Kowatch R, Findling RL; Work Group on Quality Issues: Practice parameter for the assessment and treatment of children and adolescents with bipolar disorder. J Am Child Adolesc Psychiatry 46(1):107–205, 2007. Available at: https://www.jaacap.org/article/S0890-8567(09)61968-7/fulltext. (American Academy of Child and Adolescent Psychiatry practice parameter)

Zuckerbrot RA, Cheung A, Jensen PS, et al; GLAD-PC Steering Group: Guidelines for Adolescent Depression in Primary Care (GLAD-PC), Part I: practice preparation, identification, assessment, and initial management. Pediatrics 141(3), pii: e20174081, 2018. Available at: http://pediatrics.aappublications.org/content/141/3/e20174081.long.

Readings for Patients and Families

Anglada T, Hakala SM: The Childhood Bipolar Disorder Answer Book: Practical Answers to the Top 300 Questions Parents Ask. Naperville, IL, Sourcebooks, 2008

Biegel G: The Stress Reduction Workbook for Teens: Mindfulness Skills to Help You Deal With Stress, 2nd Edition. Oakland, CA, New Harbinger, 2017

Biglan A: The Nurture Effect: How the Science of Human Behavior Can Improve Our Lives and Our World. Oakland, CA, New Harbinger, 2015

Birmaher B: New Hope for Children and Teens With Bipolar Disorder. New York, Three Rivers Press, 2004

Hinshaw SP: Another Kind of Madness: A Journey Through the Stigma and Hope of Mental Illness. New York, St Martin's Press, 2017

Jamison KL: An Unquiet Mind: A Memoir of Moods and Madness. New York, Knopf, 1995

Koplewicz HS: More Than Moody: Recognizing and Treating Adolescent Depression. New York, Berkley Publishing Group/Penguin, 2002

Lederman J, Fink C: The Ups and Downs of Raising a Bipolar Child: A Survival Guide for Parents. New York, Fireside, 2003

Miklowitz DJ, George EL: The Bipolar Teen: What You Can Do to Help Your Child and Your Family. New York, Guilford, 2008

Mondemore FM, Kelly P: Adolescent Depression: A Guide for Parents, 2nd Edition. Baltimore, MD, Johns Hopkins University Press, 2015

Papolos D, Papolos J: The Bipolar Child: The Definitive and Reassuring Guide to Childhood's Most Misunderstood Disorder, 3rd Edition. New York, Crown Archetype, 2006

Pavuluri M: What Works for Bipolar Kids: Help and Hope for Parents. New York, Guilford, 2008

Appendix B

Quick Reference Facts for the Treatment of Pediatric Mood Disorders

Manpreet Kaur Singh, M.D., M.S.

This appendix provides a quick and easy reference of facts about resilience-building interventions and medications commonly used in the treatment of pediatric mood disorders, to complement the more detailed information provided in this handbook.

General Principles About Promoting Resilience to Optimize Outcome

- Know your patient's symptoms and triggers.
- Promote a healthy diet, physical exercise, and regular sleep.
- Teach patients to train their brains using techniques such as mindfulness.
- Have patients develop a plan to manage stress.
- Continue preventive treatment for at least 2 years.
- Remember that combined medication(s) and psychotherapy and resilience-building strategies are often necessary.
- See Tables 1 through 3 below for a summary of the evidence base for some key resilience-building strategies.

TABLE 1. Nutritional interventions for youths with mood disorders

Study	Sample population and size	Intervention	Design	Outcome
Fristad et al. 2016	72 youth (7–17 years) with major depressive disorder (MDD), dysthymia, or depression not otherwise specified (NOS)	Omega-3 fatty acids (Ω3), individual-family psychoeducational psychotherapy (IF-PEP): Ω3, IF-PEP + placebo, Ω3+IF-PEP, or placebo	12-week 2×2 double-masked randomized controlled trial (RCT)	74% fidelity to IF-PEP; 77% remission to Ω3+IF-PEP. Youth with fewer social stressors responded better to Ω3 and combination vs. placebo; youth with maternal depression responded better to IF-PEP than did those without.
Young et al. 2016	72 youth (7–17 years) with MDD, dysthymia, or depression NOS	Ω3, IF-PEP+placebo, Ω3+IF-PEP, or placebo	12-week 2×2 double-masked RCT	Ω3+IF-PEP combined saw greater behavioral improvement and trajectories vs. placebo.
Fristad et al. 2015	23 youth (7–14 years) with bipolar disorder (BD) NOS and cyclothymia	Ω3, IF-PEP, Ω3 vs. placebo and IF-PEP vs. active monitoring (AM)	12-week 2×2 RCT: Ω3+IF-PEP, Ω3+AM, placebo+IF-PEP, placebo+AM	83% completed the study; side effects were uncommon and mild. Improved depressive symptoms with combined treatment vs. placebo; effect of Ω3 on depression was medium (Cohen's $d=0.48$).
Wozniak et al. 2015	24 children (5–12 years) with bipolar spectrum (including BD I, BD II, and BD NOS)	Inositol+placebo, Ω3+placebo, and Ω3+inositol	12-week double-blind, placebo-controlled RCT	54% completed the study. Combined treatment arm improved mania and depression.

Takeaway point: Combining nutraceuticals with psychotherapy may lead to better treatment outcomes.

TABLE 2. Evidence for sleep interventions in youths with mood disorders

Study	Sample population and size	Intervention	Design	Outcome
Blake et al. 2016	140 youth (12–17 years) with high levels of anxiety and sleeping difficulties but without past or current depressive disorder	Sleep improvement intervention or an active control ("study skills"); both 90-minute cognitive-behavioral and mindfulness-based group sessions over 7 weeks	7-week randomized controlled trial (RCT)	Sleep intervention showed greater improvements in subjective sleep quality, sleep-onset latency, daytime sleepiness, and anxiety (small effect) vs. control.
Hall et al. 2015	235 families of 6- to 8-month-old infants	Two-hour group teaching sessions and four support calls over 2 weeks; families were randomly allocated to intervention ($n=117$) or to control teaching sessions ($n=118$) where parents received instruction on infant safety	RCT with outcomes at baseline and at 6 weeks	Intervention showed improved baseline-adjusted parental depression, fatigue, sleep quality, and sleep cognitions; intervention also improved caregivers' assessments of infant sleep problem severity.
Hiscock et al. 2015	244 children (5–12 years) with attention-deficit/hyperactivity disorder (ADHD), most taking stimulants	Sleep hygiene practices and standardized behavioral strategies during two fortnightly consultations and a follow-up telephone call; children in the control group received usual clinical care	RCT	Intervention vs. control families reported a greater decrease in ADHD symptoms at 3 and 6 months; children's sleep, behavior, quality of life, and functioning also improved, with most benefits sustained to 6 months postintervention.

Takeaway points:
1. Treating sleep improves anxiety and ADHD symptoms.
2. If parents sleep, maybe kids can too!

TABLE 3.   Recent early-intervention randomized controlled trials to prevent depression progression in youths

Study	Sample population and size	Intervention	Design	Outcome
Schleider and Weisz 2016	96 adolescents (12–15 years) with or at risk for internalizing problems	Single-session 30-minute computer-guided mind-set intervention teaching growth personality mind-sets (the belief that personality is malleable) vs. supportive therapy control	Randomized controlled trial (RCT)	Adolescents' perceived control was strengthened; associated with increases in growth mind-sets, and linked with faster stress recovery.
Gladstone et al. 2015	400 adolescents and their parents for Competent Adulthood Transition with Cognitive Behavioral Humanistic and Interpersonal Training (CATCH-IT)	A primary care Internet-based depression prevention intervention to evaluate a self-guided, online approach to depression prevention (CATCH-IT) vs. a general health education Internet intervention	RCT	Pending.
Zatzick et al. 2014	120 adolescents (12–18 years) presenting to acute care medical settings after traumatic physical injury	Stepped collaborative care intervention targeting violence risk behaviors, alcohol and drug use, and posttraumatic stress disorder and depressive symptoms	RCT; adolescents assessed at baseline, 2, 5, and 12 months after injury	>95% retention; intervention youth had reduced weapon carrying vs. control subjects at 1 year after injury.

TABLE 3.	Recent early-intervention randomized controlled trials to prevent depression progression in youths *(continued)*		
Study	**Sample population and size**	**Intervention**	**Design**	**Outcome**
Carta et al. 2013	371 low-income mothers and their 3.5- to 5.5-year-old children	Planned Activities Training (PAT) vs. a cellular phone–enhanced version (CPAT) of the intervention; greater use of parenting strategies after treatment and at 6 months posttreatment compared with a wait-list control (WLC)	RCT of PAT vs. CPAT vs. WLC; assessed at pretest, postintervention, and 6 months postintervention	PAT and CPAT showed more frequent use of parenting strategies and more responsive parenting than WLC group; CPAT showed greater reductions in depression and stress; changes in parenting, depression, and stress predicted positive child behaviors.
Grupp-Phelan et al. 2012	204 families of adolescents presenting to the emergency department (ED) and screened for suicide-related risk factors	Short motivational interview, barrier reduction, outpatient appointment established, and reminders before scheduled appointment; vs. standard referral (telephone number for a mental health provider)	RCT: screen acceptability and mental health care linkage, change in depression 60 days after ED	Intervention group was more likely to attend a mental health appointment during follow-up.

Takeaway point: Using technology may increase engagement and improve outcome.

General Principles About Medications

- When using medications to treat mood disorders in children and adolescents, start at low doses and titrate slowly until an effective dose is reached. Weight-based dosing and gradual titration may help limit side effects, especially in young children.
- Use measurement-based care tools such as symptom severity clinical and self-report rating scales during regular follow-ups to objectively determine response.
- Manage co-occurring conditions but minimize polypharmacy, because youth are at high risk for side effects and drug-drug interactions.
- Keep in mind that offspring of parents with depression and bipolar disorder may be at high risk for developing mood disorders themselves. Prevention and early intervention are key in addressing emerging mood disorders in these high-risk groups.
- Remember that most common side effects involve the central nervous and gastrointestinal systems.

Specific Drug Class Facts

Antidepressants

U.S. Food and Drug Administration (FDA)–approved treatments for unipolar depression in youth are summarized in Figure 1.

- See Table 4 below for a summary of medications used in pediatric unipolar depression, including efficacy study results and level of evidence.
- Before starting antidepressant medications in youth, screen for bipolar disorder in the patient and his or her family.
- See Tables 5 and 6 for a summary of common side effects of antidepressants.

Acute Depression		Longer-Term	
Year	**Drug**	**Year**	**Drug**
2002	Fluoxetine (7–17 years)	None	
2009	Escitalopram (12–19 years)		

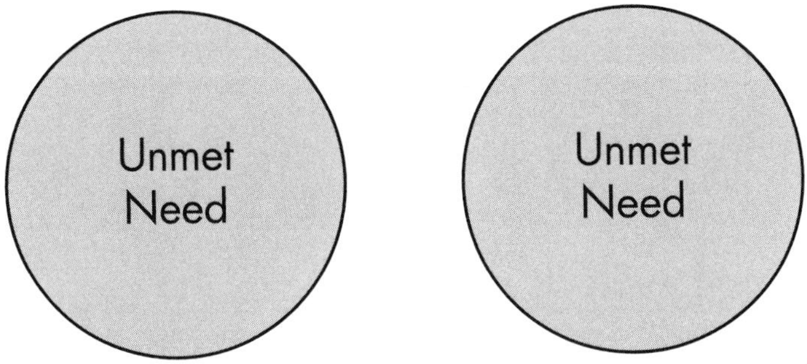

FIGURE 1. U.S. Food and Drug Administration–approved treatments for pediatric unipolar depression.

TABLE 4. U.S. Food and Drug Administration (FDA) approved, off-label, and emerging pharmacological treatments for pediatric unipolar depression

Medication	Dose range	Efficacy	Level of evidence
Fluoxetine	10–80 mg/day	4 positive studies in 6- to 17-year-olds	Randomized controlled trials (RCTs); FDA approved (Cipriani et al. 2016)
Escitalopram	10–40 mg/day	1 positive study in 12- to 17-year-olds 1 negative study in 6- to 17-year-olds	RCTs; FDA approved (Findling et al. 2013; Ignaszewski and Waslick 2018)
Sertraline	25–300 mg/day	1 positive pooled analysis in 6- to 17-year-olds	A priori pooled analysis; individual trials negative (Donnelly et al. 2006)
Citalopram	10–40 mg/day	1 negative study in 13- to 18-year-olds	RCT (von Knorring et al. 2006)
Paroxetine	10–60 mg/day	4 negative studies in 7- to 17-year-olds	RCT (Emslie et al. 2006)
Venlafaxine	37.5–375 mg/day	2 negative studies in 7- to 17-year-olds	RCT (Mandoki et al. 1997; Emslie et al. 2007)
Mirtazapine	15–45 mg/day	2 negative studies in 7- to 17-year-olds	RCT (unpublished); meta-analyses of comparative efficacy showed mirtazapine to have optimally balanced efficacy, acceptability, and safety for first-line acute treatment of child and adolescent MDD (Ma et al. 2014)
Fluvoxamine	25–300 mg/day	Positive	Open-label efficacy in pediatric dysthymia (Rabe-Jablonska 2000); no RCT data available
Vilazodone (Viibryd)	15–30 mg/day	Negative; FDA approved in adults in 2011	10-week double-blind placebo-controlled trial in 12- to 17-year-olds with depression (Phase 3) (Durgam et al. 2018); several case reports of seizures with toxic ingestion

TABLE 4. U.S. Food and Drug Administration (FDA) approved, off-label, and emerging pharmacological treatments for pediatric unipolar depression (*continued*)

Medication	Dose range	Efficacy	Level of evidence
Vortioxetine (Trintellix)	5–20 mg/day	Positive	14-day open-label extension lead-in followed by 6-month dosing study confirmed that a dosing strategy of 5–20 mg/day is safe, well tolerated, and suitable for future clinical studies of vortioxetine in pediatric patients; 12-week double-blind, placebo-controlled trial versus fluoxetine and placebo; two separate trials for children and adolescents underway
Duloxetine (Cymbalta)	30–120 mg/day	Negative	Two negative RCTs in youth MDD (Emslie et al. 2015); FDA approved in pediatric generalized anxiety disorder
Bupropion (Wellbutrin)	150–400 mg/day	Positive; not good for anxiety	Three open-label trials (Daviss et al. 2001, 2006; Glod et al. 2003; most common adverse events were insomnia and weight loss
Desvenlafaxine	25–50 mg/day	Failed	RCT compared venlafaxine with placebo and fluoxetine in 7- to 17-year-olds; participants in all treatment arms improved
Atomoxetine (Strattera)	10–80 mg/day	Negative	Seven RCTs in 5- to 18-year-olds; equally effective in reducing symptoms of attention-deficit/hyperactivity disorder in patients with or without comorbid depression (Bangs et al. 2007)

TABLE 4.   U.S. Food and Drug Administration (FDA) approved, off-label, and emerging pharmacological treatments for pediatric unipolar depression (*continued*)

Medication	Dose range	Efficacy	Level of evidence
Levomilnacipran (Fetzima)	10–40 mg/day	Unknown; FDA approved in adults in 2013 (Bruno et al. 2016)	Multisite Phase 3 study anticipated; 8-week double-blind, placebo-controlled trial comparing levomilnacipran with fluoxetine and placebo currently underway (primary outcome: change in CDRS-R); FDA approved in adults in 2013
Tricyclic antidepressants	Variable	Negative	Multiple RCTs for pediatric depressive disorders (Hazell and Mirzaie 2013)
Ketamine (Esketamine)	0.5 mg/kg infusion	Possibly positive	Open label and case reports: intravenous ketamine in adolescents with treatment-resistant depression; six infusions given over 2 weeks, with 38% response rate, including 5 responders, 3 with sustained remission at 6 weeks, and 2 who relapsed within 2 weeks (Cullen et al. 2018; Dwyer et al. 2017); multisite clinical trial for intranasal esketamine under way for acute suicidal ideation

TABLE 5.	Medication for youth depression: selective serotonin reuptake inhibitor (SSRI) side effects[a,b]			
Medication (generic)	**Trade name**	**Anticholinergic side effects**	**Sedating effect**	**Comments**
Fluoxetine	Prozac	+ (especially nausea, sexual dysfunction, anorexia)	+	U.S. Food and Drug Administration (FDA) approved; stimulating
Escitalopram	Lexapro	+	+	FDA approved
Citalopram	Celexa	+	+	Generic availability
Sertraline	Zoloft	0 (especially diarrhea and male sexual dysfunction)	+	FDA approved for teen obsessive-compulsive disorder

[a]Number needed to harm: 112.
[b]Side effects of SSRIs are serotonin selective, and they may attenuate over several weeks. In general, any SSRI may cause nausea, anxiety, agitation, anorexia, tremor, somnolence, sweating, dry mouth, headache, dizziness, diarrhea, constipation, and sexual dysfunction.

TABLE 6.   Common side effects of other antidepressant agents

Generic name/class	Side effects
Tricyclic antidepressants	Weight change, bloating, constipation, appetite loss, nausea, dry mouth, asthenia, dizziness, headache, somnolence, blurred vision, fatigue **Serious (rare):** cardiac dysrhythmia, myocardial infarction, sudden death, agranulocytosis
Venlafaxine XR	Tachycardia, hypertension, sweating, weight loss, loss of appetite, nausea, constipation, dizziness, headache, insomnia, somnolence, blurred vision, abnormal ejaculation **Serious (rare):** hyponatremia, hepatitis, seizure, neuroleptic malignant syndrome
Trazodone	Sedation, sweating, constipation, diarrhea, nausea, dizziness, headache, insomnia, memory impairment, blurred vision **Serious (rare):** Priapism in males, cardiac dysrhythmia
Nefazodone	Cough **Serious (rare):** orthostasis, liver failure, seizure
Mirtazapine	Sedation, weight gain, hypercholesterolemia, constipation, liver dysfunction, dizziness **Serious (rare):** agranulocytosis, neutropenia, seizure
Bupropion	Hypertension, tachycardia, headache, tremors, dizziness **Serious (rare):** seizure, cardiac dysrhythmia, anaphylaxis

Mood Stabilizers

Lithium

FDA approved down to age 12 years. Lithium is superior to placebo in children with bipolar disorder, with little weight gain.

Divalproex

Extended-release form showed negative results in an RCT for acute mania. Unpublished data suggest that the immediate-release form is more effective than placebo; however, it has been shown to be inferior to quetiapine and risperidone in comparative effectiveness.

Carbamazepine

Extended-release form. Open-label data showed mild to moderate improvement in pediatric mania.

Lamotrigine

Open-label studies found efficacy in pediatric acute mania, mixed mania, and depression. Maintenance randomized controlled trial showed benefit as an adjunct.

- There is at least one boxed safety warning for all mood stabilizers (see Figure 2).

Lithium	Valproate	Carbamazepine	Lamotrigine
Gastrointestinal	Gastrointestinal	Gastrointestinal	Gastrointestinal
Weight gain	Weight gain	Rash	Rash
Neurotoxicity	Tremor	Neurotoxicity	Headache
Renal toxicity	Hepatotoxicity	Hepatotoxicity	Dizziness
Thyroid toxicity	Thrombocytopenia	Thyroid changes	Pruritis
Hair loss	Hair loss	Blood dyscrasias	Dream abnormality
Cardiac toxicity	Pancreatitis	Cardiac toxicity	
Acne, psoriasis	PCOS	Hyponatremia	
Teratogen	Teratogen	Teratogen	Teratogen
	Suicidality	Suicidality	Suicidality

☐ = boxed warning in prescribing information

All mood stabilizers have at least one boxed warning.

FIGURE 2.   Mood stabilizer safety and tolerability concerns.
PCOS=polycystic ovary syndrome.

Second-Generation (Atypical) Antipsychotics

- FDA-approved agents for pediatric bipolar disorder are summarized in Figure 3.
- Most atypical antipsychotics show strong benefit-risk ratios for the treatment of mania and bipolar depression (see Figures 4, 5, and 6).
- All antipsychotics have boxed safety warnings, including risks of hyperglycemia and diabetes mellitus, requiring baseline assessment and longitudinal monitoring for the development of these problems (Figure 7).

Acute Mania		Acute Bipolar Depression		Longer-Term	
Year	**Drug**	**Year**	**Drug**	**Year**	**Drug**
1970	Lithium[a]	2013	Olanzapine + fluoxetine combination[b]	1974	Lithium[a]
2007	Risperidone[b]			2008	Aripiprazole[b]
2008	Aripiprazole[b]	**2018**	**Lurasidone[b]**		
2009	Quetiapine[b]				
2009	Olanzapine[c]				
2015	Asenapine[b]				

Unmet Need

Unmet Need

Important unmet needs—well-tolerated treatments for acute depression and maintenance.

FIGURE 3. U.S. Food and Drug Administration–approved agents for pediatric bipolar disorder.

[a]Age≥12–17 years; [b]age=10–17 years; [c]age=13–17 years.

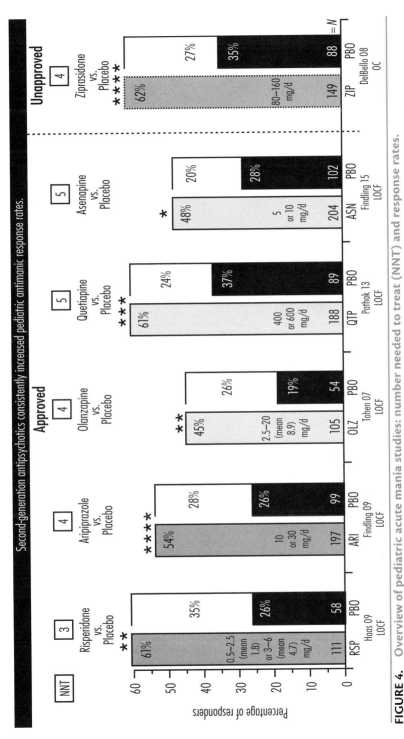

FIGURE 4. Overview of pediatric acute mania studies: number needed to treat (NNT) and response rates.

*P<0.05, **P<0.01, ***P<0.001, ****P<0.0001 vs. placebo. LOCF=last observation carried forward; OC=observed cases.

Source. Adapted from Ketter TA, Chang KD, Singh MK: "Treatment of Pediatric Bipolar Disorder," in *Advances in Treatment of Bipolar Disorders.* Edited by Ketter TA. Arlington, VA, American Psychiatric Publishing, 2015, pp. 171–198. Copyright 2015, American Psychiatric Association. Used with permission.

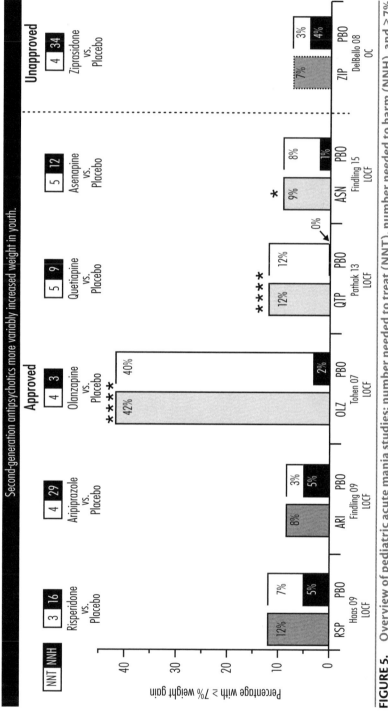

FIGURE 5.   Overview of pediatric acute mania studies: number needed to treat (NNT), number needed to harm (NNH), and ≥7% weight gain rates.

*$P<0.05$, ****$P<0.0001$ vs. placebo. LOCF=last observation carried forward; OC=observed cases.

Source.   Adapted from Ketter TA, Chang KD, Singh MK: "Treatment of Pediatric Bipolar Disorder," in *Advances in Treatment of Bipolar Disorders.* Edited by Ketter TA. Arlington, VA, American Psychiatric Association, 2015, pp. 171–198. Copyright 2015, American Psychiatric Association. Used with permission.

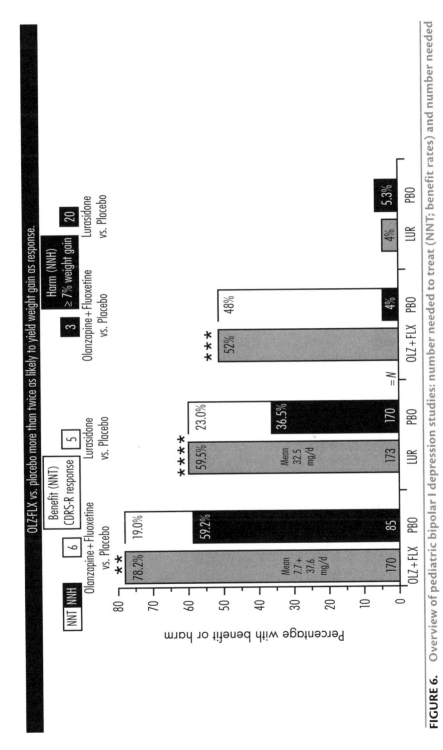

FIGURE 6. Overview of pediatric bipolar I depression studies: number needed to treat (NNT; benefit rates) and number needed to harm (NNH; ≥7% weight gain rates).

*P<0.05, **P<0.01, ***P<0.001, ****P<0.0001 vs. placebo. CDRS-R=Children's Depression Rating Scale—Revised.

Source. Data from DelBello et al. 2017; Detke et al. 2015.

First-Generation	Second-Generation
Depression	Weight gain, sedation
Akathisia	Hyperglycemia, diabetes[b]
Acute dystonia	Suicidality in age ≤ 24[c]
Tardive dyskinesia[a]	Akathisia
Weight gain, sedation	Hyperprolactinemia
Anticholinergic	Cerebrovascular in elderly[d]
Cardiac, orthostasis	Cardiac, orthostasis
Hyperprolactinemia	Tardive dyskinesia[a]
Neuroleptic malignant syndrome[a]	Neuroleptic malignant syndrome[a]
Leukopenia, neutropenia	Leukopenia, neutropenia
Agranulocytosis[a]	Agranulocytosis[a]
Cardiac/pneumonia in older adults[a]	Cardiac/pneumonia in older adults[a]

☐ = boxed warning in prescribing information

All antipsychotics have at least one boxed warning.

FIGURE 7.   Antipsychotic safety and tolerability concerns.

[a]Antipsychotic class warning/precaution.

[b]Second-generation antipsychotic class warning.

[c]Aripiprazole, quetiapine, olanzapine + fluoxetine combination (antidepressant class warning).

[d]Risperidone, olanzapine, aripiprazole.

References

Bangs ME, Emslie GJ, Spencer TJ, et al; Atomoxetine ADHD and Comorbid MDD Study Group: Efficacy and safety of atomoxetine in adolescents with attention-deficit/hyperactivity disorder and major depression. J Child Adolesc Psychopharmacol 17(4):407–420, 2007 17822337

Blake M, Waloszek JM, Schwartz O, et al: The SENSE study: post intervention effects of a randomized controlled trial of a cognitive-behavioral and mindfulness-based group sleep improvement intervention among at-risk adolescents. J Consult Clin Psychol 84(12):1039–1051, 2016 27775416

Bruno A, Morabito P, Spina E, Muscatello MR: The role of levomilnacipran in the management of major depressive disorder: a comprehensive review. Curr Neuropharmacol 14(2):191–199, 2016 26572745

Carta JJ, Lefever JB, Bigelow K, et al: Randomized trial of a cellular phone-enhanced home visitation parenting intervention. Pediatrics 132 (suppl 2):S167–S173, 2013 24187120

Cipriani A, Zhou X, Del Giovane C, et al: Comparative efficacy and tolerability of antidepressants for major depressive disorder in children and adolescents: a network meta-analysis. Lancet 388(10047):881–890, 2016 27289172

Cullen KR, Amatya P, Roback MG, et al: Intravenous ketamine for adolescents with treatment-resistant depression: an open-label study. J Child Adolesc Psychopharmacol 28(7):437–444, 2018 30004254 Erratum: J Child Adolesc Psychopharmacol 29(1):77, 2019 30585735

Daviss WB, Bentivoglio P, Racusin R, et al: Bupropion sustained release in adolescents with comorbid attention-deficit/hyperactivity disorder and depression. J Am Acad Child Adolesc Psychiatry 40(3):307–314, 2001 11288772

Daviss WB, Perel JM, Brent DA, et al: Acute antidepressant response and plasma levels of bupropion and metabolites in a pediatric-aged sample: an exploratory study. Ther Drug Monit 28(2):190–198, 2006 16628130

DelBello MP, Findling RL, Wang PP, et al: Safety and efficacy of ziprasidone in pediatric bipolar disorder. Paper presented at the 55th Annual Convention and Scientific Program of the Society of Biological Psychiatry, Washington, DC, May 1–3, 2008

DelBello MP, Goldman R, Phillips D, et al: Efficacy and safety of lurasidone in children and adolescents with bipolar I depression: a double-blind, placebo-controlled study. J Am Acad Child Adolesc Psychiatry 56(12):1015–1025, 2017 29173735

Detke HC, DelBello MP, Landry J, et al: Olanzapine/fluoxetine combination in children and adolescents with bipolar I depression: a randomized, double-blind, placebo-controlled trial. J Am Acad Child Adolesc Psychiatry 54(3):217–224, 2015 25721187

Donnelly CL, Wagner KD, Rynn M, et al: Sertraline in children and adolescents with major depressive disorder. J Am Acad Child Adolesc Psychiatry 45(10):1162–1170, 2006 17003661

Durgam S, Chen C, Migliore R, et al: A phase 3, double-blind, randomized, placebo-controlled study of vilazodone in adolescents with major depressive disorder. Paediatr Drugs 20(4):353–363, 2018 29633166

Dwyer JB, Beyer C, Wilkinson ST, et al: Ketamine as a treatment for adolescent depression: a case report. J Am Acad Child Adolesc Psychiatry 56(4):352–354, 2017 28335880

Emslie GJ, Wagner KD, Kutcher S, et al: Paroxetine treatment in children and adolescents with major depressive disorder: a randomized, multicenter, double-blind, placebo-controlled trial. J Am Acad Child Adolesc Psychiatry 45(6):709–719, 2006 16721321

Emslie GJ, Findling RL, Yeung PP, et al: Venlafaxine ER for the treatment of pediatric subjects with depression: results of two placebo-controlled trials. J Am Acad Child Adolesc Psychiatry 46(4):479–488, 2007 17420682

Emslie GJ, Wells TG, Prakash A, et al: Acute and longer-term safety results from a pooled analysis of duloxetine studies for the treatment of children and adolescents with major depressive disorder. J Child Adolesc Psychopharmacol 25(4):293–305, 2015 25978741

Findling RL, Nyilas M, Forbes RA, et al: Acute treatment of pediatric bipolar I disorder, manic or mixed episode, with aripiprazole: a randomized, double-blind, placebo-controlled study. J Clin Psychiatry 70(10):1441–1451, 2009 19906348

Findling RL, Robb A, Bose A: Escitalopram in the treatment of adolescent depression: a randomized, double-blind, placebo-controlled extension trial. J Child Adolesc Psychopharmacol 23(7):468–480, 2013 24041408

Findling RL, Landbloom RL, Szegedi A, et al: Asenapine for the acute treatment of pediatric manic or mixed episode of bipolar I disorder. J Am Acad Child Adolesc Psychiatry 54(12):1032–1041, 2015 26598478

Findling RL, Landbloom RL, Mackle M, et al: Long-term safety of asenapine in pediatric patients diagnosed with bipolar I disorder: a 50-week open-label, flexible-dose trial. Paediatr Drugs 18(5):367–378, 2016 27461426

Findling RL, Earley W, Suppes T, et al: Post hoc analyses of asenapine treatment in pediatric patients with bipolar I disorder: efficacy related to mixed or manic episode, stage of illness, and body weight. Neuropsychiatr Dis Treat 14:1941–1952, 2018 30122926

Fristad MA, Young AS, Vesco AT, et al: A randomized controlled trial of individual family psychoeducational psychotherapy and omega-3 fatty acids in youth with subsyndromal bipolar disorder. J Child Adolesc Psychopharmacol 25(10):764–774, 2015 26682997

Fristad MA, Vesco AT, Young AS, et al: Pilot randomized controlled trial of omega-3 and individual-family psychoeducational psychotherapy for children and adolescents with depression. J Clin Child Adolesc Psychol 7:1–14, 2016 27819485

Gladstone TG, Marko-Holguin M, Rothberg P, et al: An internet-based adolescent depression preventive intervention: study protocol for a randomized control trial. Trials 16:203, 2015 25927539

Glod CA, Lynch A, Flynn E, et al: Open trial of bupropion SR in adolescent major depression. J Child Adolesc Psychiatr Nurs 16(3):123–130, 2003 14603988

Grupp-Phelan J, McGuire L, Husky MM, Olfson M: A randomized controlled trial to engage in care of adolescent emergency department patients with mental health problems that increase suicide risk. Pediatr Emerg Care 28(12):1263–1268, 2012 23187979

Haas M, Delbello MP, Pandina G, et al: Risperidone for the treatment of acute mania in children and adolescents with bipolar disorder: a randomized, double-blind, placebo-controlled study. Bipolar Disord 11(7):687–700, 2009 19839994

Hall WA, Hutton E, Brant RF, et al: A randomized controlled trial of an intervention for infants' behavioral sleep problems. BMC Pediatr 15:181, 2015 26567090

Hazell P, Mirzaie M: Tricyclic drugs for depression in children and adolescents. Cochrane Database Syst Rev (6):CD002317, 2013 23780719

Hiscock H, Sciberras E, Mensah F, et al: Impact of a behavioural sleep intervention on symptoms and sleep in children with attention deficit hyperactivity disorder, and parental mental health: randomised controlled trial. BMJ 350:h68, 2015 25646809

Ignaszewski MJ, Waslick B: Update on randomized placebo-controlled trials in the past decade for treatment of major depressive disorder in child and adolescent patients: a systematic review. J Child Adolesc Psychopharmacol (July):31, 2018 30063169

Ma D, Zhang Z, Zhang X, Li L: Comparative efficacy, acceptability, and safety of medicinal, cognitive-behavioral therapy, and placebo treatments for acute major depressive disorder in children and adolescents: a multiple-treatments meta-analysis. Curr Med Res Opin 30(6):971–995, 2014 24188102

Mandoki MW, Tapia MR, Tapia MA, et al: Venlafaxine in the treatment of children and adolescents with major depression. Psychopharmacol Bull 33(1):149–154, 1997 9133767

Pathak S, Findling RL, Earley WR, et al: Efficacy and safety of quetiapine in children and adolescents with mania associated with bipolar I disorder: a 3-week, double-blind, placebo-controlled trial. J Clin Psychiatry 74(1):e100–e109, 2013 23419231

Rabe-Jablonska J: Therapeutic effects and tolerability of fluvoxamine treatment in adolescents with dysthymia. J Child Adolesc Psychopharmacol 10(1):9–18, 2000 10755577

Schleider JL, Weisz JR: Reducing risk for anxiety and depression in adolescents: effects of a single-session intervention teaching that personality can change. Behav Res Ther 87:170–181, 2016 27697671

Tohen M, Kryzhanovskaya L, Carlson G, et al: Olanzapine versus placebo in the treatment of adolescents with bipolar mania. Am J Psychiatry 164(10):1547–1556, 2007 17898346

von Knorring AL, Olsson GI, Thomsen PH, et al: A randomized, double-blind, placebo-controlled study of citalopram in adolescents with major depressive disorder. J Clin Psychopharmacol 26(3):311–315, 2006 16702897

Wozniak J, Faraone SV, Chan J, et al: A randomized clinical trial of high eicosapentaenoic acid omega-3 fatty acids and inositol as monotherapy and in combination in the treatment of pediatric bipolar spectrum disorders: a pilot study. J Clin Psychiatry 76(11):1548–1555, 2015 26646031 Erratum in: J Clin Psychiatry Sep;77(9):e1153, 2016

Young AS, Meers MR, Vesco AT, et al: Predicting therapeutic effects of psychodiagnostic assessment among children and adolescents participating in randomized controlled trials. J Clin Child Adolesc Psychol 22:1–12, 2016 27105332

Zatzick D, Russo J, Lord SP, et al: Collaborative care intervention targeting violence risk behaviors, substance use, and posttraumatic stress and depressive symptoms in injured adolescents: a randomized clinical trial. JAMA Pediatr 168(6):532–539, 2014 24733515

Index

Page numbers printed in **boldface** type refer to tables and figures.